Mosby's
Pharmacy
Technician

PRINCIPLES & PRACTICE

ELSEVIER

evolve

The Latest Evolution in Learning.

Evolve provides online access to free learning resources and activities designed specifically for the textbook you are using in your class. The resources will provide you with information that enhances the material covered in the book and much more.

Visit the Web address listed below to start your learning evolution today!

▶▶ *LOGIN:* **http://evolve.elsevier.com/Hopper/**

Evolve Student Learning Resources for Hopper: *Mosby's Pharmacy Technician: Principles and Practice* offer the following features:

- **Content Updates**
  The latest content updates from the author of the textbook to keep you current with recent developments in the field of pharmacy technician.

- **Chapter Weblinks**
  These links offer students the opportunity to check their understanding and execute the workbook web-based research assignments, plus expand their knowledge base and stay current with this ever-changing industry.

- **Internet Research Activities**
  Internet research activities for each chapter are set up to direct students toward pharmacy-specific websites.

Think outside the book... *evolve.*

Mosby's Pharmacy Technician

PRINCIPLES & PRACTICE

TERESA HOPPER, BS, CPhT

Pharmacy Technician Consultant

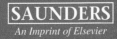

SAUNDERS

An Imprint of Elsevier

SAUNDERS
An Imprint of Elsevier

11830 Westline Industrial Drive
St. Louis, Missouri 63146

MOSBY'S PHARMACY TECHNICIAN PRINCIPLES AND PRACTICE   ISBN 0-7216-9436-5
Copyright © 2004, Elsevier Inc. All rights reserved.
Mosby is a registered trademark of Mosby Inc., used under their license.
Credit is given to Mosby Inc. for the licensed use of their name in the title.

NOTICE

Pharmacy is an ever-changing field. Standard safety precautions must be followed, but as
new research and clinical experience broaden our knowledge, changes in treatment and drug
therapy may become necessary or appropriate. Readers are advised to check the most current
product information provided by the manufacturer of each drug to be administered to verify
the recommended dose, the method and duration of administration, and contraindications. It
is the responsibility of the licensed prescriber, relying on experience and knowledge of the
patient, to determine dosages and the best treatment for each individual patient. Neither the
publisher nor the author assumes any liability for any injury and/or damage to persons or
property arising from this publication.

International Standard Book Number 0-7216-9436-5

Executive Editor: Adrianne H. Cochran
Senior Developmental Editor: Helaine Tobin
Developmental Editor: Christine Ambrose
Publishing Services Manager: Melissa Lastarria
Project Manager: Joy Moore
Designer: Amy Buxton

Printed in United States of America

Last digit is the print number: 9   8   7   6   5   4   3   2

Preface

Welcome to the World of Pharmacy Technology

You are about to embark on an exciting journey into one of today's fastest-growing fields in health care. Whether you will end up working in a hospital pharmacy, a community pharmacy, one of the large pharmacy chain stores, or another location, the knowledge you will gain from this textbook and its supplements will prepare you well for your new career. The authors and publisher have made every effort to equip you with all of the background knowledge and tools you will need to succeed on the job. To this end, *Mosby's Pharmacy Technician Principles and Practice* was designed as a fundamental, yet comprehensive, resource that also includes a companion workbook, website, and a valuable reference tool in the 2004 edition of *Mosby's Drug Consult*, which is bound free into this book. Together, these training and reference materials represent the very latest information available for preparing pharmacy technician students for today's challenging job environment.

Pharmacy technicians are increasingly called upon to perform duties traditionally fulfilled by pharmacists. This is because of new Federal regulations that now require pharmacists to spend more time with patients providing patient education. As the number of pharmacy technicians in the United States continues to grow, the need to outline a scope of practice for the pharmacy technician profession across all 50 states has become more urgent. Although there is no standardization for the qualifications and job descriptions for pharmacy technicians as of yet, this textbook covers all the theory and skills set forth by several national certifying bodies, including the Pharmacy Technician Certification Board (PTCB), the National Healthcareer Association (NHA), the American Society of Health System Pharmacists (ASHP), and the American Pharmaceutical Association (APA), the last two of which created the criteria for the Pharmacy Technician Certification Board's certification exam. These criteria are designed to help pharmacy technicians work more effectively with pharmacists, provide greater patient care and services, create a minimum standard of knowledge across all 50 states, and help employers determine a knowledge base for employment.

Organizational Structure of this Textbook

Mosby's Pharmacy Technician Principles and Practice is a reliable and understandable resource written specifically for the pharmacy technician student and for those technicians already on the job, including those who are preparing for the National Pharmacy Technician Certification exam (PCTB), or the Certified Pharmacy Technician exam (CPhT). The writing style, content, and organization guide the student to a better understanding of anatomy and physiology, diseases, and, most importantly, drugs and agents used to treat these diseases. Pharmacologic information is presented in a thorough, yet basic and concise, manner. The text is divided into five sections—General Pharmacy, Body Systems, Classifications of Drugs, Basic Sciences for the Pharmacy Technician, and Starting Your Career as a Pharmacy Technician.

Section One, General Pharmacy, provides an overview of pharmacy practice as it relates to pharmacy technicians. Highlights of Section One include history, law and ethics, drug calculations and dosage forms, abbreviations, routes of administration, filling prescriptions, over-the-counter medications, and the differences in the roles of pharmacists and pharmacy technicians. *Pharmacy Technician* is the only book on the market that devotes an entire chapter each to alternative and complementary medicine and psychopharmacology.

Section Two, Body Systems, provides a brief overview of each body system and the medications used to treat common conditions that afflict these systems. Unique to this section are detailed discussions of anatomy and physiology.

Section Three, Classifications of Drugs, discusses each major drug classification. A description of every drug classification helps the pharmacy technician student understand how similar agents work. Section Three also includes a chapter on vitamins and minerals.

Section Four, Basic Sciences for the Pharmacy Technician, includes two chapters—on microbiology and chemistry—that are indeed unique to this textbook.

Section Five, Starting Your Career as a Pharmacy Technician, offers a detailed discussion of pharmacy organizations and some forecasts regarding career opportunities for pharmacy technicians.

Distinctive Features of Our Approach

This textbook has been crafted with straightforward pedagogical features to emphasize content and engage students in the learning process. Such pedagogical features include the following:

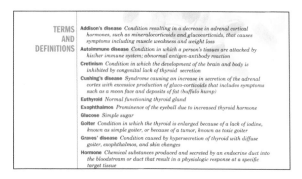

- Key terms and definitions begin each chapter, directing you to the important concepts presented in the chapter.

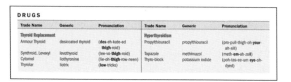

- Each chapter in Sections Two and Three provide a list of the drugs, with pronunciations, discussed in the chapter.

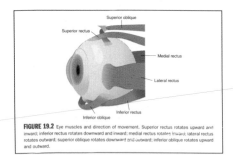

FIGURE 19.2 Eye muscles and direction of movement. Superior rectus rotates upward and inward; inferior rectus rotates downward and inward; medial rectus rotates inward; lateral rectus rotates outward; superior oblique rotates downward and outward; inferior oblique rotates upward and outward.

- Brief anatomy and physiology discussions in the body systems chapters help build a foundation for the student as to how the drugs work in the human body.

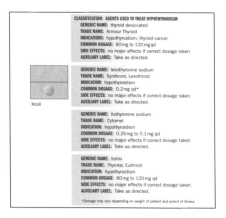

- Drug monographs that include photos of selected medications make learning drugs an easier and more meaningful task. The monographs are also good reference tools.

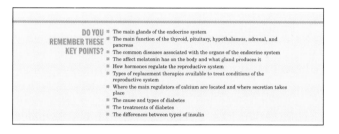

TECH NOTE! The terms *rainbow coverage* and *sliding scale* refer to the varying doses of insulin that depend on the reading of the blood glucose meter.

• Tech Notes interspersed throughout the text provide students with helpful on-the-job hints and safeguards.

• Pharmacist's Perspective boxes provide practical examples of pharmacologic principles in practice through the eyes of a pharmacist.

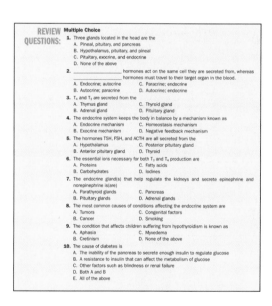

Pharmacist's Perspective
BY SUSAN WONG, PHARM.D.

Educate Oneself When It Comes to Complementary and Alternative Medicine and Health!

Many questions arise when it comes to a person's health. What is health? Some may believe that it is not getting sick, that is, staying well. Others may think it is fixing something that has gone wrong or broken. Still others believe it is maintaining overall happiness and balance. All of these play an important role in being healthy. How to do this is another story. There are four important steps:

1. A patient or customer must become a good self-observer.
2. A patient or customer must learn to recognize that he or she has control of lifestyle and choices.
3. A patient or customer must make lifestyle changes or other changes as necessary.
4. A patient or customer must follow the results of changes, as well as document and communicate them with the healthcare provider.

Your role as a pharmacy technician may be as a bridge of information between the pharmacist and the patient to help the patient become or stay healthy.

To do any and all of these things, one must first understand what makes a person tick. Over many centuries different philosophies have developed that address

health. Native Americans chewed on willow leaves for relief from pain or swelling. In Europe this eventually led to the discovery and concentration of the active component, salicin, and with a little chemistry, acetylsalicylic acid (aspirin). In Chinese medicine, a practitioner prescribes a tailored mixture or formula to cure pain and restore balance, or one can use one of the patent medicines (ready-made formulas for a general condition). Many Eastern philosophies incorporate emotional, mental, and spiritual balance into the equation. Unfortunately, how these remedies and philosophies interact may not always be clear. That is why it is important to educate oneself and communicate to others; especially important is the communication between a patient and the healthcare provider.

In the world of drugs, herbs, and nutritional supplements, it is important to clearly distinguish what types there are. Learn how each of these single or multiple agents can affect a particular situation before its use. Sometimes one therapy may counteract another or may actually augment the effects of another. This may be good or bad depending on the person's situation and overall health. Patients should keep a diary of what has been used, what they are currently using (if anything), and any questions they may have. Patients should keep track of how they feel and what may have caused it, including any prescription drugs, OTC drugs, herbs, or supplements, and let the healthcare provider know exactly what they are using. It is important to let the

Continued

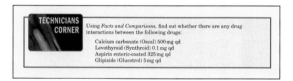

DO YOU REMEMBER THESE KEY POINTS?	▪ The main glands of the endocrine system ▪ The main function of the thyroid, pituitary, hypothalamus, adrenal, and pancreas ▪ The common diseases associated with the organs of the endocrine system ▪ The affect melatonin has on the body and what gland produces it ▪ How hormones regulate the reproductive system ▪ Types of replacement therapies available to treat conditions of the reproductive system ▪ Where the main regulators of calcium are located and where secretion takes place ▪ The cause and types of diabetes ▪ The treatments of diabetes ▪ The differences between types of insulin

• Do You Remember These Key Points? summaries direct students to each chapter's significant information.

• Review questions at the end of each chapter allow students to test their knowledge.

REVIEW QUESTIONS:

Multiple Choice

1. Three glands located in the head are the
   A. Pineal, pituitary, and pancreas
   B. Hypothalamus, pituitary, and pineal
   C. Pituitary, exocrine, and endocrine
   D. None of the above

2. _____ hormones act on the same cell they are secreted from, whereas _____ hormones must travel to their target organ in the blood.
   A. Endocrine; autocrine   C. Paracrine; endocrine
   B. Autocrine; paracrine   D. Autocrine; endocrine

3. T_4 and T_3 are secreted from the
   A. Thymus gland   C. Thyroid gland
   B. Adrenal gland   D. Pituitary gland

4. The endocrine system keeps the body in balance by a mechanism known as
   A. Endocrine mechanism   C. Homeostasis mechanism
   B. Exocrine mechanism   D. Negative feedback mechanism

5. The hormones TSH, FSH, and ACTH are all secreted from the
   A. Hypothalamus   C. Posterior pituitary gland
   B. Anterior pituitary gland D. Thyroid

6. The essential ions necessary for both T_3 and T_4 production are
   A. Proteins   C. Fatty acids
   B. Carbohydrates   D. Iodines

7. The endocrine gland(s) that help regulate the kidneys and secrete epinephrine and norepinephrine is(are)
   A. Parathyroid glands C. Pancreas
   B. Pituitary glands   D. Adrenal glands

8. The most common causes of conditions affecting the endocrine system are
   A. Tumors   C. Congenital factors
   B. Cancer   D. Smoking

9. The condition that affects children suffering from hypothyroidism is known as
   A. Aphasia   C. Myxedema
   B. Cretinism D. None of the above

10. The cause of diabetes is
    A. The inability of the pancreas to secrete enough insulin to regulate glucose
    B. A resistance to insulin that can affect the metabolism of glucose
    C. Other factors such as blindness or renal failure
    D. Both A and B
    E. All of the above

TECHNICIANS CORNER

Using *Facts and Comparisons*, find out whether there are any drug interactions between the following drugs:

Calcium carbonate (Oscal) 500 mg qd
Levothyroid (Synthroid) 0.1 mg qd
Aspirin enteric-coated 325 mg qd
Glipizide (Glucotrol) 5 mg qd

• Technician's Corners at the end of each chapter promote critical thinking skills.

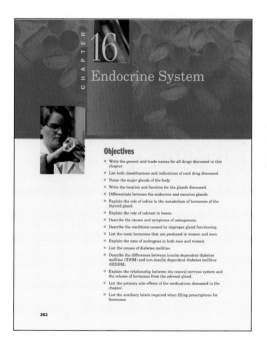

CHAPTER
16.
Endocrine System

Objectives

▪ Write the generic and trade names for all drugs discussed in this chapter.
▪ List both classifications and indications of each drug discussed.
▪ Name the major glands of the body.
▪ Write the location and function for the glands discussed.
▪ Differentiate between the endocrine and exocrine glands.
▪ Explain the role of iodine in the metabolism of hormones of the thyroid gland.
▪ Explain the role of calcium in bones.
▪ Describe the causes and symptoms of osteoporosis.
▪ Describe the conditions caused by improper gland functioning.
▪ List the main hormones that are produced in women and men.
▪ Explain the uses of androgens in both men and women.
▪ List the causes of diabetes mellitus.
▪ Describe the differences between insulin dependent diabetes mellitus (IDDM) and non-insulin dependent diabetes mellitus (NIDDM).
▪ Explain the relationship between the central nervous system and the release of hormones from the adrenal gland.
▪ List the primary side effects of the medications discussed in this chapter.
▪ List the auxiliary labels required when filling prescriptions for hormones.

262

• Attractive 4-color design makes the text inviting and information more accessible. The robust art program likewise supports the text and visually reinforces important new concepts and procedures.

Extensive Supplemental Resources

Considering the broad range of students, instructors, programs, and institutions for which this textbook was designed, we have developed an extensive package of supplements designed to complement *Mosby's Pharmacy Technician Principles and Practice*. Each of these comprehensive supplements has been thoughtfully developed with the shared goals of students and instructors in mind: producing students who are well prepared for a career in pharmacy, as well as for earning their National Pharmacy Technician Certification. These supplements and their inventive features include:

MOSBY'S DRUG CONSULT 2004

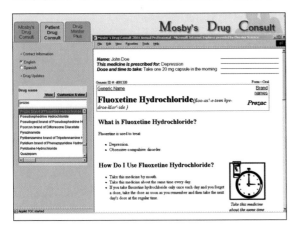

Bound free into this textbook is the 2004 version of *Mosby's Drug Consult*, a complete prescription drug annual reference tool used by physicians, dentists, pharmacists, pharmacy technicians, and other health care providers that offers more than 22,000 drug entries with generic, U.S. Brand, and international brand names. This searchable database also offers nearly 1,000 drug monographs, complete with many photos seen throughout *Mosby's Pharmacy Technician Principles and Practice* textbook, plus a *Drug Master Plus* drug interaction tool with more than 5,000 interactions that flag dangerous drug interactions and provides instant, immediately usable data, as well as *Mosby's Patient Drug Consult* with more than 1,800 patient care instructional handouts in both English and Spanish.

STUDENT WORKBOOK

Laura McBride, CPhT
Karen Snipe, CPhT, AS, BA, MAEd

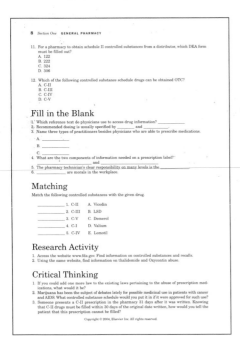

Featuring recall and application exercises to reinforce content, this workbook gives students an opportunity to test their performance skills and knowledge of cognitive content. Some of the outstanding features of this student workbook include:

• Terms and Definitions and Fill in the Blanks exercises task students specifically with using medical terminology within the context of pharmacy.

• Matching exercises provide students with essential practice in matching controlled substance drug schedules with given drug names.

• Multiple Choice and True or False questions give students an opportunity to reinforce their knowledge by distinguishing correct content from false information.

• Research Activities direct students toward pertinent websites regarding such topics as the scope of practice for pharmacy technicians and where to find information on controlled substances and recalls.

• Critical Thinking exercises task students with synthesizing their knowledge and directing it to specific situations.

• Conversion and calculation questions require students to convert measurements, thereby applying what they have learned.

INSTRUCTOR'S CURRICULUM RESOURCE WITH CD-ROM

Karen Snipe, CPhT, AS, BA, MAEd
John Albrecht, CPhT

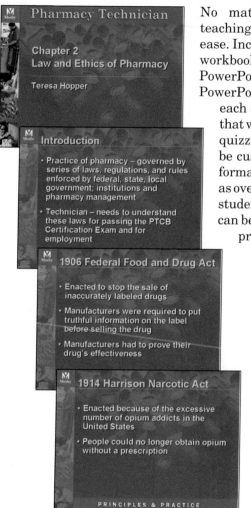

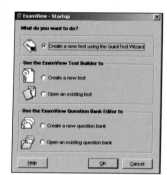

No matter what your level of teaching experience, this total-teaching solution will help you plan your lessons for lecture and lab with ease. Included in the printed materials are all answers to the textbook and workbook exercises, a printed test bank of questions, and a listing of PowerPoint slides. The CD-ROM, bound free with this item, includes a PowerPoint viewer with a comprehensive PowerPoint slide collection for each chapter, and a test bank in the ExamView test generator format that will help you easily and quickly prepare quizzes and exams. The slides can easily be customized to support your lectures or formatted within the PowerPoint program as overhead transparencies or handouts for student note-taking. Our test bank likewise can be customized to your specific teaching preparations.

EVOLVE COMPANION WEBSITE

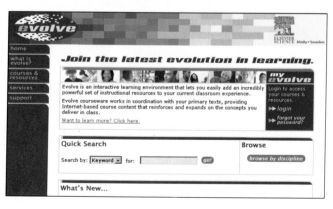

The EVOLVE Companion Website offers a resource that allows students to harness the power of the World Wide Web. Internet research activities and chapter web links offer students the opportunity to check their understanding and execute the web-based research assignments in the workbook, plus expand their knowledge base and stay current with this ever-changing industry. Students log on through the Evolve portal to complete lessons, take quizzes and exams online, participate in threaded discussions, post assignments to instructors, or chat with the instructor or fellow classmates. Instructors can download all materials available in the Instructor's Curriculum Resource.

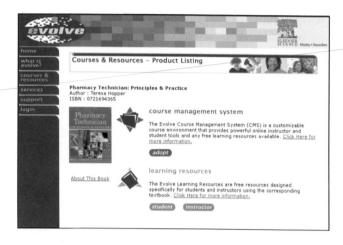

A Course Management System (CMS) is also available free to instructors who adopt the textbook. This turnkey package of Evolve Learning Resources includes program outlines for 9-, 12-, and 24-month pharmacy technician programs and individual chapter lesson plans to help instructors plan with ease. Detailed lesson plans for each chapter include pre-tests and post-tests, learning objectives, lecture outlines, suggested class and laboratory activites, teaching tips, resources, and lists of equipment needed. This web-based platform gives instructors yet another resource to facilitate learning and to make the pharmacy technician content accessible to their students. In addition to the Evolve Learning Resources available to both faculty and students, there is an entire suite of tools available that allows for communication between instructors and students, including discussion board, e-mail, chat room, and more.

To access this comprehensive online resource, simply go to the EVOLVE home page at *http://evolve.elsevier.com* and enter the user name and password provided by your instructor. If your instructor has not set up a Course Management System, you can still access all the learning resources available free with this textbook by going to *http://evolve.elsevier.com/Hopper*.

Development of This Edition

To ensure the accuracy of the material presented throughout this textbook, an extensive review and development process was used. This included several phases of evaluation by a variety of pharmacy technician instructors and experts in anatomy and physiology and pharmacology. We are deeply grateful to the numerous people who have shared their comments and suggestions. Reviewing a book or supplement takes an incredible amount of energy and attention, and we are glad so many colleagues were able to take time out of their busy schedule to help ensure the validity and appropriateness of content in this edition. The reviewers provided us with additional viewpoints and opinions that combine to make this text an incredible learning tool.

We wish to thank the following Editorial Review Team:

W. Reneé Acosta, RPh, MS
Austin Community College
Austin, Texas

James Austin, RN, BSN, CPhT
Department Chair
Pharmacy Technology
Weatherford College
Weatherford, Texas

Janet V. Cadorette, CST
Surgical Technology Department
Tennessee Technology Center at Knoxville
Knoxville, Tennessee

Jackie Cavens, RN
Ashland Technical College
Ashland, Kentucky

Michael C. Cole, MBA
Western School
Monroeville, Pennsylvania

Vince R. Druash, BS, CPhT, CMA
Program Director, Medical Assisting
Medical Careers Institute
Virginia Beach, Virginia
Formerly Senior Instructor
Pharmacy Technician School
Naval School of Health Sciences
Portsmouth, Virginia

Jill Marie Frost, BS, CPhT
Tennessee Technology Center
Murfreesboro, Tennessee

Eugenia M. Fulcher, RN, BSN, EdD, CMA
Program Director, Medical Assisting
Swainsboro Technical College
Swainsboro, GA

Robert M. Fulcher, BS, BSPh, RPh
Pharmacist-In-Charge
CVS Pharmacy
Waynesboro, GA

Lee A. Gootblatt, RPh
St. Charles Hospital
Dover, New Jersey

James J. Mizner, Jr, BS, MBA, RPh
Pharmacy Technician Program Director
Applied Career Training
Arlington, Virginia

Jahangir Moini, MD, MPH
Medical Department Chair
Florida Metropolitan University
Melbourne, Florida

Kathy Moscou, BS, RPh
Pharmacy Technician Program Director
North Seattle Community College
Seattle, Washington

Theresa A. Mozug, AS, BS, CPhT
Henry Ford Community Center
Pharmacy Technology
Dearborn, Michigan
Henry Ford Wyandotte Hospital Pharmacy
Wyandotte, Michigan

Debra L. Peelor, BS
Instructor
Bidwell Training Center
Pittsburgh, Pennsylvania

Harry E. Peery, MS, PhD candidate
Department of Pharmacology
Department of Pathology
University of Saskatchewan
Saskatoon, Saskatchewan, Canada
And
Department of Pharmacology and Toxicology
College of Pharmacy and Toxicology
College of Pharmacology
Arizona Health Sciences Center
University of Arizona
Tucson, Arizona

Michael Rais, RPh
Pharmacy Technician Coordinator
Macomb Community College
Clinton Township, Michigan

Marsha M. Sanders, RPh, BS
Jones County Junior College
Ellisville, Mississippi

Karen Snipe, CPhT, AS, BA, MAEd
Pharmacy Technician Program Coordinator
Trident Technical College
Charleston, South Carolina

Sarah Lea Welsh, BS, CPhT
Career Center of Texas—El Paso
El Paso, Texas

Mark F. Williams, BS, CPhT
Mercy College of Northwest Ohio
Toledo, Ohio

Contributors to This Edition

We extend a special acknowledgment to the following people who brought their expertise to bear by contributing content and valuable editorial input at the page proof stage:

Eugenia M. Fulcher, RN, BSN, EdD, CMA
Program Director, Medical Assisting
Swainsboro Technical College
Swainsboro, Georgia

Robert M. Fulcher, BS, BSPh, RPh
Pharmacist-In-Charge
CVS Pharmacy
Waynesboro, Georgia

Maria del Carmen Leal
Baltimore, Maryland

James J. Mizner, Jr, BS, MBA, RPh
Pharmacy Technician Program Director
Applied Career Training
Arlington, Virginia

Karen Snipe, CPhT, AS, BA, MAEd
Pharmacy Technician Program Coordinator
Trident Technical College
Charleston, South Carolina

Susan Wong, PharmD
Kaiser Permanente
Petaluma, California

Dedication

I would like to dedicate this book to the following people in my life:

My children Tracy, Jeni, Tiffy, Christo, and Ben; I'm so proud of all of you

My friends Billie, Mary, Tina, and Sue; thanks for all that you've done for me

My husband Dave, who through his perseverance and a high degree of tolerance made this book possible

Special thanks to Joni, my old friend, for your wonderful photographs

All of you are rare and exceptional people, and I'm glad to have you in my life.

Teresa Hopper

Contents

SECTION ONE General Pharmacy *1*

1 History of Medicine and Pharmacy *2*

Introduction *3*
The Medical Staff *4*
Medicine in its Infancy *4*
Ancient Herbal Remedies *6*
Medicine in the Fourteenth Century *6*
Eighteenth Century Medicine *6*
Medicine in America *6*
Changing Pharmacy *8*
Protocol *9*
Trust in Pharmacists/Trust in Technicians *9*
Technicians of the Twenty-First Century and Beyond *9*

2 Law and Ethics of Pharmacy *12*

Introduction *13*
Description of Laws *14*
Health Insurance Portability and Accountability Act of 1996 *16*
Food and Drug Administration/Drug Enforcement Agency *16*
Controlled Substances *17*
Monographs *19*
Prescription Regulations *20*
Records and Labeling Requirements *23*
State Laws *24*
Liabilities *24*
Morals Versus Ethics in the Workplace *25*

3 Pharmacy Settings for Technicians *28*

Introduction *29*
Historical Data *29*
Current Qualifications *30*
Nonjudgmental Duties *30*
Inpatient Setting Requirements *30*
Outpatient Setting Requirements *31*
Home Health Settings Requirements *32*
Mail Order Pharmacy/E-Pharmacy *32*

National Certification for Technicians *33*
Opportunities for Technicians *34*
Incentive Programs *35*

4   Conversions and Calculations Used by Pharmacy Technicians *38*

Introduction *39*
Metric System *40*
Household Measurements *40*
Apothecary System *40*
Avoirdupois System *41*
Important Differences Among Systems *42*
Writing Units Using Each System *42*
Conversions *43*
Fractions *44*
Percentages *45*
Ratio/Proportion or Formula Method *45*
Filling Prescriptions *49*
Pediatric Dosing *50*
Determining Weight *52*
Drip Rates *53*
Alligation *56*
Roman Numerals *58*
International Time *59*

5   Dosage Forms, Abbreviations, and Routes of Administration *63*

Introduction *65*
Where Did Pharmacy Abbreviations Originate? *65*
Dosage Forms *65*
Routes of Administration *73*
Other Considerations: Form and Function *79*
The Use of Additives *81*
Manufactured Products *81*
Miscellaneous Agents and Devices *83*
Packaging and Storage Requirements *83*

6   Referencing *87*

Introduction *88*
Understanding the Correct Way to Reference *88*
Main Reference Books Used in Pharmacy *89*
Learn What to Look for When Choosing a Reference Book *93*
Pocket-Sized Reference Books *94*
Journals and Newsmagazines *94*
The Internet *95*
Additional Types of Information *95*

7   Competency, Communication, and Ethics *99*

Introduction *100*
Competencies *100*
Professionalism *104*
Communication *104*
Ethics *108*
Additional Competencies *109*
Terminally Ill Patients *110*

8   Prescription Processing *113*

Introduction *114*
Processing a Script: A Step-by-Step Approach *114*
Taking in the Prescription *115*
Translation of an Order *117*
Entering the Information into the Database *118*
Filling the Script *119*
The Rights of a Patient *125*
Pharmacist Consultations: When and Who Needs Them *125*
Miscellaneous Orders *125*
Filing Prescriptions *126*
Medication Pick-Up *127*
Billing *127*
Changing Trends *127*

9   Over-the-Counter Medications and Skin Care Products *130*

Introduction *132*
Over-the-Counter Drug Considerations *133*
The Three Categories of Over-the-Counter Drugs *133*
Food and Drug Administration Regulations *134*
How a Prescription Becomes an Over-the-Counter Drug *135*
Conditions Treated with Over-the-Counter Drugs *136*
Over-the-Counter Agents: Patient Information *137*
Skin Anatomy *142*
Conditions Affecting the Skin *143*
Skin Disorders and Medications *144*

10   Complementary Alternative Medicine *151*

Introduction *152*
What is Alternative Medicine? *153*
Overview of Eastern versus Western Medicine *153*
Trends Toward Alternatives *154*
Using Traditional and Alternative Medicine *154*
The Placebo Effect *155*
Acupuncture *155*
Acupressure *155*
Ancient Chinese Medicine *155*
Art Therapy *157*
Ayurveda *157*
Biofeedback *157*
Chiropractic *158*
Crystal Healing *158*
Herbal Medicine *161*
Homeopathy *165*
Spiritual Healing *166*

11   Hospital Pharmacy *169*

Introduction *170*
Types of Hospitals *170*
Policies and Procedures *171*
Protocol *171*
Hospital Standards *172*
The Flow of Orders *172*
Responsibilities of an Inpatient Technician *174*

Aseptic Technique *175*
Intravenous Technician *176*
Intravenous Therapy and Chemotherapy Preparation *176*
Labeling *178*
Controlled Substances *179*
Additional Areas of Pharmacy *179*
Supplying Specialty Areas *181*
Nonclinical Areas the Pharmacy Stocks *182*
Patient Medication Filling *183*
Pharmacy and Nursing Staff Relationship *184*
STAT and ASAP Orders *184*
Specialty Tasks *185*

12   *Repackaging and Compounding* 187

Introduction *188*
Repackaging *189*
Compounding *192*

13   *Aseptic Technique* 205

Introduction *206*
Terminology *207*
Supplies *207*
Delivery Systems *207*
Aseptic Technique *213*
Parenteral "Syringe" Medications *216*
Compatibility Considerations of Parenteral Medications *222*
Components of an Intravenous Label *223*

14   *Pharmacy Stock and Billing* 226

Introduction *227*
Formulary *227*
Generic Versus Trade Drugs *229*
Third-Party Billing *229*
Inventory Control *235*

15   *Psychopharmacology* 243

Introduction *245*
Emotional Health *245*
Nondrug Treatments *245*
Medication Therapy *246*

SECTION TWO   Body Systems 260

16   *Endocrine System* 262

Introduction *264*
Endocrine Anatomy *264*
Description of Hormones *266*
Structure and Function of Hormones *266*
Mechanism of Action *266*
Functions of the Endocrine Glands *267*
Conditions of the Endocrine System and Their Treatments *270*

17 Nervous System 282

Introduction 284
Nervous System 284
The Neuron 287
Nerve Transmission 288
Central Nervous System 288
Peripheral Nervous System 294
Conditions of the Nervous System and Their Treatments 297
Conditions Affecting the Peripheral Nervous System 300
Disorders of the Brain and Spinal Cord 301

18 Respiratory System 313

Introduction 315
Structure of the Respiratory System 315
Respiration 317
Exchange of Gases 318
Breathing 318
Disorders of the Upper Respiratory System 320
Disorders of the Lower Respiratory Tract 321
Treatment of Respiratory Disorders 323

19 Visual and Auditory Systems 332

Introduction 334
The Eyes 334
The Ears 348

20 Gastrointestinal System 355

Introduction 357
Form and Function of the GI System 357
Auxiliary Organ Functions 361
Conditions Affecting the GI System 362
General Information 374

21 Urinary System 377

Introduction 379
Function of the Kidneys 380
Conditions Affecting the Urinary System 383
Treatments for Urinary System Conditions 386

22 Cardiovascular System 395

Introduction 397
Location and Anatomy of the Heart 397
Conditions Affecting the Heart 399
Treatments and Medications for the Cardiovascular System 404

23 Reproductive System 422
Eugenia M. Fulcher and Robert M. Fulcher

Introduction 424
Medications Related to Male Hormones 427
Medications Related to Female Hormones 431
Miscellaneous Medications Used in the Reproductive System 440

SECTION THREE   Classifications of Drugs 444

24   Antiinfectives 446

    Introduction 448
    History of Antibiotics 449
    Types of Infections and Their Treatments 451
    Antibiotic Treatments 454

25   Antiinflammatories and Antihistamines 473

    Introduction 475
    Inflammation 475
    Pain 477
    Asthma 483
    Antihistamines 486

26   Vitamins and Minerals 492

    Introduction 494
    Vitamins 495
    Minerals 502

27   Vaccines 507

    Introduction 508
    The Lymphatic System 509
    Immunizations 510

28   Oncology Agents 520

    Introduction 522
    What is Cancer? 522
    What Causes Cancer? 523
    Diagnosis of Cancer 524
    Types of Cancer 524
    Treatments for Cancer 525
    Nuclear Pharmacy Technician 532

SECTION FOUR   Basic Sciences for the Pharmacy Technician 536

29   Microbiology 538

    Introduction 540
    Charles Darwin (Evolution) 540
    The Golden Age of Microbiology 541
    Classifications of Organisms (Taxonomy) 541
    Brief History of Antibiotics 552
    Viruses 555

30   Chemistry 563

    Introduction 564
    Parts of an Atom 565
    Molecules 567
    Metabolism: Anabolism and Catabolism 568
    Amino Acids 571
    Measurements 572

SECTION FIVE   **Starting Your Career as a Pharmacy Technician** *578*

31   *Pharmacy Organizations and the Future of Technicians 580*

Introduction *581*
Organizations *581*
National Certification *583*
Two Sides of the Story *584*
The Professional Technician *584*
Less is More . . . *584*
The Possibilities . . . *585*
Getting Involved *585*

APPENDIXES *588*

A   *Abbreviations 590*
Karen Snipe

Common Abbreviations Used in Pharmacy *590*
Drug and Chemical Abbreviations *594*
Disease States *595*
Organizations *595*

B   *Top-Selling Drugs for 2002 596*
Karen Snipe

C   *Top 30 Herbal Remedies 601*
Karen Snipe

D   *Math Review for Pharmacy Technicians 602*
James J. Mizner, Jr

Proportions *602*
Percents *603*
Metric, Household, and Apothecary Conversions *604*
Units *606*
Milliequivalents *606*
Pediatric Dosages *606*
Concentration/Dilution *607*
Alligation *608*
Flow Rates *610*
Temperature Conversions *611*

E   *Health Insurance Portability and Accountability Act of 1996 (HIPAA) 612*
Eugenia M. Fulcher and Robert M. Fulcher

F   *Proper Hand Care for Medical Asepsis in Pharmacy 615*
Eugenia M. Fulcher and Robert M. Fulcher

Glossary *617*

Credits *635*

Index *637*

General Pharmacy

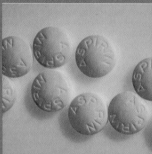

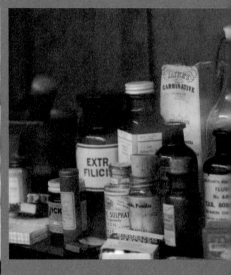

1 History of Medicine and Pharmacy

2 Law and Ethics of Pharmacy

3 Pharmacy Settings for Technicians

4 Conversion and Calculations Used by Pharmacy Technicians

5 Dosage Forms, Abbreviations, and Routes of Administration

6 Referencing

7 Competency, Communication, and Ethics

8 Prescription Processing

9 Over-the-Counter Medications and Skin Care Products

10 Complementary Alternative Medicine

11 Hospital Pharmacy

12 Repackaging and Compounding

13 Aseptic Technique

14 Pharmacy Stock and Billing

15 Psychopharmacology

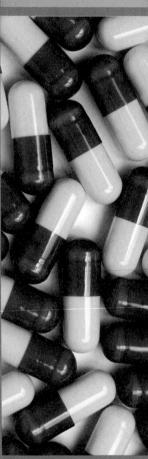

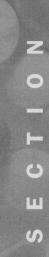
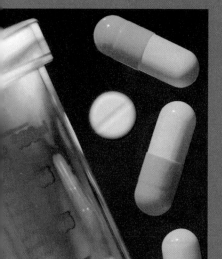
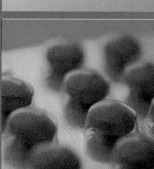
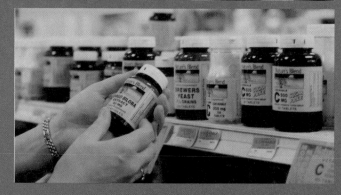
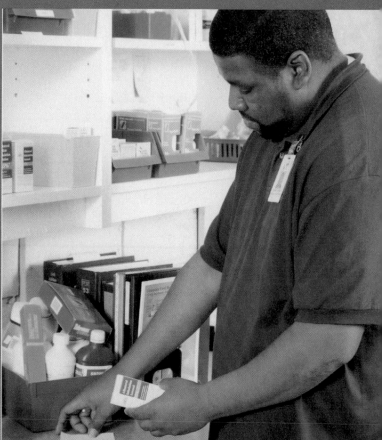

1 History of Medicine and Pharmacy

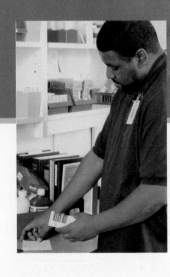

Objectives

- Discuss ancient medicine 440 BC through 1600 AD.

- List common ancient treatments that prevailed in Western civilization.

- Describe fourteenth century medicine and what effects it had on Western medicine.

- Describe eighteenth century medicine and identify influences major wars had on medicine.

- Describe the use of opium and alcohol.

- Identify the role that early pharmacists played in society.

- Describe the first technicians in pharmacy.

- Describe how the first pharmacies came about in the United States.

- List major ways pharmacy has changed over the past 100 years.

- Identify the need for protocol in the pharmacy profession.

- List major current trends in pharmacy in relation to pharmacy technicians.

- Identify the resistance to technicians that parallel historical resistance to pharmacists.

IMPORTANT PEOPLE

Aesculapius	God of medicine in Greek mythology
Aristotle	Greek scientist, philosopher
Bacon, Roger	English scientist responsible for scientific methods
Galen	Greek physician
Hippocrates	Greek physician and philosopher, considered to be the father of medicine
Mendel, Gregor	Scientist and monk
Paracelsus	Swiss physician, philosopher, and scientist

TERMS AND DEFINITIONS

Apothecary *Latin term for pharmacist*

Clinical pharmacist *Pharmacist who monitors patient medications in inpatient and some retail settings*

Drug education coordinator (DEC) *Pharmacist who helps set protocol in a hospital setting*

Dogma *Code of beliefs based on tradition rather than fact*

Inpatient pharmacy *A pharmacy in a hospital or institutional setting*

Outpatient pharmacy *Community pharmacies or pharmacies in outpatient hospital settings*

Pharmacist *Person who dispenses drugs and counsels patients*

Pharmacy clerk *Person who assists the pharmacist at the front counter of the pharmacy; the person who accepts payment for medications*

Pharmacy technician *Person who assists pharmacist by filling prescriptions and performing other nondispensing tasks*

Protocol *Set of standards written by hospital or insurance company for patient treatment*

Shaman *Medicine person who holds a high place of honor in a tribe*

Introduction

ANCIENT BELIEFS AND TREATMENTS

Medicine has been practiced for thousands of years. Archaeological discoveries have unearthed civilizations that have documented the use of minerals, animals, and plant parts to heal the sick. However, it is difficult to know exactly what people of that time believed to be true concerning death and disease. Some remedies, such as herbals, have been used throughout history. Various herbs were used for minor ailments such as intestinal problems, arthritis, gout, and others.

However, many of the popular beliefs of the past have disappeared. One such belief required that an incision be made into the skull of the diseased person. A cut was made into the skull to give the disease a portal to leave through. This type of treatment was called trephining.

Another belief surrounding healing the sick was the idea that severe illness was caused by evil spirits. To rid oneself of an evil spirit, one needed help from the respected tribal shaman. Shamans were and still are known as medicine men and women. It was believed that tribal shamans had the gift of being able to communicate with the spirits. They were connected with a special spirit who helped them render the evil spirits harmless through the use of prayer, herbs, or potions. Shamans were prevalent throughout societies in ancient times. Some still exist in various societies throughout the world. In North America, various Eskimo and Native American tribes held shamans in high esteem. Many people believed they survived their illnesses because of magical treatments, various herbs, and even quackery. Some illnesses may have been cured because of a placebo effect. Because the patient believed so strongly in the treatment rendered, his or her ailment was cured. This effect is still evident today, and there is still no conclusive explanation of why or how it works.

The Medical Staff

Aesculapius was the Greek god of medicine. His symbol—still used today to signify medicine—was a staff with a snake wrapped around it. Because snakes shed their skin, they signify new life. Treatments for illness were based on the dreams or visions of the believers. Dogmatic beliefs, such as gods being able to cause and cure illness, are based on a set of beliefs (e.g., church doctrines) set forth by authoritarians. These beliefs are based on writings from prophets rather than on hypotheses based on scientific methods.

Medicine in Its Infancy

The infancy of medicine was not a smooth road. Throughout the ages many plagues killed thousands of people. The existence of microbes, unseen by the eye, was not known to be responsible for many of the diseases that caused death and despair. Despite advancements made through early history, most remedies for physical ailments tended to be extreme in nature. Other ancient remedies have been used for hundreds of years. Prevalent thoughts included, for example, that sickness was an entity within the body that needed a means to leave the body. Another was that spirits were responsible for illness. The most common form of treatment, prayer, has still remained in many cultures as the only way to cure illness.

Hippocrates (460-377 BC) was born on the small island of Cos near Greece, and he was a third generation physician. He taught at Cos School of Medicine, which was one of the first medical schools established. He believed in the prevailing concept of that era that life consisted of a balance of four elements that were linked to qualities of good health. They consisted of wet, dry, hot, and cold. In addition, he believed that illness resulted from an imbalance of the four humors of the body system: blood, phlegm, yellow bile, and black bile. These four humors were linked to the four basic elements: blood = air, phlegm = water, yellow bile = fire, and black bile = earth. Methods used to treat imbalance of the humors included bloodletting and laxatives to help rebalance the humors. Hippocrates was responsible for many advancements in the world of medicine. Some of his observations included the effects of food, climate, and other influences on illness. He was one of the first physicians to record his patients' medical illnesses. This new way of viewing the causes of illnesses eventually led to the belief that sickness originated from something other than the supernatural, as was the belief until the time of Hippocrates.

Hippocrates believed that the spirit of the patient should be as important as the condition being treated, and he promoted being kind to the sick. He also believed in letting nature do the healing and promoted rest and eating light foods. He taught that doctors needed to bring the four humors back into balance. Most of his teachings have been documented in a collection of books called *Corpus Hippocraticum*. Although many of the writings are now believed to be from different authors, they still reflect the teachings of Hippocrates.

Today's medical schools still use the Hippocratic oath as part of their graduation ceremony. This oath, taken from the book of *Ancient Greece and Rome* by Moulton, states: "Doctors act only for the good of their patients and keep confidential what they learn about their patients." As the book explains, the Hippocratic oath outlines the physician's responsibility to the patient. Hippocrates practiced what he preached with respect to exercise, rest, diet, and overall moderation in one's lifestyle. Various records have his death at 377 BC while others record his death in 357 BC. Considering the average human lifespan was no more than 40 years at that time, living between 83 and 103 years was astonishing. Because of the many advancements he promoted in the world of medicine, it is not surprising that Hippocrates is known as the Father of Medicine.

TECH NOTE! The origin of the term "black humor" stems from the belief that too much of the black bile humor resulted in a person showing signs of melancholy.

Prior to Hippocrates and other innovative scientists, people believed that they were at the mercy of the gods or supernatural forces. One such god was Aesculapius, the god of healing, to whom temples and shrines were built to pray for health.

Later in history, the Greek philosopher and scientist Aristotle (384-322 BC) was responsible for many advancements in the areas of biology and medicine. His main area of interest was biology and the study and classification of various organisms. He classified humans as animals. Because the belief system in those times did not allow dissection of the dead, he described much of human anatomy from observations he made from dissections of other animals. This included in-depth descriptions of the brain, heart, lungs, and blood vessels.

Claudius Galen (129-200 AD) began to study medicine at the age of 16. He attended medical schools in Greece as well as the famous Alexandria school of medicine in Egypt. He later resided in Rome and was the personal physician of the Roman Imperial family. Although he was born nearly 600 years after Hippocrates, he followed many of the same beliefs, such as eating a balanced diet, exercise, and good hygiene. He contributed greatly to the study of medicine, writing more than 100 books on topics such as physiology, anatomy, pathology, diagnosis, and pharmacology. Many of his books were used in medical schools for 1500 years. He proved that blood flowed through arteries rather than air.

Philosopher and alchemist Roger Bacon (1214-1294 AD) further refined and explained the importance of experimental methods, moving even further away from the era's dogmatic beliefs.

Paracelsus (1493-1541 AD), a Swiss physician and alchemist, believed that it was important to treat illness with one medication at a time. At that time it was a common practice to give multiple remedies or large quantities of agents that had not been previously tested. Through the use of documentation of the effectiveness of each individual agent, Paracelsus was able to produce many nontoxic medications. He introduced one of the most popular tonics of that time—laudanum, which was used to deaden pain. Figure 1.1 lists major figures in early medical history.

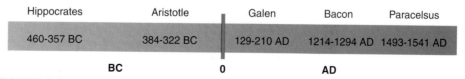

FIGURE 1.1 Time line. People who had a profound influence on medicine between 460 BC and 1500 AD.

Ancient Herbal Remedies

Over the millennia some prevalent treatments consisted of multiple mixtures of plants, roots, and other concoctions. It was also believed that digesting the type of plant that resembled the organ affected by disease could cure illnesses. For example, those with liver problems ingested a plant called liverwort (named because the leaves were shaped like a liver). Other popular treatments included using garlic for inflammation of the bronchial tubes, wine and pepper for various stomach ailments, onions for worms, and tiger fat for joint pain. It was very hard to detect which if any of the ingredients administered actually worked because many concoctions contained a multitude of ingredients.

Medicine in the Fourteenth Century

Throughout history, some popular religious beliefs revolved around the idea that evil spirits were the cause of illness in a person who had sinned. This belief may have persisted partially because no one had the slightest idea about germs or genetics. Many times, through trial and error (error sometimes causing death), certain treatments were found to be fairly effective.

Any time new theories are proposed they can be met with some skepticism and disbelief. A new hypothesis should be treated as a possible answer that has not been disproved. As new scientists emerge and new methods are devised to test hypotheses, their results give way to advancements.

Eighteenth Century Medicine

During the eighteenth century, religious leaders of the church became very active in researching medical remedies to treat the sick. It was during this period that a famous scientist and monk, Gregor Mendel, documented experiments on plants. Born in Austria, Mendel's research on generations of pea plants and other species helped determine the mechanism of how more hearty plants could be propagated. He found the basis of current understanding of genetics and how genes are interwoven into heredity. It was not until a decade after Mendel's death that his research papers made him known as the father of genetics.

Medicine in America

In early America, as new immigrants brought their families from England and other parts of the world, disease followed. Doctors were responsible for not only diagnosing the conditions but for preparing the necessary remedies to cure patients in early times. Therefore the first druggists were doctors. Disease was widespread in the colonies; many people did not survive the voyage across the sea from Europe, succumbing to diseases such as scurvy and severe intestinal infection. The main remedies used in early American history included cinchona bark (quinine) used to treat malaria, and more unconventional and dangerous treatments such as the use of mercury to treat syphilis. Many people died of mercury poisoning because of its toxicity. Hundreds of people also died of typhoid fever, malaria, diphtheria, and dysentery. The need for doctors and treatments increased dramatically. The average life expectancy was around 40 years and many families lost several children to childhood diseases for which there were no vaccines available. Most treatments were concoctions handed down through family tradition. If a person were to use a doctor, he or she would most likely be treated at home or in a doctor's office, with treatments ranging from minor procedures to surgery. There were few doctors and even fewer hospitals throughout the colonies. However, it was not until after the Civil War that a clear division between physicians and pharmacists began.

THE USE OF OPIUM AND ALCOHOL

One of the most popular tonics made for medicinal use in early America contained opium and alcohol. Its effectiveness was surpassed only by its addictiveness. This tonic was given as a sedative and to dull the sensation of pain. Paracelsus (as mentioned earlier) introduced the opium-alcohol mixture called laudanum in the sixteenth century, and it was used as a medicinal remedy. It was widely used during the Civil War not only to treat painful wounds from the battlefield but also in households throughout the United States for less severe problems and even for depression. People became addicted at an alarming rate. Even though it was well known by the eighteenth century that both opium and alcohol were addictive, alternative remedies were hard to find. Another alcohol-based liquid was absinthe. This herb (*Artemisia absinthium*) was mixed with alcohol and other additives. It was served with water and sugar to rid oneself of tapeworms.

TECH NOTE! Alcohol use has been dated back to 3500 BC in Egypt, and opium made its appearance in 5000 BC in Europe.

EARLY PHARMACISTS

The need for specialists such as veterinarians, eye doctors, and pharmacists was due to the growing population and the need for more trained medical personnel. In addition, it was becoming difficult to ship medicines to America from England as the colonies separated from England. After the Civil War, apothecaries (pharmacies) began to spring up in towns across America, manufacturing plants were built, and persons were trained to prepare medications accurately. As the physician's role moved away from distributing drugs to diagnosing disease and surgery, pharmacists moved into the role of druggist. The first pharmacy school opened in 1821 at Philadelphia's College of Pharmacy and Sciences (PCPS). It is now called the University of the Sciences in Philadelphia (USP). Through the 1800s the pharmacist compounded nearly every drug ordered by physicians. Large ornate apothecary jars called cisterns were used to store the various herbs and ingredients. The remedies were contained in medical books and read like a recipe book. Ingredients such as chalk for heartburn; rose petals for headaches; and oils, herbs, and spices filled containers in the apothecary. Of course, people could also buy other items such as personal toiletries at the nearby apothecary store. Some of the remedies of the 1800s are listed in Box 1.1.

BOX 1.1 TYPICAL REMEDIES OF THE 1800S

To stop earaches	Blow tobacco smoke into the ear.
To treat a cold	A mixture of sugar, mineral oil, sulfur, ginger, lemon, and whisky in 8 oz. water: drink and go to bed.
For baldness	Rub the head with an onion both morning and at night before bed until the skin becomes red and then rub with honey.
For worms	Take a tablespoon of molasses and mix with tin rust and ingest.

EARLY PHARMACY TECHNICIANS

The first pharmacy technicians were family members of the pharmacists who owned the corner drugstores. Their wives helped behind the counter and also waited on customers. Older children might have filled in as clerks waiting on customers or placing medication stock onto shelves. It wasn't until much later that pharmacies began to train their clerks to perform simple repetitive tasks such as filling medication drawers, profiling doctor's orders, and even compounding simple mixtures. These early clerks then moved on to become what we now call pharmacy technicians. Although the transition from clerk to technician is fairly recent in history, forecasts indicate that the pharmacy technician will play a critical role in the pharmacy setting.

THE SODA FOUNTAIN/PHARMACY IN AMERICA

Early pharmacists played a minimal role in health care. In the late 1800s and early 1900s, the soda fountain became an extension of a town's drugstore. As mineral water became known as a treatment for many different ailments, it was the natural place to store and prepare the beverages. Many of the drinks, such as carbonated drinks, required chemicals, which the pharmacist had in supply. Some of the many conditions mineral water was supposed to have cured were obesity, upset stomach, depression, and nervous disorders. Pharmacists sold phosphate sodas and ice cream favorites, worked the lunch counter, and filled the day's prescriptions. The first 7-Up drink was made with lithium and was sold from soda fountains for conditions such as gout, uremia, and rheumatism. By the mid 1800s, the soda shop/pharmacy was so popular that people came to drink the sweet concoctions whether they were ailing or not. This type of pharmacy setting undoubtedly added to the image of the friendly neighborhood pharmacist that one could trust. The stereotype local neighborhood pharmacist who wore a white jacket, packaged medications, and sometimes worked the soda machine has all but disappeared except in a few small towns in America, where a person may still fill a prescription and get an old-fashioned malt or shake.

Changing Pharmacy

Times have changed and so have the requirements of today's pharmacist. All states now require pharmacists to obtain a doctor of pharmacy degree, which requires six years of education in an accredited school of pharmacy. Required grade point averages for pharmacy school admission are rising, as is the cost of a pharmacist's education. Today's druggist (referred to more commonly as a pharmacist) also needs in-depth and broad communication skills with doctors and with customers. What has happened to the wife or child who may have helped behind the drugstore counter? Today's typical pharmacy technician (an emerging profession) is required to do an array of tasks, all of which require competency with many skills. Thus in some states, today's technicians are required to get education in addition to on-the-job training. Currently there are no nationally standardized requirements for pharmacy technicians. With the increase in available medications, the fear of interactions or wrong dosing also increases in the pharmacy setting. Technicians help the pharmacist by preparing prescriptions and compounding. In a hospital setting, also known as an inpatient pharmacy, tasks include supplying floor stock to the hospital floors, preparing parenteral medications, transcribing doctors' orders, and filling them in patients' medication cassettes. Other specialized technicians may do all the ordering of drugs and supplies. As always, filtering phone calls and the need for strong communication skills are required by the technician for both inpatient (hospital) and community (outpatient) pharmacies.

Pharmacists can specialize. For example, there are pharmacists who read patients' laboratory results to determine the level of a drug (e.g., anticoagulants or aminoglycosides) that should be dosed. Then, they are allowed to write the necessary change in medication strength based on the laboratory results. Other specialty duties include oncology pharmacists and compounding pharmacists.

Protocol

Protocol is a set of standardized rules that are agreed on within a pharmacy setting. All medical personnel must abide by the protocol of their workplace. There are assortments of people who create protocol, including pharmacists. Some hospitals have specialty pharmacists called drug education coordinators (DECs). These individuals meet to discuss various new medications that have become available. The DECs are part of a hospital committee along with physicians, dietitians, and other medical staff. Each new drug is reviewed, and it is determined whether it is a better drug and more cost effective than current medications being used. Other information that the committee takes into consideration is any new literature that drug companies produce concerning the best use of their medication. Protocol is then put in place that everyone working in the facility must adhere to. For example, if a doctor writes a prescription order for ceftriaxone every 6 hours (normally given either once or twice daily), the pharmacist on duty will call the doctor and find out whether the patient had the proper diagnosis for this dosing regimen. In another institution, the pharmacist may have the ability to change the doctor's orders when necessary as long as it is predetermined per protocol.

Trust in Pharmacists/ Trust in Technicians

Over the decades pharmacists have become known as persons who can be trusted to provide truthful information, and someone a person can be comfortable confiding in. Although some traditions do live on, times have changed concerning the role of the pharmacist. The most prevalent change can be seen in the inpatient setting of the hospital. As the competency of a pharmacist has become more "clinical," pharmacists are becoming more involved alongside doctors in the appropriate prescribing of medications and their dosages. In the community pharmacy, the major change has been in the laws governing patient consultation. All patients who are prescribed new or changed medications must be offered consultation. This is meant to enlighten the patient about the medication he or she is taking. Because of these changes in the way pharmacies function, virtually every pharmacy employs pharmacy technicians. Therefore it is important that the patient can trust a technician to provide the best care by filling the correct medication and referring the patient to the pharmacist for appropriate counsel. This takes a true commitment to the profession of pharmacy on the part of the pharmacy personnel to continue the trust that has existed between patient and health care provider. Through education, training, and good communication skills, technicians will gain the trust of the patients whom they serve.

Technicians of the Twenty-First Century and Beyond

In the new millennium with the roles of pharmacists, technicians, and clerks becoming more clearly defined, new concerns arise: We must be aware that just as the advancement of medicine through the ages met with much resistance, so has the profession of pharmacy. The changing roles of pharmacists, technicians, and even clerks have had their share of blockades, mostly from within the medical community. Some doctors are not eager to have pharmacists writing orders, even if the medications are simple in nature. Likewise, technicians have been perceived as posing a threat to pharmacy. Some pharmacists believe that technicians may take jobs away from pharmacists or increase the liability to the pharmacist if someone who is not properly trained makes a mistake. Therefore there is disparity across the United States regarding the duties of a pharmacy technician. In some states, pharmacies limit technicians' duties to a clerk level. In other states, technicians are required to be certified as pharmacy technicians before they are employed. All technicians must be aware of what is happening legislatively within their state. The federal government has not yet intervened to a high degree in the regulation of technicians.

TECH NOTE! Some states such as Florida allow pharmacists to write certain prescriptions.

Clerks' duties are also expanding and changing. In some pharmacies, clerks regularly enter new prescription orders into the computer. This task was previously done exclusively by a pharmacist or technician. The pharmacist is moving into a more highly clinical role not only counseling patients but also working with medical staff. To a degree, the technician has become what the traditional pharmacist once was—transcribing orders, pulling medications, and filling prescriptions. Finally, the clerk has replaced the early technicians. Some colleges are offering specialized training programs for pharmacy clerks. The introduction of trade/generic drug names and billing are some of the curriculum taught specifically for future pharmacy clerks. To learn more about future pharmacy see Chapter 30.

DO YOU REMEMBER THESE KEY POINTS?

- Terms and definitions used within this chapter
- Common ancient beliefs including the dogmas of those eras
- Common treatments used for conditions in earlier times
- Major persons who influenced the changes of dogmas in medicine
- The beginnings of both pharmacists and pharmacy technicians
- How the roles have changed for pharmacists, technicians, and pharmacy clerks
- New standards being required of today's technicians
- The use of protocol in setting standards in medicine and pharmacy

REVIEW QUESTIONS:

Multiple Choice

1. _____ is known as the father of genetics.
   A. Hippocrates   C. Mendel
   B. Paracelsus   D. A pharmacist

2. Which of the following choices best describes sources of materials for remedies in ancient times?
   A. Chemicals, minerals, vitamins   C. Minerals, animals, plants
   B. Minerals, animals, prayer   D. Plants, seeds, leaves

3. The best definition for dogma would be
   A. A system of beliefs that are considered the absolute truth whether it is truly wrong or not
   B. A type of herbal remedy used in ancient times
   C. A certain way of treating patients
   D. A belief that only certain treatment is proper based on religion

4. Taking new prescriptions and entering them into the computer are tasks a _____ _____ can do.
  A. Pharmacist
  B. Pharmacy technician
  C. Pharmacy clerk
  D. All of the above

5. The period of time when pharmacies were owned and run by pharmacists was
  A. After the sixteenth century
  B. After the Civil War
  C. After World War I
  D. After World War II

6. Doctors used to perform all of the following tasks except
  A. Mend farm animals
  B. Dispense drugs
  C. Prepare drugs
  D. Use prayer for healing

7. Opium and alcohol were once used to
  A. Desensitize a person from pain
  B. Help ease depression
  C. Sedate patients with minor pain
  D. All of the above

8. Apothecary means
  A. Pharmacist
  B. Pharmacy
  C. Doctor
  D. Drug

9. _____ is known as the father of medicine.
  A. Hippocrates
  B. Paracelsus
  C. Mendel
  D. Aristotle

10. Trephining was the technique of
  A. Blood letting to rid the body of toxins
  B. Prayer to rid the body of sickness
  C. Making an incision into the skull to release poison
  D. The making of opium and alcohol

True/False

*If a statement is false, then change it to make it true.

1. In ancient times, plants were the only available remedies for illness.

2. Bloodletting was a short-lived treatment because of many deaths.

3. Sometimes families of the "early" pharmacists assisted behind the counter.

4. Shamans were medicine men who communicated with the spirits.

5. The roles of technicians have changed little since their beginning.

6. Plants given to ill patients in early times resembled the organ being treated.

7. Pharmacists have very little contact with patients in today's pharmacy.

8. Only pharmacists can fill prescriptions.

9. Over the years technician's job description has remained the same.

10. The concept of the four basic elements of life (air, water, fire, and earth) was created by Hippocrates in the late 5th century.

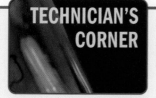

TECHNICIAN'S CORNER

Write a brief summary on the new types of advancements that are occurring in medicine today. Do any of the dogmas that plagued ancient civilizations affect current beliefs?

BIBLIOGRAPHY

Ballington DA: *Pharmacy practice,* St Paul, 1999, EMC/Paradigm.

Anderson MJ, Stephenson KF: *Scientists of the ancient world,* Springfield, NJ, 1999, Enslow.

Suplee C: *Milestones of science,* Washington, DC, 2000, National Geographic.

Narcto D: *The complete history of ancient Greece,* San Diego, 2001, Greenhaven Press.

Moulton C (ed): *Ancient Greece and Rome,* vol 3, New York, 1998, Simon & Schuster.

2

Law and Ethics of Pharmacy

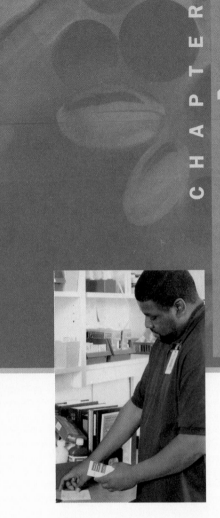

Objectives

- List the history of federal law in chronological order.

- Explain which law prevails among state, federal, and local laws.

- Define the functions of the Food and Drug Administration (FDA) and Drug Enforcement Agency (DEA).

- Describe the FDA reporting process of adverse reactions.

- Explain the necessary forms and regulations used for controlled substances.

- List the current laws pertaining to ordering stock and required record keeping.

- Explain the difference between technicians' tasks and pharmacists' responsibilities.

- Identify the major laws that technicians need to work within when performing nondiscretionary functions in a pharmacy.

- Explain how to verify a doctor's DEA number.

- List who can prescribe medications/devices.

- Define the responsibilities of pharmacy personnel as they apply to morals, ethics, and liabilities.

- Describe the implications of the new Health Insurance Portability and Accountability Act (HIPAA) laws that are in effect as of 2003.

Board of Pharmacy (BOP) *State boards that regulate pharmaceutical practice*

Drug Enforcement Agency (DEA) *Federal agency within the Department of Justice that regulates the misuse of controlled substances*

Facts and Comparisons *Reference book found in all pharmacies containing detailed information on all medications*

Food and Drug Administration (FDA) *Federal agency within the Department of Health and Human Services that regulates the manufacture and safeguarding of medications*

Health Insurance Portability and Accountability Act of 1996 (HIPAA) *Federal act for protecting patients' rights*

Legend drug *Drug that requires a prescription for dispensing*

Monograph *Medication information sheet provided by the manufacturer*

Over-the-counter (OTC) medication *Medication that can be purchased without a prescription; non-legend medications*

Physician's Desk Reference (PDR) *Reference book of medications*

Pharmacy Technician Certification Board (PTCB) *National board for the certification of pharmacy technicians*

Introduction

The practice of pharmacy is governed by a series of laws, regulations, and rules enforced by federal, state, and local government. Pharmacy is also subject to rules made by institutions and/or pharmacy management at each pharmacy site. The number of rules and regulations is staggering and most of us cannot easily decipher the legal tangle of words; however, we are required to follow these rules and regulations. Therefore this chapter presents the most basic of these laws and regulations as they pertain to pharmacy, pharmacists, and especially the technician. A good understanding of these laws is necessary to pass the Pharmacy Technician Certification Board (PTCB) examination and, more important, it is necessary to know your responsibilities when working in pharmacy. The laws are described in chronological order along with a short description of how and why each one was put into place. Common record keeping practices are covered. The legal liabilities of both pharmacists and technicians are explained. Morals and ethics are discussed at the end of this section because they play a vital role in the decisions that technicians will make in pharmacy.

Following is a list of well-known federal laws in chronological order.

Federal Laws

1906	Federal Food and Drug Act
1914	International Opium Convention 1912/Harrison Narcotic Act 1914
1938	Food, Drug, and Cosmetic Act
1951	Durham-Humphrey Amendment
1962	Kefauver-Harris Amendments (thalidomide disaster)
1970	Comprehensive Drug Abuse Prevention and Control Act
	Poison Control Act of 1970
1983	Orphan Drug Act
1987	Prescription Drug Marketing Act
1990	Anabolic Steroids Control Act
1990	Omnibus Budget Reconciliation Act (OBRA 90)
1996	Health Insurance Portability and Accountability Act of 1996

Description of Laws

The following descriptions are brief because the various acts and amendments encompass broader descriptions. Further reading is suggested to gain a deeper insight into the laws that pertain to pharmacy and patient rights.

1906 FEDERAL FOOD AND DRUG ACT

The 1906 Food and Drug Act was one of the first laws enacted to stop the sale of inaccurately labeled drugs. All manufacturers were required to put truthful information on the label before selling their drugs. Although this act was well intentioned, there were many drugs that still made their way onto the market because of continued false claims regarding their effectiveness. Additional changes were made to this act that ultimately required manufacturers to prove their drugs' effectiveness through methods such as scientific studies. These changes are summarized in the listed acts that follow. In 1970 the Food and Drug Act was rewritten to incorporate all the changes.

1914 HARRISON NARCOTIC ACT

By 1912 international meetings were being held to curb the rise in controlled substances trafficking. Limitations on opium transport and use were attempted. The Harrison Narcotic Act of 1914 was enacted because of the excessive number of opium addicts in the United States. People could no longer obtain opium without a prescription and it became harder to get.

1938 FOOD, DRUG, AND COSMETIC ACT

The 1938 Food, Drug, and Cosmetic Act was enacted because the earlier Food and Drug Act was not worded strictly enough and did not include cosmetics. False or exaggerated claims were commonly placed on a drug label, which often misled the consumer. This act defined the exact labeling for products and defined misbranding and adulteration as being illegal. The new law required drug companies to include package inserts and directions to the consumer regarding use and package inserts on drugs. All controlled substances were required to be labeled "Warning: May be habit forming." This act also provided the legal status for the Food and Drug Administration (FDA).

1951 DURHAM-HUMPHREY AMENDMENT

The 1951 Durham-Humphrey Amendment added more instructions for drug companies and required the labeling "Caution: Federal law prohibits dispensing without a prescription." Under this amendment, certain drugs require a doctor's order and supervision. This amendment also made the initial distinction between legend drugs (by prescription only) and over-the-counter medications (OTCs), which do not require a physician's order (non-legend drugs).

1962 KEFAUVER-HARRIS AMENDMENTS

The Kefauver-Harris Amendments were enacted in 1962 in an attempt to ensure the safety and effectiveness of all new drugs on the market. The burden was put on the drug manufacturing companies as the good manufacturing practices (GMPs) were put into place. The Food and Drug Administration (FDA) was placed in charge of how advertising was handled. One example of the FDA's effectiveness is illustrated by its role in preventing the sale of thalidomide in the United States. In Europe, people were taking this new medication to help them sleep. Although it was believed to be effective, it was not allowed to be sold in the United States. Meanwhile in Europe in 1962 women who had taken thalidomide while pregnant gave birth to children with severe defects including the absence of limbs. In the United States, however, very few cases occurred because of the FDA's ban on thalidomide. What the thalidomide scare did do was make consumers aware that drug companies were not doing enough to test the drugs they were marketing. More laws ensued after the thalidomide tragedy to better safeguard the public and greatly increase both time and money spent on testing a drug for its safety and effectiveness.

1970 COMPREHENSIVE DRUG ABUSE PREVENTION AND CONTROL ACT

The Drug Enforcement Agency (DEA) was formed to enforce the laws concerning controlled substances and their distribution. A stair-step schedule of controlled substances was introduced. The stair-step schedule of controlled substances requires stricter rules as the drug rating increases. Therefore a schedule V drug requires less documentation than a schedule II drug.

1983 ORPHAN DRUG ACT

The 1983 Orphan Drug Act allowed drug companies to bypass the lengthy time requirements of testing a new drug and the costs that accompanied them to provide a medication to persons who had a rare disease. Before this act, companies had no incentive to find medications and spend millions of dollars and many years of trials to treat a disease that affected a small portion of the population. Therefore many of the restrictions were waived for diseases that affected fewer than 200,000 persons in the United States. It also covered diseases that affected more than 200,000 persons if it could be proven that the cost of developing and testing a drug could not be recovered by the eventual sales.

1987 PRESCRIPTION DRUG MARKETING ACT

One of the main labeling changes that was required by the 1987 Prescription Drug Marketing Act controlled the use of drugs in animals. Until 1987, many drugs were sold OTC in feed stores for use in animals without any restrictions. This new act required the labeling "Caution: Federal law restricts this drug to use by or on the order of a licensed veterinarian." Therefore veterinarians must now write prescriptions before people can buy drugs for their animals.

1990 ANABOLIC STEROIDS CONTROL ACT

The Anabolic Steroids Control Act helped stiffen regulation on the abuse problems of anabolic steroids and their misuse by athletes.

1990 OMNIBUS BUDGET RECONCILIATION ACT (OBRA 90)

Passed by the U.S. Congress, OBRA 90 deals specifically with practicing pharmacists. The law came about because of reimbursement regulations for people who are covered under Medicaid or Medicare insurance. OBRA 90 deals with the specifics of reimbursement for medications, the bottom line that has affected pharmacy. This act states that a pharmacist must offer to counsel (at the time of purchase) all patients who receive new prescriptions. This requirement was to ensure that all medications being prescribed to patients would be investigated for any problems, interactions, possible allergic reactions, and so forth. All patients must be given information on the drug that they are taking, its name, when to take it, how long to take it, and any side effects or possible interactions. If these provisions are not met, the Board of Pharmacy (BOP) who oversees the compliance of OBRA 90 can fine pharmacies and pharmacists.

Health Insurance Portability and Accountability Act of 1996

The Health Insurance Portability and Accountability Act of 1996 (HIPAA) was a bill that has been only partially implemented. Specifically, this bill deals with a patient's right to continuance of health insurance even when changing employers. Recently, however, Congress has placed a date on many new regulations that will affect almost all areas of medicine, including pharmacy. As of April 14, 2003 major changes became required of pharmacy to ensure the rights of patients. HIPAA will affect pharmacy technicians in many ways because technicians have direct knowledge of patients' medical information on a daily basis. Most of the changes are related to implementing consent forms that will need to be signed by patients before any information can be accessed. This pertains to releasing patients' information outside the pharmacy or hospital as well as requiring consent forms within the hospital.

The effects of having to implement computer programs, generate forms, and code sensitive information relating to the patient's medical history are just some of the many changes that will shape pharmacy operations of the future. Not all changes that need to be made have been completed and many have not begun. Also the impact on the cost to health care is not fully known at this time. It is important that technicians keep abreast of all new laws such as HIPAA that come into effect in the future because they can be held liable if they do not work within these guidelines.

Food and Drug Administration/ Drug Enforcement Agency

Two government agencies that are important with respect to pharmacy are the Food and Drug Administration (FDA) and Drug Enforcement Agency (DEA). The FDA was created under the Department of Health and Human Services. The main function of the FDA is to enforce the guidelines for manufacturers to ensure the safety and effectiveness of medications. The DEA was created later under the Department of Justice. The function of the DEA is to prevent illegal distribution and misuse of controlled substances. The DEA also issues licenses to practitioners, pharmacies, and manufacturers of controlled substances. Each agency plays a different part in law enforcement, but they do work together when the DEA must get a determination on new drugs and the level at which they should be controlled.

FDA REPORTING PROCESS AND ADVERSE REACTIONS

The FDA has a toll free number (1-800-FDA-1088) for reporting any defect found in OTC medications or any drug problem of which people become aware. A technician or pharmacist also has this number available to report any problems with a drug, whether it is OTC or legend (prescription). If a product looks different from its normal package it should be reported. Adverse reactions should also be reported to the FDA and to the state's poison control center. Any medication reaction that may cause disability, hospitalization, or death should be reported along with any less disabling type of reaction such as fainting or other types of reactions that may not have been covered in the drug monograph. MedWatch is the program under the FDA that allows consumers and health care professionals to report discrepancies or adverse reactions with medications. The form for such reports may be found in the PDR and in *Facts and Comparisons*. The patient's identity is kept confidential.

Controlled Substances

Controlled substances, more commonly known as narcotics, are substances that are addictive and have a potential to be abused. Controlled substances are derived from opium or opium like substances. Opium comes from the poppy plant and is well known for its analgesic effects and its effects on mood and behavior. Opiates, such as codeine and morphine, are substances created from opium, while opioids are controlled substances that are produced synthetically in a laboratory. All opiates and opioids are addictive. When consumed over time, a person can build up a tolerance to their effects and require increased doses. Each type of controlled substances is assigned a rating that depends on its addiction potential.

REGISTRATION REQUIRED FOR MAINTAINING NARCOTICS

The DEA has three main registration forms used in the regulation of controlled substances. Only Form 224 is needed by the pharmacy to dispense controlled substances.

1. To manufacture or distribute controlled substances: Form 225
2. To run a controlled substances treatment program or compound controlled substances: Form 363
3. To dispense controlled substances: Form 224

ORDERING CONTROLLED SUBSTANCES

For a pharmacy to obtain schedule II controlled substances (C-II) from a distributor, DEA Form 222 must be filled out by the receiving pharmacist. This form must be filled out only with a pen, typewriter, or an indelible pencil. The top copy and the middle (DEA) copy with the carbon paper are sent to the supplier or manufacturer by the pharmacy receiving the drugs. The bottom copy is retained by the pharmacy. When the medication is shipped to the pharmacy, the middle (DEA) copy is forwarded to the DEA to prove that the medication is properly accounted for. When the pharmacy receives the controlled substances, the pharmacist compares the pharmacy's copy of Form 222 with the invoice and signs both. The invoice and the form are stapled together and retained for 7 years. If any error is made, the form becomes invalid but must be retained for reference; therefore you cannot erase mistakes or throw away the form. When returning any C-II drugs, the pharmacy must have the manufacturer or wholesaler fill out the same form (222) to request the controlled substance, and the pharmacy then is the provider who retains the top copy and sends the middle copy to the DEA. Other controlled substances (C-III, C-IV, and C-V) are ordered on normal invoice forms, but invoices must be filed and retained for possible DEA or state board of pharmacy inspection. These should be kept separate from other nonscheduled drugs for easy retrieval. Once the scheduled drugs are received, the invoice forms for schedules III through V must be kept for no less than 2 years.

RECORD KEEPING

There are three methods of filing controlled substances and legend drugs in a pharmacy, as shown in Table 2.1. Although federal law allows any one of these three methods to be used, a state's board of pharmacy may require a specific one.

RATINGS OF SCHEDULED (CONTROLLED) SUBSTANCES

The letter *C* (meaning controlled substance) is used in addition to Roman numerals to indicate the addictiveness or abuse potential of controlled substances. In 1970 the U.S. Congress established five levels of control based on the Potential for Abuse. The strongest in terms of abuse potential are C-I drugs. These include such drugs as d-lysergic acid diethylamide (LSD) and heroin. Pharmacies do not

TABLE 2.1 Three Methods of Filing Controlled Substances and Legend Drugs

System	Drawer 1	Drawer II	Drawer III
1	C-II separate	C-III through C-V	All other prescriptions
2	C-II separate	C-III–C-V* and all legend drugs	
3	C-II through C-V*	All other prescriptions	

*If any C-III, C-IV, or C-V controlled drugs are kept with non-controlled drugs (System 2) or mixed with C-II drugs (System 3), they must be stamped with a red "C" for easy identification. All records must be kept on site for no less than 2 years. Many states, however, have longer requirements for keeping records; remember the strictest law is the one that must be followed. When taking inventory it is necessary to have exact counts of CII controlled substances at all times. The final count can only be inventoried by a licensed pharmacist.

stock drugs in the C-I class because they have not been determined by the FDA to have any medicinal use in the United States. Therefore doctors cannot prescribe C-I drugs for their patients. All medicinal controlled substances drugs are placed in the following four categories: C-II, C-III, C-IV, and C-V. Table 2.2 shows the schedule, types of medications, and abuse potential for each level of controlled substances.

In some states C-V medications (referred to as exempt controlled substances) are kept OTC because of the low Potential of Abuse, whereas all states are required to lock up C-II drugs because of their high Potential of Abuse. However, for these exempt controlled substances there are specific rules governing the quantity kept on hand and records that need to be retained by the pharmacy on their purchase by consumers. The Attorney General has the authority to decide what schedule a drug should be placed under. The decision is made after careful consideration is given to scientific findings and input from various authorities on the possible dependency potential of each agent. Some drugs may be labeled under two different schedules because the dose may alter the dependency of the drug. Sometimes controlled

TABLE 2.2 Typical Controlled Substances

Drug Level	Type of Medication Generic Name	Trade Name	Potential for Abuse
C-II	Meperidine	Demerol	High potential for abuse; used for medicinal purposes; abuse may lead to severe psychological or physical dependence
	Codeine		
	Morphine		
	Oxycodone/APAP	Percocet	
	Opium		
C-III	Hydrocodone/APAP	Vicodin	The potential for abuse under this schedule is less than controlled substances under C-II; abuse may lead to moderate or low physical dependence or high psychological dependence
	Acetaminophen/codeine	Tylenol/codeine	
	Oxycodone/ASA	Percodan	
C-IV	Diazepam	Valium	The potential for abuse is low in comparison to schedule C-III; abuse may lead to limited physical or psychological dependence compared with C-III drugs
	Lorazepam	Ativan	
	Pentazocine	Talwin	
	Chlordiazepoxide	Librium	
C-V	Diphenoxylate/atropine	Lomotil	Low potential for abuse in relation to C-IV drugs; abuse may lead to limited physical or psychological dependence compared with C-IV drugs
	Guaifenesin/codeine	Robitussin/codeine	
	Promethazine/codeine	Phenergan/codeine	

APAP, Acetyl-p-aminophenol (acetaminophen); *ASA*, acetylsalicylic acid (aspirin).

substances can be reevaluated; for example, dronabinol was previously rated as a C-II drug but is now a C-III drug.

REFILLING CONTROLLED SUBSTANCES

There are strict guidelines on the amount of controlled substances that can be refilled. Drugs with a rating of C-III or C-IV can be refilled if indicated by the physician or authorized prescriber but only to a maximum of five times or within 6 months from the original order, whichever comes first. In addition, the amount ordered on the refills may not exceed the original order. A record must be kept of controlled substance refills indicating the pharmacist's initials and the date it was dispensed.

Monographs

Under the FDA's labeling regulations the following information must be available in monographs, also known as package inserts, because of the lack of room on the drug container. Doctors refer to this information in the *Physicians' Desk Reference (PDR)*, and it is also contained in the *Facts and Comparisons* reference book in pharmacy (see Chapter 6). All information is required to give the date of the most recent revision. As new information is found or reported, new monographs are written. Thus it is important to have an updated copy of both the *PDR* and *Facts and Comparison* in the pharmacy. If you do not have one available, you can always read the package insert from the medication container to find the most recent information. The type of information contained in a package insert follows.

DESCRIPTION

The basic description of the medication indicates the basic chemical structure, including pH, and may show the chemical structure in picture form as well. Some examples of chemical structures are given in Chapter 29.

CLINICAL PHARMACOLOGY

The clinical pharmacology section lists the drug action, drug interaction, and any other information related to the action of the medication.

INDICATIONS AND USAGE

The indications and usage section describes the specific conditions that the medication is used to prevent or treat. Some medications cannot treat the condition but are used to relieve the symtoms of the condition. Side effects of some medications are used for treating some diseases.

CONTRAINDICATIONS

The section on contraindications explains the types of people who should not use the medication. Studies have shown that certain patients such as diabetics or patients on certain medications have a severe reaction if they take the medication. Many times it includes a class of drugs to be avoided rather than one specific drug that a patient might be taking.

WARNINGS

The warnings heading lists very serious side effects of the medication and what should be done if the patient experiences such side effects. Warnings are not necessarily contraindications but fall close to that heading. The prescriber must be aware of potential problems of the drug before prescribing it to a patient.

PRECAUTIONS

The precautions section gives a list of information about possible side effects that the patient should know when taking the medication. Cautions such as "do not operate any heavy machinery" or "do not drink alcohol while taking this medication" are the types of information provided on auxiliary labels.

DRUG ABUSE AND DEPENDENCE

If patients have shown any tendency to become addicted to the medication or if the medication has been found to be abused by patients, the information should be listed in this section.

ADVERSE REACTIONS

An adverse reaction is an unexpected and possibly life-threatening reaction to a medication, such as an allergic reaction. A side effect is a possible reaction caused by the drug's action, such as drowsiness. All possible adverse reactions to the medication are listed. In addition to listing specific reactions, such as nausea, the percentage of people affected by the reaction (from reported studies) is included.

DOSAGE

The recommended dosing is indicated in this section. It usually specifies by age and/or weight the most common Strength of Drug to administer or prescribe to the patient, along with the dosing time and interval or length. It also gives suggested dosing regimens for patients with specific conditions.

HOW SUPPLIED

Information about how the medication is supplied is often given in chart format because it lists the varying strengths, amount of drug per container, dosage form, and whether it should be given any special considerations such as protection from light or storage in a refrigerator.

Prescription Regulations

WHO CAN PRESCRIBE?

The FDA and DEA have no authority in determining prescribers. Doctors and other medical prescribers are licensed by their governing bodies. The scope of practice is determined by their degree. For example, a podiatrist, a doctor of feet, can prescribe medications and devices that are used in treating foot conditions; they would not and should not be prescribing heart medication. The same is true for dentists, veterinarians, and optometrists because each are experts in their own areas and not in others. The prescribers can vary from state to state (Box 2.1), therefore the specific laws governing them are not covered. However, more states are allowing professionals such as nurse practitioners and physician assistants to prescribe a limited amount of medications and/or devices. These practitioners are required to be supervised by a physician who assumes responsibility for their prescribing methods and scope of knowledge. The standard practitioners in all 50 states are physicians, doctors of osteopathy, dentists, doctors of podiatry, and veterinary medicine. Each state also regulates whether they will accept out of state prescriptions written by practitioners who are not licensed within their state.

BOX 2.1 OTHER PRACTITIONERS WITH PRESCRIBING PRIVILEGES ACCORDING TO STATE STATUTES

Chiropractors
Nurse practitioners
Pharmacists
Physician assistants
Naturopaths

WHO CAN RECEIVE A PRESCRIPTION?

Clearly a pharmacy technician takes in prescriptions, interprets them, and fills them; the pharmacist is responsible for reviewing the prescription before dispensing. A pharmacy intern can also receive prescriptions by phone. However, it is not within the scope of the pharmacy technician, at this time, to take phone orders. Often prescriptions are called in by the doctor's office. A pharmacist must translate verbal orders into written form. Also, if a patient wants a prescription transferred to another pharmacy, this must occur between licensed pharmacists or pharmacy interns.

RECEIVING PRESCRIPTIONS FOR CONTROLLED DRUGS

Pharmacists can receive an oral prescription for a controlled drug over the phone by reducing it to written form. If the drug is a C-II substance, the pharmacist is allowed to take the order and fill the prescription following strict guidelines. The guidelines are as follows:

A. The doctor must determine that the patient needs the C-II and considers it to be an emergency with no alternative treatment possible.
B. The doctor cannot get a written prescription to the pharmacist. This may be because he or she is away from the office.
C. The pharmacist must obtain all information from the doctor, including the drug name, strength, dosage form, and route of administration. The doctor's name, address, phone number and DEA number are required.
D. The amount of the drug can only be enough to sustain the patient through the emergency period. The pharmacist should indicate on the prescription that it is being filled because of an emergency.
E. The pharmacist must make every effort to verify the doctor's authority unless he or she knows the doctor personally.
F. The prescriber has only 72 hours to produce the written prescription covering the filled script. If this is not done, the prescriber must be reported to the DEA.

PRESCRIPTION LABELS

The information on a prescription label differs from what is required on a prescription order. There are two necessary components: the pharmacy information and patient information.

Component 1
  A. Name of pharmacy
  B. Address of pharmacy
  C. Name of prescriber
  D. Date prescription was filled

Component 2
  A. Name of patient
  B. Directions

    C. Any cautions either described or provided on auxiliary labels

    D. Refill information

Special Labeling

Certain drugs require that additional information be given to a patient because of the possibility of teratogenicity (genetic harm) to an unborn fetus. These are given out by either the prescriber or the pharmacy dispensing the medication (Box 2.2).

DEA VERIFICATION

All prescribers must be registered with the DEA to write prescriptions for controlled substances. When approved, the prescribers are given a nine-character identification code. This code is different for each prescriber. There is a method of verifying DEA numbers. The first two characters are composed of letters. The first is either an A or B, followed by the first letter of the prescriber's last name. For example, for Dr. D. Wong the DEA number could begin with either AW or BW. The next seven digits are composed of numbers that are added together. Following the six steps laid out in Box 2.3, a DEA number can be verified.

CHILD RESISTANT CAPS

The Poison Prevention Act of 1970 addresses the issue of accidental poisoning of children. Most medications are required to be packaged in containers that are exceptionally hard for children to open. Hence childproof caps were created. Unfortunately they can be very difficult for some adults to open as well. Therefore some exceptions to this regulation were made because of the necessity of patients to access their medications easily (Table 2.3). In addition to these exceptions, medications can be packaged in non–child-resistant containers if certain requirements have been met. Either the prescriber, such as a doctor, will order the medication to be filled without a childproof cap or the patient will request that the medication be filled without a childproof cap. Usually this information will be put into

BOX 2.2 DRUGS REQUIRING ADDITIONAL INFORMATION

> **Estrogens**
> **Injectable contraceptives**
> **Intrauterine devices**
> **Oral contraceptives**
> **Progestational drugs**
> **Retinoids**

BOX 2.3 DEA VERIFICATION PROCESS

> Dr. Tom Johnson writes an order for Tylenol #3. The doctor's DEA number is AJ1234892.
>
> To verify physician's DEA number:
> Step 1   Make sure the first letter is either A or B
> Step 2   The second letter must be the first letter of the doctor's last name, (in this case J for Johnston)
> Step 3   Add the first, third, and fifth number in the DEA set
>   ($1 + 3 + 8 = 12$)
> Step 4   Add the second, fourth, and sixth number then multiply by 2
>   ($2 + 4 + 9 = 15 \times 2 = 30$)
> Step 5   Add the two sums together ($12 + 30 = 42$)
> Step 6   The last digit "2" from your total must match the last number in the DEA set. In this case all steps match; therefore it is a good number.

TABLE 2.3 Drugs that Can Be Packaged in Nonresistant Bottles

Drug	Dosage Form	Restriction on Strength of Drug
Betamethasone	Tab	x
Cholestyramine	Powder	x
Colestipol	Powder	x
Erythromycin (EES)	Tab, granules	x
Isosorbide dinitrate (less than 10 mg)	Sublingual, chew tabs	x
Mebendazole	Tab	x
Methylprednisolone	Tab	x
Nitroglycerin*	Sublingual	
Prednisone	Tab	x
Sodium fluoride	Package	x

*Nitroglycerin is the only medication that does not have a strength limit on filling it without a childproof cap.

the patient's medial record for future reference. Some pharmacies may require the patient to sign a release form that is kept in the patient record.

MAILING PRESCRIPTION DRUGS

It is common to mail medications through the post office or other authorized mailing system. With the introduction of online pharmacies and mail order pharmacies this option will always be available for patients. However, there are exceptions to what can be mailed. The U.S. Postal Service will not allow any controlled substances to be sent by mail. The one exception is certain veterans receiving prescriptions via the Veterans' Administration. Other postal services are not governed under the same rules as the U.S. Postal Service. However, pharmacies generally do not mail out controlled substances. When they are mailed, they must be unmarked on the outside as to what the contents are. Manufacturing mailing is somewhat different between pharmacies and the manufacturer. All medications and controlled substances are allowed to be mailed as long as the recipient (pharmacy) is registered with the DEA. All medications sent from the manufacturer to the recipient are required to be sent as registered mail with a return receipt request form. In addition, the DEA number must be part of the address label.

RECALLED DRUGS

The manufacturer must recall items that have been found to be either defective or somehow tainted. In pharmacies, there are forms used for such events. All stock must be pulled from the shelves following the guidelines of the manufacturing company. There are 3 classes of recalls:

> Class 1: The highest level of recall dealing with products that could cause serious or even fatal harm
> Class 2: The next level deals with products found to cause serious but reversible harm
> Class 3: The lowest level used for products that may have a minor defect or other condition that would not harm the patient but cannot be resold

Records and Labeling Requirements

Hospitals and community pharmacies differ in the length of time that patient records are to be kept. Both are required to keep complete and accurate records of patients. For the purpose of simplicity, outpatient (community, home health) are listed separately from inpatient (hospital) in Table 2.4.

TABLE 2.4 Required Patient Information

Type of Facility	Patient's Full Name	Prescriber's Name	Name and Strength of Drug	Date of Issue	Prescription Number	Expiration Data	Lot and Control Number of Drug	Manufacturer	Name of Drug Dispensed
Hospital	x	x	x	x	*	x	*	*	x
Community	x	x	x	x	x	x	x	x	x
Home health	x	x	x	x	x	x	x	x	x

*Gray areas represent information not transcribed onto the patient's computer record.
Each medication sent to the floor has manufacturer name, lot number, and expiration date on each unit dose medication. Hospital patients are not given prescription numbers but are listed in the computer under their medical record number and a hard copy is made daily of all their medications.

REPACKAGING

Unit dose medication that is prepared in the pharmacy requires the following record keeping rules. Technicians traditionally make most of the unit dose medications in a pharmacy setting. Any medication taken from bulk packages and placed into blister packs must have the following information on each individual label:

A. Drug name (trade/generic)
B. Strength
C. Dosage form
D. Manufacturer
E. Lot number
F. Expiration date

All information must be logged into a binder or a system that can be easily retrieved.

State Laws

Each state has its own set of laws that must be followed by pharmacists, interns, pharmacy technicians, and clerks when working in the pharmacy. It is important to know your state's regulations. All pharmacy personnel should become familiar with the laws by obtaining their state board of pharmacy's regulations booklet. You will notice that many states have laws that differ from federal law. Remember that the strictest law is the one you follow. Therefore if the FDA states that you must keep records for no less than 2 years but your state regulations require 7 years for inpatient records, then you would follow the strictest regulation, in this case your state's regulation.

Liabilities

You should also be aware of both federal and state liability laws pertaining to pharmacy technicians. There are various charges that can be made by a patient toward a pharmacy technician if the pharmacy technician caused damage because of negligence or intentional action in the workplace. A tort is causing injury to a person intentionally or because of negligence. The word *negligence* may describe an action taken without the forethought that should have been taken by a reasonable person; a mistake was made. For an intentional mistake, the penalty can range from criminal charges to the awarding of damages, which usually means that money is paid to the person or persons who were wrongly affected. A negligent mistake can affect a person's ability to continue to work as a technician and may also result in punitive damages (i.e., money).

There are many reasons mistakes happen. Some are due to excessive workload or possibly staffing shortages that can lead to a mishap and could be classified a negligent tort. Criminal behavior, such as false insurance claims or diverting drugs, could be called an intentional tort that could result in imprisonment. One of the questions you should ask your employer is if you are covered under their legal department. If a lawsuit was to be filed with you as the plaintiff, do you know who would represent you? Many companies have lawyers that represent the company, although it should not be assumed that they would represent you. If you are not covered by your employer, you may want to purchase malpractice insurance. Most technicians do not have such insurance and it is a personal preference. At the very least, be aware of what your rights and responsibilities, including legal considerations, are before entering a workplace. If any incidents should happen at work that you might be involved in or witness to, you should follow the following guidelines:

A. Review your state's regulations
B. Understand employer's rules and practices
C. Define scope of employment

In case of an "event" that takes place in the pharmacy:

A. Know who your attorney is
B. Always be careful of what you say and to whom if ever questioned by state or federal investigators pertaining to a mishap
C. Write down in-depth notes on the facts of the event and keep for reference

Morals Versus Ethics in the Workplace

One important factor that the pharmacy technician must remember is that he or she has a clear responsibility to the patient on many levels. Patients are consumers, and as consumers they have the right to receive goods that have been handled properly and are in good condition. They also trust the pharmacy personnel with their personal information, expecting that their information will be treated as confidential information and not be discussed. Many times within a pharmacy or any work setting, employees will voice their beliefs concerning various medical procedures such as abortion, surgery, or a type of treatment. These are very controversial topics and the opinions that each person has are a part of the personal morals or beliefs that the person was brought up with. Although each person has his or her own set of morals, many morals tend to coincide with others' beliefs, such as stealing is not good, and so forth.

In a workplace, however, technicians, pharmacists, and other health care workers are faced with patients who come in for help and who might have different morals. In these situations, the type of professionalism that must be shown to the patients is one's ethics. Ethics are morals in the workplace and in the public domain. When you take on the responsibility of serving the public in a setting such as the pharmacy, you take on work ethics that will guide your behavior. For instance, in a hospital setting there may be a need for medication that is used in abortions or other controversial treatments. It is the responsibility of the pharmacy staff to provide services for all patients. If you have a deeply rooted belief that you believe prohibits you from participating in servicing patients, you must bring this to the attention of your supervisor.

On a lighter side, just keeping small matters in perspective can help you decide what the right choice is in many decisions. Keeping patients' information confidential and working within pharmacy laws and guidelines including policies and procedures will ensure that patients are getting the best service possible. One should remember that pharmacists, technicians, and clerks are there to serve the patients and customers in a professional manner at all times.

DO YOU REMEMBER THESE KEY POINTS?

- Terms and definitions covered in this chapter
- Major federal laws affecting pharmacists and pharmacy
- The differences between functions of the DEA and FDA
- Filing systems required for stock and controlled substances inventory
- Filing requirements for patients' information
- Who can write a prescription
- The legal limitations of pharmacy technicians
- Labeling requirements for repackaging medications
- How to decipher a DEA number
- Types of recalls and how to handle them
- The functions and authority of the state board of pharmacy
- The difference between morals and ethics and the importance of them
- Which medications require package inserts when dispensed

REVIEW QUESTIONS:

Multiple Choice

1. The Amendment that required the labeling "Caution, Federal law prohibits dispensing without a prescription" was the
   A. Durham-Humphrey Amendment
   B. Kefauver-Harris Amendment
   C. OBRA 90
   D. None of the above

2. What does the Orphan Drug Act do?
   A. Put into effect stricter rules concerning controlled substances sales and distribution
   B. Allows drug companies to bypass lengthy testing to treat persons who have a rare disease
   C. Stops the use of drugs without a prescription in animals
   D. Ensures safety and effectiveness of manufacturing practices

3. The law that requires pharmacists to counsel patients on new medications is
   A. OBRA 90
   B. Comprehensive Drug Abuse Prevention and Control Act
   C. Prescription Drug Marketing Act
   D. Durham-Humphrey Amendment

4. The FDA's main purpose is to
   A. Make arrests
   B. Ensure that both safety and effectiveness of medications is met by manufacturers
   C. Prevent distribution and the illegal use of controlled substances
   D. Make sure all laws pertaining to physicians and pharmacists are met

5. A pharmacy that will be dispensing controlled drugs must have which one of the following forms on file with the DEA?
   A. Form 222
   B. Form 224
   C. Form 363
   D. Form 225

6. All adverse reactions should be reported to
   A. FDA
   B. DEA
   C. CIA
   D. Pharmacy management

7. The five categories of controlled substances are rated based on
   A. Cost
   B. Strength
   C. Conditions that they treat
   D. Potential for Abuse

8. Of the information contained in a monograph of a medication, which of the following statements best describes the information related to the action of the drug?
   A. Description
   B. Clinical pharmacology
   C. Adverse reactions
   D. Indication and usage

9. Of the types of health care providers that follow which one is not one of the standard practitioners that all states accept?
   A. Doctors of Podiatry C. Chiropractors
   B. Dentists D. Veterinarians

10. Which of the components listed is not required on a prescription label?
    A. Name, address, and phone number of the pharmacy
    B. Name, address, and phone number of the prescriber
    C. Date prescription was filled
    D. Any auxiliary stickers and/or warnings

True/False

*If a statement is false, then change it to make it true.

1. The thalidomide tragedy of 1962 resulted in the United States recalling the drug.
2. DEA Form 222 is used to obtain controlled substances from the manufacturer or distributor.
3. Scheduled drugs such as LSD and heroin are CI drugs and are used only in extreme cases.
4. Monographs can be found with the drug and in the *PDR*.
5. The contraindication section of the monograph explains the abuse and dependence dangers of the medication.
6. Physicians should only order medications within their scope of practice.
7. Pharmacy technicians can take oral prescriptions as long as there is a pharmacist on duty who gives permission for them to do so.
8. Only pharmacists can fill out Form 222 required by the DEA in pencil.
9. Both isosorbide and nitroglycerin can be dispensed without childproof caps.
10. A recall that is classified as Class 1 means that it is the lowest level of a recall and is used for products that contain only a minor defect.

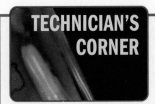
TECHNICIAN'S CORNER

Dr. Beth Golden writes an order for the following prescription:
DEA#BG1958366
Disp: hydrocodone/acetaminophen tablets #50
Sig: Take 1 tablet q8h prn severe pain
10 refills

Determine whether this DEA number is correct, and explain each step of the checking process. List how many mistakes, if any, you find on all parts of this order.

BIBLIOGRAPHY

Nielsen JR: *Handbook of federal drug law,* ed 2, Philadelphia, 1992, Williams & Wilkins.
Ballington DA: *Pharmacy practice for technicians,* St. Paul, Minn, 1999, EMC/Paradigm.
Shargel L, et al: *Comprehensive pharmacy review,* ed 4, Baltimore, 2001, Lippincott.

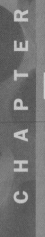

CHAPTER 3

Pharmacy Settings for Technicians

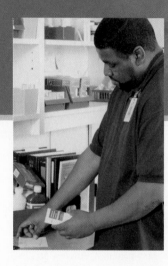

Objectives

- Discuss historical data on technicians.

- Describe current qualifications of technicians.

- Explain what the term *nonjudgmental duties* means.

- Explore various settings for technicians.

- Describe various pharmacy setting requirements as they apply to technicians.

- Describe how pharmacy has expanded onto the Internet.

- List the new position openings for technicians that are available in the health care field.

Continuing Education (CE) *Education beyond the basic technical education, usually required for license renewal*

Hyperalimentation *Parenteral nutrition for patients who are unable to eat solids or liquids*

Inpatient pharmacy *Pharmacies that supply medications for patients in hospitals or nursing homes*

National Association of Boards of Pharmacy (NABP) *National organization for members of state boards of pharmacy*

Outpatient pharmacy *Pharmacies that serve patients in their communities; pharmacies that are not in inpatient facilities*

Parenterals *All medications that are given as an injection*

Introduction

Traditionally, pharmacists worked filling prescriptions in a pharmacy, computer operators worked on pharmacy software components, and secretaries worked in the health care billing offices. The vocation of pharmacy technician began as a clerk with minimal tasks that related to understanding medications. However, healthcare is changing rapidly as are the job descriptions and educational requirements of pharmacy technicians. In this chapter, each area in the health care field pertaining to pharmacy is explored along with the necessary job qualifications and expectations. As the medical field changes and the various guidelines expand, more pharmacy technicians will be able to move into other areas of healthcare. Along with their expanding roles, the expectations of the technician's expertise will rise. Each of America's 50 states has not standardized the qualifications and job descriptions for the pharmacy technician. This is also true for pharmacists because each state has different laws to which pharmacists must adhere, although the laws do not vary as much as technicians' requirements do. Therefore each state's board of pharmacy determines what standards are and how they must be met by technicians. This one area of discrepancy is an issue that over the next decade will become more defined through the continuing efforts of the boards of pharmacy. Eventually technicians throughout the United States will become respected as pharmacy paraprofessionals.

Historical Data

Historically, technicians have answered to a variety of titles. These include pharmacy clerk, pharmacist assistant, pharmacy aide, pharmacy technician, and pharmacy helper. They have held a variety of positions. Some of the job responsibilities have been billing, ordering, stock clerk, typist, phone receptionist, troubleshooter, cashier, and errand runner. Technicians have been a part of the pharmacy field since the beginning of pharmacy, even though they were not always called pharmacy technicians (see Chapter 1). However, more recently, pharmacy managers and their respective state board of pharmacy have been attempting to classify and clearly define the role of the pharmacy technician as the needs of pharmacy change.

Current Qualifications

Each state in the United States has its own board of pharmacy that is overseen by the National Association of Boards of Pharmacy (NABP). Each state's board of pharmacy serves many functions besides registering technicians and licensing pharmacists. It also provides consumers with a way to complain or report any problems or illegal actions they have experienced in a pharmacy. The board of pharmacy also reviews and updates current rules and regulations pertaining to pharmacy practice (see Chapter 2). The NABP is currently looking into the expanded use of technicians in the pharmacy field. This examination of the current uses of technicians will no doubt reveal the skill level necessary for various types of pharmacy tasks, and ultimately changes will be made throughout each state's board of pharmacy. Boards of pharmacy may also change technician-to-pharmacist ratios in pharmacy settings.

Nonjudgmental Duties

All technicians, regardless of their title, can and do perform many types of nondiscretionary duties in the pharmacy setting. The term *nonjudgmental* can be confusing because it can be misunderstood as performing tasks that require little or no thought. This assumption is far from the truth. As the job classification of pharmacy technicians expands, so will their duties and their knowledge of pharmacology. Nonjudgmental simply means that the final approval for any task completed in a pharmacy setting must be checked and approved by a pharmacist. This limits technicians from interpreting scientific studies, counseling patients about their current or adjunct medications, and conferring with other medical personnel about proper treatments.

Inpatient Setting Requirements

Inpatient pharmacy usually refers to hospitals in which patients stay overnight or longer, depending on the procedures they require. Most departments in a hospital have medication and supplies that are specific to their department. This is supplied by the inpatient pharmacy. Therefore inpatient pharmacies traditionally have more different types of stock than outpatient pharmacies so that they can provide all the necessary supplies required of each individual department. For example, labor and delivery stocks a large amount of the drug oxytocin (induces labor), whereas the intensive care unit (ICU) and coronary care unit (CCU) require a wide variety of cardiac medications in their stock areas. The cancer units may stock high amounts of morphine and other analgesics, whereas the pediatrics department stocks many drugs in liquid form for children. Stocking all of these areas is just one of the responsibilities of an inpatient pharmacy technician.

In addition to knowing all of the various drugs, strengths, and dosage forms, the technician must be able to react on a moment's notice when emergency (stat) orders are received by the pharmacy. The dynamics of an inpatient pharmacy can fluctuate on a minute-to-minute basis depending on the flow of patients into and out of the hospital. Stat doses are to be delivered within 15 minutes to the station requesting them, such as the emergency room (ER), operating room (OR), ICU, CCU, and other departments. This duty includes preparing any intravenous (IV) solutions.

An aspect of the inpatient pharmacy is the ability to prepare parenterals, hyperalimentations, and chemotherapy. Helping the pharmacist answer phones, preparing first doses, and loading the medication drawers for patients are other tasks that the technician must be able to do competently. All patient medications are loaded into medication drawers in amounts to complete a 24-hour cycle. All documentation in the inpatient pharmacy is usually based on a 24-hour cycle for each patient. It is important to be quick, but always more important to be correct and thorough when distributing medications to patients. Another aspect of the inpatient pharmacy is the preparation of unit dose medications (see Chapter 12). There are two reasons why medications need to be repackaged:

1. The drug companies do not have the medication available in unit dose.
2. The hospital has chosen to prepare its own medication for cost-saving reasons.

TECH NOTE! The bottom line in working any area of pharmacy is "Always make sure the pharmacist has checked all drugs and/or devices before they leave the pharmacy." If this step is taken, the technician is working in the scope of practice and fewer mistakes will result.

Following are common job descriptions of inpatient technicians, along with some new responsibilities that are new additions in the pharmacy setting. The jobs listed do not require any additional educational training other than the training provided by each pharmacy setting. Most inpatient pharmacy technicians who are interested in the following areas in pharmacy will receive additional on-the-job training to prepare them for these additional tasks:

- Inventory technician—Orders all stock, takes care of billing, talks to drug representatives, and may be responsible for ordering lowest cost item.
- Robot filler—Many pharmacies are installing robots to fill patient medication drawers on a daily basis. Technicians must be trained to load these million-dollar mechanical robots and to keep them running smoothly.
- IV technician—Interprets orders and prepares all parenteral medications, both large and small volumes, including controlled substance drips, hyperalimentation, insulin drips, and any other special order IV or intramuscular (IM) drugs.
- Chemotherapy technician—Interprets orders and prepares all chemotherapeutic agents and their adjunct medications, such as antiemetics.
- Anticoagulant technician—Helps assist the anticoagulant pharmacist in contacting patients to alter their warfarin doses.
- Clinical technician—Helps assist the clinical pharmacist with tracking patients' medications. The pharmacist contacts physicians who may not be ordering formulary drugs or drugs used for specific conditions.
- Supervisory technician—Schedules other technicians. May even hire perspective technicians by reviewing their skills and backgrounds.

Outpatient Setting Requirements

Working in outpatient pharmacy is one of the most difficult tasks in pharmacy because of their front-line interaction with patients on a daily basis. This job tests communication skills and stress levels of the technicians who work with the public. There is a high volume of interacting on the telephone, taking in refill prescriptions, and answering questions pertaining to various insurances. Computer skills are often used to look up specific patient information to assist the customer over the phone or in person. Many neighborhood pharmacies fill a high volume of prescriptions on a daily basis. It is not uncommon for a midsize pharmacy to fill 300 prescriptions in a day, answer phone calls, and take care of patients' problems. In addition to filling prescriptions, the outpatient technician must be able to order stock in a timely manner. Smaller community pharmacies may keep minimal stock because of limited space and the limited variety of drugs prescribed by physicians in the area. Billing various insurance companies is another skill the outpatient technician must master. This includes knowing all of the various rules, regulations, and special codes that may accompany each prescription.

Following are the job descriptions of outpatient pharmacy technicians and a few new positions being filled by technicians in community pharmacies. Larger drug companies that are community based have seen the positive aspects of hiring technicians to fill certain positions.

- Insurance billing technician—This person must know Medicare, Blue Cross, Medicaid, and other insurance companies' guidelines.
- Retail technician—This person must have extremely good communication skills, phone skills, and prescription-filling abilities.
- Stock inventory technician—This person must know contacts for fast service, be able to get products and drugs as soon as possible (ASAP), and perform proper billing functions for the pharmacy, including processing returns, recalled drugs, and controlled substances.
- Technician recruiter—Some outpatient pharmacies and/or temporary agencies employ these technicians to recruit other technicians into their company.
- Technician trainer—Various outpatient pharmacies employ technicians to train newly hired technicians on computer programs and to master other necessary skills relevant to their specific pharmacy.

Home Health Settings Requirements

A home health pharmacy fits somewhere between inpatient and outpatient pharmacy. On one hand, the technicians usually are processing prescription medications for patients on a weekly or monthly basis, which is more similar to an outpatient setting. They prepare the drugs with the same type of labeling required for patient use. On the other hand, there are no patients, doctors, nurses, or other health care providers in the facility. Most home health pharmacies are based away from hospital sites and are not open to the public. Couriers deliver the medications to the home health clients. In addition, the prescriptions are usually packaged differently. Flat cardboard blister packs are prepared by technicians to be used by nurses who administer the drugs in the home health setting (see Chapter 12). Other technician responsibilities include preparing parenteral medications. Usually a few days' to a month's supply is filled each time instead of only 24-hours' worth, which is how the inpatient pharmacy technician loads patient medications. All medications filled for a patient at home are checked by a licensed pharmacist before they are delivered. Home health clinics also provide services for patients that are taken care of by nurses in the patient's home setting. Home health nurses may receive supplies from the pharmacy clinic, or the patient's family may pick up or have supplies delivered. Patients who may receive care at home include kidney dialysis patients receiving peritoneal dialysis and hospice patients.

Mail Order Pharmacy/E-Pharmacy

The mail order pharmacy and E-pharmacy is growing as the baby boomers reach maturity. With more medications becoming available to treat commonly acquired illnesses specific to older people, the need to expeditiously fill their prescriptions increases. There are large buildings in many industrial areas that are used to process new prescriptions and refill others. Technicians are used in these settings as well. This is a relatively new area of pharmacy that is steadily growing.

National Certification for Technicians

Another factor that must be acknowledged is the Pharmacy Technician Certification Board that gives an examination three times per year throughout all 50 states. In 1995, four major societies came together and developed guidelines for a way to gauge pharmacy technicians nationwide: The American Society of Health-System Pharmacists (ASHP), American Pharmaceutical Association (APhA), Illinois Council of Health-System Pharmacists (ICHP), and the Michigan Pharmacists Association (MPA). These four entities created the Pharmacy Technician Certification Board (PTCB) and created goals for pharmacy technicians:

- To work more effectively with pharmacists
- To provide greater patient care and service
- To create a minimum standard of knowledge
- To help employers determine knowledge base

Most states, such as Kentucky and Arizona, do not require certification of their technicians but have different guidelines for their capabilities in the pharmacy practice. For example, Arizona allows only certified technicians to compound in a retail setting. Other states, such as Texas, require certification of all new technicians but do have exemptions for certain pharmacy technicians. Alabama does not require certification, but they do require that all pharmacy technicians receive continuing education (CE) each year. It is apparent that not all states' requirements are standardized. However, most, if not all, now require technicians to have a high school diploma. It is important for each student to visit the website of his or her board of pharmacy to become familiar with the state's current laws pertaining to pharmacy technicians.

TECH NOTE! Visit www.PTCB.org to get statistics on certified technicians and to access your state's BOP for the latest laws pertaining to technicians.

Box 3.1 lists common duties, and Box 3.2 lists qualifications for technicians according to the Pharmacy Technician Certification Board (PTCB).

According to the current statistics, there are more than 200,000 technicians nationwide. Each state has different standards for their technicians, which is one reason that there is such a difference in pay for this skilled job. Many states are beginning to recognize the importance of certification to guarantee that the technicians hired are competent in all areas of pharmacy. Technicians are able to take the national examination three times a year. Once the 140-question examination is passed, the technician is certified and may use CPhT after his or her name, indicating that he or she is a certified technician. Technicians must keep their certification current by attaining 20 credits of CE every 2 years, including one

BOX 3.1 DUTIES OF A CERTIFIED TECHNICIAN

- Handling of ongoing pharmacy benefit telephone calls from members, pharmacy providers, and physicians daily under the supervision of a pharmacist
- Troubleshooting third-party prescription claims questions with an understanding of online rejections and plan parameters
- Developing and maintaining an electronic service log on all telephone calls with complete follow-up history
- Developing a trending report on the aforementioned service calls with an eye toward forecasting possible trends in pharmacy service
- Providing as-needed telephone and administrative support for the department

BOX 3.2 CHARACTERISTICS OF A CERTIFIED TECHNICIAN

- Strong organizational, prioritization, communications, and mathematics skills required
- Pharmacy Claims Processing Computer System experience preferred
- Minimum 2 years experience in a retail pharmacy setting and/or managed care/pharmacy benefit environment beneficial
- Comprehensive understanding of third-party pharmacy benefit plan parameters necessary
- Ability to understand the importance of and respect the confidentiality of all patient information
- Computer literacy with proficiency in general word processing and data entry necessary

This information was attained via the PTCB website (www.PTCB.org).

credit in pharmacy law. Currently, the national examination given by the PTCB is one of two national certifications that a pharmacy technician can obtain. The other is the Certified Pharmacy Technician (CPhT), offered by the National Healthcareer Association (NHA). More information about this credential, and schools that offer it, can be obtained at www.nhanow.com. Employers are increasingly using these credentials as a requirement for hiring technicians.

Opportunities for Technicians

Pharmacies use computers daily; therefore it is important to develop software for pharmacy personnel. Some pharmacy-related fields do require more education in specific areas such as computers. With the proper educational training such as an AS or BS in computer science, the pharmacy technician is well equipped to write software or supply support. Also, as many technicians move into the area of training technicians, their expertise may help them write curriculum, articles, and even books for pharmacy technicians. Many vocational schools hire experienced pharmacy technicians to teach students the necessary requirements to be a competent pharmacy technician. Completion of such training programs offers different degrees, such as certificates, an associate's degree (AA, AS), or a bachelor's degree (BA, BS).

There are many other positions that a pharmacy technician can fill. Following is a list of various nontraditional jobs that technicians are filling:

- Pharmacy business management operators—These pharmacy business management companies are beginning to realize the importance of knowing not only the trade and generic names of drugs but also the classifications of drugs. They are hiring technicians, rather than registered pharmacists, to help pharmacy customers over the phone, which is a cost savings for the company.
- Computer support technician (PYXIS, SUREMED)—Large companies that supply hospitals, community pharmacies, and other facilities with automated medication dispensing systems are employing technicians as support personnel.
- Software writer—With some additional computer background and/or training, some pharmacy software writers are using technicians to prepare software services. Technicians use their terminology and drug knowledge in creating new software programs.
- Authors—With some additional education background and extensive knowledge of pharmacy, technicians can participate not only in preparing and presenting CE credits but also in writing supplemental books for pharmacy technicians.

- Poison Control Call Center Operator—Some poison control centers are using technicians to triage calls coming into the 911 stations. If the call is in regard to something life threatening, then they transfer the call to a pharmacist or poison specialist. If the call is something less critical, they are authorized to take the call.
- Nuclear Pharmacy Technician—The technician may assist the pharmacist with handling and preparing doctors' orders for radioactive medications used in diagnosis and treatment.
- Director/Instructor—Pharmacy technicians can oversee technician training programs and/or instruct in schools around the country. Some require a BS degree or vocational education teaching credentials.

In addition to these positions listed, there are new positions being developed by different pharmacy settings. Although these positions may currently be nontraditional, their numbers are growing. It would not be surprising if they became commonly held positions for future technicians.

Incentive Programs

Pharmacies sometimes have an incentive program for employees who want to further their careers in pharmacy. Many pharmacists once began their careers as technicians. Many pharmacy employers usually give incentives for returning to school to become a pharmacist. They may reimburse tuition costs or give pay incentives. Whether a company does support and partially fund school programs is a consideration that should be taken when inquiring about a pharmacy position.

As the geriatric community increases in number over the next millennium so will the need for qualified medical personnel. Pharmacy technicians know much about the benefits and challenges that pharmacy has to offer. The future of technicians is still being determined, but judging from the ground currently being broken by technicians, their only limitations are self-imposed. Many pharmacy companies reimburse their technicians after they pass the PTCB examination. This is more likely to take place in states in which certification is not mandatory but preferred. Attaining increased skill levels, including becoming certified pharmacy technicians, opens more doors for technicians in pharmacy.

DO YOU REMEMBER THESE KEY POINTS?

- Various duties that pharmacy technicians can perform under the supervision of a pharmacist
- Jobs that pharmacy technicians can perform outside the pharmacy
- Where technicians can find their state's current requirements necessary to work as a pharmacy technician
- Major differences between the functions of inpatient (hospital), outpatient (community), and home health pharmacies
- New expanding areas of pharmacy, such as mail order and E-pharmacy, that are incorporating pharmacy technicians
- Duties and characteristics of national certified pharmacy technicians
- Additional degrees for pharmacy technicians that can lead them into other areas of pharmacy

REVIEW QUESTIONS:

Multiple Choice

1. Some nontraditional job areas that technicians can work in include
   A. Recruiter
   B. Pharmacy business management operators
   C. Computers
   D. All of the above

2. It is up to each state to determine the minimum requirements of pharmacy technicians and may include which of the following?
   A. Licensing
   B. Registration
   C. Certification
   D. All of the above

3. Boards of pharmacy serve what function?
   A. Licensing and registration of pharmacists and technicians
   B. Writing and enforcing the rules and regulations of pharmacy practice
   C. An avenue for consumer complaints
   D. All of the above

4. All pharmacies in their perspective states are overseen by
   A. Each state's NABP
   B. Each state's board of pharmacy
   C. Pharmacy managers
   D. Consumers advocacy groups

5. Nonjudgmental duties of a technician include all of the following except
   A. Requiring all work to be checked by a pharmacist
   B. Duties that do not require interpretation of reference materials
   C. Duties that assist the pharmacist in preparing and dispensing medication
   D. Counseling patients on all nonprescription medications

6. All of the following duties are required of an inpatient technician except
   A. Supplying stock to emergency clinics
   B. Repackaging medications into unit dose packages
   C. Helping customers with insurance claims
   D. Preparing chemotherapy

7. The job description that best describes a technician that assists in repackaging, parenteral preparation, and delivery of medications in a hospital setting is a(n)
   A. Inpatient technician
   B. Home health technician
   C. Outpatient technician
   D. Clinical technician

8. Important aspects of outpatient pharmacy is the need to keep lower levels of drugs on the shelf but in stock at all times. This is due to
   A. Lack of shelf space
   B. The need to keep employee hours down
   C. Changes in medication usage by physicians
   D. A and C

9. Companies that use technicians for assistance in medical dispensing systems in pharmacies would best describe
   A. Software writers
   B. PBM operators
   C. Inpatient technicians
   D. Computer support technicians

10. Of the following jobs, which usually require(s) additional education of a technician?
    A. Instructor of pharmacy technicians
    B. Director of a pharmacy program
    C. Software writer
    D. All of the above

True/False
*If the statement is false, then change it to make it true.

1. The NABP determines each state's regulations pertaining to technicians.

2. Technicians currently hold the same positions that they have held historically.

3. Most pharmacies that hire technicians require the same basic skills.

4. Most companies that use pharmacy technicians outside of the pharmacy require additional education.

5. Most prescription orders filled in a hospital pharmacy are for 24 hours, whereas a community pharmacy fills the full length of the prescription order.

6. Inpatient technicians assist inpatient pharmacists to monitor patients who are taking certain medications.

7. Stat doses are to be delivered within 3 minutes.

8. Technicians giving advice to a nurse on what dosage form to use for a patient in the hospital is nonjudgmental.

9. Most states require technicians to be certified.

10. Certification renewal for a pharmacy technician requires 30 hours of continuing education per year.

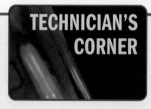

TECHNICIAN'S CORNER

Internet assignment: Log onto the Internet and visit the NABP (www.nabp.org). List their objectives and find the listing for your state and another state. Visit the two board of pharmacy sites and find the current requirements for technicians. Print out your findings and submit them to your instructor. Write a one-page summary on the differences between the two states as they pertain to the description of a pharmacy technician.

BIBLIOGRAPHY

Harteker LR: *The pharmacy technician companion,* Washington, DC, 1998, American Pharmaceutical Association.

WEBSITES

http://www.pTCB.org

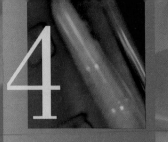

CHAPTER 4

Conversions and Calculations Used by Pharmacy Technicians

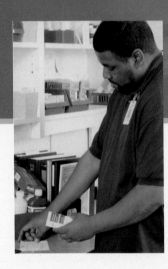

Objectives

■ Describe the differences among the following measurement systems:
- Apothecary system
- Avoirdupois system
- Metric system
- Common Household Measurements

■ Convert arabic numbers into roman numerals

■ Demonstrate the ability to convert among the following measurement systems commonly used on prescriptions:
- Metric system
- Apothecary system
- Household system

■ Use mathematical calculations to determine dosage:
- Ratios/proportions
- Fractions
- Percentages

■ Demonstrate the ability to set up equations and solve problems for:
- Determining days supply
- Pediatric dosages
- Drip rates
- Alligation
- Percent dosages

Alligation *A method of determining the needed amounts of two different concentrations to prepare a needed concentration*

Apothecary system *A system of measurement used in pharmacy*

Avoirdupois system *A system of measurement used for determination of weight*

Household system *A system of measurement commonly used for weight, volume, and length in the United States*

International time *A 24-hour method of keeping time in which hours are not distinguished between AM and PM but are counted continuously through the entire day*

Metric system *A system of measurement based on multiples of 10*

Volume *The amount of liquid enclosed within a container*

Introduction

The ability to manipulate conversions is a required competency of pharmacy technicians. It is also a foundation for filling orders and calculating doses in the pharmacy. This chapter covers the basics in conversions in pharmacy along with common mathematical problems that a technician may encounter. Although all transcribing and calculations need to be checked by a pharmacist, it is important that the technician have a good understanding to avoid medication errors. As you move through this chapter, make sure you learn each basic step before moving on to the next. Once you have a good knowledge of the basic conversions, then you can begin to work out the calculations that follow.

Pharmacy has a long history (see Chapter 1), and many of the old forms of measurement are still in use. These measurements come from different regions of the world; therefore not all units are easily converted or exact. For example, many equivalencies will be rounded to a more usable number. The pharmacy technician must be well versed in all of the different measurements. The four most common types are as follows:

1. Metric system
2. Household Measurements
3. Apothecary system
4. Avoirdupois system

All of these systems are used in a pharmacy at one time or another.

A good way to become familiar with common pharmacy measurements is to start with what you know and then slowly build on that knowledge. For example, most people are familiar with the measurement of a teaspoon. In fact, most people could gauge a teaspoonful by eye alone. Some doctors may prefer not to write instructions for 1 teaspoonful when ordering a prescription; instead you will see the measurement for a teaspoonful in one of the other three systems. The pharmacy technician must translate the doctor's orders into lay person's terms. Remember to always read what will be printed on the label to see if it makes sense. Do not assume that people understand what a milliliter or an ounce is. You must make the instructions easy enough for a child to understand. This will decrease the chance of any misreading of the label's instructions.

TABLE 4.1 Common Household Measurements

Household Measurements (Volume)	Metric (Volume)	Household
1 teaspoon	5 ml or cc*	1 teaspoon
1 tablespoon	15 ml or cc	3 teaspoons
1 cup	240 ml or cc	8 ounces
1 pint	480 ml or cc	2 cups
1 quart	960 ml or cc	4 cups
1 gallon	3840 ml or cc or 3.84 L	16 cups

*Remember that 1 ml and 1 cc contain the same amount of liquid.

Metric System

The metric system is used throughout pharmacy because of its accuracy. The units used in the metric system include milliliters (ml), cubic centimeters (cc), and liters (L) for volume; kilograms, grams (g), milligrams (mg), and micrograms (mcg) for weight; and millimeters (mm) and meters (m) for distance. It is important for a technician to know the difference between each unit given. For example, if a prescription were filled with 1 gram of drug when only 1 milligram is ordered, the patient would overdose by 1000 times the ordered dose. There is a 1000-unit difference between each measurement. This means 1000 mcg equals 1 mg.

The use of millimeters is reserved for drug calculations that are based on body surface areas and would be calculated by a physician or pharmacist using a surface area calculation chart. For most technicians, knowing the basics for volume and weight conversions is adequate.

TECH NOTE! Remember: It is very important to place the proper units (such as ml, L, mg, or g) next to the number amount. This cannot be stressed enough especially because you will be working with various systems. Putting the units on all numbers is the only way to help avoid mistakes.

Household Measurements

The most common measurement system that is still used extensively in the United States is the household system. You probably already know this system. Measurements come in a variety of units. For instance, volume refers to liquids, weight refers to dry ingredients, and length refers to distance. If you want to bake a cake, you must use utensils to measure both dry and liquid ingredients. If you carpet a room, you need to multiply width by length to get the square footage or distance. Let's review some of these measurements. The most common Household Measurement is probably the teaspoon. Other common measurements include tablespoons and cups. In Table 4.1 these common Household Measurements are listed next to some of the most common volumes written (in metric) by physicians.

TECH NOTE! If you have measuring cups and spoons in your kitchen, pull them out and convert them into milliliters and ounces. Do the same for food items on your kitchen shelf.

Apothecary System

Although the apothecary system originated in Europe, it is used throughout the medical field in the United States. The units used in this system are grains (gr)

TABLE 4.2 Apothecary Weights

Dry Weight	Fluid Weight
1 grain = 60 mg	1 dram = ℞ 60
15 grains = 1 gram	8 drams = ℞ 480
20 grains = ℈ 1	3 scruples* = ʒ 1
1 dram = ℈ 3	
1 ounce = ʒ 8 or	
= ℈ 24	
= gr 480	
= 31.1 grams	
1 pound = 16 ounces	
= ʒ 96	
= ℈ 288	
= gr 5760	
= 454 grams	

*Scruples (℈) and minims (℞) are not commonly used units.

TABLE 4.3 Conversion Table: Apothecary/Metric/Household

Apothecary Volume	Apothecary Weight	Metric Volume	Metric Weight	Common Household
ʒ 1	ʒ 1	30 ml	30 g	2 tbsp
ʒ 4	ʒ 4	15 ml	15 g	1 tbsp
ʒ 2	ʒ 2	7.5 ml	7.5 g	½ tbsp
ʒ 1	gr 60	4 ml	4 g	1 tsp
ʒ ½	gr 30	2 ml	2 g	½ tsp

and scruples (℈) for dry weight and ounces (ʒ), drams (ʒ), and minims (℞) for liquids. More common measurements include ounces and pounds. The apothecary conversions are shown in Table 4.2. When using the apothecary system, the measurement is placed before the amount; for example, 1 grain is written as gr 1. How do you write ½ grain? The most common way is gr $\overline{ss}$ ($\overline{ss}$ means ½) gr vii$\overline{ss}$ thyroid qd = 7½ grains daily.

The most common pharmacy units are converted into both metric and Household Measurements (Table 4.3). Be sure to learn these conversions before continuing.

TECH NOTE! The weight of a grain in the apothecary system may vary between 60 mg, 64 mg, and 65 mg. Why? When the grain was used in ancient times to determine weight, real grains of wheat were used, and the weight depended on that year's harvest. If the crop was good, then it took fewer grains because each one weighed more. If the crops were bad that year, then it may have taken more grains to equal the same weight. Therefore be aware that some medication labels will say that there is 60 mg/grain, whereas others might have 64 mg/grain or even 65 mg/grain. However, when performing calculations, the use of 60 mg/grain is customary.

Avoirdupois System

The avoirdupois system is another type of measurement that originated in England. It is similar to the apothecary system because it also uses grains, ounces, and pounds for weights. Table 4.4 shows the common avoirdupois weights.

TABLE 4.4 Standard Weights: Avoirdupois/Metric

Avoirdupois		Metric Equivalents
Dry Weights		
1 Pound	=	454 g
1 Ounce	=	30 g
1 Grain	=	64.8 mg
Liquids		
1 Fluid ounce	=	30 ml
1 Pint	=	473 ml
1 Gallon	=	3785 ml

Important Differences Among Systems

You should know how the metric system's units vary from other units of measure such as ounces and grains. Most of the time they convert easily, but sometimes there are variances, making conversions between measurement systems approximate in these instances. Because the metric system is the most common system used in pharmacies, it is the measurement you use when preparing a compounded drug. However, you will see differences among manufacturers' products and their weights. For example, some manufacturers consider 473 ml to equal a pint, whereas others consider 480 ml or 500 ml to equal a pint.

As shown in the following, 1 pound is equal to 454 g in metric measurements, whereas it is only 373 g in the apothecary system. Although there is some difference between systems on the exact weight, the most accepted measurement is the metric system.

2.2 Pounds = 1 kg	Metric
1 Pound = 454 g	Metric
1 Pound = 373.2 g	Apothecary
1 Ounce = 28.35 g	Avoirdupois
1 Ounce = 31.1 g	Apothecary
1 Ounce = 30 g	Metric

Writing Units Using Each System

See the following for the most common type of units used for each of the systems discussed in this chapter. Although all four systems will be used in writing prescriptions, the pharmacy primarily uses the metric system. However, regardless of which system is used in a prescription, it must be converted into Household Measurements for the patient. At the end of each section there are quick check questions to answer. The answers to these problems are at the end of the chapter.

METRIC MEASUREMENTS

1. You can use cc (cubic centimeter) and ml (milliliter) interchangeably, although ml is the preferred measurement.

1 ml	= 1 cc
5 ml	= 5 cc
100 ml	= 100 cc
1000 ml	= 1000 cc

2. Dry weights use microgram (mcg), milligram (mg), gram (g), and kilogram (kg).
3. Liquid volumes use milliliter (ml) and liter (L).

APOTHECARY MEASUREMENTS

1. Dry weights use pounds (#), ounces (℥), drams (ʒ), scruples (Ɵ), and grains (gr).
2. Liquid volume weights use fluidounces (f℥), fluidrams (fʒ), and minims (℞).

AVOIRDUPOIS MEASUREMENTS

1. Dry weights use pounds (#), ounces (oz), and grains (gr).
2. Liquid volumes use fluid ounces (foz), pints (pt), and gallons (gal).

EXERCISE 4.1 QUICK CHECK

1 dram = _____ teaspoon(s)
8 ounces = _____ cup(s)
1 gallon = _____ cup(s)
5 cc = _____ teaspoon(s)
30 ml = _____ tablespoon(s)
30 ml = _____ ounce(s)
1 gr = _____ mg
1 pint = _____ cup(s)
1 pint = _____ ml
15 tablespoons = _____ ml
1 kg = _____ g

Conversions

When converting orders, it is important to know the basics. Once you have memorized the basic units of the preceding tables and figures, then continue.

METRIC SYSTEM SLIDE

When converting metric measurements from one unit to another, you need to move the decimal either to the right or the left. All changes of the metric system involve either dividing or multiplying by 10s. The most common units used in pharmacy are kg, g, mg, and mcg. Each unit is a multiple of 1000. By moving the decimal by three spaces (to the right or left) you can change between these units. For example, changing units from 5000 mg to grams involves dividing the 5000 mg by 1000, or moving the decimal three places to the left. See the scale below. Remember, the difference between 1 kg, 1 g, 1 mg, and 1 mcg is 1000. Therefore you need to always move three decimal places in one direction or another. One of the most frustrating problems is when you can't remember which way the decimal must be moved when changing between large and small numbers or vice versa. There are two ways; choose the one that works for you and stick with it.

Method A for Determining Metric Conversions

Left				Right
Largest				Smallest
__1_____	1_____	1_____	1_____ ə	
1000 kg	1000 g	1000 mg	mcg	
(3 decimals)	(3 decimals)	(3 decimals)		
0.000000001 kg =	0.000001 g =	0.001 mg =	1 mcg	
1 kg =	1000 g =	1,000,000 mg =	1,000,000,000 mcg	

TECH NOTE!   Remember that there are 1000 g in 1 kg, 1000 mg in 1 g, 1000 mcg in 1 mg.

For the purpose of most pharmacy drug calculations, these are the only four units that you need to use. When going from large, 1 kilogram (kg), to a smaller amount, gram (g), move the decimal to the right three spaces. In the following illustration the decimal is placed in this equation to show you how to count off the right amount of spaces. Decimals are not placed at the end of a number *unless* there is a fraction, such as 1.1 kg. Decimals and periods have been a main source of mistakes in pharmacies because they can be mistaken for changing a number by a thousand. For example (0.10 and 01.) Do you know for sure what this number represents? This could have devastating effects if a medication were given to a patient and the doctor had intended 1 and not 0.1.

$$1 \text{ kg} = ? \text{ grams} \quad \rightarrow \quad 1 \text{ kg} = 1000. \text{ g}$$

Count to the right three spaces and fill in your zeros.

$$1 \text{ g} \ = ? \text{ milligrams} \quad \rightarrow \quad 1 \text{ g} \ = 1000. \text{ mg}$$
$$1 \text{ kg} = ? \text{ milligrams} \quad \rightarrow \quad 1 \text{ kg} = 1000000. \text{ mg}$$

Move three spaces to the right twice.

Method B Large Number to Small Number, Don't Divide—Multiply

When converting from large to small you multiply (use the previous ruler). When converting from small to large you divide.

TECH NOTE!   This is an easy way using the calculator to quickly get the number, but sometimes it becomes confusing—divide or multiply? When going from a **L**arger to **S**maller unit don't **D**ivide! **(LSD)**; multiply to obtain the answer instead.

Try the following three questions using your calculator. All of these are large units going to smaller units.

$$2 \text{ kg} = ? \text{ grams} \qquad\qquad 2 \text{ kg} \times 1000 = 2000 \text{ g}$$
$$2 \text{ g} = ? \text{ milligrams} \qquad\qquad 2 \text{ g} \times 1000 = 2000 \text{ mg}$$
$$2 \text{ kg} = ? \text{ milligrams} \qquad 2 \text{ kg} \times 1000 \times 1000 = 2,000,000 \text{ mg}$$

Let's go in reverse: smaller to larger using the calculator.

$$2 \text{ micrograms} = ? \text{ mg} \qquad 0.002 \text{ mg}$$
$$2 \text{ milligrams} = ? \text{ g} \qquad \tfrac{2}{1000} = 0.002 \text{ g}$$

EXERICISE 4.2 QUICK CHECK

> Use both previous methods and see which one works best.
> You receive a doctor's order for 0.88 mcg of levothyroxine.
>> How many milligrams is this equivalent to?
>> How many grams?
>> How many kilograms?
> Both weight and volume are calculated the same way. Practice on small numbers until becoming comfortable with this conversion.

Fractions

Rarely will you receive an order in fraction form that you need to convert; however, you should know how to do this in case the need should ever arise. It is a simple two-step process to convert simple fractions into percentages. For example, $^6/_9$ converted into a percentage requires dividing 6 by 9 and multiplying this by 100 to get the percentage. Remember that a percentage is always a portion of 100. $^6/_9 = 0.66 \times 100 = 66.6\%$ or rounded up would be 67%. To convert a decimal into a percentage you simply multiply by 100 because decimals are just a different representation of a percentage or part of 100. For example, 1.5 is the same as 150%. If you are converting a fraction from grains into milligrams, however, you multiply by 60 rather than 100 because there are 60 milligrams per grain. For example, if you receive an order for $^1/_{150}$ gr of nitroglycerin SL (sublingual) tablets you first divide 1 by 150, then multiply by 60 to get the answer of 0.39999..., which would be rounded up to 0.4 mg.

Percentages

Percentages represent a portion of 100. This means 10% is the same as 10 g in 100 ml of solution or other product. All percentages must be converted into the metric system, then they can be changed into any other system if necessary.

Let's try some conversions. Convert the following fractions into percentages:

1. $0.125 = $ _____%	Answers:	1. 12.5%
2. $2.5 = $ _____%		2. 250%
3. $\frac{3}{10} = $ _____%		3. 30%
4. $\frac{5}{20} = $ _____%		4. 25%
5. $0.0125 = $ _____%		5. 1.25%

Ratio/Proportion or Formula Method

When technicians compound certain products, they may be required to solve problems using ratios, which can be considered parts or fractions. For example, a concentration of 1:1000 means there is 1 part to 1000 parts or 1 g of drug in 1000 ml of solution. If you receive an order for 5% hydrocortisone and you have 1:1000 concentration in stock, you can use a simple two-step ratio/proportion to solve the problem.

EXAMPLE 4.1 RATIO/PROPORTION

Step 1
5% is equivalent to 5 g per 100 ml or 5000 mg per 100 ml. This can be reduced to 50 mg/ml. Your stock solution is 1 g in 1000 ml or 1000 mg in 1000 ml, which can be reduced to equal 1 mg/1 ml.

Step 2
Subtract what you have from what you need to find the final volume or strength. In this case it would be:

5 g (needed) − 1 g (have) = 4 g needed to prepare the final product per 100 ml

About 90% of the orders you will encounter in the pharmacy will be ratio/proportion equations. This is a three-step process. One of the first rules to remember is to filter out the unnecessary information. Second, find what strength you have in stock and what strength you need (what the doctor is ordering). Finally, set up the equation and double check the calculations. There are two methods to use: method A (ratio/proportion) (have = need) or method B (formula) using $\frac{D}{H} \times Q$ = medication to give, where:

D = Desired dose
H = Have in stock
Q = Quantity on hand

For each of the following examples, both types of calculations are used. Try to solve the problems using both methods, and use what works best.

For other medication orders, finding the answer may not be as simple. For example, if a drug is ordered that does not easily convert, these two methods can be used. The most important point to remember is to place the correct units into the correct position. Try both methods and choose the one that makes more sense to you.

EXAMPLE 4.2 RATIO/PROPORTION

Order: Prepare 240 mg of a drug using the pharmacy stock concentration of 80 mg/4 ml.

Method A: (Have = Need)

In this case, you need to determine how many milliliters of the stock solution are needed to fill the 240 mg order. Write your stock or given concentration on the left and your needed amount on the right. Make sure your milligrams and milliliters match across from one another. Then cross multiply by the quantity on the side of the x, then divide by the numerator of your concentration, and you'll have your necessary milliliters to draw from the vial.

$$\frac{80 \text{ mg}}{4 \text{ ml}} = \frac{240 \text{ mg}}{x}$$

$$960 = 80x$$

$$\frac{960}{80} = \frac{80x}{80}$$

$$12 \text{ ml} = x$$

Answer: You will need to withdraw 12 ml of solution to equal 240 mg of drug.

Method B: D/H × Q = Medication to give

Using a different method, you can set up the equation as the desired amount (240 mg) over the stock strength (80 mg) times the quantity of the stock volume (4 ml) as shown below:

$$\frac{240 \text{ mg}}{80 \text{ mg}} \times 4 \text{ ml} = 12 \text{ ml}$$

EXAMPLE 4.3 RATIO/PROPORTION

Method A: (Have = Need)

Order: You need to prepare 1 pint of 40 mcg medicated lotion. How many milliliters of the stock solution 5 mcg/ml will it take to prepare the final product? Write your stock or given concentration on the left and your volume needed on the right. Make sure your milligrams and milliliters match across from one another. Don't forget to cross multiply and divide by the quantity on the side of the x and you'll have your necessary volume to draw from the container.

$$\frac{5 \text{ mcg}}{1 \text{ ml}} = \frac{40 \text{ mcg}}{x}$$

$$40 = 5x$$

$$\frac{40}{5} = \frac{5x}{5}$$

$$8 \text{ ml} = x$$

Answer: You need a total volume of 8 ml of drug mixed into the lotion to equal 1 pint. To determine 1 pint (30 ml/ounce; 8 ounces/cup; 2 cups/pint; so 30 ml × 16 oz = 480 ml). Therefore you subtract the amount of drug to be added from the total volume:

$$480 \text{ ml} - 8 \text{ ml} = 472 \text{ ml}$$

Answer: You will add 8 ml of drug to 472 ml of lotion to get a 40 mcg bottle of lotion.

Method B: D/H × Q = Medication to Give

Using a different method, you can set up the equation as the desired strength (40%) over the stock strength (5%) times the volume of the stock strength (1 ml). Remember when setting up Method B the units must match in the fraction as shown below:

$$\frac{40\%}{5\%} \times 1 \text{ ml} = 8 \text{ ml}$$

Answer: You will need to convert the pint the same way as indicated previously, and you will end up with the same answer.

EXAMPLE 4.4

You receive an order for clindamycin 450 mg q 12 hr. To set up your equation you need to know what you have on hand. Clindamycin is available in different sizes, but all of them have the same concentration. The strength for clindamycin is 150 mg/ml. For each of the milliliters in the vial there is 150 mg of drug (clindamycin). We now have all the components we need to begin.

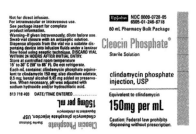

Method A (Have = Need)

What you have = What you need

$$\frac{150 \text{ mg}}{1 \text{ ml}} = \frac{450 \text{ mg}}{x \text{ ml}}$$

You are solving for x because you don't know how much clindamycin to draw up into a syringe. To solve for x, you *cross multiply and divide*.

$$\frac{150 \text{ mg}}{1 \text{ ml}} \times \frac{450 \text{ mg}}{x \text{ ml}}$$

$$\frac{1 \text{ ml} \times 450 \text{ mg}}{150 \text{ mg}} = x$$

$$x = 3 \text{ ml}$$

Method B (D/H × Q)

$$\frac{450 \text{ mg}}{150 \text{ mg}} \times 1 \text{ ml} = 3 \text{ ml}$$

In this case the desired amount of drug is 450 mg; the stock on hand is 150 mg per 1 ml. When laid out in this linear fashion, the amount needed is 3 ml. This can be confirmed by multiplying 3 ml × 150 mg = 450 mg.

EXAMPLE 4.5

You receive an order for 0.5 mg of alprazolam (Xanax) 1 to 2 tabs qhs × 7 days prn insomnia.
You only have 1-mg tablets in stock.
How many tablets are needed to fill this order?

Method A (Have = Need)

$$\text{What you have} = \text{What you need}$$

$$\frac{1 \text{ mg}}{1 \text{ tab}} = \frac{0.5 \text{ mg}}{x \text{ tabs}}$$

In this case, multiply the answer by the maximum dosage ordered (1 mg), then multiply it by 7 days.

$$\frac{1 \text{ mg}}{\text{tab}} = \frac{0.5 \text{ mg}}{x \text{ tabs}} = 0.5 \text{ tabs}$$

$$0.5 \text{ tabs} \times 2 \text{ tabs} = 1 \text{ mg tablets}$$

$$1 \text{ mg tab} \times 7 \text{ days} = 7 \text{ tablets}$$

Give 7 tablets with the following instructions:
Take ½ to 1 tablet at bedtime for 7 days as needed for insomnia.

Method B (D/H × Q)

$$\frac{0.5 \text{ mg}}{1 \text{ mg}} \times 1 \text{ tablet} = 0.5 \text{ tablets}$$

$$0.5 \text{ tabs} \times 2 \text{ tabs} = 1 \text{ mg tablets}$$

$$1 \text{ mg} \times 7 \text{ days} = 7 \text{ tablets}$$

Give 7 tablets with the following instructions:
Take ½ to 1 tablet at bedtime for 7 days as needed for insomnia.

TECH NOTE! Remember, you have to fill the prescription for the maximum amount ordered. In this case the patient could take up to one tablet each night.

EXAMPLE 4.6

You receive an order for erythromycin 200 mg/5 ml suspension.
Give 150 mg every 6 hours per day × 10 days.
   1. How many milliliters of suspension will be given per dose?
   2. How many milliliters of suspension will be given per day?
   3. How many milliliters of suspension will be given over the course of the treatment?
   4. How much suspension will be discarded, if any?

To Solve:
You have on hand 200 mg/5 ml. You need 150 mg/x ml (x ml = the volume).

Answer to question 1
Using Method A

$$\frac{200 \text{ mg}}{5 \text{ ml}} = \frac{150 \text{ mg}}{x \text{ ml}}$$

$$x = 3.75 \text{ ml per dose}$$

Using Method B

$$\frac{150 \text{ mg}}{200 \text{ mg}} \times 5 \text{ ml} = 3.75 \text{ ml per dose}$$

Answer to question 2

Multiply the dose by times per day.

3.75 per dose × 4 doses = 15 ml

Answer to question 3

This requires a straight multiplication to get the answer.

15 ml (per day) × 10 (amount of days) = 150 ml over 10 days

Answer to question 4

This requires subtraction of the total volume minus the used portion.

Erythromycin suspension 200 ml − 150 ml = 50 ml will be discarded

EXERCISE 4.3 **QUICK CHECK**

You receive an order for erythromycin 1.5 g dose stat to the hospital floor. You have 500 mg tablets in stock. How many 500 mg tablets will you need to fill this order? How many would you need for 3 doses?

EXERCISE 4.4 **QUICK CHECK**

Order #1: Metoprolol tartrate (Lopressor) 100 mg tablet twice a day for 30 days. You have 50 mg tablets. How many tablets will it take to fill this 30-day supply?

Order #2: Ranitidine 75 mg syrup at bedtime. You have 1 pint of a 15 mg/ml bottle available. How many milliliters will it take to fill a 30-day supply? Do you have enough?

Try both methods for each of the problems listed previously.
Determine which method you find simpler to use, then stick with that style.

TECH NOTE! Always pay attention to the dosage form. If you have a capsule, you cannot take 1½, but you can with a scored tablet. Also remember not all tablets can be split.

Filling Prescriptions

Following are more examples of basic calculations using ratio/proportion. When filling an oral tablet prescription using a different strength than what was ordered, use the following technique to determine the correct quantity.

EXAMPLE 4.7 DETERMINING QUANTITY

You need to fill cimetidine 600 mg tid (3 times a day) × 30 days.
You have 400-mg tablets.

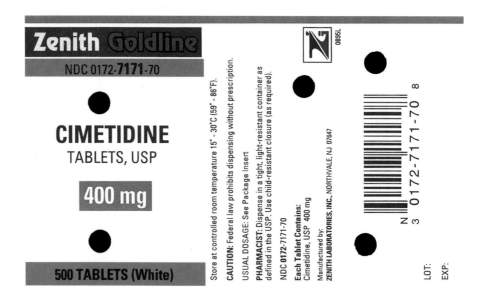

How many 400 mg tablets will you need to fill this order?
To solve:

$$600 \text{ mg} \times 3 \text{ doses} = 1800 \text{ mg per day}$$

$$\frac{1800 \text{ mg per day}}{400 \text{ mg}} = 4.5 \text{ tabs per day}$$

$$4.5 \text{ tablets (per day)} \times 30\text{-day supply} = 135 \text{ tablets to fill this order}$$

Directions: The label would read:

Take 1½ tablets three times daily for 30 days

Pediatric Dosing

Many prescriptions are filled daily for children, and it is extremely important that the parent understand how much medicine to give the child. When the strength needed cannot be measured with a teaspoon or is an odd amount, droppers must be used. Various measuring devices that can be used to deliver suspensions are shown in Figure 4.1. The pharmacist, not the technician, should show the parent of the patient how to measure the correct amount.

TECH NOTE! This is how to remember kilogram conversion: Your weight is more than cut in half when put in kilograms (2.2 lb = 1 kg). If you weighed 200 lb, you would weigh 90.0 kg.

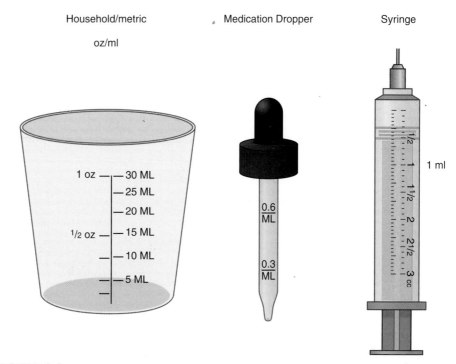

FIGURE 4.1 Three common liquid measuring devices: 30-ml cup, dropper, and oral syringe.

EXAMPLE 4.8 PEDIATRIC DOSAGE CALCULATION

You receive an order for carbamazepine suspension. Below is an example of what you have in stock.

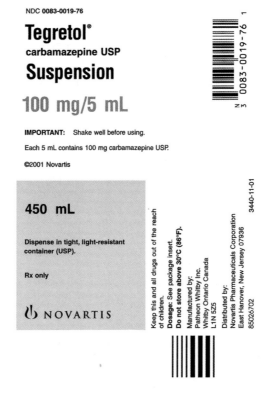

You receive an order for carbamazepine suspension. Below is an example of what you have in stock.

In stock: carbamazepine 100 mg/5 ml bottle of 450 ml.

Order: carbamazepine 250 mg tid (3 times a day) po (by mouth)

1. How many milliliters are needed per dose?
2. How many milliliters are needed per day?
3. How many doses can be taken from the 450 ml bottle?

To solve, use either method A or method B explained previously:

Answer to question 1

Using method A:

$$\frac{100 \text{ mg}}{5 \text{ ml}} = \frac{250 \text{ mg}}{x \text{ ml}}$$

$$\frac{1250}{100} = \frac{100 \text{ x}}{100}$$

$$x = 12.5 \text{ ml per dose}$$

Using method B:

$$\frac{250 \text{ mg}}{100 \text{ mg}} \times 5 \text{ ml} = 12.5 \text{ ml per dose}$$

Answer to question 2

$$12.5 \text{ ml (per dose)} \times 3 \text{ (times per day)} = 37.5 \text{ ml per day}$$

Answer to question 3

If we have 450 ml of carbamazepine (Tegretol), divide by 12.5 ml = 36 doses

Determining Weight

Because all manufacturers provide proper dosing regimens based on kilograms, it is necessary to convert pounds into kilograms. Because most people do not know their weight in kilograms, they will provide their weight in pounds. Therefore the pharmacy technician will need to convert the patient's weight. Although the steps are simple, it is important to remember that there are 2.2 pounds per kilogram.

16 ounces = 1 lb
2.2 pounds = 1 kg

To determine how many kilograms there are in 1 lb, divide.
To determine how many pounds there are in 1 kg, multiply.

EXAMPLE 4.9   CONVERTING WEIGHT AND DETERMINING PEDIATRIC DOSAGE

The pharmacy receives an order for a baby girl weighing 7 pounds.
The order calls for 20 mg/kg/dose.
This means for every kilogram the child weighs, she should receive 20 mg of medication.

To solve:

1. $$\frac{2.2 \text{ lb}}{1 \text{ kg}} = \frac{7 \text{ lb}}{x \text{ kg}}$$

   $$\frac{7 \text{ lb}}{2.2 \text{ lb}} = 3.18 \text{ kg}$$

2. Now multiply the weight in kilograms by the recommended dosage.

   $$20 \text{ mg} \times 3.18 \text{ kg} \times 1 \text{ dose} = 63.6 \text{ mg/dose}$$

EXAMPLE 4.10 CONVERTING WEIGHTS

Determine the total amount of drug to be given per day and then per dose.

For the same baby given in Example 4.9, we now have an order for 60 mg/kg/day to be given q 8 hr. To figure out the problem, first multiply the milligrams of medicine by the weight of the child in kilograms to obtain the daily amount. Then divide by the number of doses per day.

60 mg × 3.18 kg = 190.8 mg/day

190.8 mg/day divided by 3 doses = 63.6 mg/dose

EXERCISE 4.5 QUICK CHECK

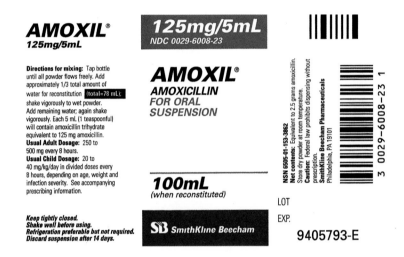

You receive an order for a pediatric patient.

Baby, male   Weight 23 lb

Sig: Give amoxicillin suspension 30 mg/kg/day in divided doses q 8 hr.

1. What is the weight of the baby in kilograms (rounded to the nearest tenth)?
2. What is the dose per day based on the baby's weight?
3. What is the strength of a single dose?
4. How many ml are to be given with each dose?

TECH NOTE! When rounding off numbers, complete all of the calculations, and then round at the very end if instructed to do so by the pharmacist. If you round off at each step, your answer will not be as accurate.

Drip Rates

Hospital pharmacy technicians deliver a 24-hour supply of intravenous (IV) solutions to the nursing stations daily, so the nurses can administer them to their patients. Most IV piggybacks are smaller IV solutions that are given over 30 to 60 minutes. Large volume medications need to be given at a slow rate because veins can only handle a small amount of volume. For large volume drips, the pharmacy technician must be able to calculate the volume needed to last over a certain amount of time, or he or she may need to calculate how much longer a currently hanging IV solution will last. Depending on the order received, the technician must be able to manipulate the numbers to determine this information. This will ultimately determine the amount of IV solution to be prepared that will last for 24 hours (Figure 4.2).

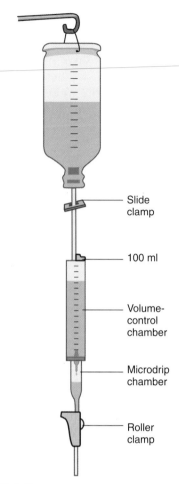

Slide
clamp

100 ml

Volume-
control
chamber

Microdrip
chamber

Roller
clamp

FIGURE 4.2 Intravenous (IV) drip system.

TECH NOTE! Here is a hint for determining drops. Remember drops are written as gtt. Amounts differ between dropper sizes. There are about 60 drops in 5 ml (cc). Also, drops can be intended for drip rates. The amount of drops per milliliter depends on the tubing.

These calculations involve determining:

1. The right amount of drug that is to be given over time
2. The amount of time left until an IV runs out
3. The amount of drug needed to last a certain time

Basic conversions are as follows:

Time: 1 hour = 60 minutes, 24 hours = 1 day
Volume: ml, gtt

This will be determined by the size of tubing used to deliver the medication. We will be using a common drop factor (DF) to determine the volume. The drop factor is given on each set of tubing. If you have a tubing set that states 10 gtt/ml, this is the drop factor and will be used to determine the rate.

EXAMPLE 4.11 CALCULATING DRIP RATES

You receive an order for a 2-L bag to be given over 24 hours. Your tubing says it delivers 15 gtt/ml. What are the drops per minute? To find this out we have to prepare the problem.

Steps involved in determining drops per minute:

1. What is the drop factor? *15 gtt/ml*
2. What will be the milliliters per hour?

$$\frac{2000\ ml}{24\ hours} = \frac{83.3\ ml}{hour}$$

(24 hours/day)

3. What will be the milliliters per minute?

$$\frac{83.3\ ml}{60\ minutes} = \frac{1.38\ ml}{min}$$

(60 minutes/hour)

4. What will be the drops per minute?

$$\frac{1.38\ \cancel{ml}}{min} \times \frac{15\ gtt}{\cancel{ml}} = \frac{20.7\ gtt}{min}$$

EXAMPLE 4.12 DETERMINING DROPS PER MINUTE

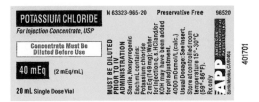

Order: 1500 ml of 20 mEq KCl for 12 hours. The tubing size is 20 gtt/ml
How many drops per minute will be delivered?

Answer:

$$\frac{1500\ ml}{12\ hours} = \frac{125\ ml}{hr}$$

$$\frac{125\ ml}{60\ min} = \frac{2.08\ ml}{min}$$

$$\frac{2.08\ \cancel{ml}}{min} \times \frac{20\ gtt}{\cancel{ml}} = \frac{41.66\ gtt}{min}$$

EXAMPLE 4.13 DETERMINING VOLUME BASED ON DROPS PER MINUTE

Administer to patient 3-L total parenteral nutrition (TPN) bag to be given over 24 hours. Tubing size delivers 15 gtt/ml.
How many milliliters per minute are being delivered to the patient?
How many drops per minute will be delivered?
Determine ml/hour:

$$\frac{3000\ ml}{24\ hr} = 125\ gtt/min$$

Determine ml/min:

$$\frac{125\ ml/hr}{60\ min} = 2.08\ gtt/min$$

Determine gtt/min:

$$2.08\ gtt/min \times 15\ gtt/min = 31.2\ gtt/min$$

EXAMPLE 4.14 DETERMINING DROPS PER MINUTE BASED ON VOLUME AND DROP FACTOR

How many gtt/min would an IV deliver to a patient receiving 40 ml/hr using a 20 gtt/ml set?

Determine the ml/min: 40 ml/hr divided by 60 min = 0.666 ml/min
Determine the gtt/min: 0.666 gtt/min × 20 gtt/ml drop factor = 13.33 or 13 gtt/min

TECH NOTE! Technicians and pharmacists do not determine the size of the tubing. This is predetermined by the doctor's orders to the nurse.

EXERCISE 4.6 **QUICK CHECK**

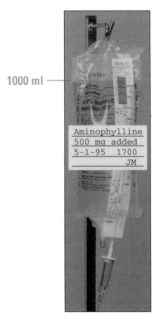

1000 ml

Aminophylline
500 mg added
5-1-95 1700
JM

Order: Patient to be given aminophylline 500 mg in 1000 ml over 24 hours. The drip rate is 25 gtt/ml. What is the flow rate in gtt/min? How many milliliters would be delivered per hour?

TECH NOTE! A large-volume bag can hang for a maximum of 24 hours before it must be changed to prevent microbial growth.

Alligation

Alligation is used when you need to prepare (compound) percent strength that you do not have in stock. To make this strength, you need to use two other strengths to attain the correct one. For example, if a doctor orders 20% KCl but you only have 10% and 50% on hand, calculate the amount of each solution to attain a 20% solution. This can be done using any two strengths as long as only one is less than the final solution. This means you cannot make a 20% solution from a 5% and a 10% because both are less than the needed amount. However, you can make a 10% solution from a 5% and a 70%. Also, water is another element you might use as one of the solutions. The percentage of water is considered 0%. Let's begin by working with these numbers.

Problem: You have in stock a 70% solution and a 20% solution. How much of each do you need in order to create 1 liter of 40% solution?

This is as simple as tic-tac-toe, following these basic rules:

1. Draw a tic-tac-toe board.

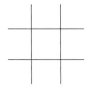

2. Place your desired strength in the middle square.

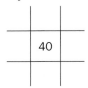

3. Put your high strength solution in the top left square.

4. Put your lower strength solution in the bottom left square. If you are using water, you will place a zero in this square.

5. Take the difference between top left square and middle square number, and place the new number in bottom right square. Do the same with the bottom left number, and place this result in the top right square.

$$40 - 20 = 20$$

$$70 - 40 = 30$$

6. Create a fraction by adding the two new figures (top and bottom right squares) together for a common denominator. Place the top right number over the denominator and do the same for the bottom right number.

$$\frac{20}{20 + 30} \qquad \frac{30}{20 + 30}$$

7. Divide out each fraction, and then multiply by the total volume you need.

$$\frac{20}{50} \times 1000 \, ml = 400 \, ml$$

$$\frac{30}{50} \times 1000 \, ml = 600 \, ml$$

8. Check your answer by adding the two parts. They should equal the total volume.

400 ml

600 ml
_____
1000 ml

Answer: 400 ml of the 70% solution, and 600 ml of the 20% solution will prepare 1 liter solution of 40%.

TECH NOTE! Do not read your answer diagonally. Read your answer straight across!

EXERCISE 4.7 QUICK CHECK

Prepare a 20% KCl 500 ml from your stock of 5% and 70% KCl.

Roman Numerals

The number system commonly used in the United States is the Arabic system, consisting of the numbers 1, 2, 3, and so forth. This system is not always used by physicians when ordering medications. Instead they may use Roman numerals indicating a quantity of tablets or capsules to be filled or to order the strength of medication. When adding Roman numerals, begin with I to III, then write IV (1 less than 5) to equal 4. Repeat the process at 9 by writing IX (1 less than 10) to equal 9. In the same way, if you were to write 49, you would write IL (1 less than 50) to equal 49. See the following for a comparison of Roman numerals and Arabic numbers.

Roman Numerals	Arabic Numerals	Roman Numerals	Arabic Numerals
I	1	XI	11
II	2	XIX	19
III	3	XX	20
IV	4	L	50
V	5	C	100
VI	6	D	500
VII	7	M	1000
VIII	8		
IX	9		
X	10		

Rules for Determining Roman Numerals

1. When a numeral is repeated, its value is repeated.
    Example: II = 2
2. A numeral may not be repeated more than three times
    Example XL = 40, not XXXX
3. V, L, and D are never repeated. LL is incorrect.
4. When a smaller numeral is placed before a larger numeral, it is subtracted from the larger numeral.
    Example: XC = 100 – 10 = 90
5. When a smaller numeral is placed after a larger numeral, it is added to the larger numeral.
    Example: CL = 100 + 50 = 150
6. V, L, and D are never subtracted. LC is incorrect.
7. Never subtract more than one numeral
    Example: 8 = VIII not IIX
8. When subtracting, only use a numeral before the next two higher-value numerals. For example, use I before V and X, X before L and C, and C before D and M.

EXAMPLE 4.15 WORKING WITH ROMAN NUMERALS

When working with Roman numerals, remember that if a larger number is placed in front of a smaller one, you must add both to determine the value.

$$XV \quad X(10) + V(5) = 15$$

However, if there is a smaller number placed before a larger number, then you must subtract.

$$IX \quad X(10) - I(1) = 9$$

EXERCISE 4.8 QUICK CHECK

Determine the following:
- a. XIV = _____
- b. XC = _____
- c. CIV = _____
- d. XL = _____
- e. VIII = _____
- f. C = _____
- g. IV = _____
- h. LX = _____
- i. IX = _____
- j. III = _____
- k. X = _____
- l. XI = _____
- m. XXXIX = _____
- n. VII = _____

International Time

In hospital settings, international time, also known as military time, is used exclusively. Because orders are written 24 hours a day, a system is needed to ensure that all medical-related caretakers understand exactly when the order was written and when the medication or treatment is to take place. The system is based on 100. Starting with the first hour of the day, the clock begins at 0100 (1 AM) through 2400 or 12 midnight (Figure 4.3). It is easy for most people to use this system through 1200 (noon), but then it can get confusing. As the clock hands begin to make their second trip around the face of the clock, the numbers continue on. For example 1300 is 1 PM; 1400 is 2 PM. When orders are received by the pharmacy, the date and time need to be checked against previous orders to ensure that the most recent order is in effect. By using this system there is never any question as to when an order was written or which order supersedes another.

EXERCISE 4.9 QUICK CHECK

Fill in the blanks:

From 0800 to 1500 hours is _____ hours.

A dose given at 0600, 1400, and 2200 hours is _____ hours apart.

A dose given at 0005, 1430, and 2045 would be given at _____ , _____ , and _____ on a 12-hour clock.

Write 4:20 PM, 7:15 PM, and 12:00 AM in international time: _____ _____ _____ .

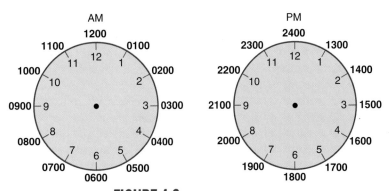

FIGURE 4.3 Military time clock.

DO YOU REMEMBER THESE KEY POINTS?

- The basic measurements of the metric, apothecary, and avoirdupois systems
- The primary system used in pharmacy is the metric system
- How to convert metric numbers from kilograms all the way to micrograms
- All measurements must have units attached to keep them straight
- How to convert pounds into kilograms and vise versa
- Double checking calculations is important before preparing medications
- How to determine how long an IV solution will last
- When to use ratio/proportion and the steps involved in both methods shown
- When to use alligation and how to set up the equation
- How to convert Roman numerals to Arabic numbers

REVIEW QUESTIONS:

Convert the following units into percentages.

1. 1/5 _____
2. 0.25 _____
3. 10/25 _____
4. 2.275 _____

Convert the following fractions of grains into milligrams.

5. 1/300 gr _____
6. 1/150 gr _____

Write the Arabic numbers in Roman numerals and Roman numerals in Arabic.

7. 20
8. 50
9. 100
10. 59
11. 2
12. CXL
13. XC
14. XXXIV
15. XIX
16. VIII

Convert the following metric units into the units indicated to the right.

17. 5 cc = _____ teaspoon
18. 15 cc = _____ teaspoon
19. 30 ml = _____ teaspoon
20. 1000 ml = _____ liter
21. 2 kg = _____ lb
22. 1 mcg = _____ mg
23. 1000 mg = _____ g
24. 900 ml = _____ ounce
25. 0.25 L = _____ ml
26. 0.25 mg = _____ mcg

Solve the following drug orders. Be sure to show your work. Use the following conversions.

qd = daily
bid = 2 times daily
tid = 3 times daily
qid = 4 times daily
po = orally/by mouth
IV = intravenous

27. You receive the following order: Cimetidine 300 mg tab qid × 30 days. You have cimetidine 150 mg in stock. How many tablets will you need to fill this order?
28. Make a tobramycin IV 60 mg q 8 hr in D5W 50 ml. You have tobramycin 40 mg/ml in 2-ml vials. How much will you need in milliliters?
29. Make a vancomycin IV 750 mg q 12 hr in D5W 250 ml. You have vancomycin 1 g/20 ml vial. How much will you take from the 1-g vial?
30. Make a 10% NS solution 1 L. You have 5% and 50% NS bags only. How much of each solution will it take to make a 10% NS 1-L bag?

31. Make amino acids 30% solution 0.5 L. You have 70% amino acids and sterile water in stock. How much of each solution is required to prepare a 30% solution?

32. Convert the following ratios into grams over milliliters.
   a. 1:10
   b. 2:100
   c. 1:1000
   d. 100:100
   e. 100:100,000
   f. 2:10,000

33. Prepare 5-ml of a 1:1000 epinephrine solution. You have 1:1000/ml stock solution. What will be the amount of epinephrine (in milligrams) in 5-ml?

34. Dispense ibuprofen liquid 40 mg/kg/day, give qid. You have ibuprofen liquid 100 mg/5 ml in stock. How much will this patient receive per dose if the patient's weight is 10 lb? How much liquid is needed to fill a 7-day supply?

35. Administer 500 ml heparin to be given over 20 hours. Tubing size delivers 10 gtt/ml. How many gtt/min are being delivered to the patient?

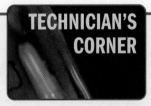

TECHNICIAN'S CORNER

A compounding order comes to the pharmacy with the following directions:
Gentamicin 15 mg/ml dispense 5 ml ii gtt os bid
You have a 5-ml bottle of gentamicin ophthalmic drops 40 mg/ml in stock. You must decrease the concentration from 40 mg/ml to 15 mg/ml using sterile water.

ANSWERS TO QUICK CHECK EXERCISES:

ANSWERS TO QUICK CHECK 4.1

1. 0.8 tsp or 1 tsp
2. 1 cup
3. 16 cups
4. 1 tsp
5. 2 tbsp
6. 1 oz
7. 60 mg
8. 2 cups
9. 480 ml
10. 225 ml
11. 1000 g

ANSWERS TO QUICK CHECK 4.2

0.00088 mg
0.00000088 g
0.00000000088 kg

ANSWERS TO QUICK CHECK 4.3

3 tablets = 1500 mg or 1.5 g
3 tablets × 3 doses = 9 tablets

ANSWERS TO QUICK CHECK 4.4

Order 1: 120 tablets
Order 2: 150 ml; yes, because there are 480 ml in one pint

ANSWERS TO QUICK CHECK 4.5

Baby weighs 10.5 kg
Dose per day: 315 mg/day
Single dose: 105 mg
ml per dose: 4.25 ml

ANSWERS TO QUICK CHECK 4.6

The flow rate is 17.36, or 17 gtt/min
41.66, or 42 ml/hr

ANSWERS TO QUICK CHECK 4.7

115.38 ml, or (115 ml) of the 70% solution
384.61 ml, or (385 ml) of the 20% solution

ANSWERS TO QUICK CHECK 4.8

a. 14
b. 90
c. 104
d. 40
e. 8
f. 100
g. 4
h. 60
i. 9
j. 3
k. 10
l. 11
m. 39
n. 7

ANSWERS TO QUICK CHECK 4.9

a. 7 hr
b. 8 hr
c. 5 minutes after midnight; 2:30 PM; 8:45 PM
d. 1620; 1915; 2400

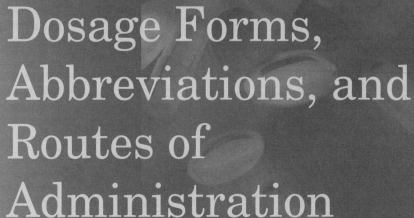

CHAPTER

5

Dosage Forms,
Abbreviations, and
Routes of
Administration

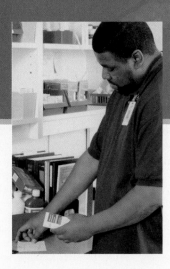

Objectives

- List at least three reasons why certain drugs need to be given by certain routes.

- Discuss the different components of medications and how that affects their bioavailability and pharmacology.

- List the most common routes and dosage forms of drugs.

- List the different dosage forms of common drugs and their storage requirements.

- Describe why additives are necessary in the production of medications.

- Define the common abbreviations for extended-release agents.

- Explain basic storage requirements of various dosage forms.

Dosage forms	Abbreviation	Main routes of administration	Abbreviation
Buccal tablet	buccal	Right ear	AD
Capsule	cap	Left ear	AS
Chewable tablet	chew tab	Both ears	AU
Cream	cr	Gastrostomy tube	GT
Elixir	elix	Intradermal	ID
Enema	enema	Intramuscular	IM
Enteric coated tablet	EC tab	Intravenous	IV
Gelatin	gel	Intravenous piggyback	IVPB
Gel cap	cap	Nasal gastric	NG
Inhalent	inh	Nasal gastric tube	NGT
Liquid	liq	Right eye	OD
Lotion	lot	Left eye	OS
Lozenge	loz	Both eyes	OU
Metered dose inhaler	MDI	Orally or by mouth	PO
Ointment	ung, oint	Rectal, per rectum	PR
Patch, transdermal	top	Subcutaneous	SQ/SC
Powder	top	Topical	TOP
Spray	spry		
Sublingual	sl		
Suppository	supp		
Suspension	susp		
Syrup	syr		
Tablet	tab		
Tincture	tinc		
Troche	troches		
Vaginal tablet	vag tab		
Vaginal cream	vag cr		

Absorption *The taking in or incorporation of a chemical agent across natural barriers in the body system*

Bioavailability *The amount of drug that reaches its intended destination by being absorbed into the bloodstream*

Bioequivalence *The difference between a drug that is manufactured in a different dosage form or by a different company; includes the rate of absorption, distribution, metabolism, and excretion*

Distribution *The ability of a drug to pass into the bloodstream*

Excretion *The process of elimination of medicinal agents*

Half-life *The amount of time it takes a chemical to be decreased by one half*

Inhale *To breathe in, directions used for inhaler*

Instill *To place into; instructions used for ophthalmics or otics*

Metabolism *Process that breaks down drugs for excretion*

OTC *Over-the-counter medications; do not require a prescription*

Parenteral *Medication given by injection*

Pharmacokinetics *The life of the drug, which includes absorption, metabolism, distribution, and excretion*

Introduction

For a technician to become proficient, it is necessary to interpret orders correctly. Although it may be true that many doctors' handwriting is referred to as "chicken scratch," it is the responsibility of the pharmacy to interpret and clarify orders if necessary. Many of the abbreviations that are used in prescribing medication look very much alike. For instance, mg (milligram) can look much like mcg (microgram) when written quickly. In this chapter we explore the common abbreviations seen in pharmacy as they apply to dosage forms and routes of administration. We also take a look at many examples of prescriptions to interpret them and understand how they are filled by the pharmacy. In addition to learning various routes of administration, we cover the many different types of dosage forms that are available and the reasons why they are necessary.

Where Did Pharmacy Abbreviations Originate?

Much of the terminology in pharmacy and medicine comes from the Latin and Greek languages. Because pharmacy began in Europe, most of the abbreviations have their origins in a foreign language. The use of Latin and Greek has remained into the twenty-first century with little change. Although these abbreviations tend to be confusing at first, they serve an important function. For example, if each pharmacy used its own terminology, it would be virtually impossible for one pharmacy to fill another pharmacy's prescriptions. Therefore the medical community uses terms in Latin and Greek. These serve as a universal language that all medical doctors, nurses, pharmacists, technicians, and other medical personnel can understand. The ability to clarify doctors' orders is still a real dilemma in the United States. The amount of errors caused by doctors' poor handwriting and by mistranscribing of orders by pharmacists and technicians is of great concern. It is therefore very important for the pharmacy staff to interpret doctors' orders correctly. This can be a time-consuming element of pharmacy that conflicts with the requirements of most pharmacies because patients want their medications quickly. This leaves the pharmacy staff little time to confer or call on all orders that seem unclear; however, this is what must happen if errors are to be avoided. When writing out the various abbreviations, be sure to write as neatly as possible because other technicians and pharmacists will be reading your writing. Scrolls, stylized, or fancy lettering can easily seem to represent the wrong meaning. The pharmacy technician must learn all of the dosage forms and their abbreviations to decipher doctors' orders (see Terms and Abbreviations at the beginning of the chapter).

Dosage Forms

A dosage form refers to the means by which a drug is available for use, or the vehicle by which the drug is delivered. With individual packaging, the dosage form is given on the package. For example, it may be a tablet or capsule. However, there is more than one type of tablet and capsule. Tablets come in a wide variety of shapes and sizes. For example, they come scored or unscored and coated or uncoated (Figure 5.1). Much of what determines the dosage form of a medication is determined by the drug's effectiveness. For instance, heparin (an anticoagulant) is available only in parenteral (intravenous [IV] or subcutaneous [SQ]) form because it becomes ineffective if taken by mouth because of the effect of stomach

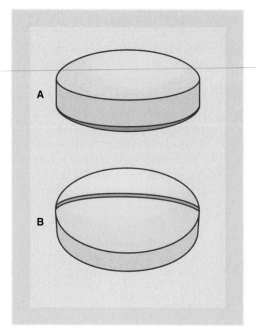

FIGURE 5.1 **A,** Unscored tablet. **B,** Scored tablet.

acids on the drug. Manufacturers prepare certain medication with the ability to release the active ingredient over an extended period. This allows the patient to take the medication less often, which increases compliance. Another consideration is given to the person taking the drug. This includes age and condition of the person. If the prescription of acetaminophen (Tylenol) is intended for a child, that dosage form should be available in liquid if at all possible for ease of administration. The following list of dosage forms gives a brief explanation of their differences. All the different forms can be broken down into three major categories that are composed of subcategories:

1. Solids: Tablets, chewable tablets, enteric coated tablets, extended release agents, capsules, caplets, lozenges, troches, implant capsules, patches
2. Liquids: Syrups, elixirs, sprays, inhalants, emulsions, suspensions, solutions, enemas
3. Semisolids: Cream, lotions, ointments, powders, gelatins, suppositories

SOLIDS

Solid agents can be contained in various packages and administered by almost all routes except parenterally. The following brief descriptions give a glance at the wide variety of solids available.

Tablets

There are hundreds of types of tablets that range in size, shape, color, thickness, and composition. The most common type of tablet contains some type of filler. These fillers are composed of inert substances (no active ingredient) that serve to fill space or cover the tablet (sugar coatings). Sugar coatings improve taste and color or cover unpleasant odors. Finally, certain additives may be used to improve the absorption and/or distribution throughout the body. There are tablets that are made to be administered sublingually (under the tongue) or vaginally. Also, some tablets come scored to allow the dosage to be cut in half if needed. Chewable tablets are convenient for persons who have difficulty swallowing tablets and for children who are unable to swallow large tablets. Other tablets are enteric coated (EC) to help protect the drug through the acidic environment of the stomach until it reaches

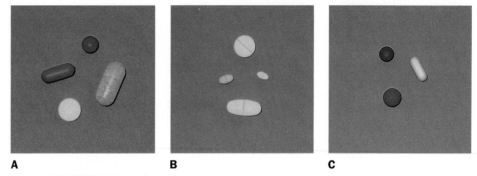

FIGURE 5.2 **A,** Plain tablets. **B,** Scored tablets. **C,** Enteric-coated tablets.

the more alkaline intestine. In other cases, the protective covering may delay the release of the drug while it is traveling through the stomach so that it will not irritate the stomach. Extended-release–type dosage forms are made to control the amount of drug distributed over a set time. See Figure 5.2 for examples of tablets.

Many medications have both extended-release forms and regular forms. It is important to know which form the doctor has ordered. Abbreviations for agents that release medication over long periods are as follows:

CD   Controlled-diffusion
CR   Continuous/controlled-release
CRT Controlled-released tablet
LA   Long acting
SA   Sustained-action
SR   Sustained/slow-release
TD   Time-delay
TR   Time-release
XL   Extra-long
XR   Extended-release

EXAMPLE 5.1 TABLETS

Aspirin tablets (OTC), Aspirin tablets EC (OTC), Nifedipine (prescription [RX]), Nifedipine XL (RX)

TECH NOTE! Dosage forms that are especially made to release over time should not be crushed or broken into two. This would alter the delayed process.

TECH NOTE! Some companies have their own unique names for extended-release agents. For example, Slo-Bid is a theophylline agent that is released over 12 hours, which is why they have named it Slo-Bid (taken only twice daily).

Capsules and Caplets

Capsules are a dosage form in a gelatin container. Caplet dosage forms are closely related to tablets, but they are smooth and are therefore easier to swallow. The word *caplet* refers to the shape of the tablet. Capsules can have either a hard or soft outer shell. Hard capsules' shells are composed of sugar, gelatin, and water. Their color is determined by the manufacturer and is used primarily for identification. Another type of capsule is the pulvule, which is shaped slightly different for identification purposes. Spansules are capsules that can be pulled apart to sprinkle the medication onto food for children, making it easier to administer.

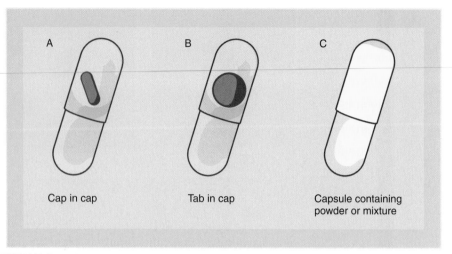

FIGURE 5.3 Different types of capsules. (Courtesy Amanda Sunderman, St. Louis, MO.)

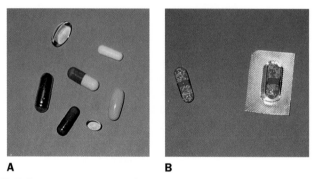

FIGURE 5.4 Types of capsules. **A,** Capsules. **B,** Extended-release capsule.

Because of the many sizes available in capsules and caplets, they can be produced to administer medication in many ways. For example, as seen in Figure 5.3, these capsules can be made to lock to different degrees and can even hold a smaller capsule inside. The reasons behind this manufacturing decision is to determine the best absorption and distribution of the medication. The main difference between capsules and caplets is that capsules can be pulled apart. More medications are being prepared as caplets to ensure that they are tamper proof. See Figure 5.4 for examples of capsules.

EXAMPLE 5.2   CAPSULES AND CAPLETS

Acetaminophen caplets (OTC), Omeprazole capsules (RX).

Lozenges/Troches
Lozenges and troches are other forms of tablets that are not meant to be swallowed but dissolve in the mouth, which releases the medication more slowly. Many cough drops come in this type of package. Lozenges are similar to hard candy. Troches are larger than normal-size tablets and are flat; they usually have a chalky consistency in order to dissolve in the mouth.

EXAMPLE 5.3   LOZENGES AND TROCHES

Lozenge, cetylpyridinium chloride (Cepacol) (OTC); Troche, clotrimazole (RX)

Implants

A special type of capsule can be implanted under the skin and left in place for up to 5 years. This type of capsule comes in a set of six, each containing progestin, which acts as a contraceptive. The medication is released in a stair-step method starting with the highest amount of drug released in the first year, then tapering down from there to a minimum level that is maintained throughout the remaining time.

Patches

Patches are solid pieces of material that hold a specific amount of medication to be released into the skin over time. These are convenient dosage forms because they are easily administered and eliminate possible upset stomach. Anginal medication transdermal patches can be placed on the chest once daily. Some motion sickness patches can be applied and left in place for up to 3 days. Duragesic, a chronic pain medication, is a transdermal patch with a 3-day delivery time.

EXAMPLE 5.4 PATCHES

Nitroglycerin patches (RX), scopolamine transdermal patches (RX), fentanyl patch (Duragesic) (RX)

LIQUIDS

Liquids are composed of various solutions as outlined later. Their names relate to the types of liquid with which the medication is mixed. Depending on the type of taste, speed of action, or route of administration intended, a physician can choose the best agent for the job. Liquids can be administered by all routes, which makes them a popular choice. For example, enemas are liquid-filled bottles with a dispensing top that can be placed into the rectum to administer the solution into the lower intestine. This works very well for cleaning out impacted intestines. Other liquids are used in eye and ear products, which are used to treat a variety of conditions. Solutions also can be used topically to treat skin conditions.

Syrups

Syrups are sugar-based solutions that have medication dissolved into them, which improves the taste of the drug. Syrups tend to be thicker than water.

EXAMPLE 5.5 SYRUPS

Vicks syrup (OTC), metaproterenol syrup (RX)

Elixirs

Elixir agents contain dissolved medication in either an alcohol base or water and alcohol (hydroalcoholic) base. The alcohol usually covers up the bad taste of the drug. Unlike syrups, elixirs have the same consistency as water.

EXAMPLE 5.6 ELIXERS

Dimetapp DM Elixir (OTC), theophylline Elixir (RX)

Sprays

Sprays are composed of various bases such as alcohol or water in a pump-type dispenser. Sprays are available for use in products such as nasal decongestants and sunscreens. There is also a nitroglycerin translingual spray used under the tongue for relief of anginal pain.

EXAMPLE 5.7   SPRAYS

Oxymetolozone (OTC), nitroglycerin (Nitrolingual) (RX)

Inhalants and Aerosols

Certain patients need to be able to get medication directly to the source of inflammation, such as the bronchial tree. Because these areas are so small, the particles must be extremely fine to reach these areas effectively. Inhaler agents come in a variety of forms, but all must be able to be easily inhaled into the lungs. Common devices of this type, available OTC, are vaporizers and humidifiers that distribute medications by adding agents to a container located on the device. In a hospital, respiratory therapists use nebulizers to give breathing treatments to patients, but patients can also use nebulizers at home if they are trained. Anesthetics come in solutions that are inhaled and are administered during surgery by an anesthesiologist. Many of the prescribed inhalants contain drugs that treat asthma and allergies. These agents are called metered dose inhalers (MDIs) and dispense a specific amount of drug with each puff or inhalation. Some aerosols are used to deliver medication into the nasal passages, whereas others are inhaled orally. For orally inhaled agents, although the sizes of the particles are extremely small, unless the patient uses this device correctly much of the drug is swallowed rather than inhaled into the lungs where it is needed.

EXAMPLE 5.8   INHALANTS

Primatene Mist aerosol (OTC), Albuterol MDI (RX)

TECH NOTE! Most inhalants are propelled out by the use of various gases. In the past, most propellants contained chlorofluorocarbons (CFCs), which have been found to destroy the ozone. When the ozone is decreased, ultraviolet light is allowed to enter the atmosphere at levels that are known to cause skin cancer. Because of this finding (years ago), new guidelines have been put into effect to switch over to another source of propellant. The replacements for CFCs must not harm the environment or alter or destroy the medication.

Emulsions

A mixture of water and oil may be used with an emulsifier to bind the two together. There are many different types of emulsifiers depending on what the manufacturer is preparing.

TECH NOTE! An emulsifier is a substance that binds an oil to a water base. It binds to both of them and holds them together. For example, take a look at mayonnaise. It is composed of oil and water and uses egg yolks as an emulsifier, which allows the product to form a smooth consistency.

Oil can have water as a base; in some cases, water is contained in an oil base. Although most emulsions are used topically, there are a few parenteral emulsion agents that can be given, such as lipids, also known as fat, which are used for nutritional parenteral feedings. Various types of emulsion preparations can be administered topically, orally, and even parenterally.

EXAMPLE 5.9   EMULSIONS

Simethicone drops (OTC), Milk of Magnesia (OTC)

Suspensions

Suspensions are liquids that have very small, solid particles suspended in the base solution. Certain active ingredients are found to be unstable when dissolved in a solution, but are stable in a suspension form. Also, they can be used orally by children and seniors because these patients can take the medication more easily. OTC products that are suspensions have a "Shake Well" ancillary label that is easily seen on the front of the bottle and in the directions. In the pharmacy setting, depending on the age and weight of the child, suspension dosages can be altered by either adding more or less sterile water to the powder product. It is important that suspensions are mixed properly before dispensing and that auxiliary labels are attached that instruct the patient to shake well before using and that include the date of expiration.

Suspensions are also used in the eye and ear, rectally, and even parenterally.

TECH NOTE! It is always important to shake most suspensions before using. One exception is some types of insulin suspensions that should be rolled, not shaken.

EXAMPLE 5.10 SUSPENSIONS

Prednisolone ophthalmic suspension (RX), amoxicillin suspension (RX) (All antibiotic suspensions are available by prescription.)

Enemas
Enemas may be administered for two different reasons—retention or evacuation. They can be used to deliver medication to the body, bypassing the stomach while being absorbed. Conditions such as colitis (inflammation of the intestines) can be treated with agents in this manner to reduce the swelling. The most common reason for enemas, however, is to evacuate the lower intestine for a variety of reasons such as preoperative care (for example, to prepare for surgeries involving the intestine), or for women about to give birth. These types of enemas can be administered from prefilled squeeze bottles. There are enemas available OTC that are used strictly for the relief of constipation. However, because of the dramatic effects of enemas, it is usually not recommended by physicians as the first line of treatment. Enemas come in a water base that is faster acting than an oil base. The typical amount of time it takes enemas to work is less than 10 minutes.

EXAMPLE 5.11 ENEMAS

Fleets enema (OTC)

SEMISOLIDS

Semisolid agents are somewhat different in their composition than liquids or solids. Although they contain both, they are normally meant for topical application. Examples include creams, lotions, ointments, gels, paste, and suppositories.

Creams
Creams usually have medications in a base that is part oil and part water and is meant for topical or local use. When an emulsifier is added, the water and oil will stay bound together. They are easily massaged into the skin and do not leave a heavy, oily residue. They can also be used vaginally or in the rectum.

EXAMPLE 5.12 CREAMS

Hydrocortisone cream 1% (OTC)

Lotions
Lotions are thinner than creams because their base contains more water. They penetrate well into the skin and do not leave an oily residue after application.

EXAMPLE 5.13 LOTIONS

Jergens lotion (OTC), Hydrocortisone lotion 2.5% (RX)

Ointments

Ointments contain medication in a glycol or oil base, such as petrolatum. These work very well on a skin surface to cover an area while keeping out moisture. Ointments can be used rectally, topically, and ophthalmically.

EXAMPLE 5.14 OINTMENTS

Hydrocortisone ointment 2.5% (RX), erythromycin ophthalmic ointment (RX)

Gels

Gels contain medication in a very viscous (thick) liquid that easily penetrates the skin and does not leave a residue. Many sunscreens come in this dosage form. Medications for various skin conditions are available in gels as well.

EXAMPLE 5.15 GELS

Naftifine gel (RX), Bullfrog gel (OTC), Oragel (OTC)

Pastes

Pastes contain a lesser amount of liquid base than solids. They are used for topical application and are able to absorb skin secretions unlike other topical agents.

EXAMPLE 5.16 PASTES

Zinc oxide paste (RX)

Suppositories

Suppositories can be used both rectally and vaginally. They have several advantages over other dosage forms. Rectal suppositories bypass the stomach, which is important if the patient has nausea and vomiting. They can relieve these symptoms without requiring an injection, which is much more invasive. They also are good for relief of constipation. Vaginal suppositories are used mostly to treat infections of the vaginal area without having to involve other systems, such as the stomach.

EXAMPLE 5.17 SUPPOSITORIES

Bisacodyl suppositories (OTC), promethazine suppositories (RX), miconazole vaginal suppositories (RX)

Powders

Powders do not fit neatly into semisolids. Powders are solids, yet they are packaged in some forms that allow them to be sprayed similar to liquid dosage forms. Therefore they have been included in the semisolids section. One of the main uses of powders involves decreasing the amount of wetness of an area. Most antifungal foot agents are available in powdered forms to keep the area as dry as possible, decreasing the ability of the fungus to thrive. They can also be spread over a wide area if needed.

EXAMPLE 5.18 POWDERS

Tolnaftate powder (OTC), nystatin (Mycostatin) powder (RX)

Although there are many other types of dosage forms that can be made by manufacturers or by compounding pharmacies, the various types covered in this chapter are the most commonly seen in pharmacy. Because the types of dosage forms are kept in their respective areas in the pharmacy, it is important for the technician student to be familiar with the dosage forms to find them in the pharmacy. Table 5.1 lists the most common dosage forms and their routes of administration.

The advantages and disadvantages of each type of route of administration determines the doctors' final decisions as to what type of agent their patients should receive. The following describes each route and its pros and cons.

Routes of Administration

BY MOUTH OR ORAL

A positive aspect of taking tablets or capsules or any agent by mouth (PO) is the convenience of the drug to the patient. Most can be carried along throughout the day in a handy bottle. Tablets and capsules do not need to be measured, which increases their ease of use, and most oral forms are much less expensive than other alternatives. Oral medications are systemic, which means they are dispersed throughout the whole body. They are also one of the safer ways to take medication because if too much is given, there is time to react before the drug begins to work. The downside of these drugs is that they do not work as quickly as parenterals; they take anywhere from 30 minutes to 1 hour to become active. This can be important, for instance, if the medication is intended for pain relief. Also, some drugs cannot be taken orally because they are not as effective. This is due to the acid pH of the stomach, which breaks down some substances and makes certain medications of little use.

CAPSULE SIZES

There are different sizes and types of capsules as seen in Figure 5.5. They vary in color, transparency, and identifying marks. The larger half of the capsule is known as the body and the shorter half is known as the cap. Many companies produce a hard-shelled capsule that does not come apart to ensure that it is tamper resistant. Not all capsules are meant to be swallowed. Instead, specific dosages of medications are held inside the capsule. These can be sprinkled onto food or into liquid for administration. An example of this is Theo-Dur Sprinkles.

SUBLINGUAL AND BUCCAL AGENTS

Although there are not many medications available at this time in the form of sublingual (SL) or buccal agents, the few that are commonly used are extremely effective. Nitroglycerin is the most commonly used sublingual tablet that treats anginal attacks. Angina is a common heart ailment that affects millions of people with symptoms that include shortness of breath and pain in and around the chest cavity. Nitroglycerin sublingual tablets bypass the long trek through the gastrointestinal (GI) system and are absorbed readily into the bloodstream. This speeds up its action to a few minutes as opposed to the longer time requirement of oral agents. Buccal agents are another type of dosage form. These oral tablets are placed between the gums and cheek where the medication penetrates the mouth lining and then enters the bloodstream.

RECTAL

Rectal (R) agents are used for many different reasons; an example is a person who is vomiting and cannot take oral medications. Suppositories or rectal creams can

TABLE 5.1 Common Abbreviations Used with Dosage Forms

Abbreviation	Route of Administration	Specific Site of Action	Dosage Forms
PO	Oral	Absorbed into bloodstream	Tablet Capsule Solution Syrup Suspension Powder Elixir Tincture Troche
SL	Sublingual	Under the tongue	Tablet Sprays
Buc	Buccal	In the cheek	Lozenge/Troche
R	Per rectal	Rectum	Suppository Solution Enema Ointment
IV	Intravenous	In the vein	Solution/Suspension
IM	Intramuscular	In the muscle	Solution/Suspension
SQ	Subcutaneous	Under the skin	Solution/Suspension
IT	Intrathecal	In the spine	Solution
IA	Intraarterial	In the artery	Solution
TOP	Epicutaneous or percutaneous	On the skin surface	Ointment Cream Paste Powder Spray Solution Lotion
	Transdermal	On the skin surface	Patch Disc
OS, OD, OU	Ophthalmic	Eye	Suspension Ointment Solution Lens
AS, AD, AU	Otic	Ear	Suspension Solution
NAS	Intranasal	Nose	Solution Spray Inhalent
Inh	Inhalent	Mouth	Solution Aerosol
Va	Per vagina	Vagina	Solution Ointment Foam Gel Suppository Sponge
Urethral	Urethral	Urethra	Solution Suppository

Number	Quantity	Example
000	1.37 ml	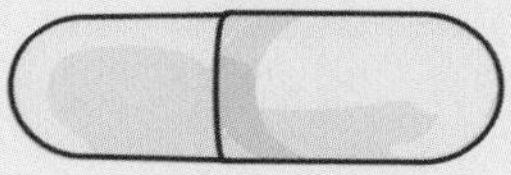
00	0.95 ml	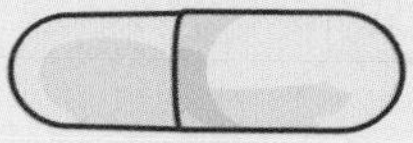
0	0.68 ml	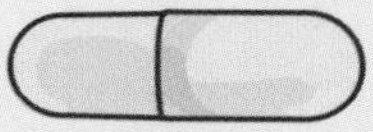
1	0.5 ml	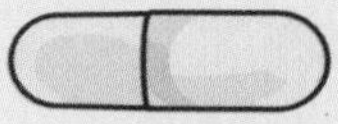
2	0.37 ml	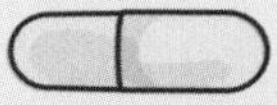
3	0.3 ml	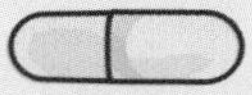
4	0.2 ml	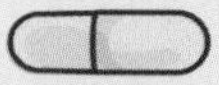
5	0.13 ml	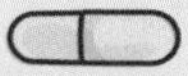

FIGURE 5.5 Different sizes of capsules. There are eight sizes available; each holds a specific volume, each holding a specific amount of medication. The size numbers are 5, 4, 3, 2, 1, 0, 00, 000—5 being the smallest and 000 being the largest.

be used to treat the patient. There are different preparations depending on what result is desired. To reduce inflammation, either ointments or creams can be used in addition to suppositories. These types of drugs work on a specific site rather than systemically. However, for treating nausea or motion sickness, a systemic-acting suppository can be used. Other agents include solutions that are also used locally for various reasons, usually to clear the intestines of fecal material. The downside is that most people do not feel comfortable using suppositories. Also, the actual amount of drug absorbed is not as predictable as with those medications taken orally.

TOPICAL

There are many different preparations of topical (TOP) treatments. The effects of topical preparations range from systemic to localized for rashes. The skin is the largest organ of the body because of its large surface area. Also, there are many portals through which drugs can pass into the body via the skin. Openings include sweat glands, hair follicles, and other small openings in the pores of the skin. There are agents that fight skin infections, inflammation, and ultraviolet rays of the sun. Topical agents work at the site of action, which makes them very effective. In addition manufacturers have created topical treatments that work systemically, such as medications for the heart, blood pressure, hormonal replacement, motion sickness, and smoking cessation (to stop) agents. These are prepared in a variety of dosage forms from ointments to patches or small disks that can be applied to the skin. The medication is absorbed through the pores into the bloodstream where it begins to work. An advantage of topical agents is the ease of application for the patient. Many topical medications act rapidly at the site of application to relieve itching or inflammation. Patches can be worn all day, which increases patient compliance because they do not have to remember to take the medication at various times during the day. In fact, some patches, such as those for motion sickness, can be applied and left in place for days. The downside of topicals is that they may cause a reaction; therefore many agents cannot be given by this route of administration. Because patches are relatively new on the market, they tend to be a little more expensive than their counterpart, the oral medications.

PARENTERAL: INTRAVENOUS, INTRAVENOUS PIGGYBACK, INTRAMUSCULAR, SUBCUTANEOUS

The word *parenteral* comes from Greek and means "side of intestine" or "outside the intestine," which is where oral medications travel. There is a wide range of parenteral dosages and sites where these agents can be given. The most common parenteral medications are given intravenously, or into the veins; intramuscularly, into the muscles; or subcutaneously, under the skin. See Figures 5.6 and 5.7 for types of containers for injectable medications. Very small gauge needles are used, and the lengths depend on the sites being injected. There are clear benefits

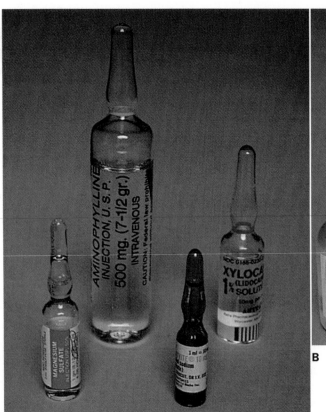
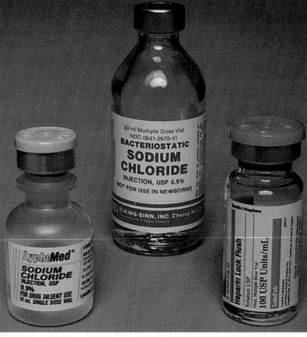

FIGURE 5.6 A, Medication in ampules. **B,** Medication in vials.

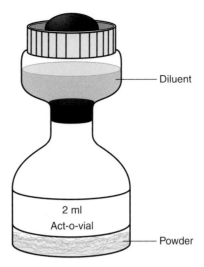

FIGURE 5.7 This type of vial stores the diluent at the top of the vial and the powder at the bottom. When the rubber top is pushed, the diluent is forced down into the vial where the two ingredients are mixed.

to this type of administration, such as the speed of action. Parenteral medications such as insulin have allowed millions of people who suffer from diabetes to inject themselves daily, thus allowing them to live more normal lives. In addition, parenteral drugs work faster than those given by the oral route. This is important for emergency situations, for those who are unconscious or combative, or for those who are unable to swallow. Also, smaller doses are needed because of the high bioavailability of the agents injected. The disadvantage of parenterals as a group is the increased risk of infection. Any drug injection must be done using as sterile a technique as possible to avoid introducing any microbes into the body. Also, any injection is much more expensive than other routes of administration because of the required preparation and administration by trained personnel. Another downside is that, because it works quickly, once the drug is injected there is little time to alter its course if an allergic reaction should take place or too much drug is given. See Figure 5.8 for examples of a large-volume IV and an IV piggyback (IVPB) drug.

EYE/EAR/NOSE

There are a wide variety of agents used for treating a large assortment of conditions affecting eyes, nose, and ears. A consideration that must be remembered when preparing and filling prescriptions for agents that treat the ear or eye is that doctors often use eye solutions to treat ear conditions; however, because the eye is sterile, ear solutions cannot be used to treat eye conditions. Therefore all eye agents are sterile. Otics (ear preparations) are not necessarily sterile because they treat the ear canal and do not penetrate a sterile environment. The pharmacy technician may prepare ophthalmics in a laminar flow hood (see Chapter 13) using aseptic technique. It is important to remember that all ophthalmics need to be kept sterile. For the eye, ear, and nose there are different types of agents used, including ointments, solutions, and suspensions. Most treatments of the ear are for clearing up an infection or cleaning out ear wax buildup. Most nasal sprays are used to treat symptoms of colds and allergies, whereas eye treatments are for infections, inflammation, and conditions such as glaucoma (increased pressure of the eye). These types of dosage forms work on a specific site rather than involving the whole body. They can be administered with ease because of the small package size of the drug. Instructions for both eye and ear preparations

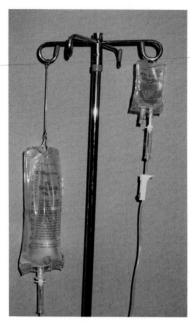

FIGURE 5.8 On the left is a large-volume IV. On the right is an IVPB.

should say *instill* rather than *take* or *put.* The main disadvantage is that solutions used for the eye, if not kept sterile, can introduce bacteria into the area being treated. Also, ophthalmics do not last as long as other treatments because of the blinking of the eye and tearing, which washes away the medication. Therefore dosing times may be more frequent. In addition, most opthalmic ointments make it hard to see clearly.

INHALANTS inh

Many people suffer from lung diseases and use inhalants to treat these conditions. Gases such as oxygen mixed with anesthetics are used to keep patients asleep during procedures as well. Dosage forms may be limited; however, they are very effective if used properly. For patients suffering from conditions such as asthma, bronchitis, or emphysema, a metered dose inhaler (MDI) is often used. There are agents that open the passageways (bronchodilators) to the lungs and those that can be used afterward to prolong the effectiveness of the bronchodilators. For more chronic or severe conditions, corticosteroids are also available in MDIs.

A positive aspect of inhalants is that most aerosols come in handheld units, are convenient for carrying, and may be used when the need arises. The onset of action for these types of agents is relatively quick and can make an extreme difference in a person's ability to breath comfortably. The downside is that, if not used properly, little if any of the drug is able to get into the lungs. It is important to breathe in as the inhaler is activated, and it is necessary to always shake inhalers before administering. Respiratory solutions that are packaged in unit dose ampules deliver a specific amount of drug per treatment.

TECH NOTE!   To determine how much medicine is left in an inhaler, float the container in water. If it sinks, it is full; if it floats on top of the water, it is empty. If the container is half submerged, it is about half full.

MISCELLANEOUS ROUTES

Other routes include vaginal or urethral dosage forms. These are suppositories, ointments, foams, and gels. These types of delivery systems are used for treatment of infections and inflammation and, in the case of vaginal foams, for birth control. Although there are clear advantages in using these agents, such as bypassing a systemic effect and affecting the specific site, they are not necessarily easily applied and can be somewhat uncomfortable.

TECH NOTE! Remember that suspensions and inhalers always need to be shaken before using. This is done to evenly distribute the drug throughout the liquid to attain an even dosage of drug.

Other Considerations: Form and Function

Dosage forms are created based on the results from many clinical trials that delve into the pharmacokinetics of the medication or the function of the drug in experiments.

PHARMACOKINETICS

Pharmacokinetics is a (all inclusive) word that represents many different components concerning the actions of a drug. For example, from the time a person takes a tablet, various considerations are examined, such as levels of drug in the blood and tissues; the absorption or movement of the drug throughout the body; and the overall distribution, metabolism, and excretion of the drug. This includes the reaction of the drug with other drugs to see what may change in the course of its time in the body. As these components are tested and refined, the eventual result is a dosage form that is tailor made to work at its optimal level, which is determined by pharmacokinetics with patient compliance in mind. Patient compliance is the level at which patients will or will not take their scheduled drugs (see Chapter 7). If a manufacturer can effectively make a drug that can be taken once daily rather than several times a day, the odds that the patient will take the medication as directed are increased.

Other areas in a drug's overall pharmacokinetics or life of the drug includes the drug's bioavailability, half-life, bioequivalence, and excretion. Each of these areas are discussed briefly.

ABSORPTION

Medications are specifically made to get through natural body barriers such as the skin, stomach, intestines, blood-brain barrier (surrounding the brain), and other membranous tissues. How well the drug passes through these barriers is one factor that determines its ultimate effectiveness. Some considerations include whether the barrier is a lipid base (fatty) or not. Membranes surrounding organs, such as the intestine, have a variety of proteins and other structures implanted in a membranous protective structure that act as receptor sites. Important chemicals and drugs are able to pass a lock and key mechanism by latching onto receptive sites that allow the chemical or drug to pass into the organ to reach the final site of action intended for the drug. An example of this action is shown in Figure 5.9.

DISTRIBUTION

After the absorption of a medication, it is distributed throughout the body from the bloodstream into tissues, membranes, and ultimately organs of the body. Not

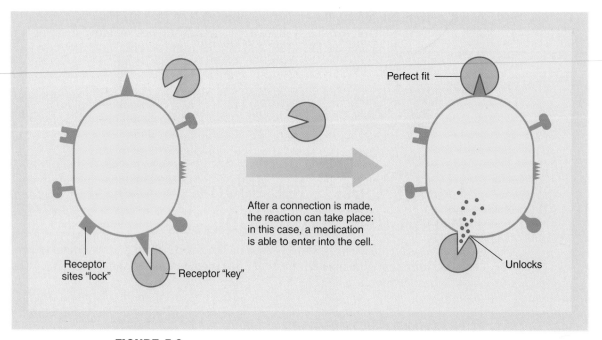

FIGURE 5.9 Lock and key mechanism allowing absorption to take place in a cell. These common reactions take place naturally throughout the body. Only after the correct receptor makes a connection with the matching receptor site will the cell allow a reaction to take place. Medications often mimic this natural mechanism.

all systems are affected equally by the drugs administered, with some areas not allowing the drugs to infiltrate as rapidly as other areas. The distribution of a drug is therefore not necessarily equal throughout the whole body.

METABOLISM

As the drug is being distributed throughout the body, some of the drug reenters the bloodstream and ultimately ends up in the liver where most metabolism takes place. Metabolism changes the chemical structure of the original drug. Agents can be altered in the liver to produce a more effective chemical agent (called prodrug) or can be made less toxic or effective. Some drugs can go directly from the GI tract to the liver where the drug's active ingredient is lessened before it enters the bloodstream. This alters the available drug at the site where it is needed. However, many drugs do not undergo any change at all and are excreted from the body in the same form in which they started. There are different influences that can alter metabolism such as age, gender, genetics, diet, and other chemicals ingested.

EXCRETION

Excretion is the last phase of a drug's life in the body. Although excretion usually is associated with urination, it is important to know that there are many ways that a drug can be excreted from the body. In addition to excretion via the kidneys, drugs may also be expelled via the feces, exhalation, sweat glands, and even breast milk in women who are breast-feeding. Urination and bowel movements are by far the most common methods of excretion. Less common methods such as through breast milk must be considered when a doctor prescribes a drug. For the doctor to give an appropriate drug, all drugs must be tested by the manufacturer for excretion into breast milk and the results reported in the package insert. All information concerning the proper dosing and pharmacokinetics are listed in several reference books (see Chapter 8) and drug package inserts.

BIOAVAILABILITY

Bioavailability is the proportion of the drug that makes it to its destination and is available to the site of action for which it was intended. Drugs that are intended for a certain organ or tissues in the body must pass many different obstacles such as stomach acids, which may break down any substance in the stomach. Many drugs travel into the liver before they have a chance to be absorbed into the whole system. This "first pass" can therefore metabolize the drugs and lower their bioavailability before the drug arrives at the site of action.

HALF-LIFE

Half-life refers to the measurement of the time it takes the body to break down and excrete one half of the drug. For example, if a person takes a medication that has a half-life of 10 hours, this means that in 10 hours one half of the drug will be gone, and in another 10 hours another one half of the remaining drug will be gone. This is an important factor in the creation of all drugs because this information tells the manufacturer how long it takes the body to rid itself of the drug. If a person takes too much medication or takes doses too close together, the liver or kidneys can have toxic build up of the drug, which can be dangerous to the patient.

BIOEQUIVALENCE

Bioequivalence is the comparison between drugs either from different manufacturers or in the same company but from different batches of drug. This is an important aspect of a drug because patients assume that every tablet they take is exactly the same as the one before and that all are the exact strength as listed on the label. Generic drug manufacturers strive to achieve the same equivalence as brand name manufacturers so that they can compete with the original manufacturer. Most of the final metabolism of a drug takes place in the liver. This is the body's final processing center that extracts toxins and unwanted chemicals from the body and forwards them onto the excretion (in the kidneys) process. The liver works very hard but can only process so much within a given time. Persons suffering from any type of liver damage must be monitored closely when taking various medications to ensure that toxic levels are not present in the liver.

The Use of Additives

All medications are prepared with some sort of additive for many different reasons, as shown in Table 5.2. These include adding coloring for better appearance of the product and flavorings to cover taste and/or smell. Many times fillers are used to increase the size of the medication because there may be such a small amount of drug that it otherwise would be hard, if not impossible, to handle. There are many different types of preservatives. Each prevents certain microbes from affecting the drug. In this way, the shelf life after the drug is obtained by the patient is prolonged. Other types of additives include those that increase the dispersing of the drug once it reaches the intestines and others that release the medication much slower over a longer period. Again, many components that go into preparing dosage forms are done for the patients' convenience. Patients are more likely to take medication once or twice daily as opposed to multiple times per day.

Manufactured Products

After learning how many different routes of administration there are and the dosage forms used, you may think that is all there is. The ever-changing world of

TABLE 5.2 Description of Additives

Type of Additive	Example of Chemical	Reason
Weak salt acid/base	Hydrochloric acid	Helps dissolve drug easier once it arrives in the GI system
Preservative	Phenol	Increases shelf life
Sweetener	Sucrose	Improves taste
Flavoring	Cherry	Improves taste
Coloring	Yellow dye No. 5	Improves visual appeal
Buffer	Sodium acetate	Adjusts pH
Antifungal	Benzoic acid	Prevents fungal growth
Base	Petrolatum	Main component to which medication is added for ointments and creams
Filler	Starch, powdered cellulose	To increase size of dosage form

TABLE 5.3 Description of Dosage Forms

Dosage Form	Types	Result
Oral tablet	Layered	Slow release
	Film coated	Protects against stomach acid
	Extended release	Releases medication slowly
	Compressed	Hard dissolves slower, soft dissolves faster
Coated tablet	Sugar and colored	Protects drug, covers taste
	Caplet	Hard capsule-shaped tablet
	Colored	Appearance
	Gel	Smaller than a capsule, easier to swallow
	Enteric coated	Delayed release, easier to swallow
	Dissolving	Dissolve in the mouth on contact
Sublingual/buccal	Soft compressed	Dissolve in mouth
Chewable tablet		Chewed
Capsule	Gelatin cover	Allows for pharmacy compounded agents, easy to swallow
	Spansule	Capsule holds small pellets or beads
	Pulvule	Manufacturer prepared (bullet shaped)
	Dry fill	Filled with powder
Hard gelatin		Filled with a tablet inside
		Filled with pellets
		Filled with another capsule
Soft gelatin	Wet fill	Filled with a liquid
Injectable vial		Filled with paste
	MDV	May be used more than once (see Figure 5.6)
	SDV	Must be discarded after one use (see Figure 5.6)
	Act-o-vial	Rubber stopper is pushed releasing diluent into powder product (see Figure 5.7)

MDV, Multiple-dose vial; *SDV,* single-dose vial.

drug manufacturing has made available many different choices and has turned a simple compressed powder, known as a tablet, into a intricate, complicated, and highly structured format. A tablet is not just a tablet nor a capsule merely a capsule. As seen in Table 5.3, there are many different types of dosage forms depending on the desired effect of the drug in question. All types of dosage forms must be approved by the Food and Drug Administration (FDA) (see Chapter 2). This includes constant testing of the product from batch to batch to ensure continuity of the medication. Injectable dosage forms are discussed further in Chapter 13.

Miscellaneous Agents and Devices

OCULAR INSERTS (FOR THE EYE)

Ocular inserts are a new treatment for glaucoma. Lenses are inserted into the eye that release a continuous amount of drug over time.

INJECTABLE FORMS

There is an assortment of long-acting parenterals that can be used in place of daily dosing such as medroxyprogesterone acetate (Depo Provera) for birth control, which must be injected every 3 months. Other parenteral medications include haloperidol decanoate, which is used monthly for antipsychotic episodes, and the steroid dexamethasone, which is given intramuscularly every 1 to 3 weeks per doctor's orders.

Packaging and Storage Requirements

Medications are packaged according to manufacturers' specifications to ensure the effectiveness and shelf life of the drug. It is extremely important for the technician to learn the various storage requirements of medications. Listed in Table 5.4 are some examples of storage requirements for various drugs along with any special considerations. All medications have a package insert that describes the storage and stability of the drug. Technicians should become familiar with this type of information.

TABLE 5.4 Examples of Storage Requirements

Medication	Location	Considerations
Suppository	Drug shelf or refrigerator	Meant to melt at body temperature
Latanoprost	Refrigerator	Stored in the refrigerator (2°C–8°C) until opened; may be kept up to 6 wk at room temperature after opening
Metronidazole IV	At room temperature	Most premade IV medications are stored in the freezer until thawed for use; store at 15°C–30°C and protect from light
Vaccines	Refrigerator	Kept in the refrigerator (2°C–8°C)
Insulin	Refrigerator	Although insulin is kept in the refrigerator, it may be be kept at room temperature for up to 1 mo
Penicillins (Wycillin, Bicillin)	Drug shelf or refrigerator	Must be stored in refrigerator after reconstitution
Mannitol	At room temperature	Mannitol crystallizes at room temperature; temperature of drug must be raised before using

DO YOU REMEMBER THESE KEY POINTS?

- Various routes of administration
- Terms and definitions relating to pharmacokinetics
- Abbreviations for the routes of administration
- Reasons why different routes are used to administer drugs
- Form and function of medications
- Storage requirements of medications
- FDA guidelines for proper manufacturing practices
- Types of additives used in manufacturing dosage forms and the reasons behind them
- How different dosage forms affect pharmacokinetics
- The types of natural barriers that medications must pass before becoming bioavailable
- The importance of a drug's half-life

REVIEW QUESTIONS:

Multiple Choice

1. Why are sublingual tablets better when relieving anginal attacks than traditional tablets?
   A. They are smaller.
   B. They bypass the stomach entering the bloodstream for quicker relief.
   C. They are cheaper.
   D. Both A and C.

2. Why do manufacturers make dosage forms that work over a longer time?
   A. To cut down on the cost of making the drug
   B. To save time preparing each dose
   C. To enable the patient to take the medication less often
   D. To meet FDA standards

3. Preservatives are often added to medications to
   A. Increase their shelf life
   B. Decrease the possibility of contamination
   C. Cut down on the cost of having to make large amounts of the drug
   D. Both A and B

4. Often, parenteral medications are used because
   A. They work fast.
   B. They bypass the stomach acid secretions.
   C. The patient is unable to take medication by mouth.
   D. All of the above.

5. The definition for pharmacokinetics can be best described as
   A. The processing of a drug by the body
   B. The absorption of a drug
   C. The pharmacy aspect of a drug
   D. The testing of a drug

6. An advantage of taking medications orally is/are
   A. Lower cost
   B. Easier to take than other routes
   C. Less chance of infection with oral dosage forms
   D. All of the above

7. The organ that performs most of the metabolism of a drug is
   A. The kidney
   B. The blood
   C. The stomach
   D. The liver

8. If a drug has a half-life of 20 hours, this would mean that
   A. Half of the drug would be gone in the first 20 hours, followed by the second half in 20 more hours.
   B. The drug will only last half as long as needed.
   C. The drug will lose half its strength in half of 20 hours.
   D. The drug will lose half its strength in 20 hours, followed by half of the remaining strength in the following 20 hours, and so forth.

9. Of the body areas listed here, which one is not a common route for excretion?
   A. Intestines
   B. Kidneys
   C. Mouth
   D. Skin

10. Both dyes and sugars are used in preparing medications to
    A. Improve looks and taste
    B. Improve taste and shelf life
    C. Improve sales
    D. All of the above

True/False
*If the statement is false, then change it to make it true.

1. Medications for the ear can also be used for the eye.

2. Depending on the type of rectal medication given, they can work both systemically or locally.

3. Parenterals are only used in emergency rooms.

4. A bioequivalent generic drug means it is equivalent to the brand name drug for effectiveness.

5. Phenol is used in making drugs because of its taste properties.

6. Both fungus and bacterial contamination can occur if medications are not stored properly.

7. Some medications require tests to determine if the liver is clearing medications appropriately.

8. Ophthalmic medications can be delivered in lenses.

9. Capsules can be manufactured to hold smaller capsules or tablets.

10. Pharmacy technicians are not responsible for making errors if the doctor's handwriting is illegible.

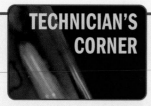

TECHNICIAN'S CORNER

The following examples list the proper way to transcribe orders along with an example of a prescription order for that route. Using these as a guideline, answer the question at the end of this Technicians Corner.

Remember that physicians may write either in upper or lower case for these orders:

1. Oral routes, written PO
   PO = by mouth
2. Rectal routes, written PR
   PR = Per rectal
3. Topically, written TOP
   TOP = To be applied to the surface of the skin
4. Ophthalmic, written OD, OS, OU
   D = right, S = left, U = both
5. Otic, written AD, AS, AU
   D = right, S = left, U = both
6. Parenterals; written either IV, IM, SQ, or ID
   IV = Intravenous
   IM = Intramuscular
   SQ = Subcutaneous (also written SC)
   ID = Intradermal

Question

A patient brings in the following prescription. Transcribe this order into lay person's terms, and list any auxiliary labels that should be adhered to the prescription. Finally, list any questions that you may have about the order and whom you would ask.

Acme Doctors
1000 Meca Way
St. Louis, IL
ph: 555-555-5555

Patient name: _l. Seenell_

Address: _____ Date: _____

℞:

  Cortisporin susp. 10ml
  iii gtts os qd tg

_____
Dr. Signature

Refills: 0   DEA # _____

BIBLIOGRAPHY

Ansel HC, Allen LV, Popovich NG: *Pharmaceutical dosage forms and drug delivery systems,* ed 7, Baltimore, 1999, Lippincott Williams & Wilkins.

Brown M, Mulholland J: *Drug calculations,* ed 6, St Louis, 2000, Mosby.

Drug facts and comparisons, ed 53, St Louis, 1999, Wolters Kluwer.

Mosby's Drug Consult, St Louis, 2004, Elsevier.

6 Referencing

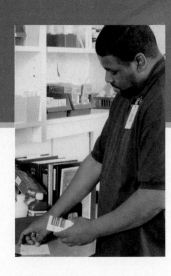

Objectives

- Demonstrate the appropriate way to reference drugs and other information.

- Describe the information contained in the following reference books:

   American Hospital Formulary Service Drug Information (AHFS DI)

   Drug Topics Red Book

   Facts and Comparisons (F&C)

   Goodman & Gilman's The Pharmacological Basis of Therapeutics

   Handbook on Injectable Drugs

   Ident-A-Drug Handbook

   Mosby's Drug Consult

   Physicians' Desk Reference (PDR)

   Remington's Pharmaceutical Sciences: The Science and Practice of Pharmacy

- Explain the specialized reference books necessary in hospital pharmacy.

- List other types of referencing materials in addition to books.

- Explain the importance of journals and news magazines as they pertain to pharmacy and continuing education.

Introduction

Reference books are some of the most important tools that are used in pharmacy. Doctors, nurses, and other health care professionals call the pharmacy daily to ask questions concerning various medications. Pharmacists rely on good reference books to help give the correct information to the caller. Although a few of the books in pharmacy are highly technical, most give basic information on drugs. Knowing which book to choose for referencing and how to access the information is an important skill for both pharmacists and technicians. This chapter covers the popular books that most pharmacies stock. In addition, other types of referencing materials that can be of help specifically to the technician are listed.

Understanding the Correct Way to Reference

Before you begin to look for information, some key points should be taken into consideration. First, what exactly are you looking for? Do you need to know the generic drug name only, interactions, classification, or maybe what the drug looks like? Let us begin with the making of a drug to learn the importance of each one of these components.

When a new drug is in the experimentation phase, the creators or the company give the drug a name based on its chemical attributes. Later, when the drug is approved through the Food and Drug Administration (FDA), a monograph is created to include the classification, indication, and important findings such as side effects that were reported during the testing phase. The classification is important because it puts the drug into the proper category based on its chemical actions. Many times drugs within the same class act the same way if they are taken with other drugs. This information can assist the pharmacist in knowing whether an adverse reaction might occur. The indication lists the main conditions that this chemical is used for. The founding company also gives the chemical a trade name. Many times names are closely related to the chemical name but not always. For example, atenolol is a generic name and is classified as a beta-blocker.

TECH NOTE! Technically, all generic drug names are spelled in lower case as opposed to trade or brand names, which are capitalized, for example, atenolol (generic) and Tenormin (brand).

Most of the chemical names for beta-blockers end in *-olol*. Each drug company produces monographs, also known as package inserts, that list pertinent information.

Most reference books that pharmacists use list trade and generic names of drugs, indications, classifications, possible contraindications, and dosage strengths, and dosage forms. When studies are completed and all the data has been analyzed, a list of contraindications is made by the manufacturing companies. This list identifies types of persons who should not be given the medication. Reasons may range from certain serious drug-drug interactions to conditions that conflict with the action of the drug.

Technicians also must be at ease using reference books in the pharmacy. Good reference books have a section on how to use the text. This is an important step with which all users should become familiar. Knowing how to use books allows the technician to find the correct information in a timely manner.

Main Reference Books Used in Pharmacy

Although there are many different types of reference books available, this chapter covers only the most common types seen in a pharmacy setting. There are many good reference books available to both technicians and pharmacists. Determining which book to use depends on what information you need and how easy it is to find in a book.

FACTS AND COMPARISONS

Facts and Comparisons (F&C) is one of the "bibles" of pharmacy. This reference book was first published in 1946 and was created for quick and accurate reference and drug comparison. Because of its vital information and the ease of use, it is used in most pharmacies. There are five sections to *F&C* as shown in Table 6.1.

TECH NOTE! As of 2001, *F&C* is now published by Lippincott Williams & Wilkins, and the sections within the reference book have been changed; however, they still may be purchased either as hardbound books or as an unbound book that can be updated monthly.

TABLE 6.1 Sections in *Facts and Comparisons*

Sections in Order of Reference	Contents of Each Section	Specific Information
Section 1	Index	Generic and trade names
Section 2	Keeping up	Orphan, investigational, and temporary listings
Section 3	Drug monographs	14 chapters of drug descriptions
Section 4	Drug identification	More than 250 drugs are shown in color
Section 5	Appendix	Dosage calculations and list of manufacturers

At the front of each F&C classification section there is extensive information on various aspects of the class of drugs. Included under each drug listing are indications for use. There is also a chart that lists all of the dosage strengths, dosage forms, sizes, and manufacturers. Most pharmacies carry the unbound book to allow for monthly updates. F&C answers most questions for the pharmacist.

PHYSICIANS' DESK REFERENCE

The *Physicians' Desk Reference (PDR)* is a very popular book found in most doctors' offices and pharmacies. It has been in publication for more than 50 years. There are six sections in the *PDR,* as shown in Table 6.2

Each drug referenced in the *PDR* has a complete description of the drug, including its chemical structure, study results, and so forth. This book is a compilation of package inserts, which are small printed information packets that are inserted or attached to each drug as it leaves the manufacturer. Package inserts can be very hard to read. Although most pharmacies have a *PDR,* it is used mostly by physicians and again it lists only FDA-approved drugs that the manufacturers choose. This book is not as important in a pharmacy setting as it is in a physician's office. It does, however, contain useful drug manufacturer contact information such as addresses and phone numbers.

DRUG TOPICS RED BOOK

One of the longest published reference guides is *Drug Topics Red Book,* often known as *Red Book.* This book is a good source of information pertaining to drug costs. There are 10 sections in the newer *Red Book,* as outlined in Table 6.3. Community pharmacies, rather than hospital pharmacies, are more likely to use this book.

Red Book contains valuable information in the form of quick referencing charts that technicians can use, such as drugs that should not be crushed, sugar-free and alcohol-free drugs, and drugs excreted in breast milk. In addition, *Red Book* includes convenient tables showing pharmacy calculations and dosing instructions converted into Spanish. Although *Red Book* has an extraordinary amount of information, it is not an easy book to reference without knowing the abbreviations for the drug sections (Table 6.4). An added feature of *Red Book* is a listing

TABLE 6.2 Sections of *Physicians' Desk Reference*

Sections in Order of Reference	Contents of Each Section	Specific Information
Section 1	Manufacturer indexing	Lists address and phone number
Section 2	Generic and trade names	Serves as an index for referencing manufacturers
Section 3	Product category index	Products are listed by classification or method of action
Section 4	Product identification guide	Drugs shown in color
Section 5	Product information	Most FDA-approved drugs
Section 6	Diagnostic product information	Information on drug products used as diagnostic agents
Miscellaneous section	Miscellaneous information	Drug information centers listed, key to controlled substances, key for FDA pregnancy ratings, US FDA telephone directory, and poison control centers

FDA, Food and Drug Administration.

TABLE 6.3 Sections in *Drug Topics Red Book*

Sections in Order of Reference	Contents of Each Section	Specific Information
Section 1	Emergency information	Lists address and phone number
Section 2	Clinical reference guide	Quick guide listings for sugar-free and alcohol-free products, sulfite-containing drugs, drugs that cannot be crushed, and so forth
Section 3	Practice management and professional development	Disease management programs, listed in alphabetical order with address and phone number
Section 4	Pharmacy and health care organizations	Lists 25 major organizations including ASHP, NABP, and American Association of Colleges of Pharmacy, no technician organizations listed
Section 5	Drug reimbursement information	State Aids Drug Assistance Programs listed for all states; lists Medicaid upper limit prices and rules on what units each type of drug must be billed
Section 6	Manufacturer/wholesaler information	Address and phone number for manufacturers, wholesalers, OBRA '90 participating manufacturers (by identification number), and returned goods policies
Section 7	Product identification	Color photos of limited drugs; also includes look-a-like, sound-a-like drug names list
Section 8	RX product listings	Contains "Orange Book," which lists generic drug, manufacturer, NDC number, AWP, DP, and OBC
Section 9	OTC/non-drug products listing	This section lists drugs by generic name or trademarked name and contains HRI, UPC, NDC, AWP, and SRP
Section 10	Complementary/herbal product referencing	A short listing of popular herbal remedies along with a listing of those that may be contraindicated, those that require supervision by medical personnel, and interactions; followed by a list of both scientific and common herbal names

ASHP, American Society of Health-systems Pharmacists; *NABP,* National Association of Boards of Pharmacy; *OBRA '90,* Omnibus Budget Reconciliation Act of 1990; *RX,* prescription; *NDC,* national drug code; *AWP,* average wholesale price; *DP,* direct price; *OBC,* Orange Book code; *OTC,* over-the-counter; *HRI,* health-related item; *UPC,* universal product code; *SRP,* suggested retail price.

of all nontraditional Doctor of Pharmacy (PharmD) programs, along with requirements and current enrollment numbers. This is information that few, if any, other books contain.

MOSBY'S DRUG CONSULT

Mosby's Drug Consult is a full drug reference first published in 1991 to provide practitioners with complete, unbiased drug information. Since it is organized alphabetically by generic name, it is easy to quickly find key information.

Each monograph includes a key information section at the beginning listing approved indications, drug classes, pregnancy category, FDA approval date, DEA class, orphan drug status, and if it is included on the WHO formulary. A product listing table at the end of each monograph lists all the dosage forms and sizes, the manufacturer, the average wholesale prices (AWP), and the NDC codes. Therapeutic equivalency ratings (orange book ratings) are also indicated when appropriate. A CD-ROM is included with the book that includes a drug interaction tool and patient education handouts in English and Spanish.

AMERICAN HOSPITAL FORMULARY SERVICE DRUG INFORMATION

Used mainly by hospitals, *American Hospital Formulary Service Drug Information (AHFS DI)* gives a comprehensive listing of approved formulary drugs, their uses, adverse reactions, and other pertinent information. This information is derived from experts in the fields of medicine, pharmacy, and management.

Formularies are lists of approved uses of medications. The criteria for a formulary include the best use of a drug based on effectiveness of the drug, cost, and other factors. A hospital pharmacist usually provides drug education for doctors, nurses, and other ancillary staff to identify the drugs that are on the hospital's formulary. Doctors should stay within their institutions' formulary guidelines when ordering drugs.

UNITED STATES PHARMACOPOEIA DRUG INFORMATION

United States Pharmacopoeia Drug Information (USP DI) comes as a set of three volumes. Volume 1 gives drug information, including labeled and unlabeled uses for the drug. Volume II helps the pharmacist in advising patients about their medications. Volume III covers both state and federal requirements such as how the drug must be stored, and so forth.

IDENT-A-DRUG

Ident-A-Drug lists both tablet and capsule identifications. Most tablets and capsules have a code or number stamped onto them by the manufacturer for identification purposes. *Ident-A-Drug* is the most extensive reference book available with more than 7000 listings. The drugs are not listed by pictures but by identifiable codes, colors, shapes, and whether the tablet is scored. Once these are identified, the book provides the manufacturer, generic and brand names, strength, and use of the drug. This type of referencing comes in handy when patients do not know what drug they are taking but have a capsule or tablet of the drug to show. Emergency departments often have a patient who has overdosed on a drug but cannot identify it. If one tablet or capsule is brought in with the patient, it can probably be identified by the pharmacy using this book. Although some books such as *F&C* do have some pictures of tablets and capsules, these are not extensive and are not the first choice to use in identifying a drug.

THE INJECTABLE DRUG HANDBOOK

Mostly used in the hospital setting, *The Injectable Drug Handbook* is able to reference the compatibility of various agents given parenterally. Although technicians cannot relay information from this book to doctors or nurses, they can find the information and have it ready for the pharmacist. In this way, they can facilitate a rapid response from the pharmacy to the necessary medical personnel.

LESS COMMONLY USED HANDBOOKS

The Pediatric Drug Handbook
American Drug Index
Goodman & Gilman's The Pharmacological Basis of Therapeutics
Handbook of Non-Prescription Drugs
Martindale's Extra Pharmacopia
Remington's Pharmaceutical Sciences: The Science and Practice of Pharmacy

TECH NOTE! Hospitals or pharmacies that work extensively with pediatric and/or geriatric patients may use these types of handbooks more often. Specifics concerning each of the books listed previously or discussed in this chapter are outlined in Table 6.5. This includes how often the reference books are updated along with which professionals most often use them.

In addition to these well-known books, there are many specialty reference books such as those on lactating mothers, psychotropic medications, and antibiotics. Many pharmacies keep a wide range of these types of reference books.

Learn What to Look for When Choosing a Reference Book

At times, technicians need to use reference books to find out more information on a drug or for billing purposes. Knowing the proper book to reference is important not only for the correct information but also for saving time and avoiding frustration.

TECH NOTE! If a technician needs to find a drug price and manufacturer for a drug such as atenolol (Tenormin) and only the brand name of the drug is known, a book such as *PDR* is not helpful because the drugs are listed by manufacturer. *Red Book* is the book to look in to find price, but drugs are not listed in order by trade names. Therefore a reference book such as *F&C* that references drugs by both trade and generic name is the book to use in this situation.

The books listed previously are all large reference books that are provided for the staff in the pharmacy. If you choose to buy your own reference books for home use or pocket versions for use at work, there are some basics you should consider. If

TABLE 6.4 Main Attributes of Various Reference Books

Reference Book	Who Uses Information	Updated
Facts and Comparisons (F&C)	Pharmacy	Yearly (hardbound) Monthly (unbound)
Physicians' Desk Reference (PDR)	Physicians, pharmacy	Yearly
Drug Topics Red Book	Outpatient pharmacy	Yearly
Goodman & Gilman's The Pharmacological Basis of Therapeutics	Pharmacy students, and practicing physicians, and RPhs	Every 5 years
Remington's Pharmaceutical Sciences: The Science and Practice of Pharmacy	For RPhs, physicians, and medical scientists	Every 5 years
United States Pharmacopoeia Drug Information (USP DI)	Pharmacy	Yearly
American Hospital Formulary Service Drug Information (AHFS DI)	Pharmacy	Yearly
Injectable Drug Handbook	Inpatient pharmacy	Yearly
Pediatric Handbook	Pharmacy	Yearly
Geriatric Handbook	Pharmacy	Yearly

RPh, Registered pharmacist.

your main use of the book will be to determine generic and trade names, indications, and side effects, then a book such as *F&C* is a good choice. As pharmacies update their stock, you might be able to get a free copy of *F&C*. Also, check at bookstores for the previous year's edition. They can be sold at a decreased price and contain most of the information you require. You might check other book companies for similar information. There are many reference books that contain the same type of information as *F&C*. Another consideration may be the size of the reference book. For instance, although *F&C* is a very complete and up-to-date book, it is rather large and will not fit in your pocket for easy access; however, there is a pocket version available. Other publishers also offer pocket versions of books.

Stay away from books that only reference drug names one way (only trade or generic names) because this can become time consuming. Most drugs have many names depending on the drug company that manufacturers them. If you are going to keep the book at home or in your office, you might be looking for a larger book. If your space is limited, you may be more interested in a small book. Remember with the smaller books that either there will be less information provided or the print may be harder to read. If you are going to purchase a reference book at a bookstore, take a wide variety of drug names with you to reference in the store. If the book has all the drugs you are looking for and is easy to read, you will use the book more often.

Pocket-Sized Reference Books

Technicians traditionally have not carried pocket versions of drug books. As roles expand at work, the pharmacy technician needs to have his or her own reference books. Some manufacturers produce small pocket versions of trade/generic name drug books, but the drugs listed are often limited to their drug line only. It is becoming more important for technicians to carry a good pocket guide of not only trade and generic names but also of the drug classifications, indications, and side effects. Thus it is important to check out as many pocket versions as you can to see what works for you. One of the best books to keep is one in which a drug can be looked up either by trade or brand name without having to check the index. The cost of these pocket handbooks range between $20 and $40. The downside is that they are all softbound and will need to be updated yearly to incorporate new drugs or discontinued ones. The upside is that most of the drugs remain the same year after year.

Palm pilots are becoming more popular and more economical. It is possible to download *F&C* and other reference materials onto a palm pilot for easy access. Palm pilots are small enough to be carried in a coat pocket or purse. However, it is still one of the more expensive ways to attain reference materials. As technology advances, the prices of these handheld devices will decrease, making it more affordable.

Journals and Newsmagazines

Nearly every pharmacy subscribes to journals and newsmagazines that pertain to pharmacy. These can be extremely informative to the pharmacy technician. When a technician becomes nationally certified, he or she must complete continuing education (CE) units and may at some point use these journals for completing some if not all the necessary units. Journals offer CE at a reasonable cost; in addition, they allow the technician to keep up on the most recent drugs that are coming into pharmacy. Journals and newsletters may be published monthly, bimonthly, quarterly, or even weekly. They contain articles on new drugs, technicians, the future of pharmacy, and various legislative changes that may be

TABLE 6.5 Types of Journals and Pharmacy Magazines Available

News Magazine	Journal	Published	CE Included	Website	Association
AAPT		6 times yearly	Yes	www.pharmacytechnician.com	Yes
Computertalk		6 times yearly	No	www.computertalk.com	No
Drug Topics		Monthly	Yes	www.drugtopics.com	No
NPTA		6 times yearly	Yes	www.pharmacytechnician.org	Yes
Pharmacy Times		Monthly	Yes	www.pharmacytimes.com	No
The Script		Monthly	No	www.pharmacy.ca.gov	No
US Pharmacist		Monthly	Yes	www.uspharmacist.com	No
	AJHP	24 times yearly	Yes		Yes
	ASHP	6 times yearly	Yes	www.ashp.org	Yes
	Pharmacy Technology	6 times yearly	Yes	www.jpharmtechnol.com	No

AAPT, American Association of Pharmacy Technician; *NPTA*, National Pharmacy Technician Association; *ASHP*, American Society of Health-System Pharmacists.

taking place. The information they can give you on the field of pharmacy can be very beneficial. There are many different journals, newsletters, and magazines to choose from. Another source of journals that technicians may not see in the pharmacy setting are those written by pharmacy technician associations. These are geared specifically toward technician issues. Table 6.6 provides a sample of the types of journals and pharmacy magazines available.

The Internet

Referencing should not be limited to books alone. The Internet has a lot of information; however, it is up to the reader to determine whether the information is reliable and accurate. Finding websites at universities and through publishing companies is a good way to look for information. Going to personal websites may give you a person's perspective but may not provide medically sound information.

Pharmacy organizations have websites on the Internet and many have weekly news boards that reference important information concerning pharmacy. Because so much is happening in pharmacy today, much of the information cannot be included in journals. The news links are listed on the website. This is a valuable tool used to keep members updated with accurate information. Also, these association sites have links to other pharmacy sites that may be of interest. Pharmacy associations may also offer Internet areas where the user can have questions answered by other members.

Additional Types of Information

In addition to large desktop books, pocket handbooks, journals, and the Internet, there are other types of information that can keep you current and on the cutting edge as a pharmacy technician. Joining an association can be very rewarding, and serve as good source of information, and a way to network. Currently the following associations provide continuing education and information for technicians:

National Pharmacy Technicians Association (NPTA)
American Association of Pharmacy Technicians (AAPT)
American Society of Health-systems Pharmacists (ASHP)
American Pharmaceutical Association (APhA)

All of these organizations offer a great way to stay up to date on new drugs, devices, and current and future pharmacy issues. In addition, they usually offer a vehicle to order pharmacy technician certification review books and other reference books, sometimes at a reduced membership rate. These can be found on their websites or at their bookstores (this information may be found at their seminars). The information and support they can provide is only limited by how much they are used. Also, many pharmacist associations such as ASHP and APhA and their chapters do have a technician division that allows technicians an avenue for learning new information. It is important to inquire about your local pharmacy associations to see what they have to offer. Some technician divisions are very active in bringing CE courses to technicians and host various functions for networking and unifying pharmacy technicians from different types of pharmacies.

TECH NOTE! Before you join an association, check out their website for information on how involved they are with their technician members. Many associations do not have a technician division or offer CE classes specifically for technicians. Currently, only one association is run by technicians and allows only technicians as members; this is NPTA. They have yearly seminars and a bimonthly journal containing CE and other useful information pertaining specifically to technicians.

Seminars and CE dinners, provided by pharmacy associations, are sponsored mostly by drug companies and are another good source of information on drug topics, new drugs, and more. You do not need to be a member of an association to attend but the cost usually is lower for members. Although seminars normally are held once or twice yearly depending on the association that is putting on the seminar, CE dinners may be hosted monthly by the local chapter of an association. At seminars, many of the technician classes include math, aseptic technique, the future of pharmacy technicians, law updates, and more. Monthly CE dinners or events usually have a limited amount of space available and, depending on the drug company sponsoring the event, there may be a speaker and a meal for either a low cost or no cost. These costs are usually predetermined by the association's chapter. All of these seminar classes and CE dinners can be used toward CE credit for pharmacy technicians.

DO YOU REMEMBER THESE KEY POINTS?

- The major sources of information that a technician most often uses in pharmacy
- The benefits of joining a pharmacy association
- Why CE is an important factor for pharmacy technicians
- The key attributes of each of the books explained in this chapter
- Other sources available to technicians in addition to books, journals, and magazines
- Types of information that a technician must keep up on in pharmacy
- The difference between organizations and associations outlined in this chapter

REVIEW QUESTIONS:

Multiple Choice

1. Which of the books listed provides package inserts from manufacturers?
A. *F&C*
B. *Goodman & Gilman's The Pharmacological Basis of Therapeutics*
C. *Red Book*
D. *PDR*

2. Which book(s) listed below is(are) the best source for locating manufacturer addresses?
A. *Red Book*
B. *PDR*
C. *Goodman & Gilman's The Pharmacological Basis of Therapeutics*
D. *F&C*
E. A, B, and D

3. If you need to look up the average wholesale price (AWP) of a drug, the best source to look in is
A. *American Drug Index*   C. *Red Book*
B. *F&C*   D. A journal

4. The book that comes both hardbound and loose-leaf to allow for monthly updates is
A. *F&C*
B. *Red Book*
C. *Goodman & Gilman's The Pharmacological Basis of Therapeutics*
D. None of the above

5. The most widely used reference book in pharmacy is
A. *Goodman & Gilman's The Pharmacological Basis of Therapeutics*
B. Dictionary
C. *Remington's Pharmaceutical Sciences: The Science and Practice of Pharmacy*
D. *F&C*

6. A major pharmacy technician association run by technicians for technicians is
A. ASHP   C. APhA
B. NPTA   D. All of the above

7. If you need to identify a specific tablet or capsule only by the markings and color, you will look in
A. *F&C*   C. *American Drug Index*
B. *Ident-A-Drug*   D. None of the above

8. The best way to choose a reference book is to
A. Ask a friend
B. Choose the largest book because it will be the most comprehensive
C. Choose the least expensive
D. Choose one that you can easily use and covers the areas that you are interested in

9. One alternative to buying books is to
A. Wait until the pharmacy is going to throw out an old version
B. Check for lower prices as a member of an association
C. Use the Internet for information and read journals that your pharmacy provides for employees
D. Both A and C

10. All of the following books are updated at least yearly except
A. *F&C*
B. *Red Book*
C. *Goodman & Gilman's The Pharmacological Basis of Therapeutics*
D. *PDR*

True/False

*If a statement is false, then change it to make it true.

1. Classification and indication mean the same thing.

2. If a drug is contraindicated, it is not available in the United States.

3. Monographs for a specific drug are produced after the experimentation phase and after approval from the FDA.

4. A palm pilot is a device that allows referencing materials to be downloaded for individual use.

5. Technicians can take CE only through pharmacists' journals.

6. The Internet has information that is incorrect and should not be used as a source.

7. Technicians do not need to use reference materials in a pharmacy.

8. Many pharmacy associations have technician divisions for members.

9. One of the best reasons to join an association and get involved is to network.

10. Technicians are not expected to keep up with current medications or pharmacy trends.

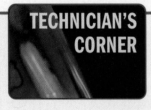

TECHNICIAN'S CORNER

A patient comes into the pharmacy holding one capsule of medication that he or she needs to have refilled. The patient wants to know the price of the medication and whether it is available as a liquid. The capsule is white and has the markings "Watson 369" on one side and "5 mg" on the opposite. What is this drug and what is it used for? Also list the AWP, NDC number, and dosage forms.

BIBLIOGRAPHY

Billups NF, Billups SM: *American drug index,* Philadelphia, 2002, Lippincott Williams & Wilkins.

Blumenthal M: *Handbook of non-prescription drugs,* ed 11, Washington, DC, 1997, American Pharmacists Association.

Drug facts and comparisons, ed 53, St Louis, 1999, Wolters-Kluwer.

Drug Topics Red Book, ed 102, Montvale, NJ, 1998, Medical Economics.

Gennaro A: *Remington's pharmaceutical sciences: the science and practice of pharmacy,* ed 18, Easton, PA, 1990, Mack.

Hardman JG, Limbird LE, editors: *Goodman & Gilman's the pharmaceutical basis of therapeutics,* ed 8, New York, 1990, Pergamon.

Mosby's Drug Consult, St Louis, 2004, Elsevier.

Therapeutic Research Center Faculty, editors: *Ident-a-drug,* Stockton, CA, 2001, Therapeutic Research Center.

Trissel, L: *Handbook on injectable drugs,* ed 9, Bethesda, MD, 1996, American Pharmacists Association.

US pharmacopoeia, ed 18, Rockville, MD, 1995, US Pharmacopeial Convention.

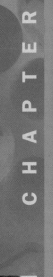

7

Competency, Communication, and Ethics

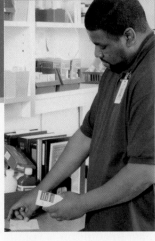

Objectives

- List the primary responsibilities of a pharmacy technician.

- Differentiate between morals and ethics.

- Define communication.

- Describe the importance of good communication skills.

- Explain the current trends toward dealing with the reduction of medication errors.

- List examples of ways pharmacy technicians can lessen errors in the workplace.

- Give an example of resolution techniques when dealing with irate patients.

- Explain the main psychological steps through which a terminally ill patient proceeds.

- Provide examples of situations in which pharmacy technicians must use their communication skills, ethics, and competencies.

Communication *The ability to express oneself in such a way that one is readily and clearly understood*

Competency *The capability or proficiency to perform a function*

Confidentiality *To keep privileged customer information from being disclosed without the customer's consent*

Ethics *The values and morals that are used within a profession*

Morals *Ethics; honorable beliefs*

Nationally Certified Technician *Proficient in minimum standards set by the Pharmacy Technician Certification Board*

Professionalism *Conforming to right principles of conduct (work ethics) as accepted by others in the profession*

Protocol *Code of behavior; procedure*

Introduction

As the number of pharmacy technician jobs increases in many different areas of pharmacy, so will the number of applicants for those positions. As the population grows older, use of prescription medications also continues to grow. Therefore more technicians are needed to help fill those prescriptions. In addition, as pharmacists are becoming more involved in patient care (consulting with patients, conferring with physicians, and helping to make decisions in clinical aspects of patients' prescribing), pharmacy technicians are taking over the traditional role of a pharmacist. In addition to filling prescriptions, technicians also work in many other areas of pharmacy practice (see Chapter 3). The technician who can function in more areas of the pharmacy is more valuable as an employee; however, this alone does not guarantee a long-lasting career. There are several factors that must be considered before a person can be considered a competent employee, specifically whether he or she meets the state's regulations (i.e., certification and registration) as a pharmacy technician. This chapter reveals the major competencies required of a pharmacy technician, which include communication skills and ethics. In addition, this chapter covers the rights of a patient and identifies the five stages of a terminally ill patient.

Competencies

REGISTRATION AND CERTIFICATION

Meeting the specific guidelines of state regulations is the single most basic requirement of a pharmacy technician. Each state has a Board of Pharmacy that institutes regulations for pharmacy technicians. Regulations can be found on each state's respective website. More states are requiring registration of technicians. Registration is an important tool for pharmacy management to ensure that each technician has a clean background to work in the pharmacy environment. By doing a simple fingerprint background check, the hiring pharmacy gains a measure of confidence in the pharmacy technician candidate; however, it is not a measurement of the competency of the technician. Thus certification is being used in more states and will most likely be used soon in some form or another throughout all 50 states. Presently there is only one certification examination, which is nationally administered. Administered three times per year, it tests on all areas of pharmacy and encompasses all types of pharmacy practice.

Registration and certification help pharmacy management to more easily choose the most competent technician to fill the position. Of course, these alone do not necessarily cover all skills required of a competent technician. Thus a probationary period is imposed to assess the pharmacy technician daily. The following sections describe the areas of competency that, if met, increase the prospective pharmacy technician's chances at being chosen for a pharmacy position.

LAWS AND PROTOCOL

Knowledge of pharmacy law is essential before working in a pharmacy environment. The basics are listed in Box 7.1 (for more examples see Chapter 2). Federal laws govern all 50 states. Each state also has specific laws, regulations, and guidelines that pertain to pharmacy practice and are governed by their boards of pharmacy.

Each pharmacy has a binder of policies and procedures (P&P) that are the protocol of the pharmacy. These standards pertain to the use of medications, inventory, order of operations, work schedules, and specific tasks required of pharmacy staff. Other information that can be found in this binder are guidelines pertaining to job duties, employee benefits, job orientation, training, and evaluation methods. These policies are developed by management and are updated regularly. In addition to this information, procedures that must be followed to report errors, discrepancies, or other areas of concern that may arise are outlined. This is an important tool that every pharmacy technician should become acquainted with as a component of professional behavior.

MEDICATION ERRORS

One of the functions of the Food and Drug Administration (FDA) is to protect the consumer against harmful medications and devices. This includes medication errors

BOX 7.1 EXAMPLES OF FEDERAL LAWS GOVERNING PHARMACY

- Required prescription label information: pharmacy name, address, and phone; patient name; prescription number; name of drug; strength; dosage form; quantity; date filled; doctor; refills; expiration date; and pharmacist's initials. If a technician fills the prescription, he or she must also initial label.
- Required prescription information: doctor's name, address, and phone; patients name; name of drug; strength; dosage form; quantity; date written; refills; doctor's DEA number; and signature.
- Verbal orders: Only a registered pharmacist within the pharmacy can take a doctor's verbal orders for prescriptions.
- Patient consultation: Only a registered pharmacist can give advice or consult a patient about his or her medications.
- Unit dosing: Proper documentation of a medication includes manufacturer, lot number, expiration date, dosage form, quantity prepared, date, technician's initials, and pharmacist initials. On each unit dose label, the following information must show: drug, strength, dosage form, manufacturer facilities lot, and expiration date.
- Controlled substances: Only a registered pharmacist can sign controlled substances into the pharmacy inventory or send them back to the manufacturer. Within a hospital, only pharmacists, pharmacy technicians, nurses, and doctors may sign controlled substances into stock.

that may originate within hospitals, clinics, doctors' offices, and pharmacies. According to current information provided by the FDA, medication error is the top cause of injury and death in the United States. A 1999 report issued by the Institute of Medicine estimated that up to 98,000 people die in hospitals yearly from medication errors. This statistic tops death rates linked to breast cancer, motor vehicle accidents, and acquired immunodeficiency syndrome (AIDS). The cost of errors can reach the astounding amount of $75 billion annually. Because of these shocking numbers, decreasing medication errors has become a hot issue and has received the attention of all agencies and organizations that are linked to medicine and consumer information services. Some of these agencies are listed in Box 7.2. All of these agencies can be accessed on the internet to keep updated on new policies and practices that are currently being implemented across the United States.

The FDA and other agencies have proposed specific avenues and guidelines that will ultimately decrease drug errors to the consumer. The medical community and consumers have an avenue to report errors called "Med Watch." Information given is not meant to punish the person or place blame but to look into the reason behind the error in hopes that change may be implemented to prevent future errors.

Errors can occur almost anywhere and at any time (Table 7.1). Errors that occur in hospital pharmacies and pharmacies outside the hospital directly affect the performance of the pharmacy technician. There are common reasons why errors occur, such as stressful job environment resulting from understaffing, increased work load, and lack of training. Types of errors that can occur within the pharmacy are listed in Table 7.2.

Pharmacy technicians can prevent all the examples of errors listed in Table 7.2 by taking certain steps. The misconception that pharmacists can and will catch every mistake that a pharmacy technician makes is dangerous.

The following section outlines necessary competencies that every pharmacy technician must know about and continually strive to increase their knowledge of to lessen the possibility of errors.

Doctors' Orders

It is important to know normal dosing of medications and those that are abnormal. A strong knowledge of generic and trade drug names and their strengths can

BOX 7.2 AGENCIES THAT TRACK MEDICATION ERRORS

FDA	Federal Drug Administration
AMA	American Medical Association
JCAHO	Joint Commission on Accreditation of Hospital Organizations
ASHP	American Society of Health-System Pharmacists
AHRQ	Agency for Healthcare Research and Quality
CDER	Center for Drug Evaluation and Research

TABLE 7.1 Places Where Errors Can Occur

Location	Example of Type of Error That Might Occur
Hospitals/clinics	Dosing medications
Pharmacies	Wrong dosing information, drug interactions, wrong drug
Nursing homes	Dosing side effects, overdosing or underdosing
Doctors' offices	Poor doctor-patient communication, improper diagnosis
Patients' homes	Skipped dosing times, wrong dose taken, overdose

TABLE 7.2 Types of Errors That Can Occur In the Pharmacy

Type of Error	Example of Errors Made by Technicians
Lack of or incorrect communication	Poor telephone message
Errors in repackaging medications	Wrong drug name or unit dose medication
Poor procedures or techniques	Poor aseptic technique used preparing drug
Poor training or knowledge	Improper calculations used in compounding
Poor doctor's handwriting	Assuming a drug name in error
Poor use of abbreviations	Transcribing an assumed drug abbreviation in error
Poor written directions for medication use	Typing a label based on assumption of doctor's poorly written prescription
Similar sounding drug name	Pulling wrong drug to be dispensed

enable the pharmacy technician to catch a possible prescribing mistake. All orders that are difficult to read should be brought to the pharmacist's attention before filling the prescription. Often the wrong medication is dispensed because of the physician's poor handwriting. Both pharmacists and technicians may pull the wrong medication based on an assumption of what the order says.

Aseptic Technique

Daily preparation and compounding of various medications requires knowledge of aseptic technique. Although pharmacists are responsible for all medications dispensed from the pharmacy, they cannot watch every pharmacy technician every moment of the day to ensure that proper procedures are used. Competent pharmacy technicians have learned how to use aseptic technique and why it is important to cultivate their skills. Pharmacy supervisors regularly take samples of compounded intravenous drugs and send them to the laboratory to be tested for microbial growth. Because each sample has the name of the pharmacy technician who prepared it, this information may be used to assess his or her performance.

Sound Alike, Look Alike Drugs

Drugs whose names are spelled similarly but are totally different classes of drugs have been the cause of many medication errors. For example, quinidine and quinine have been mistaken for one another. Quinidine is for the heart, whereas quinine is for malaria. It can be even more confusing when the drugs are similar not only in name but also in the condition that they treat. For example, the drugs amrinone and amiodarone are used for various heart conditions, and their names sound and look very much alike.

Manufacturers who package several different drugs have been known to package all of their products in similar colored packaging with similar print size and font for the cost savings. For example, unit dose packages of the generic version of promethazine 25 mg and promethazine 50 mg have the same packaging (font size, color, and package size) and can be easily confused if the technician is pulling a dose in a hurry. These types of errors have been documented over the years by the FDA. The FDA and others are encouraging drug companies to package their medications in packages that are markedly different (such as using various colors and different print) to further distinguish each individual drug name and strength for easy identification.

Because most drugs are kept on the pharmacy shelves in alphabetical order by generic name, a drug can be accidentally mistaken for another drug with a similar spelling. Each pharmacy must take steps to prevent this from happening by identifying these medications. For example, hydralazine and hydroxyzine are similarly sounding drugs and are close to one another on the shelf.

TECH NOTE! One way to decrease errors is to read prescription labels three times. First, when pulling the drug from the shelf to fill an order, check the prescription against the drug label. Next, as you prepare the prescription, check the name of the drug, strength, and dosage form against the medication you have chosen. Finally, check the drug as you move it over to the pharmacist for final checking. It works!

Professionalism

Pharmacy technicians are paraprofessionals and may be thought of as assistants to pharmacists. Because of the vast changes that have taken place during the last decade, pharmacy technicians are moving into an emerging field of pharmacy. As technicians assume more roles, such as clinical pharmacy technicians, inventory specialists, nuclear medication technicians, and other specialized roles, they must be knowledgeable in many areas of pharmacy. More technical colleges are offering associate degrees for pharmacy technicians. The field of pharmacy technician is becoming a profession. According to the American Medical Association (AMA), pharmacy technician was the top new profession in 2001.

Although it is good that the job of a pharmacy technician is beginning to be thought of as a profession, there is a difference between a profession and professionalism. A profession is a job, occupation, or line of work that becomes a career. Professionalism is conforming to right principles of conduct (work ethics) as accepted by others in the profession. It takes time, hard work, and consistency to be respected as a professional. Because of the increasing depth of education and training that a pharmacy technician needs, pharmacy technicians of today are the first generation of pharmacy technician professionals. If certain responsibilities are not met, they will remain pharmacy assistants and not professionals in the eyes of other health care professionals. In addition to meeting state requirements, behavior, attitude, and interpersonal skills are measures of professionalism. Pharmacy technicians deal daily with patients, pharmacists, doctors, and nurses. How they handle themselves in various situations reveals their competencies in the pharmacy and their personal maturity. Probably one of the most prevalent concerns of pharmacy managers and pharmacists is the need for pharmacy technicians who are competent in the area of communication.

Communication

Pharmacy technicians communicate every day with family, friends, strangers, acquaintances, and customers that they help (Figure 7.1). People depend on good communication skills to get a job; to buy products; and to have needs, wants, and concerns presented to others. Communication is defined as the ability to express oneself in such a way that one is readily and clearly understood; however, one of the major complaints from customers and managers is the lack of good communication skills. Most schools do not teach students to be good communicators; however, virtually all jobs require good communication skills. One of the most important areas in which effective communication is needed is in the pharmacy and other health care settings because life and death issues are often faced there. Good communication skills include diplomacy, compassion, sensitivity, responsibility, tact, and patience. Communication skills, or interpersonal skills, can also be referred to as the ability to relate to another person, verbally or nonverbally.

Every person takes his or her health seriously. Going to the doctor is not enjoyable but is done out of necessity. Feeling sick or unable to perform normally does

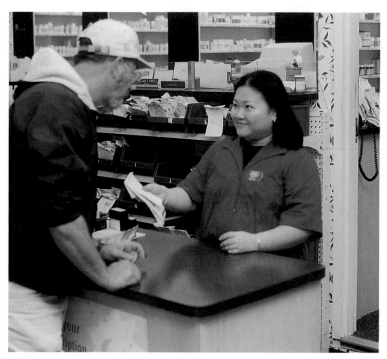

FIGURE 7.1 Technicians must be sensitive when helping patients.

not put people in a happy mood. After visiting the doctor, a person may have to start taking medication or add another medication to the many that they are already taking. On arrival to the pharmacy, the first person the customer may have to interact with is the pharmacy technician. It is this up-close-and-personal interaction that reveals the best and worst communication skills of the pharmacy technician. There are several areas to consider when assessing interpersonal skills, such as the different ways in which we communicate.

WAYS TO COMMUNICATE

Body Language

Have you ever heard the phrase "Actions speak louder than words"? Many people make an instant judgment of others within the first 30 seconds of meeting. This is true with respect to the pharmacy setting too. The primary goal of pharmacy personnel is to help people, which can be accomplished by being in a friendly manner and remaining calm. Facial expressions can show many different emotions, thoughts, and biases. As a professional, it is imperative that the only body language that should be conveyed is that of a helpful and concerned pharmacy staff member. A professional should not bring his or her outside personal problems to work. Stress manifests in various ways such as frowning, tensing the shoulders, biting one's lip, raising eyebrows, folding arms, placing hands on hips, or other idiosyncrasies that each person is aware of in himself or herself. If and when stress begins to transform into body language, it is time to take a step back and maybe a deep breath to bring oneself back into focus (Box 7.3).

Listening Skills

Listen, listen, and listen. Sometimes just listening to a person is all that is required. If a customer is angry about the medication, regardless of the problem, just listening can ease the person's frustration. Rather than trying to beat the person to the next sentence and telling the person that he or she is wrong, try to listen until the person is finished and empathize with the dilemma. Most people know a problem with medication is not the fault of the pharmacy technician, but they want to be heard. A professional does not allow himself or herself to be directed by another person's inappropriate behavior. Pharmacy technicians must remember the final outcome and behave professionally.

Phone Skills

Pharmacies receive phone calls every few minutes. If there are multiple lines, the phone can ring almost constantly. This can lead to several problems. For example, most people do not want to be placed on hold, but it is often necessary. It is not acceptable for a customer to be placed on hold and then forgotten. When answering the phone, it is best to identify oneself, place the customer on hold, and check back every minute or so just to let the customer know that he or she is not forgotten. Customers are calling about medications, and often these are essential medications that are extremely important. They must be treated with respect and courtesy (Box 7.4).

Appearance

Pharmacy technicians must interact daily with all types of customers or patients. In addition to customers, they must interact with nurses, doctors, and hospital staff. Knowledge, behavior, and good communications skills are essential to be considered a professional. But all of these attributes are inadequate if the pharmacy technician is not dressed professionally. A well-groomed person conveys self-confidence and professionalism. Of course, this should not be the only goal of the pharmacy technician; however, pharmacy protocol usually outlines what is acceptable and unacceptable with regard to uniform, shoes, hair, jewelry, and other miscellaneous items. Consider the message conveyed to customers when the pharmacy technician that takes the prescription has messy hair, too much makeup, a nose ring, and tattoos. Does this convey professionalism? Probably not, which is why the management of most pharmacies frowns on facial jewelry, an unkempt appearance, and visible tattoos.

BOX 7.3 EXAMPLE OF NEGATIVE BODY LANGUAGE

Ms. Lehman walks up to the counter to have her prescription filled and asks whether it can be done within 5 minutes because her bus will be leaving. Pharmacy technician John rolls his eyes and shakes his head in disbelief that everyone thinks that he or she should not have to wait. He turns and walks away without saying a word.

Alternate response: John shows concern for Ms. Lehman and tells her they will fill her prescription as soon as possible. John can ask the pharmacist to please fill the prescription as quickly as possible.

BOX 7.4 EXAMPLE OF UNACCEPTABLE PHONE ETIQUETTE

Patient: Hello, I'm calling because my medication looks different than before and I need to know if it's the same drug or not.

Pharmacy technician: Would you please hold?

Patient: No, I need to know now because . . .

Pharmacy technician: (places the patient on hold and forgets to get back to them)

Alternate response: The technician waits to hear the patient's response to the question. When the patient says she cannot wait, the technician waits to hear why, then proceeds to help her.

Good Writing Skills

One of the daily duties of a pharmacy technician is to answer the phones; talk to patients, nurses, and doctors; and take messages when the pharmacist is busy. It may seem simple to just write a question down quickly on a note pad, but if done poorly it can lead to improper communication or possibly an error. For example, if a nurse calls the pharmacy with a question about a drug interaction, it is

Pharmacist's Perspective
BY SUSAN WONG, PHARM D

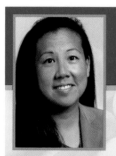

In recent years, there has been a national shortage of medical professionals, especially pharmacists and nurses. In some states, recent legislation has been approved to help pharmacies deliver better service in a timely manner. This will allow pharmacists to spend more time counseling patients. As an example in California, more technician support for pharmacists is allowed (up to two technicians to work with each pharmacist in certain situations—the technician to pharmacist ratio.) Now the challenge will be to find enough qualified technicians to work in the pharmacies. More emphasis will be placed on competency, communication, and ethics/professional behavior as the growth and expansion of the pharmacy technician role continues.

As mentioned in a previous chapter, the technician role has evolved from a clerical role to a more technical one behind the scenes, helping pharmacists provide medicines to those who need it. The technician is part of the team, not an individual practitioner. It is important that the technician be willing and competent to work anywhere from the front line helping customers to working behind the counter with the pharmacist answering phones, assist in filling prescriptions, preparing intravenous (IV) admixtures, and so on. Being competent in as many skills as possible is what sets the technician apart as a valued team member. Together, under the guidance and supervision of licensed pharmacists, this team will function as a well-oiled machine. This will allow efficiency on the job, delivery of world class pharmaceutical care, and personal job satisfaction.

Competency and Communication

Hallmark to excelling in competency on the job is communication skills. Accuracy and interpersonal (or "people") skills are absolutely necessary in the medical world. Clear, precise, legible information is required—look at it as if you won't have a second chance to fix a mistake. This might sound extreme but if a mistake results in a bad outcome, such as death, you will not have a second chance to fix it. This is also where the saying "do unto others as you would have them do unto

you" applies. Always remember there are two sides to every story. Don't be quick to judge a person by their words or actions. Many people, be they sick or well, professional colleagues or customers, handle stress in different ways. Treat them with respect as if you were interacting with other family members. I've always found that if you listen to them, they will listen to you. Some people are confrontational, but don't let them get the best of you, always take the high road. If the low road is taken, then they've won, haven't they?

Ethics

Ethics and high moral standards are always essential to doing a job well. In addition to knowing right from wrong, confidentiality is imperative. Breaking confidentiality with any customer information when not for work purposes is grounds for termination. Again, think about what it would be like if you were standing in the other person's shoes—most people would not want their own personal or medical information being shared either with strangers or with people they know. Keep your ethics and moral standards high, and you will always succeed.

Professionalism

Lastly, one might ask what exactly is professional behavior? It includes all of the information presented in this chapter. It also includes other aspects one might not always think about. Always remember, no matter who your employer is, the pharmacy technician will always be a reflection of the person or company for whom he or she works. The professional dress code should always be honored. Expressing one's individuality is not a bad thing, but save it for your personal time. Leave the fads at home, cover the midriff or tattoos, save excess jewelry for later. One's behavior, even on your own time, can be a reflection of your personal or professional affiliations. For example, involvement with a professional organization is a prime opportunity to network with your peers. If one's own behavior is inappropriate, it may be observed and possibly remembered for the future. This might have negative consequences on your future (e.g., future job prospects). Always aim for the high road! ∎

BOX 7.5 EXAMPLE OF POOR WRITTEN COMMUNICATION SKILLS

> Nurse Black calls and wants to know if the two drugs that she is about to administer are compatible. She's in a hurry. Joe North, CPhT, scribbles down the question but does not get the nurse's name or extension. By the time the nurse calls back to contact the pharmacist, the dose is late and the patient has been in pain while waiting.
>
>   Alternate response: The technician, Joe North, tells the nurse he will ask the pharmacist to call her back, then proceeds to ask her name, station, extension, and patient's name and medical record number.

imperative that the technician write down all of the pertinent information. Make sure that the following information is spelled correctly:

- Nurse's name
- Floor location and extension in a hospital setting, or the physician's office in a community pharmacy
- The purpose of the call written in a concise question
- The time of the call
- The initials of the technician who took the call

Only then can a pharmacist quickly and easily relay the correct information to the appropriate person. If your handwriting is illegible, it can cost time and possibly result in a preventable error. There is no excuse for poor handwriting. This is one of the reasons that doctors are now moving to electronic medication ordering. Thousands of preventable errors can be overcome through the use of computer ordering (Box 7.5).

Ethics

The morals that children are raised with stem from their family's beliefs in what is right and wrong. These morals and values extend throughout a lifetime and are passed to the next generation. Ethics are slightly different than morals, yet they are just as important. Ethics are the values and morals that are used within a profession. Each person has his or her own morals concerning issues such as abortion, and those morals can affect the ethics of a person in a professional situation. For example, if delivering medication used in performing abortions goes against a technician's morals, it may affect work ethics because the technician is required to deliver medications to customers as prescribed regardless of personal beliefs. The technician should not make a judgment about the patient. If a technician does not deliver the medication, he or she is not performing the assigned duties, which is a violation of professional duties. Most people can separate their own morals from work ethics and are able to do their job without believing that they have betrayed their belief system. This is a delicate topic for some and it must be addressed before taking a position that may bring up problems later.

TECH NOTE! Remember that working ethically is doing what is right for the patient, not what is right for you.

CONFIDENTIALITY

Confidentiality is another aspect of working ethically. The definition of confidentiality is to keep privileged information about a customer from being disclosed without his or her consent. This includes information that may cause the patient embarrassment or harm. Patients have a right to privacy concerning their

BOX 7.6 EXAMPLE OF BREACHING CONFIDENTIALITY

> Ms. K has cancer. Two pharmacy technicians discuss her condition and the medications that she is taking. A co-worker of Ms. K overhears this information and tells her employer.

medications, treatment, or any aspect of their healthcare. Confidentiality is the basis of HIPAA in the pharmacy (See Appendix E). These new laws affect all areas of medicine, including pharmacy, concerning issues of obtaining, transferring, and accessing patient information. Changes have been made throughout all medical facilities and medical information centers that will limit access to patient information in charts and computer bases. Any information concerning a patient will need the patient's approval before it is released to any third party, including insurance companies, doctors, and pharmacies. Because pharmacy technicians and other health care professionals have access to a patient's condition, medications, and other personal information, it is their responsibility to keep the patient's information confidential (Box 7.6).

Additional Competencies

TYPING

The speed required by most pharmacy employers does not exceed 35 words per minute (WPM), but a technician who has speed and a good knowledge of medication is cherished within the pharmacy setting. The number of prescriptions processed per day in a pharmacy directly relates to the speed of the typist. This makes a fast and accurate pharmacy technician typist a much sought-after commodity.

COMPUTERS

One of the requirements imposed on pharmacies by the federal government is the reduction of pharmacy errors. This has influenced pharmacies to use computers for dispensing medications and keeping inventory. Dispensing medication systems accurately count and dispense medications and directly have led to a decrease in the rate of errors. Although these systems increase accurate dosing, human error still occurs. Nothing replaces the knowledge of a skilled pharmacy technician to actively decrease error rates.

REPORTS

Many pharmacies expect technicians to prepare various reports. Knowledge of computers and programs such as Microsoft Word and Excel can make a technician a valuable asset to the pharmacy. Because all pharmacies have integrated computers into their ordering, filling, and documentation procedures, it is a necessity that technicians be computer savvy.

ORDERING SUPPLIES

The task of ordering stock usually falls on a specific person within the pharmacy, although everyone should know how to order stock when necessary. Learning how to order stock, return expired or damaged stock, and handle recalled items are among the duties in which pharmacy technicians should be competent.

Additional skills in which a pharmacy technician should be competent are listed in Box 7.7. Also listed in this box is the chapter in this book where further

BOX 7.7 ADDITIONAL PHARMACY TECHNICIAN COMPETENCIES

Conversions and calculations	Chapter 4
Dosage forms, abbreviations, and routes of administration	Chapter 5
Referencing	Chapter 6
Prescriptions	Chapter 8
Inpatient pharmacy	Chapter 11
Repackaging and compounding	Chapter 12
Aseptic technique	Chapter 13
Pharmacy stock and billing practices	Chapter 14

information can be found. Each chapter should be read before the completion of a pharmacy technician program. Of course, nothing supplements skills better than working in a pharmacy and learning firsthand the skills necessary to become a well-rounded pharmacy technician.

Terminally Ill Patients

Special consideration should be given to those patients who are terminally ill. This can prove difficult. Although each person deals with his or her own mortality differently, there are "normal" progressive steps that people experience. The five stages that terminally ill patients experience are as follows:

Stages	Example
Denial	"This can't be happening. . . ."
Anger	"It isn't fair. I don't deserve this. . . ."
Bargaining	"Please make me better and I promise. . . ."
Depression	"I will never be able to see you again. . . ."
Acceptance	"I can do this, everyone does. . . ."

Normally the first stage is denial. This is a defense mechanism in which the situation does not seem real. Perhaps the reality is too harsh for the person to accept. The next stage is anger. Sometimes a feeling of unfairness may be felt in this stage. Bargaining usually follows anger. The person makes promises to himself or herself or to a higher power in the hope of a miracle. Depression may take over at this point when the realization sets in that nothing is going to change concerning the prognosis. The final phase is acceptance, in which the person concedes to his or her own mortality and prepares for eventual death.

Each of these stages can manifest at any time and last for different lengths of time. Therefore it is important that the technician be compassionate to the patient's situation. Most health care workers do not hesitate to help a dying patient; however, the problem is how to identify these patients. Unfortunately, unless the patient decides to share this information, the pharmacy staff does not necessarily know. There are medications that indicate an advancing medical condition. These include pain medications, such as fentanyl patches or morphine; however, these drugs do not identify definitively a fatal condition. Therefore the pharmacy technician must be objective about each person who enters the pharmacy and realize that he or she does not know what each person is experiencing.

If people are treated equally regardless of their disposition, then the pharmacy technician is behaving appropriately and professionally. The pharmacy technician can influence the development of a positive atmosphere within the pharmacy setting. Allowing customers to express frustration, being a good listener, and doing one's best to help people is what being a professional is all about.

DO YOU REMEMBER THESE KEY POINTS?

- The difference between registration and certification
- The benefits of certification
- Federal laws that pharmacy technicians should know
- Protocol and where to find it within the pharmacy
- Information contained in the policies and procedures binder
- The major causes of medication errors
- The agencies that track errors
- Examples of how a pharmacy technician can decrease errors
- The difference between profession and professionalism
- The difference between morals and work ethics
- Five ways to communicate
- The importance of confidentiality
- Examples of additional competencies of a pharmacy technician
- The five stages of a terminally ill patient

REVIEW QUESTIONS:

Multiple Choice

1. Of the skills listed, which one is not a competency required of a pharmacy technician?
   A. Providing prescription label information
   B. Transcribing doctors' orders
   C. Consulting a doctor to clarify orders
   D. Preparing unit dose medications, including documentation

2. Of the information listed, which one is not normally contained in the policies and procedures binder within the pharmacy?
   A. Work shifts
   B. Job duties
   C. Employee benefits
   D. Insurance forms

3. Which of the statements is not true pertaining to medication errors?
   A. As many as 98,000 people die yearly because of medication errors.
   B. Costs resulting from drug errors can reach $75 billion annually.
   C. As of 2002, the FDA has just begun to gather information on drug errors.
   D. Deaths caused by drug errors surpass deaths caused by AIDS, auto accidents, and breast cancer.

4. Pharmacy technicians can decrease errors in all of the following ways except
   A. Bringing prescriptions that are difficult to read to the pharmacist's attention
   B. Writing notes or messages clearly
   C. Using good communication techniques
   D. Relying on the pharmacist to catch mistakes

5. The best definition for communication is
   A. Talking between two people
   B. Telling information to another person
   C. Expressing oneself in a way that is understood by another
   D. Winning an argument

6. Communication skills involve all of the following except
   A. Body language
   B. Listening
   C. Talking loudly
   D. Appearance

7. Concerning confidentially, which of the following statements is the most correct?
   A. Patients never have to worry about anyone talking about their personal health information.
   B. Patients give up their rights to confidentially when they are admitted into a hospital.
   C. Pharmacy technicians do not have access to patient information other than their current drugs.
   D. All health care workers are responsible for keeping patient information confidential.

8. Of the skills listed, identify the important ones.
   A. Computer skills
   B. Inventory skills
   C. Aseptic technique skills
   D. All of the above

9. Which of the following stages of a terminally ill patient is not one of those outlined in this chapter?
   A. Denial
   B. Anger
   C. Bargaining
   D. Psychosis

10. Of the statements listed, which one is not true concerning technician-to-patient interaction?
   A. Treating all patients equally is best.
   B. Using compassion and patience is important.
   C. Calling security immediately when a patient becomes angry.
   D. Calling the pharmacist for assistance if a patient insists on speaking with one.

True/False

*If a statement is false, then change it to make it true.

1. Registration and certification are both done by each state's Board of Pharmacy.

2. Only the FDA keeps information pertaining to drug errors.

3. Both consumers and health care workers can report drug errors to Med Watch.

4. Drug errors are likely to occur any time and any place.

5. All persons who are in the profession of pharmacy technician are automatically professional.

6. Facial jewelry, tattoos, and brightly colored hair on health care workers does not exhibit a professional appearance.

7. *Morals* and *ethics* are exactly the same.

8. Confidentially is something that only doctors and nurses need to worry about.

9. If pharmacy technicians are registered, this means they have had background checks done.

10. Only pharmacists should talk to angry patients.

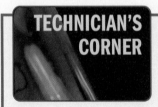

TECHNICIAN'S CORNER

Go to the FDA website at www.fda.gov and find the area in which medication errors can be reported. Download the form used and attach it to one of the many incident reports that have come into the FDA from either a consumer or health care professional.

BIBLIOGRAPHY

Koln, Linda T., Corrigan, Janet M., and Donaldson, Mike S: *To err is human: building a safer health system.* books.nap.edu/books/030906837/html/R1.html (accessed March 2, 2003).

Manual for pharmacy technicians, ed 2, Bethesda, MD, 1998, American Society of Health-System Pharmacists.

Nordenberg, Tamar: *Make no mistake: medical errors can be deadly serious.* www.fda.gov/fdac/features/2000/500_err.html (accessed March 2, 2003).

Western Career College curriculum, Sacramento, CA, Western Career College.

WEBSITES

www.fda.gov — Food and Drug Administration

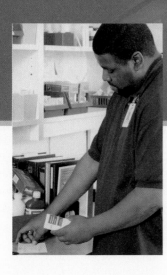

8 Prescription Processing

Objectives

- Describe the responsibilities of a technician filling prescriptions.
- List the necessary information required for prescriptions and labels.
- Demonstrate the ability to prioritize the filling of prescriptions.
- Differentiate filling methods between controlled substances and noncontrolled substances.
- Describe laws pertaining to the technician's responsibilities when filling prescriptions.
- Differentiate between inpatient and outpatient information requirements.
- List the types of automated machines used in filling prescriptions.
- Explain steps in reducing medication errors.
- List the rights of a patient.

Introduction

Filling a prescription is one of the most important and commonly performed duties of a technician, regardless of the setting. The art of transcribing doctors' writing into lay terms can sometimes be frustrating if not impossible. However, with time and experience, a good technician can easily determine whether or not he or she can process a prescription quickly or if assistance from the pharmacist is needed. Often the pharmacist cannot decipher the doctor's writing either. In this case, the pharmacist is responsible for calling the physician and asking for clarification of the prescription, also known as the script. Whether a technician is working in a hospital or community pharmacy, the process of reading a doctor's orders and the documentation of that order is much the same.

This chapter first explores the various methods by which a prescription can arrive in a pharmacy and the fundamentals of reading a prescription. Then the chapter explores what to look for, how to fill, file, and, finally, how to resolve discrepancies. In addition, the most common types of medication errors and how the technician can avoid some of the more common pitfalls are discussed. As with any skill, practice makes perfect.

Processing a Script: A Step-by-Step Approach

There are five basic steps for filling a prescription. Four of these relate directly to the technician; the fifth relates directly to the pharmacist. Although these steps may seem simple, they require complete presence of mind and concentration. Within each step there are several important points to remember that have been outlined in this chapter. The five steps include the following:

1. Taking in the prescription
2. Translating the prescription
3. Entering information into the computer system
4. Filling the script
5. Patient counseling*

*Counseling may be done by a registered pharmacist or pharmacist intern.

Taking in the Prescription

There are various methods by which a prescription can arrive in a pharmacy. A prescription can be in the form of a written order that is on a conventional prescription pad listing the doctor's information. A prescription can be carried into the pharmacy by hand or be faxed from the doctor's office to the pharmacy. Computer generated prescriptions are becoming more common. Prescriptions written in this way may be provided to the patient on discharge from the hospital or physician's office.

TECH NOTE! Prescriptions may be faxed to a pharmacy. However, it is a good idea for the pharmacist to know the prescriber who will be faxing prescriptions, because forgery is more likely to occur otherwise.

Prescriptions can be called into the pharmacy; the pharmacist transcribes the verbal order onto a blank prescription pad. Technicians should be aware of their state's specific rules for taking a called-in prescription. The most commonly followed rules are shown in Box 8.1.

PRESCRIPTION INFORMATION

Outpatient Setting

If the order is written by a physician or other authorized person, it will usually be hand carried to the pharmacy by the patient. Therefore the person at the take-in counter will be the first one to handle the script. This is usually the clerk or technician who is on duty. It is important to ensure that the correct information is listed on the prescription. Table 8.1 lists the information that should be on a prescription presented to the pharmacy for filling. Additional information, such as information regarding allergies, is usually needed for a new patient. This information is placed into the computer system for future reference.

It is important for the patient to know his or her medical record number if the patient is a member of a health maintenance organization (HMO) or the specific medical coverage information. For a prescriber, the Drug Enforcement Agency

BOX 8.1 COMMONLY FOLLOWED RULES FOR TAKING IN PRESCRIPTIONS

Call-In

Calling in a prescription can be done by a doctor, nurse, physician's assistant, or a person designated by the doctor.

Taking a prescription over the phone must only be done by a registered pharmacist or pharmacist intern (in some states).

Fax

Faxed original copies are mostly used by hospitals but are becoming more common in community pharmacies. Schedule II medications, if faxed, must have a written prescription at the pharmacy in 72 hours.

Walk-In

Most prescriptions in a community pharmacy are walked into a pharmacy by the patient or the patient's relative. In hospitals, discharge orders are usually sent to the pharmacy via pneumatic tube system or hand delivered by staff or volunteers. In an outpatient dispensing pharmacy of a hospital, prescriptions are handled in the same manner as a community pharmacy.

TABLE 8.1   Important Patient Information

Patient Information	Provider's Information
Name	Name
Phone number and address	Phone number and address
Insurance information, if applicable	Provider's license number
Age or date of birth	Provider's DEA number if applicable
	Name of medication
	Strength
	Dosage form
	Route
	Quanitity
	Route of administration
	Sig
	Refill information
	Provider's signature
	Date written
	"Brand necessary" if brand name drug is desired

TABLE 8.2   Necessary Patient Information in a Hospital Setting

Patient	Prescriber
Patient name	Name of medication
Medical record number	Strength
Room number	Route of administration
	Dosage form
	Sig (route and frequency)
	Provider's signature
	Date and time written

Other important information

Allergies	Diagnosis
Weight	
Age	
In pediatrics and geriatrics, the height and weight of the patient is needed for dosage calculations.	

(DEA) number is necessary if a controlled drug is being dispensed. In addition, a controlled drug must be written in either ink or indelible pencil. See Chapter 2 for more information on DEA numbers.

Inpatient Setting

In a hospital setting, the information required on a prescription is different. If the doctor works for the hospital, the license number and DEA number are on file. Therefore it may not be necessary for the doctor to write out as much information. The same is true for the patient because that information is also more readily available. The information that is required for in-house scripts is shown in Table 8.2.

TECH NOTE! An order written in the chart of a hospital patient is considered a legal prescription once signed by the prescriber.

Because most dosing is set on a 24-hour period, the doctor writes only the actual dose to be given daily. For example, a multivitamin written as 1 qd (daily) will be loaded into the patient's medication tray every 24 hours and will continue until the doctor writes D/C (discontinue). Exceptions to this are orders for antibiotics, which usually have an automatic stop date.

Translation of an Order

When reading an order that is very hard to decipher, make sure you look at the whole order. For instance: Do you know what clinic the order came from? Can you make out the strength or dose? What is the route of administration? How often is the medication being ordered? What is the dosage form? Are there refills? If you are having a hard time reading the order, but you can see that the drug strength is 0.125 mg and it is to be taken daily, this limits the types of possible medications because of the strength and the dosing time. It may become clear to you what the order is for. Of course the bottom line is, if you are in doubt, ask another person such as the pharmacist.

TECH NOTE! When you ask someone to decipher a drug or instruction, do not first tell him or her your thought. This can inadvertently make that person see it the same way. Simply ask, "What does this look like to you?" If the answer matches yours, then you have an unbiased opinion. However, if you are not sure, ask the pharmacist to call the doctor to confirm the prescription.

WHEN TO ASK FOR HELP

When a job relies on reading another's handwriting and the handwriting is poor, it is common to need assistance in interpreting the writing. However, each person filling scripts is under intense pressure to fill them quickly, and this can lead to "guessing" at an order and then filling it. The following example is to help you feel comfortable in asking for help.

EXAMPLE 8.1 ASK FOR HELP

A patient's prescription is filled inappropriately with a strength of medication higher than ordered. She is admitted to the hospital suffering from a stroke. The probable cause is determined to be error in medication. Because the technician did not ask for help in deciphering the script and the pharmacist did not question the technician, the following occurred:

- The costs of the hospital stay for 3 days: $15,000
- Cost of litigation: $40,000
- Settlement amount: $100,000
- Overall stress and hardship on those involved in the case: ? (Varies for each person)
- The pharmacist's license was revoked for 6 months and a fine was imposed

If the technician had asked the pharmacist for help, the pharmacist could have called the doctor who wrote the prescription and asked for clarification, and the order would have been filled correctly—time, 45 minutes. Was it a good idea to make an assumption when filling the script? It is evident that the best way to deal with a questionable script is to inquire further rather than make quick judgments and run the risk of errors.

- Fact: Most court cases will favor the patient and award him or her with cash settlements.
- Fact: Most errors require a minimal amount of time to correct.
- Fact: Most errors are due to the technician and pharmacist trying to hurry.

Bottom line: Whenever in doubt always ask for help.

TECH NOTE! As physicians begin to move into the paperless writing of prescriptions, it is hoped that these difficult tasks will be a thing of the past. More and more hospitals are using preprinted order forms, and some have begun to use handheld computers capable of transferring a prescription to the pharmacy.

Entering the Information into the Database

OUTPATIENT SETTING

Once you have correctly read the doctor's order or prescription, it is then entered into the computer terminal (Figure 8.1). In a community pharmacy setting, the technician usually does this. The computerized label is checked against the prescription after it is filled. Two labels are always discharged from the printer; one is placed on the vial for dispensing and the other is placed on the back of the original prescription. Both copies must be initialed by the pharmacist. Most pharmacies today copy prescriptions to the computer for verfication. If a change must be made, the pharmacist can easily access the terminal and make the change to the order. At the time of consultation, the pharmacist also finds out which other medications the patient is taking.

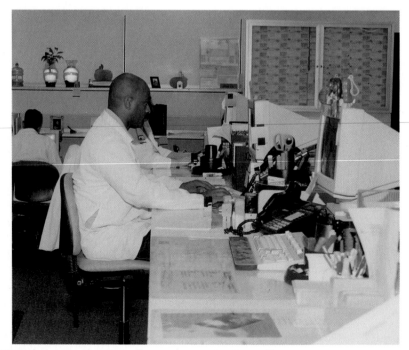

FIGURE 8.1 Technicians may enter information into the computer system in many pharmacy settings.

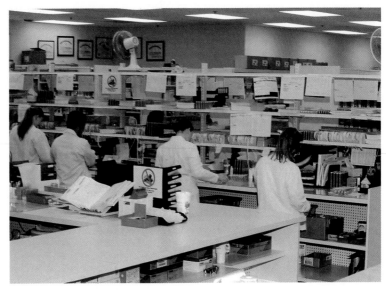

FIGURE 8.2 Technicians filling prescriptions.

INPATIENT SETTING

In a hospital, it is uncommon to have a technician enter new prescriptions into the computer. A pharmacist most likely has this responsibility. In a hospital there are multiple orders sent on the admission of a patient and throughout the patient's hospital stay. Because all orders have to be verified by a pharmacist, it saves time if he or she inputs the order and the technician fills the order. If the pharmacist enters the order, he or she only has to check the technician's work once rather than twice—after the technician enters the order and after the technician fills it. In addition, most computers have a built-in system that alerts the person entering prescriptions that a drug interaction can occur. A technician cannot handle interaction problems; a pharmacist must initiate a phone call to the physician for an order change if necessary.

Filling the Script

After the prescription label is prepared, it is matched with the original order and sent to the counter for filling (Figure 8.2). Again, the technician (in most settings) receives the order. It is important that from the beginning the technician pay close attention to the prescription he or she is filling because this is where many mistakes can be avoided. Following these 10 simple yet important steps may prevent the technician from making a grievous error:

1. Check the label on the stock bottle and the NDC number in the computer against the original prescription for confirmation of the order.*
2. Pull the appropriate medication from the shelf.*
3. Measure or count out the necessary amount of the medication.
4. Fill the vial with the medication, taking care not to touch the medication.
5. Make sure that the lid is the appropriate type and affixed properly onto the vial.
6. Apply the labels onto the vial and back of the prescription.*
7. Place the technician's initial on the bottom right hand side of all labels printed.
8. Apply any necessary auxiliary labels to the vial.
9. Put the medication on top of the original prescription.*

*The technician should check the medication against the script and/or against the label at these points.

10. Pass it onto the pharmacist for final inspection. Usually the pharmacist on duty signs in to the computer with his or her initials that will appear on the prescription label.

CHECKING THE LABEL AGAINST THE SCRIPT

When the label is passed along with the original script, it must be checked many times before it ever reaches the patient. The technician should hold the original script next to the label and check for any apparent errors or discrepancies.

TECH NOTE! If the order does not seem right, it probably is not. Ask for assistance if you cannot put your finger on what is wrong.

Look at the name of the drug, the strength or dose, dosage form, amount, and the sig (directions). Make sure all information matches.

PULLING THE CORRECT MEDICATION

You will leave the counter to get the medication from the shelf. When doing this, make sure that you take the label with you for two reasons:

1. You do not forget what you are looking for (which cuts down on time spent).
2. Once the bottle of medication is found, compare the label information to the bottle, checking the name, strength, and dosage form as well as the NDC number on refills.

TECH NOTE! When checking the dosage form, do not make assumptions. It is easy to assume that a spansule is the same as a capsule (they look similar); however, they are different.

COUNTING AND FILLING THE MEDICATION

After the technician locates the medication, removes it from the shelf, and returns to the counter, the script is filled.

TECH NOTE! Keep medications away from one another on the counter when filling to prevent grabbing the wrong bottle.

Again, you should check your label and script against the medication bottle for accuracy. If the order calls for a bottle of #100, check to make sure that the manufacturer's package size matches your order. For example, many times bottles hold different amounts. Although there are various ways to count medications, many pharmacies still use counting trays, in which case it is best to count by multiples of five. Another way to count is with a device that uses a beam of light. As the light is broken, the digital counter adds another tablet or capsule on the monitor. High-technology filling is now done by semi-automated to automated machines. These range from Baker Cell systems to large hospital computer dispensing systems. Dispensing systems are discussed later in this chapter.

PRESCRIPTION LIDS AND AUXILIARY LABELS

Once the vial is filled with the medication, the appropriate lid is applied to the vial. As the average human life expectancy increases, there is a growing segment of the population that is older than 70 years. Two of the problems that accompany aging are decreasing dexterity and strength. As most of us have experienced, there is a safety lid that even Godzilla cannot remove! It is not surprising that many older patients do not wish to have safety lids on their medication. By law it is

TABLE 8.3 Exceptions for Safety Caps*

Drug	Dispensed Without Safety Lid	Reason
Nitroglycerin	Never has a safety lid	For emergencies
Isosorbide SL	May be dispensed without a safety lid	For emergencies
All other medications	If documented via doctor's request on prescription or patient's request documented in computer or in hard copy	Any conditions

SL, Sublingual.
*Refer to the Poison Control Act of 1970 for all exceptions.

important that the pharmacy use safety lids in all cases except for a selected few. These are outlined in Table 8.3.

Most patients receive childproof caps; however, there are many older patients or those with disabilities who cannot manipulate prescription lids. If a waiver is signed by the patient or his or her physician has requested no childproof caps, then the cap is replaced with a snap-on lid. This is listed on the patient information in the computer for future reference.

APPLYING THE LABEL

When labeling a bottle, it is important to remember professionalism. A torn or crooked label should not be placed on a medication bottle. No one wants to believe that the prescription was put together in a rush, but rather with care and concern. When filling a prescription for a full bottle, such as cough syrup, you can place the label over the existing bottle's label, making sure not to cover the lot number and expiration date. If the medication has to be counted, the medication should be poured into an appropriate-sized bottle.

Sometimes labels must be cut down in size because of lengthy directions. For example, a tapering dose of prednisone is a typical challenge, but it is possible to fit these labels onto a vial even if you must use a vial that is larger than normal to accommodate the label. Care should be taken when cutting a label so that it will not be apparent to the patient. Also, the label must not cover any important print. In addition, auxiliary labels, when required, must be placed onto the bottle so that the patient can easily read the instructions. Many computer systems have a labeling system that allows the following information to be printed on one sheet:

- The prescription label
- A duplicate copy to be placed on the original hard copy
- Billing information
- Auxiliary labels

Once a prescription is entered into the computer system, the instructions and necessary information are printed out on labels. Most labels contain pre-printed information that is required by law, which consists of the following:

- Name, address, and phone number of pharmacy
- A prescription number, given automatically by the computer
- Patient name
- Drug, strength or dose, dosage form
- Manufacturer's name if not dispensed in manufacturer's bottle
- Instructions
- Date filled
- Refill information
- Prescriber
- Expiration date if not dispensed in the manufacturer's bottle

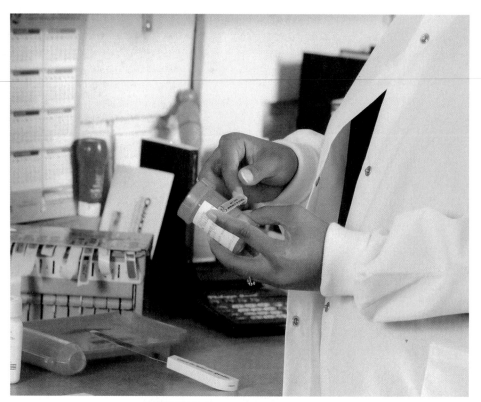

FIGURE 8.3 Applying auxiliary label.

TECHNICIAN'S INITIALS

All orders filled by a technician should be initialed by him or her as the prescriptions are filled per state law. This is important for several reasons. The pharmacist who will give the final check-off now knows that the prescription is filled. If the pharmacist has any questions, he or she knows whom to ask. Finally, if there should be an error, the technician can be notified and learn from that error. In addition, the pharmacist must always sign off after completion. There are some computer systems that have the pharmacist's initials printed on the label which is acceptable to most state boards of pharmacy.

AUXILIARY LABELS

All necessary auxiliary labels must adhere to the vial in a neat manner (Figure 8.3). These labels are normally printed out along with the label, making it very easy for the technician. However, it is still important to know what medications need special auxiliary labels because not all pharmacies have this ability. If many auxiliary labels are printed out, it is necessary to choose the most important ones that can easily fit on the medication bottle.

TECH NOTE! Rest auxiliary labels on top of the cap or lid of the medication so that the pharmacist can easily select which ones to affix to the bottle.

For the technician to know which medications require an auxiliary label, he or she must know the drug's classification, interactions, and side effects. Remembering a few common rules will help with the most general auxiliary labels (Table 8.4). For the most part, it takes time and experience to learn which auxiliary labels are the best. However, it is ultimately up to the pharmacist to choose which labels

TABLE 8.4 Commonly Used Auxiliary Labels for Side Effects

Medication	Most Common Auxiliary Label
Contraceptives	Take as directed
NSAIDs	May cause dizziness/drowsiness
	Take with food
Narcotics	Do not drink alcohol and/or drinking may increase the effects of the drug
Macrolides	Take on an empty stomach
	Take with plenty of water
Antibiotics	Take until gone
Sulfa	May cause sensitivity to light
	Take on an empty stomach
	Take with plenty of water
Warfarin	Do not take aspirin

NSAIDs, Nonsteroidal antiinflammatory drugs.

to place on the prescription bottle. Be sure to read auxiliary labels before adhering them to the bottle because many different instructions are colored the same and may appear similar.

THE PHARMACIST'S FINAL INSPECTION

The last step in filling scripts is placing the filled vial, along with the medication container taken from the shelf, on top of the original prescription and passing it to the pharmacist for final inspection. Give the order one more inspection to ensure that the patient's name on the script matches the label and all other information is correct. Only then should you pass the medication to the pharmacist and begin the next order.

It may seem as though all of these steps would take a long time; however, it takes only a few moments. Another important aspect of filling a prescription is to remember not to fill more than one prescription at a time; this is an invitation for error! You can pull several orders, giving each a double check for accuracy, but then place them back away from the prescription you are filling.

If a new stock bottle is opened to fill an order, it should be marked across the front with an X (in pen) to alert fellow employees that this is not a full bottle. Do not cover NDC number or expiration date with the mark. When the bottle is finally returned to stock, the next person pulling the bottle will know it is a partial. If a full bottle is needed, he or she will choose an unmarked one. The overall time that a prescription is in the hands of the pharmacy technician is not very long, which is why it is so important to make each moment count when trying to fill a flawless prescription.

COMPUTER DISPENSING SYSTEMS

Another type of prescription filler besides the traditional pharmacist or technician is the emerging computer system (Figure 8.4). New and improved versions become available every year. Pharmacy personnel must become comfortable with manipulating these devices because they are here to stay. The two major versions of dispensing systems are those made for filling outpatient prescriptions and those used in hospitals. Because of many differences between the two pharmacy settings and because each pharmacy has different requirements, the computer systems used in each one must be made to specifically handle their needs. Because of this, most manufacturers of automated systems offer various components to fit each pharmacy's specific needs.

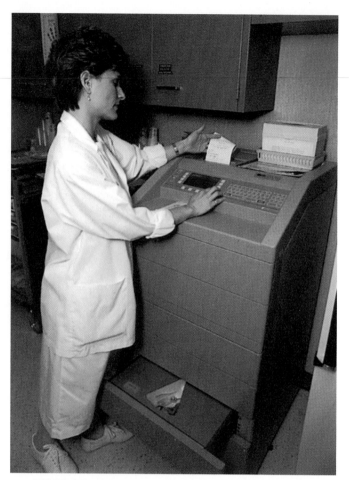

FIGURE 8.4 Inpatient automated dispensing system.

BOX 8.2 ADVANTAGES OF COMPUTER DISPENSING SYSTEMS

Speed up dispensing medication	As the prescription is entered into the computer system, the information is transferred to the dispensing system.
Cut down on errors	The proper amount of tablets or capsules is then dispensed into a container.
Inventory control	Medication can be scanned to keep accurate count of inventory. Daily printouts can be used by a technician or pharmacist to help the inventory technician keep the correct amount of drug on the shelf.

Outpatient Dispensing Systems

Many chain pharmacies are using automated dispensing systems for three primary reasons: to cut down on errors, to increase productivity, and for inventory control (Box 8.2). The only current disadvantage is the high cost. However, because of new laws that require pharmacies to decrease medication errors, pharmacies are slowly converting to these types of systems.

Inpatient Dispensing Systems

Most hospitals use some type of computerized dispensing system because it is important that medication be available around the clock. Although many inpatient pharmacies are open 24 hours a day, 7 days a week, staffing is limited throughout the night, and computer dispensing systems can help reduce staffing needs.

Medical personnel such as doctors or nurses should only be able to access stocked medications. Another major use of automation in hospital systems is to regulate controlled substances and track their movement.

A system that is being incorporated into some hospital pharmacies is the robot-type dispensing machine. This machine uses mechanical arms to scan bar codes on each unit-dosed medication to identify the correct dose. (Dose information is fed into it by computer input from the pharmacist or technician.) It fills each patient's medication cassette with 99% accuracy. Once the medication is filled, the cassette is delivered by the technician, who will bring back the previous day's cassette for the next day's filling.

The Rights of a Patient

When a technician takes on the role of prescription filler, it is very important that he or she always remembers the rights of a patient. A good mind set is to think of yourself as the recipient of the medication that you are preparing. Checking the prescription at least three times during the filling process helps ensure accuracy. The rights of the patient are as follows:

1. The right dose
2. The right medication
3. The right route
4. The right time
5. The right price
6. The right dosage form
7. The right patient

Pharmacist Consultations: When and Who Needs Them

As the patient's medication is being entered into the computer system, one of the functions of pharmacy tracking is to determine whether it is a new prescription or a refill. First-time prescriptions are usually flagged in some manner so that they come to the attention of the pharmacist. If flagging is not automatic, it is up to the individual pharmacist to check the computer system for this information. If the script is a new one, a sticker is placed on the medication bag indicating to the technician or clerk that the patient needs a consultation. It is a federal law that, with all new prescriptions or changes in an existing prescription, a patient must be offered consultation. They can refuse consultation, but it must be offered per the Omnibus Reconciliation Act of 1990 (OBRA '90) (see Chapter 2). At this time, the pharmacist looks into the records of the patient to determine whether there are any possible "red flags," and explains the instructions to the patient and any side effects that he or she might encounter. At this time, the patient can also inquire about any questions or concerns specific to the medication.

Miscellaneous Orders

Unlike first-time prescriptions, refills and transferring prescriptions can be done by technicians, clerks, and pharmacy interns over the phone as outlined in the following. Although these guidelines are federally enacted, they may be stricter depending on each pharmacy's protocol.

REFILLS

A pharmacy technician may phone and receive authorization for a prescription refill. When a patient calls in a prescription refill or a request is faxed, the following information is necessary:

1. Patient's name
2. Home phone number
3. Prescription number
4. Name of the medication, strength, quantity, and Rx number
5. Prescription number

ZERO REFILL REORDERS

Many pharmacies have an additional phone request line for prescriptions that have run out of refills. Typically, the patient should allow 2 days to get proper authorization from the prescriber, and technicians are able to perform this task under the pharmacist's direction.

TRANSFERS

A pharmacist may transfer a previously filled prescription from one pharmacy to another. Most state Boards of Pharmacy (BOPs) prefer to allow transfers of a prescription to occur only one time; however, federal law stipulates that controlled substances may only be transferred one time. Always be aware of your Board of Pharmacy laws. In general the following applies:

- A pharmacy technician may assist the pharmacist in the transfer of a prescription.
- Under the supervision of the pharmacist, the technician may fax a copy of the prescription to another pharmacy. The pharmacist directs the technician on what information may be needed from the receiving or transferring pharmacy.

Filing Prescriptions

Although times have changed with use of computers, it is still necessary to follow through on the manual filing of hard copy prescriptions. After the computer entry is made, the prescription makes its way down the filling counter, and all steps are completed, the hard copy must be filed for future reference. The law states that all prescriptions must be kept on file for a period of at least 3 years. This is done by using the prescription number. On the back of the prescription is a copy of the label used on the dispensed drug, along with the initials of the technician or pharmacist who filled the order. In addition, some states require that all controlled substances (Schedules III–IV) that are filled together or with other prescriptions must be stamped with a red "C" 1 inch down on the right hand side of the prescription label to make it easier to find. The location of the stamp may differ depending on state law. All Schedule II medications must be filed seperately. Other filing guidelines are discussed in Chapter 2. Usually, all prescriptions are filed at the end of the day. They are filed in small packets that are clearly marked on the outside with the date for easy reference. These are all kept on the pharmacy premises. In addition to the hard copy, the computer copy indicates whether a drug is a controlled substance and lists all the other information required by the federal and state regulations. At the end of the workday, back-up copies are usually made of all the orders in the system in case of a computer crash.

Medication Pick-Up

Patients can wait for their prescription, have it delivered, or pick it up another day. Occasionally, a patient has a relative pick up a prescription. For these cases a note should be made in the computer listing the person or persons who are authorized to pick up another's prescription. Regardless of who picks up the prescription, it is important to ensure that the right person gets the right medication. Therefore all identification should be checked against the prescription before releasing the medication. In the case of a controlled substance, if the person picking up the medication is not the patient, they must show identification to the clerk or technician and sign for it. All third-party prescriptions must have the signature of the receiver. Also, it is good professional practice to ask for identification on all Schedule II controlled substance prescriptions.

Billing

The billing portion of processing a prescription varies depending on what type of coverage the patient has, if any. If the patient does not have coverage, there is no additional paperwork to fill out because the patient simply has to pay full price for the prescription. Most people have some type of coverage. Each type of insurance has its own limitations and conditions. Each pharmacy is responsible for contacting the coverage program. For more information see Chapter 14.

Changing Trends

Interpreting, transcribing, producing labels, filling, and checking are the "meat and potatoes" of the pharmacy business. Laws such as OBRA '90 require that consultations be given to patients. The increasing age and population of Americans has moved the pharmacist away from the filling counter to interacting more with patients and prescribers. Because of this nationwide change, the technician has been placed on the front line. This responsibility requires the technician to fill prescriptions as quickly and with the same accuracy as a pharmacist. Technicians must also know their limitations at all times. In addition to these capabilities, many technicians are in charge of the billing process and must be acutely aware of the policies and procedures of their pharmacy and how to process various insurance claims. Patients expect perfection when it comes to their medications and proper billing practices. This weight clearly falls on the technician filling the orders as well as the pharmacist in charge. It is a responsibility that should never be taken lightly, and one that requires continued education in all areas of pharmacy practice.

DO YOU REMEMBER THESE KEY POINTS?

- The various ways a prescription can be submitted to the pharmacy for processing
- The steps involved in filling a prescription
- Who can call in a prescription
- Who can transfer a prescription from one pharmacy to another
- The differences between information on inpatient and outpatient prescriptions
- What type of patient information is needed in different pharmacy settings

- The importance of knowing when and why to ask for help from a pharmacist
- The number of times a pharmacy technician should check a prescription while filling it
- The necessary authorization to use snap-on caps rather than childproof caps
- The auxiliary labels needed for the medications outlined in this chapter
- Why computer dispensing systems are used
- The rights of a patient
- When patient consultations are done and who is authorized to do them
- How to process refills
- Requirements of filing prescriptions (hard copies)
- Patient requirements for picking up medication at the pharmacy

REVIEW QUESTIONS:

Multiple Choice

1. Of the methods listed, which are the acceptable forms of receiving a prescription?
   A. By mail
   B. In person
   C. Called in
   D. Both A and B
   E. All of the above

2. The best times to check for errors on a script while filling are
   A. When the order is first received, during filling, and after filling
   B. While filling the order, after filling, and when handing to the patient
   C. When checking the original order against the label, against the stock bottle before filling, and before filling the vial and labeling
   D. Before applying the label, before applying the auxiliary labels, and before giving it to the pharmacist

3. Of the information listed, which is vital information needed from a patient before filling his or her prescription?
   A. Full name
   B. Address
   C. Insurance number or medical record number
   D. All of the above

4. When in doubt as to the directions on a prescription, it is best to
   A. Call the doctor's office immediately
   B. Try your best to decipher the order
   C. Ask the pharmacist for help
   D. Ask a pharmacy clerk for help with interpretation

5. Of the reasons listed, which is/are the main reason/s for using automated dispensing systems in a community pharmacy?
   A. To increase the accuracy of filling prescriptions
   B. To help control inventory
   C. To decrease the time it takes to fill an order
   D. All of the above

6. What information is not needed from a prescriber on a prescription order?
   A. Sig
   B. Refills
   C. Manufacturer
   D. Date written

7. Which of the medications listed does not require a safety lid?
   A. All heart medication
   B. All diabetic medication
   C. Nitroglycerin sublingual tablets
   D. Acetaminophen (Tylenol)

8. Of the information listed, which is not necessary on a prescription label?
   A. Date filled
   B. Expiration date
   C. Prescriber
   D. Patient's home address

9. Which one of the rights listed is not considered a right of a patient?
   A. The right to the correct drug
   B. The right to the correct price
   C. The right to the lowest price
   D. The right to the correct strength

10. Of the following basic steps required in filling a prescription, which is not the responsibility of the technician?
    A. Filling the prescription
    B. Translation of a prescription
    C. Consulting the patient
    D. Entering the information into the database

True/False

*If a statement is false, then change it to make it true.

1. When a technician fills a script, only the pharmacist's initials should appear on the prescription bottle.

2. New prescriptions can either be called or walked into a pharmacy by the patient for filling.

3. When scripts are written by a physician for a patient in the hospital, it is not necessary for the order to be presented on a prescription pad.

4. Technicians regularly enter hospital orders and may call the doctor for additional information.

5. All prescriptions must have safety lids per federal law.

6. Most pharmacy labeling programs print out a second label to be placed on the back of the hard copy prescription.

7. Technicians need to sign their initials or last name on all prescription labels before passing them on to the pharmacist for a final check.

8. Antibiotics typically receive an auxiliary label "Take until gone" to ensure that the patient finishes the course of antibiotic treatment.

9. OBRA '90 ensures that technicians can handle drugs.

10. Technicians cannot take prescription orders over the phone.

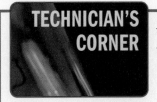

TECHNICIAN'S CORNER

You fill a prescription with the wrong drug. The error is not caught until later that evening when the prescriptions are being filed. What do you do?

BIBLIOGRAPHY

Nielsen R, James JD: *Handbook of federal drug law,* ed 2, Philadelphia, 1992, Williams & Wilkins.

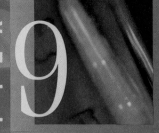

CHAPTER 9

Over-the-Counter Medications and Skin Care Products

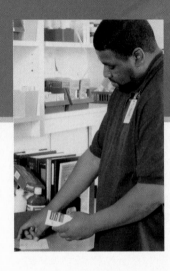

Objectives

- Describe why over-the-counter (OTC) medications are popular.
- List considerations that should be made concerning the use of OTC drugs.
- List the three categories used by the Food and Drug Administration (FDA) for OTC drugs.
- Describe FDA regulations concerning the manufacturing of OTC drugs.
- Explain how legend drugs become OTC drugs.
- Describe the various types of conditions that OTC medicines treat.
- List major components of skin anatomy.
- List the types of agents used to treat skin conditions.
- Determine the right strength of sunscreen necessary to protect skin from ultraviolet rays.
- Define the various forms of acne.
- Describe psoriasis and the types of medications used to treat this skin condition.

TERMS AND DEFINITIONS

Analgesic *A drug that relieves pain by reducing the perception of pain*

Antiinflammatory *A drug that reduces swelling, redness, and pain, and promotes healing*

Antipruritic *A drug that relieves itching, usually an antihistamine or an antiinflammatory drug*

Antiseptic *A substance that slows or stops growth of microorganisms on surfaces such as skin*

Antitussive *A drug that can decrease the coughing reflex of the central nervous system (CNS)*

ASA *Acetylsalicylic acid (aspirin)*

Bulk forming *Fiber used as a stimulant to the intestines or to cause a feeling of fullness to decrease appetite*

Desquamating *A normal process of shedding the top layer of the skin, also known as exfoliation*

Expectorant *A drug that induces coughing up mucus from the lungs*

Keratolytic *A drug that causes shedding of the outer layer of the skin*

OTC *Over-the-counter; does not require a prescription*

Prophylaxis *Treatment given before an event to prevent the event from happening*

Protectant *A substance that acts as a barrier between the skin and an irritant*

Pruritis *Itching*

ROA *Route of administration*

Rx *Legend drug; a prescription drug*

Sunscreen *A substance that protects the skin from ultraviolet (UV) light, which causes sunburns; skin protectant factor (SPF) rates effectiveness*

TABLE 9.1 Common Over-the-Counter Preparations

Brand Name	Generic Name	Classification	Brand Name	Generic Name	Classification
Fever/Pain Products			**Cold/Cough Products**		
Tylenol	Acetaminophen	Antipyretic/analgesic	Robitussin	Guaifenesin	Expectorant
			Benylin	Guaifenesin/ dextromethorphan	Expectorant/ antitussive
Fever/Pain/Inflammation Products					
Bayer	Aspirin	NSAID, analgesic	Benadryl	Diphenhydramine	Antihistamine
Motrin, Advil	Ibuprofen	NSAID	Sudafed	Pseudoephedrine	Decongestant
Excedrin	Aspirin/caffeine /acetaminophen	NSAID (migraines)	**Nasal**		
			Neosynephrine	Phenylephrine	Vasoconstrictor
Sleep Aids			Allerest	Naphazoline	Decongestant
Benadryl	Diphenhydramine	Histamine blocker, sedative, antihistamine	**Eye (Ophthalmic) Products**		
			VasoClear	Naphazoline	Decongestant

NSAID, Nonsteroidal antiinflammatory drug; *guaif,* guaifenesin.

TABLE 9.1 Common Over-the-Counter Preparations—cont'd

Brand Name	Generic Name	Classification	Brand Name	Generic Name	Classification
Sore Throat Products			**Intestinal Products**		
Cepacol	Dyclonine	Analgesic	Metamucil	Psyllium	Fiber
Chloraseptic	Benzocaine	Topical anesthetic	Imodium A–D	Loperamide	Antidiarrheal
Stomach Products			**Anticonstipation**		
Pepcid AC	Famotidine	H$_2$ antagonist	Senokot	Senna extract	Laxative
Zantac-75	Ranitidine	H$_2$ antagonist	Dulcolax	Bisacodyl	Laxative
Tagamet-HB	Cimetidine	H$_2$ antagonist	**Miscellaneous Products**		
Milk of Magnesia	Magnesium hydroxide	Antacid, laxative	Compound W	Salicylic acid	Exfoliate (warts/corns)
Tums	Calcium carbonate	Acid neutralizer/ calcium supplement	Calamine	Calamine	Antipruritic
			Tinactin	Tolnaftate	Antifungal
			Lotrimin	Clotrimazole	Antifungal
			Monostat	Miconazole	Antifungal
			Preparation H	Hydrocortisone	Antihemorrhoidal

NSAID, Nonsteroidal antiinflammatory drug; *guaif,* guaifenesin.

Introduction

If you walk into a shopping center or your corner drugstore, you will see the massive number of over-the-counter (OTC) medications that are ready to be picked off the shelf for personal use. There are no prescriptions necessary or questions to answer to get these drugs. Most consumers give no thought to purchasing several different drugs to keep at home for themselves or their family. One could almost say they are common staples of a home medicine cabinet just as staples are kept on hand in the kitchen. A basic shopping list may include items such as flour, sugar, eggs, acetaminophen (Tylenol), cough syrup, and ibuprofen (Motrin).

Since the mid-1980s, there has been a sharp increase of OTC drugs available to consumers. Studies have shown that more than 50% of medications purchased are OTC drugs. It is increasingly important for consumers to learn about appropriate dosages and proper use of these medications. Although federal law requires that pharmacists counsel patients receiving new prescriptions, OTC medications do not fall into this category. However, when counseling a patient, the pharmacist should ask what OTC medications he or she is taking and tell the patient what types of OTC drugs to avoid. The ability to buy drugs off the shelf can translate into substantial savings for consumers. This is only one of the many reasons why people want to buy their own medications. During the past two decades, the number of OTC medications available has increased to several hundred. Drug companies know that customers want more drugs available to them. Following are three reasons why consumers use OTC products:

1. Consumers want to save money on OTC medication as opposed to using many expensive prescription drugs. Money is saved because they do not have to make doctors' appointments, which involves the costs of the office visit and missed time at work.
2. Consumers want to be involved in their own treatment; OTC medications give them this capability.
3. OTC medications are more easily obtainable than prescriptions because the many stores that carry OTC medications usually have longer hours than do traditional pharmacies.

These are just three reasons that OTC medications are appealing to consumers. There are some important considerations that should be taken into account when purchasing OTC medications.

Over-the-Counter Drug Considerations

When patients decide to treat themselves, there are important factors that should be taken into account. First, there are a wide variety of drugs from which to choose. Therefore correctly identifying the cause of the problem is the first step. If the self-diagnosis is wrong, the OTC medication may mask the underlying condition from which the person is suffering. For example, if a person suffers from diarrhea and purchases an antidiarrheal medication, the diarrhea may cease for a short time, but the underlying cause could be something more serious that should be diagnosed by a physician. Ultimately, this can cost the person more money, or worse, in the long run. Many hospital stays have been attributed to patients' misuse of drugs, both OTC and prescription. Most people have not been trained to scrutinize OTC medications. This includes checking the drugs at home on a regular basis for expiration dates. Another overlooked aspect of buying OTC drugs is tampering; these drugs are sitting out where anyone can tamper with them. In a past incident, several people were the victims of a person who tampered with Tylenol. Since that time, manufacturers have taken steps to assure consumers thattheir medications are safe by adding tamper-proof wrapping. Consumers should check for any tampering before purchasing. Although there is only a slight risk, it is possible for someone to tamper with the product.

Most OTC medications do not recommend dosages for any child younger than the age of 2 years of age. Thus parents should consult with their pediatrician before giving children any medication purchased OTC, especially any child younger than 2 years. In addition to these considerations, children with colds may develop ear infections and other conditions that warrant seeing a pediatrician for an appropriate prescription medication. Important considerations that consumers should think about before buying and using OTC medications follow:

- Various OTC medications have identical ingredients; however, consumers often purchase a more expensive name brand, not knowing that they are getting the same medication as the less expensive generic form.
- Manufactures may swap "like ingredients" without notifying the consumer. The label will show the change. This is overlooked many times by a consumer because they do not read the labels carefully, if at all.
- No adverse reaction reports are required. They are required for all prescription drugs.
- Caution should be used if the person is on a special diet, has allergies, is a diabetic, or is on other medications that may interact.
- Extra care should be taken when purchasing medication for babies or young children; consumers should know and follow guidelines on the safety of agents based on the child's age. This includes topical agents.

The Three Categories of Over-the-Counter Drugs

Although OTC medications may seem harmless, they can be deadly if taken inappropriately or if the person has a life-threatening allergic reaction. There are additional side effects that one may experience from OTC medications, such as interactions with prescription medications. Before OTC medications are allowed to enter the market, the Food and Drug Administration (FDA) classifies them according to one of the following three categories:

1. Safe and effective for the claimed therapeutic indication
2. Not recognized as safe and effective

3. Additional data must be acquired to determine whether the drug is safe and effective

Food and Drug Administration Regulations

To determine what category future drugs fall into, the FDA regulates five major areas concerning the safety of OTC medications. These five areas are the following:

1. Purity
2. Potency
3. Bioavailability
4. Efficacy
5. Safety and toxicity

PURITY

The purity of a product represents the lack of contamination from environmental factors of the chemical (drug) contained in the product. Few agents are pure, because many medications are prepared on a large scale and dust particles are present in the mix. A certain amount of dust is allowed by government standards. Purity is also affected by other additives, such as those listed in Box 9.1. Various ingredients are also used in the preparation of medications to increase the size of the medication, to decrease absorption, and to make them taste better.

POTENCY

The potency of a medication refers to the strength of the drug. This measurement is done by chemical analysis and is measured in grams, milligrams, or micrograms. If the drug cannot be measured in a laboratory by the same methods, then it is tested on research animals and the strength of the drug is measured in units. Examples of these medications are shown in Box 9.2.

BIOAVAILABILITY

Bioavailability is the percentage of a drug that is both absorbed and transported to the site of action. Because of variances in absorption, the amount of drug that

BOX 9.1 TYPES OF PRODUCT ADDITIVES

Fillers	Enable manufacturers to make tablets or capsules large enough to ingest
Dyes	Used to color tablets and coatings for appearance
Solvents	Mixtures used along with chemical agents as a dissolvent
Buffers	Used to adjust the pH of a medication
Waxes	Used to mold various medications such as suppositories

BOX 9.2 MEDICATIONS MEASURED IN UNITS

Heparin	25,000 units per milliliter
Insulin	100 units per milliliter
Injectable penicillin	100,000 units per milliliter

is able to enter the bloodstream can differ. The total bioavailability is measured by the concentration of the drug in the blood or tissue at a specific time of administration.

EFFICACY

Efficacy is the ability of the drug to produce the desired chemical change in the body. Clinical trials of the drug, which include the use of a placebo, are conducted to judge the effectiveness. Many variances may affect the end results. These variances are due to other influences on a person, such as unknown health conditions, age, weight, lifestyle, gender, and genetic influences.

SAFETY AND TOXICITY

Safety and toxicity represent opposite effects of a drug being studied. After the drug is administered to test subjects, the number of adverse or undesirable effects are recorded. Laboratory animals are often used as test subjects in the beginning stages of trials, and it is sometimes impossible to know what effects might occur in humans. In later years of the studies, published results include effects of drugs on pregnancy and other outside influences that cannot be replicated in a laboratory. All drugs can be toxic if not taken correctly. The difference between dosages that produce toxic effects and those that produce desirable effects is documented. This difference is referred to as the "margin of safety." If a dose of a drug falls into the margin of safety, it is considered a "therapeutic dose." Even so, before a drug is considered safe, the potential for adverse effects must be compared with the benefits.

How a Prescription Becomes an Over-the-Counter Drug

The amount of research that takes place before putting out a new OTC drug is extensive. The FDA must approve all new drugs entering the marketplace and has strict guidelines in place. The same standards of safety and effectiveness that are placed on legend drugs (those requiring a prescription) are also used to approve OTC drugs. The FDA uses three phases of testing as criteria for minimum standards of a new product or of a product that is going to be marketed as an OTC drug, as shown in Box 9.3.

A monograph is information about a drug that includes descriptive information about clinical trials, all side effects of the agent, appropriate dosing based on symptoms/disease state, and all types of reported interactions.

BOX 9.3 THREE FOOD AND DRUG ADMINISTRATION PHASES OF OVER-THE-COUNTER DRUG APPROVAL

Phase 1	Advisors evaluate the agent in question as to whether it is safe and effective when taken by the consumer/patient.
Phase 2	A final review is done on the ingredients of the agent in question. The public is able to give feedback. All data is taken into account such as any new findings.
Phase 3	After sufficient evidence is presented and all aspects of the agent are exhausted, the final monograph is published.

If the agent meets all the criteria, it is approved as an OTC medication. If the agent is already approved as a prescription drug and the manufacturer wants it to be changed to an OTC drug, it does not require further testing. However, the drug does need to be considered safe enough to self-administer before marketed as OTC. Many agents that have gone into the OTC section also continue to be marketed as legend drugs. The difference is the strength of the drug. For instance, ibuprofen is available OTC in 200-mg tablets; however, if 400 mg, 600 mg, or 800 mg are needed, a prescription (Rx) is required. The same is true for many other agents such as ranitidine HCl (Zantac: 75 mg OTC, or 150 mg and 300 mg Rx).

The FDA is also in charge of all recalls. They inspect manufacturing facilities to make sure they are adhering to good manufacturing practices. Manufacturers must show a consistency between batches of drugs on a day-to-day basis. If they cannot, then the product cannot be distributed. There are cases of OTC medications being taken off the market as well.

Conditions Treated with Over-the-Counter Drugs

There are hundreds of OTC medications available and more are being added monthly. Table 9.2 lists some of the most common OTC medications, the symptoms they treat, and the most popular routes of administration. As new medications enter the market as OTC drugs, the routes of administration for consumers to choose from will increase. For example, many analgesics are becoming available as topical patches, and many sore throat remedies are being produced as chewing gum.

TABLE 9.2 Common Types of Over-the-Counter Products*

Type of OTC	Symptom Treated	ROA
Analgesics	Pain	Orally, topically, rectally
Antiinflammatory	Inflammation/arthritis pain	Orally
Antipyretics	Fever	Orally, rectally
Antiarthritics	Joint pain/inflammation	Orally, topically
Antihistamines	Congestion, sneezing	Orally, inhalation
Headache products	Pain	Orally
Sleep aids	Insomnia	Orally
Expectorants	Productive cough	Orally
Cough suppressants	Dry cough	Orally, inhalation
Colds/flu	Inflammatory	Orally, inhalation
Sore throat products	Pain	Orally
Sunscreens	Preventative sun barrier	Topically
Sunburn products	Pain/inflammation	Topically
Antacids	Indigestion	Orally
Antispasmodic	Indigestion	Orally
Antidiarrheals	Diarrhea	Orally, rectally
Laxative	Constipation	Orally, rectally
Antiacne	Pimples	Topically
Antibiotics	Prevent infections	Topically
Antifungals	Dry flaking skin and pain due to fungus	Topically
Cold sore preparations	Painful canker sores	Topically
Wart removal	Skin growth	Topically

OTC, Over-the-counter; *ROA,* route of administration.
*Other topical OTC products are listed later in this chapter under skin care products.

Table 9.2 lists some samples of the types of conditions that people can treat for themselves. Within each category, there are a multitude of medications from which to choose. Because of the magnitude of OTC medications available, it is impossible to cover them all. Therefore only major OTC medications used by consumers are covered.

Over-the-Counter Agents: Patient Information

This section contains a sample of common OTC agents. Included are the symptoms, generic and trade names, and indications. Some agents have added notes that are commonly seen on the product labels, which patients should read before taking the drug. Reference your pharmacy drug handbooks for further information on these and other OTC drugs.

ANALGESICS AND ANTIPYRETICS

Analgesic and antipyretic agents help reduce or relieve pain (analgesic) and fever (antipyretic). Acetylsalicylic acid, usually known by the more common generic name aspirin, has added effectiveness as an antiinflammatory agent. Aspirin also decreases clumping ability of platelets; therefore it is also used as a prophylaxis to decrease the risk of blood clotting in heart disease and stroke. Examples are shown in Table 9.3.

Common Patient Information

Children and teenagers should avoid taking aspirin for chickenpox or flu symptoms without consulting a physician because aspirin has been associated with Reye's syndrome.

TECH NOTE! Reye's syndrome is a rare condition that can affect both children and teenagers who have an active case of chickenpox or influenza (flu). The symptoms include vomiting, lethargy, delirium, and coma. Permanent brain damage can occur and it can be fatal. Although the percentage of fatalities is less than 20%, it is safer to avoid the possibility of such adverse effects.

ANTIINFLAMMATORIES

Agents that treat inflammation are referred to as nonsteroidal antiinflammatory drugs (NSAIDs). They reduce pain by decreasing inflammation of soft tissue muscle strain. NSAIDs are also used as antipyretic and analgesics, as seen in Table 9.4.

Common Patient Information

Do not take this medication if you are allergic to aspirin. May cause drowsiness. May upset stomach, take with food or milk. Do not take if you are in the last trimester of pregnancy.

TABLE 9.3 Analgesics and Antipyretic Products

Condition	Product	Dosage Forms
Fever/pain	Acetaminophen (Tylenol)	Tab, cap, liq supp
Fever/pain	Aspirin (Bayer, Alka-Seltzer)	Tab, cap, powder
Fever/pain	Ibuprofen (Motrin)	Tab, cap, liq
Pain/arthritis	Capsaicin (Zostrix)	Top

Tab, Tablet; *cap,* capsule; *liq,* liquid; *top,* topical; *supp,* suppository.

TABLE 9.4 Antiinflammatory Products

Condition	Product	Dosage Forms
Inflammation/pain	Ibuprofen (Motrin, Advil)	Tab, liq
	Naproxen sodium (Aleve)	Tab, susp
	Ketoprofen (Orudis KT)	Tab, cap

Tab, Tablet; *liq*, liquid; *susp*, suspension; *cap*, capsule.

TABLE 9.5 Decongestant Products

Condition	Product	Dosage Forms
Common cold/allergies	Oxymetazoline (Afrin)	Spray
	Phenylephrine (Neo-Synephrine)	Spray
	Normal saline (Ocean)	Spray
Common cold	Pseudoephedrine* (Sudafed)	Tab, cap, liq
	Clemastine (Tavist)	Tab, liq

Tab, Tablet; *cap*, capsule; *liq*, liquid.
*Pseudoephedrine (Sudafed) is a decongestant and is less likely to cause drowsiness. It is used exclusively as a decongestant, not for allergies.

TABLE 9.6 Antihistamine Products

Condition	Product	Dosage Forms
Congested nose, sinus	Chlorpheniramine (Chlor-Trimeton)	Tab, cap
	Diphenhydramine (Benadryl)	Tab, cap, liq
	Loratadine (Claritin)	Tab, cap

Tab, Tablet; *cap*, capsule; *liq*, liquid.
*These agents also come in many combinations with agents that treat cough, fever, and pain.

TECH NOTE! Agents used to treat arthritis are also used to treat common inflammation and pain. Aspirin still is one of the best OTC treatments for arthritis.

ALLERGY AND COLD AGENTS

For the relief of the common cold there are decongestants (Table 9.5) and antihistamines (Table 9.6) available. These agents dry out mucous membranes and open airways. Persons suffering from severe allergies may require prescription medication. For mild allergies the antihistamines available are normally very effective. Decongestants can be easily absorbed topically through nasal application. Because they cause vasoconstriction, they reduce congestion. Allergies require antihistamine agents.

TECH NOTE! Decongestants can interact with antidepressants. Patients using certain antidepressants and those with heart conditions should not use decongestant agents without the knowledge of their physician.

ANTIHISTAMINES

Antihistamines are used with allergic symptoms. The action is to block histamine (H-1) that causes allergic reactions.

A common side effect of first-generation antihistamines is sleepiness. Many different types of these agents are available OTC. Second-generation agents do not cause drowsiness, but require a prescription.

DECONGESTANTS

Decongestants are indicated for stuffiness and congestion of the nasal passages and sinuses. Decongestants act to open these passages and allow the release of mucous. Decongestants used for chest congestion permit the coughing up of phlegm. Decongestants are available both in prescription and OTC preparations.

Common Patient Information
May cause drowsiness.

TECH NOTE! Diphenhydramine (Benadryl) and chlorpheniramine (CTM) (Chlor-Trimeton) are anti-histamines that cause drowsiness. These agents should not be taken with alcohol because alcohol may intensify the effect. Patients suffering from glaucoma should not use these agents without their physicians' knowledge.

HEADACHE PRODUCTS

Depending on the severity of a headache, there are many OTC medications that can be tried. Those agents listed under analgesics are mostly used for pain. Some agents contain other additives such as caffeine that can help treat more severe headaches (Table 9.7). However, if a person suffers from severe migraines, usually a prescription drug is required.

INTERACTIONS BETWEEN ASPIRIN AND OTHER AGENTS

Aspirin has many interactions that are important to note because they can result in an adverse effect to the patient. Provided in Table 9.8 is a list of common interactions between various types of medications and aspirin. Interactions are not necessarily dangerous, but they can alter the absorption or metabolism of one of the two agents being taken concurrently. Many times patients do not familiarize themselves with these types of interactions, which is why patient consultation is very important and is a federal law. If a patient ever asks for advice from a technician or clerk, he or she must be referred to the pharmacist for advice. It is important that technicians know these interactions so that they can alert the pharmacist if they notice a possible interaction within the patient's prescriptions or medication orders.

TECH NOTE! Activated charcoal can be used to treat an overdose of aspirin. It decreases the absorption of aspirin.

TABLE 9.7 Headache Products

Condition	Product	Dosage Forms
Severe headache/migraine	ASA/caffeine/acetaminophen combination (Excedrin)	Tab Caplet
	ASA/calcium carbonate combination (Bayer Women's Aspirin Plus Calcium)	Caplet
	Acetaminophen/caffeine combination (Excedrin Tension Headach [aspirin free])	

ASA, Acetylsalicylic acid (aspirin); *tab,* tablet.

TABLE 9.8 Common Interactions between Aspirin and Other Medications

Drug	Common Use of Drugs	Results of Drug and ASA
ACE inhibitors	Treat high blood pressure	Effects may be decreased.
Alcohol	Lifestyle choice	May increase bleeding and risk of GI ulcer.
Antacids	Upset stomach	Decreases effectiveness of aspirin.
Anticoagulants	To reduce the possibility of blood clots	May prolong or increase bleeding.
β-blockers	To treat hypertension	Effects may be decreased.
CAIs (Diuretics)	To decrease edema (fluid buildup)	Toxication of aspirin may occur.
Corticosteroids	Antiinflammatory	Decreases effectiveness of aspirin.
Loop diuretics	To reduce fluid retention	Effects may be decreased.
Methotrexate	To treat certain skin conditions/cancer	Effects may be increased and excretion decreased.
NTG	To decrease angina (chest pain)	May result in hypotension.
NSAIDs	To treat inflammation, pain, fever	Effects may be decreased.
Spironolactone	To reduce edema	Effects may be decreased.
Sulfonylureas/insulin	To lower glucose (diabetes)	May increase the effects of these agents.
Valproic acid	To treat seizures	May decrease excretion, increasing potency of valproic acid.

ACE, Angiotensin-converting enzyme; *GI*, gastrointestinal; *CAI*, carbonic anhydrase inhibitor; *NTG*, nitroglycerin; *NSAID*, nonsteroidal antiinflammatory drug.

TABLE 9.9 Anti-Insomnia Products

Product	Dosage Forms
Diphenhydramine HCl (Benadryl)	Tab, caplet, liq
Diphenhydramine citrate/APAP (Excedrin PM)	Tab, caplet
Doxylamine succinate (Unisom Nighttime Sleep Aid)	Tab

Tab, Tablet; *liq*, liquid; *APAP*, acetaminophen.

SLEEP AID

Many people suffer from insomnia. Almost all OTC medications used to treat insomnia are a form of diphenhydramine or magnesium salicylate (Table 9.9). These agents can be used for transient insomnia, which is considered a short-term sleeping problem (nonchronic). Diphenhydramine is the most commonly prescribed agent ordered in hospitals to help patients sleep.

Common Patient Information

May cause drowsiness. Avoid alcoholic beverages while taking this medication. Do not take this product without consulting a physician if you are taking sedatives or tranquilizers. Do not use if you have asthma, glaucoma, emphysema, or an enlarged prostate. For chronic insomnia, a physician should be consulted.

COUGH

The cold and flu section is one of the largest; many manufactures offer the same type of ingredients in different proportions (Table 9.10). For congested coughs, expectorants should be used to cough up phlegm. For dry nonphlegm-producing coughs, a cough suppressant is best.

Common Patient Information

Do not take this product without consulting a physician if you are taking sedatives or tranquilizers. Do not use if you have asthma, glaucoma, emphysema, heart problems, or an enlarged prostate.

SORE THROAT PRODUCTS

Sore, scratchy, and dry throats usually arise from a cold or flu. They can be treated with many different agents available as OTC medications (Table 9.11). If a sore throat continues without relief, a physician should be seen to rule out an infection. A sore throat can be a symptom of a streptococcal bacterial infection, also known as strep throat. Strep throat should be treated with antibiotics. However, while the patient is on antibiotics he or she may also relieve throat pain with various syrups and sprays. The various agents used in these agents include menthol, alcohol, and benzocaine.

STOMACH REMEDIES/ANTACIDS

Several classes of medications are used to treat the common upset stomach (Table 9.12). Histamine-2 (H_2) antagonists are used to decrease acid secretion, which helps to decrease what is commonly known as heartburn. Proton pump inhibitors work differently than H_2 antagonists to relieve acid secretions. Although both work directly on the lining of the stomach, they each target different receptors. Antacid agents are used to balance the pH level in the stomach, which ultimately helps decrease heartburn. Each medication is effective in its own way.

Common Patient Information

For short-term relief of heartburn. If problems persist see your physician. May be taken without regard to meals.

TABLE 9.10 Cold and Cough Products

Condition	Product	Dosage Forms
Congested cough	Guaifenesin/pseudoephedrine (Robitussin PE)	Tab, liq, syr
	Guaifenesin (Robitussin)	Tab, cap, syr
Dry cough	Guaifenesin/dextromethorphan (Robitussin DM)	Liq, syr

Tab, Tablet; *liq*, liquid; *syr*, syrup; *cap*, capsule.

TABLE 9.11 Sore Throat Products

Condition	Product	Dosage Forms
Sore throat	Benzocaine (Chloraseptic)	Lozenges
	Dyclonine HCl (Cepacol)	Lozenges
	Dyclonine/alcohol (Sucrets)	Lozenges

TABLE 9.12 Stomach Products/Antacids

Condition	Product	Dosage Forms
Heartburn	Cimetidine (Tagamet-HB)	Tab, liq
	Ranitidine (Zantac-75)	Tab
	Famotidine (Pepcid-AC)	Tab
	Nizatidine (Axid-AR)	Tab
Antacids	Calcium hydroxate (Tums)	Chewable tab
	Aluminum hydroxide/magnesium hydroxide/simethicone (Mylanta)	Tab, liq, gelcap

Tab, Tablet; *liq*, liquid.

TECH NOTE! Chronic pain in the stomach may be an ulcer caused by *Helicobacter pylori* (a bacteria) that causes the symptoms of heartburn. If the problem persists for more than 2 weeks, it is better to seek advice for a possible underlying problem.

INTESTINAL REMEDIES

Remedies for intestinal discomfort and pain resulting from constipation, diarrhea, or gas (flatulence) are listed in Table 9.13. Agents to stimulate the intestinal tract vary, but most contain either an oil or saline solution that irritates the lining of the bowels and encourages the reflex action required to move the bowels. For diarrhea, an anticholinergic agent (one that dries out membranes) or a fiber such as psyllium powder works to either dry out or absorb the excess water, creating bulk in the intestinal track. Loperamide works well for immediate results. Psyllium (Metamucil) is a good natural choice that many doctors recommend. For the treatment of gas, simethicone is the most commonly used agent, although there are other products available such as α-d-galactosidase (Beano) or simethecone (Gas-X). These agents neutralize the production of gas, which is created as a byproduct from bacteria that reside in the intestines.

Common Patient Information

Laxatives: Do not use in the presence of abdominal pain, nausea, or vomiting. Do not use longer than one week. Loperamide: May cause drowsiness or dizziness. May cause dry mouth.

TECH NOTE! Gas can be very painful and embarrassing but is not life threatening, whereas both diarrhea and constipation can have severe outcomes if they are not controlled. Babies can die of dehydration because of excess loss of electrolytes through watery stools. In extreme cases, constipation can cause a bowel rupture, which requires surgery to repair. Psyllium is the only agent that can be used for both constipation and diarrhea because it works as a bulk-forming agent. It is also a natural agent and has been noted to reduce cholesterol.

Skin Anatomy

The skin, also known as the integumentary system, is the largest organ of the body. It includes the skin, hair, and all tissues below the surface of the skin down to the muscle. Skin is one of the most abused organs of the body system. It holds up through weather, detergents, scratches, cuts, and bruises, and it repairs itself time and time again. Like other organs, it must be nourished, oxygenated, and taken care of. In return, it functions to protect the body, regulate temperature, and act as a sensor to stimuli.

On top of the skin are layers of keratin, which help protect the layers below. The two layers beneath the keratin are the epidermis and the dermis. Below the dermis lies the subcutaneous layers of fat that insulate the body, keeping it warm.

TABLE 9.13 Intestinal Products

Condition	Product	Dosage Forms
Constipation	Combination stimulant (Ex-Lax)	Tab, chew tab
Stool softeners	Docsuate sodium (Colace)	gelcap
Diarrhea	Loperamide (Imodium A–D)	Tab, cap, liq
Flatulence	Simethicone (Mylicon)	Tab, chew tab, liq
Irregular bowels	Psyllium (Metamucil)	Powder

Tab, Tablet; *cap*, caplet; *liq*, liquid.

Skin also protects the body from bumps and falls and is a food reserve in case of emergency. The epidermis does not have blood flow of its own; instead it receives nutrition from the tissues surrounding it. The dermis is much thicker than the epidermis and acts as a support system for the outer layer and holds the nerves, blood vessels, and other connective tissue (Figure 9.1). Also, the skin has the ability to absorb moisture and medications. Diabetics inject insulin subcutaneously (SC) under the skin, which means the needle penetrates through the subcutaneous layer. Another route of administration is the intradermal (ID) route, in which the needle penetrates between the dermis layer. An intramuscular (IM) dose requires penetrating through the subcutaneous layer and into the muscle layer.

Conditions Affecting the Skin

There are many different types of agents that can be used to treat skin conditions. The cause of the problem and what the physician wants the agent to do determines what the physician prescribes. Table 9.14 lists common dosage forms and the type of conditions that they can treat.

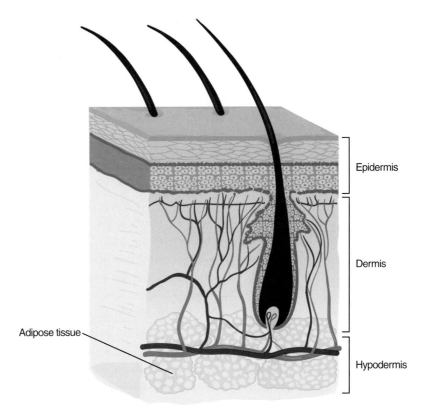

FIGURE 9.1 Anatomy of the skin. The three major layers of the skin.

TABLE 9.14 Over-the-Counter Skin Products

Dosage Forms	Indications
Creams*	Dry, scaling, pruritic areas, thickened areas
Ointment*	Dry, scaling, pruritic areas, thickened areas
Lotions/gels	Hairy areas, lesions that ooze, wet areas
Sprays*	Acute weeping lesions

*Creams, lotions, and gels are absorbed through the skin; ointments and sprays remain on top of the skin to prevent moisture from evaporating.

Skin Disorders and Medications

When unknown skin problems arise, a proper diagnosis may include a physical assessment, family history, drug history (including OTC medications used), laboratory tests, and possibly a biopsy. Sunburn and acne are two very common skin conditions that are often treated at home.

SUNSCREEN SKIN PROTECTANT FACTOR GUIDE

Skin protectant factor (SPF) agents come in topical form and prevent sunburn. Ultraviolet alpha (UVA) rays and ultraviolet beta (UVB) rays are the two main wavelengths of solar rays that are of concern. Both affect the healthiness of the skin. These alpha and beta rays given off by the sun penetrate the earth's atmosphere and the skin layers. UVA rays can enter into the dermis layer. Although UVA rays do not cause the skin to redden, these rays cause premature aging of the skin and possible changes in the cells deoxyribonucleic acid (DNA) where it is absorbed. If the skin is left unprotected, the UVB rays cause erythema and even blistering of the skin. This is what is normally seen as sunburn.

Constant overexposure to the sun over time raises the likelihood of mutations within the structure of the DNA from both UVA and UVB rays. When this happens, cancer can occur as well as discoloration of the prematurely aged skin. The chemical responsible for skin color is called melanin, which is present in different amounts over the body surface. The lighter the skin tone, the more protection needed. This is because the sun's rays affect lightly pigmented skin cells more readily. To protect oneself from both of these harmful ultraviolet rays, the proper amount of SPF must be worn. There are two types of protectants: sunscreens and sun blocks. Sunscreens protect the skin from UVA and UVB rays by allowing the skin protectant to absorb the ultraviolet rays, rendering them harmless. Sun blocks work by reflecting the ultraviolet rays. Ultimately, the best protection one can provide the skin is a sunblock/sunscreen combination. To judge how much protection is needed, divide the amount of time it takes you to burn. If you wear a sunscreen with an SPF of 20, then it will take you 20 times longer to burn. For example, say it takes you only 10 minutes to burn in the sun. If you apply a sun block of SPF 20, multiply that by the time you take to burn (10 minutes) and your coverage would last about 200 minutes, or about 3.2 hours. It is necessary to reapply based on the type of activity in which you are participating. For swimmers, there are water-resistant and waterproof agents that increase longevity of the product from 40 to 80 minutes, respectively, before it must be applied again.

Sunscreen

The sun's ultraviolet rays are always present, even on cloudy days. To protect oneself, it is important to know how the sun affects the skin. Following the previous guide, it is possible to choose the best coverage for specific skin types, as shown in Box 9.4. See Table 9.15 for sunscreen indications.

BOX 9.4 SUNSCREEN PRODUCTS

Action	Block or absorb UVA and UVB sun rays
Products	Hawaiian Tropic
	Bullfrog
	Sundown
Indications	See Table 9.15

TABLE 9.15 Skin Protectant Factor Guide for Application of Sunscreen

Skin Type	Skin Characteristics After 10 Min Sun Exposure	Suggested Minimum Coverage
I	Burns easily/rarely tans	20 to 30 SPF
II	Burns easily/tans minimally	12 to 20 SPF
III	Burns moderately/tans gradually	8 to 12 SPF
IV	Burns minimally/tans well	4 to 8 SPF
V	Rarely burns/always tans	2 to 4 SPF
VI	Never burns/deeply pigmented	None

SPF, Skin protectant factor.

ACNE DEVELOPMENT AND TREATMENT

Acne affects not only teenagers but adults as well. In most cases acne is caused by hormonal changes, which is why it is so prevalent in teenagers. However, genetics can influence acne too. The old belief that eating too much candy or greasy foods such as fries causes acne is incorrect. These foods do not cause acne, although it can worsen existing acne.

The skin has glands that have different functions. Hormones have an ability to enlarge the glands of the skin. Two of the most productive glands are the sweat glands and sebaceous glands. Sweat glands are regulators of temperature. As people sweat, the water evaporates and cools the body. The sebaceous glands are responsible for the production of skin oil called sebum. The oily layer it produces protects and lubricates the skin. When sebum production increases and traps bacteria at the base of the hair follicle, the likelihood of acne increases (Figure 9.2). The only treatment for acne is to keep the skin clean and free

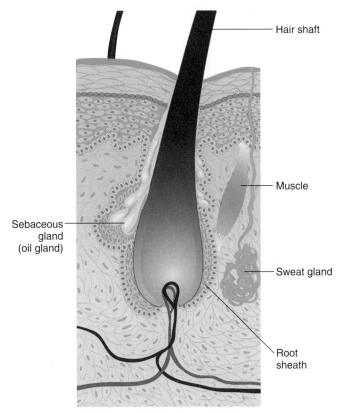

FIGURE 9.2 Diagram of sebum skin pore. Location of hair follicles and surrounding region.

from bacteria, decrease the sebum production, and finally remove dead skin (Table 9.16).

Acne can be classified into the following two groups:

1. Noninflammatory
2. Inflammatory

Acne has various forms, and each is treated differently. An assessment should be made to determine what type of agent should be used to treat the sores. In treating noninflammatory acne, a mild medication can be used, such as keratolytics. These agents dry oily skin, remove dead skin, and fight bacteria. Examples include salicylic acid and benzoyl peroxide.

Painful, swollen pustules are usually present on the face in inflammatory acne. Benzoyl peroxide is the most common OTC product recommended to help dry out the sores, called pimples. More severe inflammatory acne may require the use of antibiotics in addition to keratolytics. More powerful topical agents may be required. Antibiotics include tetracycline, erythromycin, and clindamycin (also in topical form). Topical agents include retinoic acid medications such as isotretinoin (Accutane) and tretinoin (Retin A). These agents increase the growth of skin around the acne areas, which allows the infected cells to fall away as new cells replace them. With this type of treatment, the acne may seem to worsen initially but usually improves over several weeks.

MISCELLANEOUS SKIN CONDITIONS

Most skin conditions can be divided into the following two categories:

1. Noninfectious inflammatory conditions
2. Infectious inflammatory conditions

There are many products available that work well in treating mild skin conditions, although if the symptoms continue, it is recommended that the patient visit a physician. Infectious inflammatory conditions are much more serious because they can be transferred from person to person; therefore a physician should be seen immediately for the proper treatment. If a patient is unsure of what the skin condition is, it is best to visit a physician for the proper diagnosis (Box 9.5).

TABLE 9.16 Acne Treatments

Product	Trade Name	Dosage Forms
Benzoyl peroxide	Clearasil Max Strength	Cream
	Oxy 10 Cover	Cream
	Oxy 5	Lotion
	Dry and Clear	Lotion

BOX 9.5 Common Noninfectious Conditions and Their Definitions

Condition	Defined
Urticaria (hives)	Usually caused by an allergic reaction
Eczema (red skin rash)	Allergic reaction
Psoriasis (plaques, scaly skin)	Genetic in nature
Seborrheic dermatitis (rash)	Possible allergic reaction affecting the scalp area; color usually ranges from red to brown
Atopic dermatitis (rash)	Associated with allergic reaction, may be genetic

HIVES/INFLAMMATION

Topical agents can be used for hives and other skin rashes that cause inflammation of the skin resulting from severe itching (Table 9.17). For conditions such as psoriasis, a doctor should be consulted. Prescription agents must be used and are discussed later in this chapter.

INFECTIOUS INFLAMMATORY SKIN CONDITIONS

Warts

Skin irritation can arise from viral warts. Warts are contagious, although most disappear on their own within 6 months. Corns need to be cut off or topical agents used to soften and remove the dead skin (Table 9.18). If a person is infected with genital warts, a physician should be seen for appropriate treatment.

Athlete's Foot

Athlete's foot causes dry, cracked skin; pain; and irritation. Athlete's foot is caused by fungus. It can be spread by contact from shower floor surfaces and sharing socks. Antifungals that kill the fungus are used to treat athlete's foot; they are usually in powder or spray form (Table 9.19). Keeping the feet dry and in comfortable shoes helps prevent athlete's foot. Other fungal infections treated with antifungals are jock itch and ringworm.

Canker Sores

Canker sores, located in the soft tissue of the mouth, usually inside the cheek, are small topical ulcers. They tend to disappear within 2 weeks but can be very painful (Table 9.20).

TABLE 9.17 Antiinflammatory Products

Product	Trade Names	Dosage Forms
Calamine/diphenhydramine	Caladryl	Lotion, cream
Hydrocortisone		Cream, ointment

TABLE 9.18 Products to Treat Warts

Product	Trade Names	Dosage Forms
Salicylic acid	Wart Off	Liquid
	Compound W	Liquid

TABLE 9.19 Products to Treat Athlete's Foot

Product	Trade Names	Dosage Forms
Tolnaftate	Tinactin, Aftate	Cream, soln, spray, oint, powder
Undecylenic acid	Desenex	Oint, cream, powder, spray powder
Clotrimazole	Lotrimin	Soln, lotion, cream

Soln, Solution; *oint,* ointment.

TABLE 9.20 Canker Sore Products

Product	Trade Names	Dosage Forms
Phenol, camphor, and miscellaneous additives	Campho-Phenique	Gel

TABLE 9.21 Antibiotic Products

Product	Trade Names	Dosage Forms
Bacitracin	Bacitracin	Oint
Neomycin	Neomycin	Oint
	Myciguent	Cream
Polymyxin B, neomycin, bacitracin	Neosporin	Oint, cream

Oint, Ointment.

TABLE 9.22 Agents Used to Treat Psoriasis

Product	Trade Name	Dosage	Potency
Dexamethasone (Rx)	Decaderm	Cream, ointment	Low
Betamethasone benzoate/valerate (Rx)	Uticort/Valisone	Cream, ointment	Medium
Fluocinonide (Rx)	Lidex	Cream, ointment	High
Betamethasone (Rx)	Diprosone, Topicort	Cream, ointment	High
Bethamethasone dipropionate (Rx)	Diprolene	Cream, ointment	High

Rx, Prescription.

TOPICAL ANTIBIOTICS

Abrasions, small cuts, and scrapes are easily treated with topical antibiotics available in OTC products. The wound should be cleaned properly and then treated with one of the agents listed in Table 9.21.

PSORIASIS

Psoriasis is a genetic skin condition that cannot be cured and may last a lifetime. The onset of this painful disorder is usually during the teen years, but can occur later in life. This condition is not contagious, although the lesions appear inflamed. Most affected areas are around the joints, limbs, neck, and even scalp. More potent drugs are used on psoriasis such as corticosteroids (Table 9.22). These relieve inflammation and pruritic dermatosis and act as a vasoconstrictor. Agents used to treat psoriasis require a physician's prescription.

In addition to these medications, sometimes the patient is given sunlight treatments to cause sunburn of the skin and subsequent peeling. The mechanism of action of potent corticosteroids is the suppression of T cells and other constituents that cause inflammation and an increase in cell growth. Thus these agents must be used very carefully because they impede the immune system.

DO YOU REMEMBER THESE KEY POINTS?

- The responsibility of the patient to know what type of OTC product that he or she is taking
- The problems associated with more drugs becoming OTC
- Guidelines regulated by the FDA for a legend drug to become an OTC product
- Guidelines regulated by the FDA for the manufacturing practices of OTC products
- Terms and definitions associated with OTC products
- Why consumers desire to diagnose and treat themselves
- The difference between generic and trade drugs

- The three categories of OTC products
- Main interactions between aspirin products and other medications
- The importance of skin protection against UVA and UVB rays
- The most common treatments for conditions covered in this chapter

REVIEW QUESTIONS:

Multiple Choice

1. All of the medications listed are H_2 antagonists except
   A. Cimetidine (Tagamet)
   B. Famotidine (Pepcid)
   C. Loperamide (Immodium)
   D. Ranitidine HCl (Zantac)

2. Which of the areas listed are not regulated by the FDA?
   A. Purity
   B. Bioavailability
   C. Color and texture
   D. Potency

3. Children under the age of _____ do not have recommended dosages listed on OTC products.
   A. 1 year
   B. 2 years
   C. 5 years
   D. 8 years

4. Which of the following is not one of the FDA's three categories used to rate drugs that manufacturers want to enter the marketplace?
   A. Not safe and effective
   B. Safe and effective
   C. Cost
   D. Needs more research

5. Fillers are used to
   A. Make the drug taste better
   B. Change the pH
   C. Change the shape
   D. Make the tablet larger

6. The best definition for the word efficacy is
   A. The ethical use of drugs
   B. The ability of a drug to produce the desired chemical change in a person
   C. The laboratory testing phase of a drug to determine its effectiveness
   D. The results seen in a person's illness

7. Two major OTC agents for use as nasal decongestants are
   A. Oxymetazoline and acetaminophen
   B. Oxymetazoline and phenylephrine
   C. Phenylephrine and dyclonine
   D. Dyclonine and pseudoephedrine

8. The skin has many functions. Which one of the following is not one of its main functions?
   A. Regulates temperature of the body
   B. Acts as a sensor to stimulus
   C. Protects the internal organs from the elements
   D. All of above are main functions

9. Which of the following drugs cannot be used as an antiinflammatory?
   A. Aspirin
   B. Ibuprofen (Advil)
   C. Acetaminophen (Tylenol)
   D. Naproxen sodium (Anaprox)

10. The OTC product most commonly used for insomnia is
    A. Aspirin
    B. Ibuprofen
    C. Diphenhydramine
    D. Chlorpheniramine

11. The terms UVA and UVB relate to the
    A. Amount of sun that a person can withstand
    B. Ultraviolet rays of the sun
    C. Wavelength of rays emitted from the sun
    D. Both B and C

12. If you burn easily and rarely tan when out in the sun and you decide to use an SPF of 10, how long can you be out in the sun before you would need to reapply the lotion?
    A. 10 minutes
    B. 100 minutes
    C. 1 hour
    D. 10 hours

True/False

*If a statement is false, then change it to make it true.

1. Drug manufacturers can swap or replace "like ingredients" without notifying the public.
2. Betamethasone (Diprolene) is a high-level corticosteroid that can be used for skin conditions such as psoriasis.
3. The skin is the largest organ of the body.
4. UVA rays cause what is known as sunburn of the skin, whereas UVB rays cause deep changes in the skin that result in premature aging.
5. Athlete's foot is caused by a bacteria.
6. Acne is caused by hormone levels, not eating habits.
7. The epidermis contains the blood vessels and nerves that nourish the skin.
8. Waterproof sun lotion increases the longevity of effectiveness by 40 minutes.
9. Psoriasis is an infectious, inflammatory condition of the skin.
10. The most used OTC agent for acne is tetracycline.

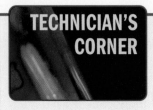

TECHNICIAN'S CORNER

1. A patient comes into the pharmacy asking for a drug that is sold OTC and can only remember the name of the ingredient benzoyl.
   How do you answer this question?
   Where is this product found?
2. A patient comes in with a toddler and asks what type of stool softener to use for her baby because she has not had any bowel movements and is very cranky.
   How do you answer this question?
   What will you tell the patient?
3. A patient comes up to the counter with two bottles of cough syrup, guaifenesin/pseudoephedrine (Robitussin PE), and guaifenesin/dextromethorphan (Robitussin DM) in hand. She wants to know the difference between them.
   How do you answer this question?
   At what point would you call in the pharmacist?

BIBLIOGRAPHY

Drug facts and comparisons, ed 53, St Louis, 1999, Wolters Kluwer.
McCuistion L, Gutierrez K: *Real world nursing survival guide: pharmacology,* Philadelphia, 2002, WB Saunders.

10

Complementary Alternative Medicine

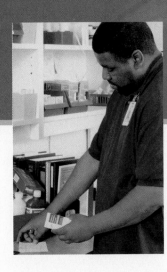

Objectives

■ Define the term *alternative medicine*.

■ Differentiate between Eastern and Western medicine.

■ Describe why alternative medicine has become popular.

■ Explain what is meant by the *placebo effect*.

■ Describe the following treatments and the belief systems of each:
Ancient Chinese medicine
Acupressure/acupuncture
Aromatherapy
Art therapy
Ayurveda
Biofeedback
Chiropractic manipulation
Crystal/gemstone therapy
Herbal remedies
Homeopathy
Spiritual healing

■ Identify common herbal preparations and their common uses.

AGENTS COVERED IN THIS CHAPTER

Common name	Species
Aloe vera	*Aloe vera* Liliaceae
Black cohosh	*Cimicifuga racemosa*
Chamomile	*Matricaria recutita*
Feverfew	*Tanacetum parthenium*
Garlic	*Allium sativum*
Ginger	*Zingiber officinale*
Gingko	*Gingkgo biloba*
Ginseng	*Panax quinquefolius*
Goldenseal	*Hydrastis canadensis*
Hawthorn	*Crataegus laevigata*
Purple coneflower	*Echinacea purpurea*
Milk thistle	*Silybum marianum*
St. John's wort	*Hypericum perforatum*
Valerian	*Valeriana officinalis*

TERMS AND DEFINITIONS

Antiemetic *Agent that stops nausea and vomiting*

Antihypertensive *Agent that decreases blood pressure*

Ayurveda *A holistic medical system originating in India*

Chiropractic *Manual manipulation of the joints and muscles*

Diagnosis *A doctor's assessment of the cause of a condition*

Fat soluble *Drugs that are absorbed into the body's fat layer*

Herbs *Any herbaceous plant consisting of fleshy stems*

Homeopathy *A system of therapy based on the belief that medicinal substances that cause a specific symptom can be used to treat an illness that yields the same symptoms.*

Legend drug *Medication that requires a prescription*

OTC *Over-the-counter medication*

Placebo *Inert compound thought to be an active agent*

Synthetic *Medication made in a laboratory*

Tincture *Plant extract mixed with alcohol*

Introduction

This chapter covers the current views on complementary alternative medicine in the United States, including the origins of various nontraditional therapies from Eastern and Western cultures. This chapter also explores the reasons why nontraditional therapies have become popular and how they are being integrated into traditional medicine. Descriptions of more extreme alternative treatments are presented, ranging from crystal therapy to spiritual healing. In addition, the placebo effect is discussed. An in-depth review of herbal remedies is presented using examples of top selling herbs such as gingko, feverfew, and ginseng. Common uses and known interactions of these herbs are covered. Finally, the type of information that the technician should know about herbal remedies and vitamin supplements when helping customers in the pharmacy is discussed.

What is Alternative Medicine?

To find out the meaning and scope of alternative medicine, one must first define traditional medicine. Traditional medical treatment includes medication prescribed by physicians, consisting of common agents or treatments for medical conditions. This includes doctor visits, possibly followed by radiographic examinations, laboratory tests, or other tests to enable the physician to make a correct diagnosis. Traditional medicine includes the use of legend (prescription) and over-the-counter (OTC) medications. Follow-up visits ensure the success of the treatment, and regular visits monitor the patient's condition.

The alternative approach might consist of visits to a chiropractor, homeopathic doctor, or other practitioner, followed by treatments used within those specific areas of study. These treatments might include herbs, acupuncture, acupressure, or yoga. Many alternative approaches have been in existence for thousands of years, whereas traditional medicine has existed for only a few hundred years. Nevertheless, traditional medicine is the standard for the Western world today.

Alternative medicine has been viewed as ineffective, ancient, and more closely related to superstition than "real" medicine. Many alternative treatments were thought of as extreme measures taken only by those who have lost all hope of recovery using traditional methods. The more controversial types of nontraditional medicine and therapies became labeled "alternative medicine" and were grouped with ancient remedies such as Ayurveda and Chinese medicine. These controversial therapies included treatments such as hydrotherapy and crystal, spiritual, and magnetic healing. However, alternative medicine is now making a comeback. Why? This chapter answers this question and explains the considerations that must be given to both traditional medicine and complementary alternative medicine. Ten popular alternative treatments are also discussed.

Overview of Eastern versus Western Medicine

Eastern medicine includes treatments originating from Eastern Asia, parts of Arabia, India, Japan, and other Far East countries. Over the centuries, advancements made from each of these cultures has helped lay the foundation for Western medicine. As medicinal knowledge was gathered over the ages, it was transcribed and translated into other languages and was subjected to further experimentation. European scientists added their own herbal remedies to the growing list of herbal treatments made from varieties of plants indigenous to their terrain.

With the invention of the first microscope in the 1600s, scientists had new pathways to explore. This was the beginning of the Golden Age of Microbiology. Scientists were able to peer through crude lenses to view tiny microbes. Illnesses that were once thought of as caused by evil spirits were now identified and treated. As science advanced through the age of antimicrobial therapy, it was possible to produce chemical agents that could produce a predetermined specific action within the body. This "magic bullet" is another important aspect of Western medicine. Western medicine has been influenced by thousands of years of experimentation gathered from many different cultures.

Western medicine has omitted all cultural superstition and has relied on scientific methods to prove effective treatments. Some of the most powerful drugs have come from ancient herbal remedies or are derived from the plants used in those remedies. For example, digoxin, one of the most prescribed heart drugs in the geriatric community, has its origins in the 1700s. It is made from the plant foxglove, and cannot be manufactured synthetically. Digoxin helps the heart beat in slow yet strong beats and is used to treat many people who have congestive heart failure. Homeopathy was first practiced in the late 1700s when diseases were treated with herbals that caused symptoms of illness when given to healthy people. Homeopathy is based on "like treating like" in disease vs. medication. Plant derivatives that are used in Western medicine include quinine for malaria, psyllium for high cholesterol and bowel regularity, and reserpine for high blood pressure.

Trends Toward Alternatives

For thousands of years, practitioners of Eastern philosophy took the whole person into consideration in making a proper diagnosis and plan of treatment. This holistic approach included the person's diet, dreams, and even smell. According to the World Health Organization (WHO), it is now estimated that alternative medicine is used by more than 70% of the world's population. Most of the countries that use alternative medicines are developing countries. These cultures use herbs as their main form of treatment because they cannot afford or obtain traditional medicine. Also, they believe in their herbal remedies.

Starting in the 1980s Eastern medicine, specifically herbal remedies, became popular in the Western world. Because herbs are not considered a form of traditional medication treatment, they became grouped with all types of nontraditional remedies that were considered ineffective, including crystals and aroma-, hydro- and sound therapy. However, during the past two decades, many of these nontraditional methods of treatment have become commonplace in the Western world. Consumers spend millions of dollars annually on alternative treatments. Until recently, most traditional practitioners have discounted all types of nontraditional or alternative medicine. However, if there were no truth to any of these alternative medicines, then why is interest still growing within the American people?

Although Western medicine can be given credit for extending life well beyond the once-average age of 45 years, the overall wellness of the whole person has been left somewhere in the dust of the speeding "magic bullet." Because of current lifestyles, stresses, and emerging diseases, people are becoming aware that traditional medicine has its limitations. As one ages, one's body experiences more age-related problems, such as diabetes, dementia, and strokes. As new medicines are produced by drug manufacturers, the risk of side effects and the rising cost of drugs can lead a person to try alternative medicine. Also, many manufacturers of herbal remedies and other therapies claim they can increase the lifespan in good health. This claim is sometimes enough for consumers to give these therapies a try. Another reason alternatives to traditional medicine are becoming more popular is that many times they claim to treat extreme illnesses. A person diagnosed with a cancer for which there is no current medication or therapy available may seek alternatives for treatment.

Using Traditional and Alternative Medicine

In the 1990s alternative therapies were a topic of discussion within the traditional medical community. As medical practitioners researched the types of treatments used by their patients, it was necessary to put together a list of all types of known alternative treatments. The National Center for Complementary and Alternative Medicine (NCCAM) was formed in the early 1990s to deal with these issues. The three main goals of the NCCAM are to do research on alternative treatments, train individuals who are interested in learning techniques, and provide the consumer with information on the various types of therapies available. NCCAM has identified and classified various therapies and continues to receive funding from the U.S. government for more research. More than half of the medical schools in the United States are currently offering classes on alternative medicine. Areas of study include supplement therapy, such as vitamins and minerals; herbal medicine; spirituality; acupuncture; and homeopathy.

The term *complementary* is used concurrently with *alternative* because nontraditional therapies have found a place alongside traditional medicine. Therefore the term *complementary alternative medicine* is an accurate description of how these two forms of treatment are being used together. More doctors, nurse practitioners, and other healthcare providers are suggesting herbal treatments and nondrug alternatives in place of, or concurrent with, traditional treatments. Nondrug alternatives may include remedies such as biofeedback, massage, and meditation. Self-hypnosis has been clinically found to reduce surgical pain in patients. Acupuncture has been used in hospitals to treat adolescent patients. Some types of complementary therapies are listed in Table 10.1.

The Placebo Effect

One must consider the effectiveness of placebo drugs when discussing nontraditional medication. A placebo is an inert drug, meaning it contains no active ingredients. Therefore its ability to help a patient recover from illness or to decrease pain is based on the power of the patient's belief that the medication worked. Many people believe so strongly in certain remedies or therapies that it is hard to determine whether the therapy or the belief of the patient is the likely cure. Through extensive double-blind tests, more information is becoming available as to whether various treatments and herbals are truly effective. Double-blind tests are conducted in which both the patient and the treating physician are not told whether the patient is receiving the investigational drug or a placebo (inert drug). In this way the patient's bias cannot influence the findings and should give a clearer picture as to whether the drug is working or if positive results are due to the placebo effect.

Acupuncture

Acupuncture has been used for thousands of years with extensive studies in both the Eastern and Western world. It is used for conditions such as chronic pain, depression, addiction, and other ailments. It is based on the Chinese belief that the body is made of energy channels. When these channels become blocked, sickness may result. The use of needles at specific points throughout the body are thought to release these channels, bringing the body into harmony once again.

Acupressure

Acupressure is closely related to acupuncture because it also uses specific energy points across the body. Instead of using needles, pressure is applied by hand to the specific point to unblock the channels. Insurance companies are beginning to pay for acupuncture and acupressure treatment if recommended by a physician for the treatment of pain. Classes are available on acupressure so that one can perform the technique on oneself.

Ancient Chinese Medicine

For more than 4000 years, Chinese medicine has been a well-known art based on years of trial and error. Although herbal remedies might readily come to mind

TABLE 10.1 Twelve Alternative Treatments

Type of Treatment	Description of Alternative Treatment
Acupuncture	Acupuncture is based on the meridians in the body. These lines are believed to carry energy to specific parts of the body. When they become blocked, illness or pain can occur. The practitioner relieves blocked pathways with the use of needles.
Acupressure	Acupressure is based on the same principles as acupuncture. Instead of using needles to unblock the pathways carrying energy, the practitioner uses his or her hands to apply pressure to specific points on the body.
Aromatherapy	Using the nasal senses, various blends of fragrances bring about relief of certain ailments. Both herbs and perfumes are used. Mostly oils are used because they are considered more healing than the whole plant or portions of plants.
Art therapy	Art therapy is based on psychoanalysis and how the mind can manifest specific images. These images then can be expressed in drawings or paintings, hopefully stimulating enlightenment. Then the patient can work on the problem through feedback.
Ayurveda	Ayurveda is based on the spiritual side of the body and all that affects the body, including the environment, emotional stability, and physical health. Practitioners find ways to change what is necessary to enable the patient to be more in tune with the world. This includes various postures, meditation, and massage. Changing habits is a large part of this treatment.
Biofeedback	Biofeedback is a learned technique that enables self-control of various physiological responses of the body. This includes both voluntary systems and involuntary systems of the body. A practitioner teaches it only until the patient is proficient in using the technique.
Chinese	Chinese medicine is based on the body spirits of the yin (meaning man) and yang (meaning woman) that are acknowledged as having similar elements yet are different in order. Therefore each is treated differently. Diagnosis is based on the person's dreams, tastes, sensations, smell, and other senses. Various types of treatments are used, including herbal remedies and acupuncture.
Chiropractic	Chiropractic treatment is based on the belief that the realignment of the body, specifically the spine, can remedy certain conditions. Periodic adjustments are usually required to align the spine and various joints throughout the body. In this way pressure and/or pain is relieved.
Crystal healing	Continual use of various stones and gems are required to produce healing. Practitioners of crystal healing place specific stones on parts of the body for certain lengths of time to draw out disease. Patients are taught which types of stone can be used for their healing abilities.
Herbal remedies	Medicinal purposes of herbs have been learned through historic literature and by word of mouth. Trial and error are the main guidelines of herbal treatments if used without consultation from an authority, such as a practitioner who has a legitimate degree in herbal use. Currently, many herbal agents are being tested, and testimonials of both side effects and interactions are being compiled for reference.
Homeopathy	Homeopathy is the traditional belief that "like cures like". Various types of toxins are mixed in extreme dilutions to the point at which they are often undetectable by scientific means. This minute amount of the same disease from which the patient is suffering allows the patient's body to fight the illness.
Spiritual healing	In the belief system of spiritual healing, the patient's treatment is attained through prayer of the practitioner and patient. The practitioner claims to be a pathway for divine intervention. Recovery is instantaneous and no follow-up visits are necessary.

when the topic of Chinese medicine is discussed, it involves much more than the use of herbaceous plant parts. The heart of Chinese practice is the yin and yang, which represents both male and female entities, respectively. The ancient Chinese belief contends that although men and women are made of the same substances, their spirits are different, and therefore appropriate treatment is different. Female spirits are thought of as a darker color, which coincides with the earth, whereas male spirits are lighter like the color of the sky.

Practitioners conduct an examination by asking about the patient's dreams, strange tastes, or smells experienced. Also, a visual examination of the skin and voice tone is performed. Once the diagnosis is completed, the practitioner may prescribe the necessary treatment that could include a variety of herbs, minerals, and/or vegetables. Herbs are used extensively in Chinese medicine and can treat more than one ailment at a time. For example, goldenseal may be used for headaches, allergies, and infections concurrently. Also, various herbal plants have the ability to work for or against a specific physiological condition, such as either raising or lowering blood pressure levels, depending on the person's condition. Herbs and other remedies are used in Chinese medicine to cure the body of the original illness and to prevent future problems. Chinese medicine is still in use today; many healthcare providers, including pharmacists, take classes based on Chinese knowledge of herbs and their medicinal uses.

Art Therapy

Art therapy became popular in psychology in the late 1960s. Psychiatrists had patients who were mentally disturbed or traumatized draw their feelings on paper if they were unable to discuss problems verbally. It was a way for patients to express themselves, relieve anxiety, and begin on the road to recovery. It can be used for simple stress relief therapy or as therapeutic treatment for persons suffering from life-threatening illnesses, such as cancer. Patients may gather in groups or individually with a practitioner who guides them through the techniques of both mental and visual awareness concerning their disease state or condition. This type of therapy is meant to supplement talking.

Art therapy is used extensively in children with autism or other psychological conditions, and is now used for many types of treatment in adults as well. Various forms of expression include painting, working with clay, making facial masks, and batiking. A master's degree is offered in this area of study through various colleges. Other art therapies include music, poetry, drama, and dance. The National Coalition of Creative Arts Therapies Association (NCCATA) offers information on these types of therapies and schools for training.

Ayurveda

Ayurveda is an ancient Indian approach to medicine still practiced today. Dating back thousands of years, Ayurveda is based on the person knowing the spiritual self. This knowledge encompasses the body and all that affects it. With an insight into the various effects of outside influences on the body's spirit, it is possible to make assumptions. One can predict whether something will have a positive effect or negative effect on the body. For example, certain colors, sounds, clothing, and other environmental stimuli are taken into consideration. The types of food and herbs that are consumed also play a role in the overall health of the person. These assumptions are then applied to both physical and spiritual activities of the ill person. Based on the type of personality of the subject, the practitioners suggest ways to alter food and/or lifestyle to both cure and prevent illnesses. This form of treatment exists today in many parts of the world. Medical schools teaching this approach are located in India. Courses in Indian medicine are also offered in various medical schools in the United States.

Biofeedback

Biofeedback has been around for approximately 50 years and has been proven to be effective for treatment of stress, hypertension, and other conditions. Biofeedback uses the patient's mental ability to alter vital signs such as blood pressure, heart rate, and even the gastrointestinal (GI) activity. The body is divided into two types of movement, voluntary and involuntary. Voluntary movements include the musculoskeletal system and involve purposeful actions such as walking, sitting, standing, and bending over. People have control over these functions on a daily basis; therefore to adjust behavior does not take much conscious effort. However, with biofeedback one is also taught the ability to mentally tap into and alter involuntary bodily functions, such as heart beat, breathing, and digestion. These functions do not normally require conscious thought.

Biofeedback is usually taught by an instructor who uses electrical leads that provide a readout of data. Patients are hooked up to monitors that allow them to see what their bodies are experiencing. A monitor can show the activity of a specific organ. For example, the instructor might have the patient alter the heart rate to a certain level through concentration. When that level is reached, a new level is set. Gradually, the person is able to adjust body functions as needed without the use of a monitor. Biofeedback is a way of connecting the mind to the body. Patients are supposed to practice these techniques often for full effects. Biofeedback is used as an alternative for medication for anxiety, low back pain, neuromuscular dysfunction, tension headaches and other conditions. It is partially covered by many insurance companies with a doctor's approval. Once the technique of biofeedback is perfected, it can be done at any time without supervision.

Chiropractic

Chiropractic therapy is an orthopedic approach to treating pain resulting from misalignment of the bones. It began in the late 1800s when it was believed to cure deafness in a man after his back popped into correct alignment. It is believed that certain changes in the skeletal structure interfere with the nervous system and other organ systems. The treatment given to a patient by a chiropractic doctor is referred to as *manipulation*. Treatment can include hands-on adjustments of the spine or joints and application of massage and heat therapy. Research has proven that some forms of manipulation can be helpful, specifically manipulation of the lower back. Although use of chiropractic therapy is on the rise, various forms of treatment are somewhat controversial. Some doctors promote the use of manipulation of certain parts of the skeletal structure, whereas other physicians believe it may be harmful. This is especially true when chiropractors have been used to manipulate skeletal structures to cure infections or treat conditions such as hearing loss or diabetes.

There is much skepticism about the ability of manipulation to treat many common illnesses, and studies are being done to find out exactly what therapy works and why. Practitioners must attend an accredited school to become a Doctor of Chiropractic (DC). Many insurance companies cover chiropractic treatment based on scientific evidence and referrals from a physician such as an orthopedic doctor. Chiropractic therapy usually takes many sessions of treatment.

Crystal Healing

There is a belief that various stones and gems have the ability to heal certain illnesses (Table 10.2). Many practitioners of crystal healing believe in chakras, which is a type of force field found in a person's aura. It is believed that when a person's chakras are blocked, the wellness of the individual is affected. The chakras are broken into seven different locations throughout the body. Each location has a specific function. Stones or gems are related to each of the seven locations. For example, the fifth chakra is located in the ear, nose, and throat. The function of this location is communication. A blue-colored stone is indicated if this area of the

TABLE 10.2 Examples of Stones with Healing Abilities

Stone	Color	Use
Amethyst	Purple	Relieve stomach problems
Green aventurine	Green	Cure viruses
Blue aventurine	Blue	Relieve congestion
Green fluorite	Green	Relieve menopause or PMS
Black onyx	Black	Alter bad habits

PMS, Premenstrual syndrome.

body is blocked. It is believed that roundness or nonroundness of the stone influences its effectiveness. When stringing stones to wear around one's neck, it is recommended that stones be strung on silk only. Gemstones should be free from cracks or other impurities.

There are no degrees offered in crystal healing. No studies have confirmed its ability to overcome illness. Patients and practitioners rely on testimonials from believers. Nevertheless, this type of treatment has a large following. Many books can be obtained describing the effectiveness of gemstones and crystals. One only needs to explore the Internet to see the endless list of websites available to consumers.

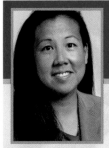

Pharmacist's Perspective
BY SUSAN WONG, PHARM.D.

Educate Oneself When It Comes to Complementary and Alternative Medicine and Health!

Many questions arise when it comes to a person's health. What is health? Some may believe that it is not getting sick, that is, staying well. Others may think it is fixing something that has gone wrong or broken. Still others believe it is maintaining overall happiness and balance. All of these play an important role in being healthy. How to do this is another story. There are four important steps:

1. A patient or customer must become a good self-observer.
2. A patient or customer must learn to recognize that he or she has control of lifestyle and choices.
3. A patient or customer must make lifestyle changes or other changes as necessary.
4. A patient or customer must follow the results of changes, as well as document and communicate them with the healthcare provider.

Your role as a pharmacy technician may be as a bridge of information between the pharmacist and the patient to help the patient become or stay healthy.

To do any and all of these things, one must first understand what makes a person tick. Over many centuries different philosophies have developed that address health. Native Americans chewed on willow leaves for relief from pain or swelling. In Europe this eventually led to the discovery and concentration of the active component, salicin, and with a little chemistry, acetylsalicylic acid (aspirin). In Chinese medicine, a practitioner prescribes a tailored mixture or formula to cure pain and restore balance, or one can use one of the patent medicines (ready-made formulas for a general condition). Many Eastern philosophies incorporate emotional, mental, and spiritual balance into the equation. Unfortunately, how these remedies and philosophies interact may not always be clear. That is why it is important to educate oneself and communicate to others; especially important is the communication between a patient and the healthcare provider.

In the world of drugs, herbs, and nutritional supplements, it is important to clearly distinguish what types there are. Learn how each of these single or multiple agents can affect a particular situation before its use. Sometimes one therapy may counteract another or may actually augment the effects of another. This may be good or bad depending on the person's situation and overall health. Patients should keep a diary of what has been used, what they are currently using (if anything), and any questions they may have. Patients should keep track of how they feel and what may have caused it, including any prescription drugs, OTC drugs, herbs, or supplements, and let the healthcare provider know exactly what they are using. It is important to let the

Continued

Pharmacist's Perspective—cont'd

medical doctor, pharmacist, chiropractor, herbalist, nutritionist, or anyone who is involved in the patient's health and well being know what he or she is taking. Healthcare providers may not know exactly how some things interact but they will find out for the patient before they recommend its use.

In Western medicine, drugs are highly refined chemicals (both of plant and synthetic origin) that are taken for a specific purpose or endpoint. They have been extensively studied and documented in the scientific literature. These drugs are available mostly as single-agent pills or capsules. There are also multiple-agent compounds designed to work together on one symptom or take care of many symptoms. There are new ways of getting those medicines into the body such as injections or shots; skin patches; creams, lotions, and ointments; inhalers; suppositories when the patient cannot swallow or keep things down; drops for eyes, ears, and nose; and drops or liquid to swallow. All of these dosage forms have developed in the last 10 to 50 years and are designed to get the medicine to exactly where it is needed. This allows a smaller effective dose with fewer side effects.

Just because a drug can be bought OTC does not mean that it is the best thing to use. For example, the asthma inhalers that can be bought OTC certainly work, but can cause some serious side effects in people with a heart condition or anxiety. Always consult the pharmacist if the patient is not sure. It is really important that the patient gets the right kind of drug in the right form and that the patient knows why, when, and how to use it.

For herbs, a similar situation exists in which there are single-agent herbs and multiple-agent formulas that work for different ailments. Fortunately, most are available in an oral form that can be swallowed or taken as a tea or infusion. Unfortunately, herbals are not as closely regulated in the United States as drugs are. Drugs are much more rigorously tested and take longer to reach the market. On the other hand, herbs have been used for centuries, even millennia, to heal and cure patients when used correctly. The patient must be aware of the exact genus and species of herb to ensure the right effect. Similarly named herbs can have very different effects. Be aware of where the active agents are derived from—roots, leaves, berries, and tree bark. Also of importance for some herbs is when they are harvested: spring and fall harvests may have very different chemical characteristics. Always be aware of the labels. Read and learn about exactly what the patient needs and how to take herbs. Use reputable sources and standardized extracts (standardized to known active ingredients) when buying herbs.

Food and dietary supplements are similar to herbs in that they are much less regulated than the drugs. We all know we need certain foods, vitamins, and minerals to survive. Too much or too little can adversely affect health. Different diets can rob patients of certain essential nutrients, so it is best for the patient to check with the physician/consultant before starting a diet. Most people who follow a well-balanced diet do not need additional supplements. Others who may have chosen certain vegetarian diets or weight loss diets may be missing some nutrients and need supplements. Remember that different types or amounts of exercise can affect one's diet and nutrient needs.

For example, osteoporosis can occur in men but is most commonly seen in women. A well-balanced diet with plenty of exercise can help prevent long-term detrimental effects. Some people take calcium supplements to augment their bone and mineral stores. The normal recommended daily allowance (RDA) for calcium in adults is about 1200 mg. By taking calcium supplements of 1000 to 1500 mg per day, a healthy adult can avoid detrimental bone loss. Recently there was a new and innovative supplement that hit the market that is not a pill but a chocolate-flavored chew. It provides 500 mg of calcium just like old-fashioned oyster shell calcium but in a candy-like form. Sounds good, doesn't it? In the fine print, there is also a tiny amount of vitamin K added in. For those folks on a closely monitored blood-thinning agent to prevent strokes, this could be really bad news. Even this tiny amount of vitamin K can counteract the good effects of a blood-thinning agent and put a patient at risk for developing a stroke.

Green tea also has high amounts of vitamin K that can counteract blood-thinning agents. As people get older and try to take better care of themselves, they could be doing harm if they don't pay attention to what they take and how.

In today's medicine we really don't know how the Western philosophy of treating illness and promoting health interacts with the Eastern philosophy. A few terms to think about follow:

- Allopathy—a system of medical practice making use of all measures that have proven value in the treatment of disease
- Homeopathy—a system of medical practice that treats a disease especially by the administration of minute doses of a remedy that would in healthy persons produce symptoms similar to those of the disease
- Vegetarianism—the theory or practice of living on a diet made up of vegetables, fruits, grains, nuts, and sometimes animal products (e.g., milk, cheese, eggs)
- Nutriceuticals/nutritional supplementation—whole foods, vitamins, minerals, enzymes, amino acids, phytochemicals, and other natural resources that are designed for use in the immune systems, the inner healing force

Continued

- Herbal or botanical medicine—plants or plant substances that are used for medicinal purposes or crude drugs of vegetable origin used for the treatment of disease states, often of chronic nature, or to attain or maintain a condition of improved health
- Phytotherapy—the use of vegetable drugs in medicine
- Aromatherapy—the treatment of medical conditions with the aromatic essential oils of fragrant herbs
- Ayurveda—a holistic medical system that covers all aspects of heath and well-being (physical, emotional, mental, and spiritual). It includes methods of healing from diet, herbs, exercise, and lifestyle regimens such as yoga and meditation and is based on a person's dominant *dosha,* one of three body/personality types
- Traditional Chinese medicine—a system of acupuncture, herbs, and diet based on the parallelism and synchronicity of events in the inner and outer world of the human organism; based on a person's Tao (one of five archetypes that symbolize human character or personality types); the five organ networks and their climates; and finally the balance (yin/yang) between Qi (the life force), blood (governing the tissue), and moisture (governing the internal environment)

Lastly, age, gender, and body type can all affect how a body responds to what is put in it. It is well known in Western medicine that pediatric (0 to 18 years old) and older patients (60 to 65 years and older) tolerate medications differently because of natural metabolic changes. Lifestyle issues such as smoking and alcohol use also affect responses to medicines. Medication doses are adjusted according to these factors and to the desired endpoints. It might be safe to infer that these changes may have similar effects when using Eastern medicines and therapies as well. Patients must be very careful before starting any new therapies and consult experts if necessary.

It is important for all patients to keep track of any and all agents they put into their bodies. They need to educate themselves on health and how they choose to maintain it. Patients should always inform their healthcare providers of any herbal remedies they are taking. This decreases the probability of a drug-drug or drug-food interaction. ■

Herbal Medicine

Although herbal remedies have been in existence for thousands of years (see Chapter 1), this basic therapy has gained renewed popularity during the past decade. It is expected to grow even more in the coming years because of many factors, such as the increasing age of the population and the increasing costs associated with traditional health care and medications. It is important to know various interactions between legend drugs, OTC drugs, and herbal remedies. Most people believe that it is not important to notify their physician or pharmacist that they are taking herbals because they believe them to be natural and therefore not harmful. However, there are many documented reports of harmful interactions between natural products, legend drugs, and OTCs.

Many of the drugs used in traditional medicine today are medications derived from herbs. The main difference is that extensive testing and documentation has preceded their use. Through testing, specific chemicals have been isolated in many herbal plants. Those chemicals that have proven effectiveness against certain conditions are then synthetically made in a laboratory if possible. Therefore most American medicine discovered from plants does not incorporate the whole plant or even parts of them. Also, over time, if literature has proven their effectiveness, they are subjected to the regulations enforced by the Food and Drug Administration (FDA). However, the FDA does not regulate herbs because they are considered a nutritional supplement.

This section discusses some of the more popular herbs and the caution that should be taken before self-administration. Because many herbs have been used in different cultures for thousands of years, they often have many different names. For example, *Echinacea* is also known as black sampson, sampson root, narrow leafed purple coneflower, and red sunflower.

Scientific nomenclature is a method of naming plants by grouping them together using a series of guidelines. Taxonomy guidelines are based on structure of the plants and is determined by scientists. Taxonomy is the science of categorizing and naming new species. Because most of the use, documentation, and naming of herbaceous plants has historically taken place in Europe, the use of Latin in naming new species has become the standard.

HERBAL TREATMENTS

One of the most popular herbal agents is a succulent plant called aloe *(Aloe vera)*. Many different species are used to produce agents to treat minor burns, acne, and various skin irritations. If taken internally, aloe vera works as a laxative and is also used for bleeding ulcers. Dosage forms are gels, powder, capsules, tonic, and juice. Pregnant women should not take aloe vera internally.

Black cohosh *(Cimicifuga racemosa),* from the family Ranunculaceae, is primarily used for hormone replacement. Other indications are rheumatism and cough; it can also be used as an insect repellent (called bugbane). Short-term studies have concluded that black cohosh is safe if used for short periods. There have not been extensive scientific studies done on this agent. It is important not to confuse black cohosh with similar sounding herbs, such as blue or white cohosh. These are not used for the same purpose and have different interactions with other medications.

Chamomile is from the family Asteraceae and has more than 20,000 known species. The species of *Matricaria recutita* is used for motion sickness, flatulence, and GI disturbances. In the topical form it is used for open ulcers, hemorrhoids, and other inflammation of the skin. When taken orally, it has been documented to cause emesis, and if used topically one should keep the medication away from the eyes because it can cause irritation. Oral chamomile is contraindicated in pregnancy and (because of lack of testing) during lactation. It has also been reported to worsen asthma attacks. Chamomile has several interactions with anticoagulants, benzodiazepines, and central nervous system (CNS) depressants. Most of these interactions can cause an additive effect of the medication if taken with chamomile.

Feverfew is also derived from the family of Asteraceae (Compositae). The species *Tanacetum parthenium* is used for many different ailments including fever, headaches, GI upset, arthritis, and asthma. It can be used in both topical and oral form. In the oral form, feverfew is known to cause irritation of the mouth and tongue and a variety of GI upsets such as nausea, vomiting, and diarrhea. There have been reports of side effects, such as increased bleeding, when taken with anticoagulants. Nonsteroidal antiinflammatory drugs (NSAIDs) may decrease the effects of feverfew.

Garlic is from the family Amaryllidaceae (Liliaceae) and is most well known as a common herb used in most kitchens in America. Although it is known for its wonderful flavor, it has medicinal uses as well. The species *Allium sativum* has several uses that range from stress relief to an anticancer agent. Some people use garlic to treat high blood pressure, colds, and flu, and for overall wellness. Although garlic is safe most of the time, it is important not to overmedicate because it has been reported to cause adverse side effects such as heartburn, GI burning, and even a kill-off of normal intestinal flora. (This normal flora of the gut is necessary for breakdown of food and some vitamin absorption.) Garlic should not be used medicinally when taking anticoagulants because it may increase bleeding. It should not be taken by diabetics because it may interact with ongoing medication therapy, such as insulin or hypoglycemic agents. Persons suffering from GI disorders should beware of possible interactions with garlic use.

Ginger is from the family Zingiberaceae, known as the ginger family, and has 1000 species. The species *Zingiber officinale* is known for its antiemetic and antivertigo properties and is used in GI upset and other GI conditions, including bleeding, flatulence, stomachache, diarrhea, and more severe conditions such as malaria and cholera. Like garlic, ginger has been shown to have interactions with anticoagulants, producing possible increased bleeding. It also may interact with GI medication such as histamine-2 (H$_2$) antagonists (ranitidine) and proton pump inhibitors (omeprazole). Use of barbiturates with ginger may increase the effects of such agents. Ginger may also affect blood pressure medication, cardiac drugs, and diabetic agents.

Gingko biloba is the only remaining species of the family Ginkgoaceae and is sometimes referred to as a living fossil. Its most popular use is to treat poor circulation, but it is also used for asthma and other less documented uses, such as regulating blood pressure, improving liver function, increasing memory, and treating heart disease. Some drug interactions include increased bleeding when taken with anticoagulants and increased blood pressure when taken with antihypertensive medications. Persons suffering from bleeding disorders, epilepsy, or infertility should avoid gingko. Many medicinal herbs are made from different parts of a plant; therefore it is important to know what part of the plant is used for which type of condition. Primarily, the gingko leaf is used as the medicinal agent, but seeds are also available. Studies have not shown their effectiveness, but it is known that raw seeds can be dangerous if taken orally.

Ginseng is from the family Araliaceae. Ginseng species *Panax quinquefolium* is widely used for overall wellness, including boosting the immune system. It is also used for other ailments such as inflammation and depression and as a diuretic. Ginseng's drug interactions include decreasing the effectiveness of anticoagulants and altering the effectiveness of some cardiac agents, diuretics, diabetic agents, and antidepressants.

Goldenseal is from the family Ranunculaceae, known as the buttercup family. The species *Hydrastis canadensis,* when taken orally, is used for GI conditions, inflammatory conditions, and painful menstruation. Topically, it has been used for dandruff, eczema, and itching rashes. Goldenseal has been reported to have interactions with H$_2$ antagonists (ranitidine), blood pressure medication, anticoagulants, and CNS sedating drugs.

Hawthorn is available in many different preparations depending on the part of the plant used; however, all are members of the family Rosaceae (the rose family). The species *Crataegus laevigata* is mostly used to increase blood circulation and improve heart conditions, although studies have not conclusively proved its effectiveness. However, hawthorn has been reported to have possible interactions with various cardiac agents such as vasodilators, antiarrhythmics, antianginal agents, and antihypertensive drugs. It also may interact with CNS depressants.

Purple coneflower is in the family Asteraceae or Compositae depending on the species used. The species *Echinacea purpurea* has common uses that include treating colds and infections and use as a general immune booster. Therefore persons on any type of immunosuppressive agents should be aware that *Echinacea* might alter the effects of such agents. In addition, diabetics and any people who have a condition that involves the immune system should not take *Echinacea* because this herb may worsen the problem.

Milk thistle is from the family of Asteraceae or Compositae. The species *Silybum marianum* is used primarily for liver conditions. Like several other herbs, various parts of the plant are used. The effect varies depending on what part is used. Unlike many other herbs, milk thistle does not have any reported major contraindications and is one of the few herbs that is used intravenously for mushroom poisoning.

St. John's wort comes from the Clusiaceae family. *Wort* means "flower" in Old English, not to be confused with *wart*, which is a viral growth on the skin. There is more literature on the effectiveness of this herb than on many others. Some of its uses include improvement of sleep disorders, anxiety, agitation, depression, and fatigue. Care should be taken if using St. John's wort with other herbs that increase sedation, such as valerian. There are many documented interactions with medications such as antianginal agents, antidepressants, and anticoagulants.

TABLE 10.3 Common Uses and Cautionary Notes for Herbals

Herb	Species	Various Uses	Caution
Black cohosh	*Cimicifuga racemosa*	Menopause, PMS	Should not be used if pregnant Studies not complete
Chamomile	*Matricaria recutita*	GI upsets, skin conditions	Should not be used if pregnant Safe if used in small quantities and short term
Feverfew	*Tanacetum parthenium*	Migraine	Should not be used if pregnant
Garlic	*Allium sativum*	Antiinfective, antibiotic	Safe if used in small quantities
Ginger	*Zingiber officinale*	Motion sickness	Safe if used in small quantities
Ginkgo	*Ginkgo biloba*	Increase circulation	Should not be used if pregnant
Ginseng	*Panax quinquefolius*	Stress relief	Safe if used in small quantities
Goldenseal	*Hydrastis canadensis*	Urinary tract infections	Should not be used if pregnant or if hypertensive problems exist
Hawthorn	*Crataegus laevigata*	Chest pain, increases blood flow	Studies not complete
Purple coneflower	*Echinacea purpure*	Antiinfective, antibiotic	Studies not complete because of the many different species and parts of herbaceous plant used
Milk thistle	*Silybum marianum*	Liver and spleen	Safe if used in small quantities
St. John's wort	*Hypericum perforatum*	Antidepressant	Safe if used in small quantities
Valerian	*Valeriana officinalis*	Sleep aid	Safe if used in small quantities

GI, Gastrointestinal; *PMS*, premenstrual syndrome.
*Various species are used; some side effects may differ depending on species.

Valerian is from the family Valerianaceae. The species *Valeriana officinalis* is used mostly for sleeplessness and depression. Because of its strong ability to induce sleepiness, it should not be taken with alcohol, barbiturates, benzodiazepines, or any other sedative type of medication. It may increase the effects of such drugs and/or their side effects.

It is important to know the family name of the herb in case of possible unwanted interactions or reactions. For instance, if someone is allergic to corn, then any herbal drug from the same family may cause an allergic response. Therefore all herbs from this family should be avoided. There are several herbal books that can be referenced to determine which family an herb is from. Knowing the species of the herb is also important because species can vary even if they are closely related (Table 10.3). Some studies have been completed on only one of many species of herbs used to prepare herbal supplements.

It is also very hard for the correct or safe dosages to be used because the ingredients of each batch of herbs can vary widely. Therefore the strength of each tablet or capsule may vary from one production lot to another. The time of harvesting, which parts of the plants used, concentrations, and consistency in the method of preparation can alter their effectiveness.

TABLE 10.4 Herbal Preparations

Dosage Form	Route of Administration	Ingredients	Use, Strength, Onset of Action
Syrups, diluted; tinctures	Internal	Alcohol, glycerin	Usually this is a potent form
Tablets, capsules	Internal	Powdered	Slower to act; these are broken down in the stomach
Teas	Internal	Syrups, sweeteners	Better tasting when sweeteners added; teas are stronger than tablets, capsules
Aromatic solutions, baths	External	Scented water	Used to treat skin conditions and burns
Oils	External	Extracted oil from herbs	Used for sore muscles and skin conditions
Compresses, salves	External	Made from teas, salves from herbal oils	A cloth soaked in herbal tea is applied to skin site; used for bruises, cramps, and so forth

HERBAL PREPARATIONS

How herbs are prepared can determine the strength of the active chemicals. Herbs that are brewed for teas are usually more potent than those prepared in capsule form. Teas can be prepared by various methods. Infusions consist of pouring hot water onto the herbs and letting them brew (steep) for a few minutes, decoctions are herbs that are simmered over heat in water for 15 to 20 minutes, and cold infusions are left to soak in cold water over many hours. Various methods are suggested depending on the type of herb being prepared (Table 10.4). Medical schools are including studies of herbal remedies because of their prevalence and possible benefits when used correctly along with traditional medicine.

Homeopathy

Homeopathy, translated from Greek, simply means "like suffering." The premise of homeopathy is the belief that "like cures like." It is also referred to as the law of similars. It is believed that if a small amount of the substance that caused a person's disease or condition is consumed, it will enable the body to fight off the disease. In the late 1700s, homeopathy was made well-known by Samuel Hahnemann, a German physician. After ingesting a small amount of quinine, he showed symptoms of having malaria, the disease that quinine cured. Over time he perfected the necessary minute amount of agent that was needed to bring about cure rather than disease. Homeopathy made its way to the United States in the 1800s and was a popular treatment. Although homeopathy has remained a popular form of treatment in parts of Europe, it became an alternative treatment in the United States. It has, however, regained some popularity over the last decade along with all other forms of alternative medicine.

There are thousands of homeopathic remedies, but only one right one for each illness; therefore homeopathic doctors must know what will work for their patient. Unlike herbs and other alternative treatments, the FDA oversees the manufacturing of homeopathic drugs. They are in the same category as OTC medications. Although more medical schools are offering classes on homeopathic medicine, it is still somewhat controversial in the traditional medical community.

All drugs are prepared following guidelines in the Homeopathic Pharmacopoeia of the United States (HPUS). Many of the remedies include herbal treatments. The process of preparing homeopathic agents involves blending and condensing the main ingredients, followed by diluting the active ingredients, and finally preparing the dosage form. The dilution of these active ingredients renders a trace amount of the agent that can equal as little as one part per million. Many times this minute amount is so small that it cannot be detected by chemical analysis.

More information on homeopathic medicine can be obtained from The National Center for Homeopathy. Although most homeopathic agents are available OTC, there are homeopathic practitioners that can oversee treatments. Various credentials are available, such as DHANP (Diplomate of the Homeopathic Academy of Naturopathic Physicians), DHt (Diplomate in Homeotherapeutics), and CCH (Certified in Classical Homeopathy).

Spiritual Healing

Although religion is a strong belief of many cultures and millions of people, most people do not seek out medical help from their local church or spiritual healer. Nevertheless, this type of alternative medicine has grown over the past few decades into a multimillion dollar business. Known by such terms as "airy-fairy" and "quackery" in the medical community, spiritual healing claims to be a real science that uses "holy" alchemy. By using various rituals and prayer, the healer (also known as an alchemist) claims to cure both physical and mental disease by the laying on of hands. These spiritual healers claim to become the catalyst between the Holy Spirit and the sick person, which allows them to heal by using this channeled energy. This form of therapy is considered by many physicians and scientists as a testimonial of the power of the placebo effect.

There are Internet schools and long distance learning institutes that train one to become a spiritual healer. No conclusive studies have been conducted that can validate any claim made by this type of medicine. Cases are based on individual testimonials from people who claim its effectiveness.

TECH NOTE! As the popularity of alternative therapies increase, the medical community must meet the responsibilities of keeping up on information about such therapies. Increased use of herbal remedies may have a great impact on medication interactions because herbal remedies have a direct effect on other drugs being prescribed for or bought over-the-counter by the patient. It is important for the technician to know the most common interactions between common herbal remedies and legend drugs. In this way the technician is able to assist the pharmacist in identifying persons who may want or need counseling. One of the most prevalent interactions is the side effect of increased bleeding when taking certain herbals with anticoagulants. This is a potential life-threatening side effect, especially for patients for whom anticoagulants are prescribed to prevent strokes. If a patient asks about herbal medications, the best advice is to tell them to talk to the pharmacist or to their physician. Letting a patient know that many herbal drugs can cause interactions with other drugs is a responsible answer; however, the technician should never comment on any specifics even if they have in-depth information. Keeping current on new scientific findings is important in case any major side effects or contraindications are found.

DO YOU REMEMBER THESE KEY POINTS?
- The difference between Eastern and Western beliefs concerning medicine and healing
- Why alternative medicine is becoming more popular
- What NCCAM's function is concerning alternative medicine
- How the placebo effect fits into the healing process
- What the major alternative therapies are and how they work

■ The current regulations pertaining to herbal remedies
■ How people feel about informing their physicians about taking herbal medicines
■ The main uses for the herbal medications covered
■ How different dosage forms of herbal medications are used when prepared in different forms
■ How homeopathy originated and the belief systems behind it

REVIEW QUESTIONS:

Multiple Choice

1. Of the following statements regarding biofeedback, which is *not* true?
   A. It is used to treat low-back pain.
   B. Treatment may be partially covered by insurance companies.
   C. The patient is able to adjust his or her body functions to a degree.
   D. It must be used with supervision from a biofeedback therapist.

2. Chamomile would most likely be used to
   A. Treat an upset stomach
   B. Relieve stress
   C. Increase circulation
   D. All of the above

3. Art therapy is often used for all of the following conditions or patients except
   A. Severe illnesses
   B. Children with autism
   C. Persons who have a difficult time communicating
   D. For persons with an artistic ability

4. Homeopathy is known as the law of similars, which can be best described as
   A. Taking a similar drug that works but at a much reduced cost
   B. Taking a drug that is similar to legend drugs but does not require a prescription
   C. Taking a drug that causes the same illness as the one you are trying to cure
   D. Taking a drug that causes a similar reaction to traditional agents

5. The herb that is known to increase circulation and memory is
   A. Garlic
   B. Goldenseal
   C. Ginger
   D. *Gingko biloba*

6. Which of the remedies listed is regulated by the FDA?
   A. Herbal agents
   B. Homeopathic agents
   C. Healing gemstones
   D. Acupuncture

7. *Echinacea purpurea's* most common use is
   A. As an immune builder
   B. To treat GI conditions
   C. To treat skin conditions
   D. As an antioxidant

8. *Silybum marianum* is commonly known as _____ and is most commonly used as
   A. Ginger, motion sickness
   B. St. John's wort, depression
   C. Milk thistle, liver and spleen conditions
   D. Garlic, antiinfective

9. Garlic has been shown to
   A. Interact with anticoagulants
   B. Increase flatulence
   C. Affect blood pressure medication
   D. Both A and C

10. The one drug classification that has unwanted interactions with many herbal drugs is
    A. Antiulcer agents
    B. Anticoagulants
    C. Vitamins
    D. Heart medications

True/False

*If a statement is false, then change it to make it true.

1. Acupuncture is used in hospitals within the United States to help relieve pain.
2. *Gingko biloba* is the last remaining species of the Ginkgoaceae family.
3. Ayurveda is an old Chinese form of medicine no longer in use.
4. Chinese philosophy relies on the belief of spiritual healing.
5. Herbal drugs are safe because they are natural.

6. Ingesting herbal tea is less potent than taking tablets or capsules.

7. Acupressure uses the same techniques as acupuncture.

8. The NCCAM's main purpose is to inform the public about herbal remedies.

9. The terms *alternative* and *nontraditional* medicine describe all forms of treatments other than the commonly used methods of Western physicians.

10. When taking any herbal agent, it is important to know the species name in case of possible allergic reactions to the specific species.

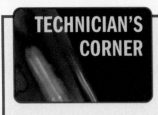

TECHNICIAN'S CORNER

1. A customer walks into your pharmacy and inquires about which herbal remedies are good for colds. What should you tell the customer?

2. An elderly customer suffering from the flu asks you if it is okay to take garlic tablets with her warfarin? What do you know about drug interactions (if any) between these two agents, and what should you tell the customer?

BIBLIOGRAPHY

Faelten S, editor: *Women's choices in natural healing,* Emmaus, PA, 1998, Rodale Press.
Freeman LW, Lawlis FG: *Complementary & alternative medicine,* St Louis, 2001, Mosby.
Loecher B, Altshul O'Donnell S: *Women's Choices in Natural Healing,* Emmaus, PA, 1998, Rodale Press.
Skidmore-Roth L: *Handbook of herbs & natural supplements,* St Louis, 2001, Mosby.

C H A P T E R

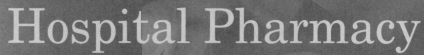

11

Hospital Pharmacy

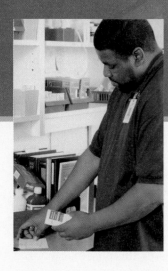

Objectives

- Define the most common tasks performed by hospital pharmacy technicians.

- Differentiate between pharmacy stock and central supply stock.

- Identify hospital units according to their specialty.

- Explain why hospitals use military time instead of standard time.

- Explain the functions of various hospital pharmacies.

- List the patient information required for processing orders.

- Describe the functions of satellite pharmacies.

- Recognize the differences in floorstock depending on the area of the hospital.

- List special unit services and the type of stock they require.

Introduction

Probably one of the most challenging areas to work in as a technician is a hospital pharmacy. The dynamics of this environment can be both exhilarating and exhausting, depending on the circumstances. Because hospitals are not as abundant as community pharmacies, there are fewer job openings for pharmacy technicians in hospitals. However, because of the changes in the pharmacist's role within the hospital setting, more highly skilled technicians are required. Pharmacists once made all intravenous (IV) antibiotics, chemotherapy drugs, and large-volume parenterals in addition to other inpatient tasks. Because of the increase in patient census and the need for pharmacy interventions and evaluations as they pertain to patient profiles, pharmacists do not have time to perform many important tasks they once performed. Technicians have taken over these tasks, which include preparing IV medications, loading patient medication drawers, and entering patient data into the computer systematically. As the health care industry continues to change and improve, so will the vital roles that pharmacy technicians play in providing health care services.

Types of Hospitals

Depending on the function of the hospital (facility), patient populations vary. The size of a hospital may be thought of as the number of beds available for patient use. Many small cities or towns may have small facilities with a bed capacity of 50 or less. Larger urban areas have facilities that can range from 50 beds to more than 250 beds. Other factors that differentiate hospitals from one another are their capabilities for diagnosis, surgery, and outpatient services. For instance, many hospitals do not have computed tomography (CT) scanners, which are very large and expensive; patients needing CT scans are sent to another hospital to have procedures performed or diagnostic examinations done.

Another important difference between hospitals is the layout of their pharmacies. Many older hospitals may have one central inpatient pharmacy that is responsible for supplying the entire hospital and all clinics. Larger hospitals or those with specialized areas may have a central pharmacy and smaller satellites located at various points throughout the facility. For instance, a large teaching

TABLE 11.1 Example of Various Sizes and Types of Hospitals

Types of Hospitals	Bed Capacity	Usually One Pharmacy	Central Pharmacy and Satellites	Each Pharmacy Independent from One Another	Type of Care Given
Small	25–50	X			Limited, minor surgeries; critical care is temporary
Medium-sized	50–100	X			Most surgeries, both CCU and ICU
Large	100+	X	X	X	Treats most conditions, PT, ICU, CCU, may have specialty areas such as burn or pediatric units
Teaching	100+	X	X	X	Covers all conditions and has specialty areas for teaching purposes; trains MDs and other healthcare providers
Institution	10–100	X		X	Care ranges from treating severe emergencies to continuing treatment but may also triage to a larger facility that specializes in a particular area; found in prisons, mental facilities, etc
Convalescent or long-term care	100+	X			Depending on the type of convalescent home, the level of care given may vary; some patients are sent to a hospital for surgery and recovery, then are sent back to their main resident home

CCU, Coronary care unit; *ICU*, intensive care unit; *PT*, physical therapy; *MD*, medical doctor.

facility may have specialized areas of treatment such as pediatrics, burn units, intensive care units (ICUs), and cancer units. Because of the large volume and specialty of the medications needed for these areas, they may have very small pharmacies that stock specific medications to speed up the turn-around time of a medical order. Listed in Table 11.1 are hospital facilities and types of pharmacy layouts.

Policies and Procedures

All pharmacies have a policies and procedures (P&P) handbook that outlines the facility's rules; these rules apply to all pharmacy employees. The information contained in the P&P binder concerns daily work routines, benefits, emergency situations, mandatory training, and other important and useful information. Technicians should be familiar with their facility's P&P handbook.

TECH NOTE! Ask for the P&P binder on your internship to familiarize yourself with specific rules and regulations of the pharmacy.

Protocol

Protocol is another term used to define the guidelines within the hospital setting, such as the type of medications that are available for dispensing. These rules must be constantly enforced and updated. A committee composed of pharmacists, doctors, nurses, other health care workers, and administrators meet to discuss appropriate changes to the protocol. Their purpose is to choose the best medicine for patients at the best cost. A drug education coordinator is a pharmacist who helps educate the health care providers about the changes in protocol concerning drug coverage and also helps the hospital pharmacy implement these changes. Not all hospitals have the extra help needed to perform these duties; therefore the tasks of the drug education coordinator may fall onto the staff pharmacists or pharmacy manager.

Hospital Standards

All hospitals must meet both federal and state guidelines if they are to be reimbursed for patients that have Medicare or Medicaid insurance coverage. Various agencies such as the Department of Public Health ensure that hospitals meet all standards of safe operation. The Board of Pharmacy may inspect all pharmacies to ensure that all personnel are working within legal guidelines. It has the authority to impose fines on any pharmacy not in compliance with current laws and can close noncompliant pharmacies.

TECH NOTE! All pharmacists and technicians must have their license, registration, and/or certification visible for inspection by the Board of Pharmacy at all times.

The following are some of the agencies that govern the operations of hospitals:

- Joint Commission on Accreditation of Healthcare Organizations (JCAHO). Hospitals pay a fee for JCAHO accreditation. This inspection is done every 3 years and is conducted over a 2-day period. JCAHO inspects only hospital pharmacies, not community pharmacies.
- Health Care Financing Administration (HCFA). Programs include Medicare, Medicaid, and HIPAA (see Chapter 14).
- Department of Public Health (DPH). Runs more than 300 programs. Linked to HCFA and Medicare and Medicaid Standards.
- Board of Pharmacy (BOP). Developing, implementing, and enforcing standards for the purpose of protecting the public.

The Flow of Orders

When a doctor visits a patient in the hospital and writes medication orders for the patient, it is equivalent to a prescription. The order is written on a doctor's order sheet and is placed in the patient's record. This record contains all of the medical records written by medical staff and remains in the patient care area where the patient is admitted. The unit clerk or nurse periodically checks all records for new orders that need to be sent to various areas of the hospital. These include dietary restrictions to be sent to dietary, laboratory test requests to be sent to the laboratory, and orders for medications to be sent to the pharmacy. It is important that the doctor, nurse, or unit clerk include all the necessary information on the patient's admitting record and subsequent medication orders to ensure that the orders are filled correctly. This includes the patient's full name, date of birth, medical record number, room number, diagnosis, weight, and, of course, drug allergies. See Figure 11.1 for a visual representation of the flow of orders.

Although many hospital pharmacies are not open to the public 24 hours a day, orders arrive at the pharmacy around the clock, 365 days a year. There are various methods that are used to send orders. One is a pneumatic tube system that allows a person to send orders and other small items by way of an air-propelled system. In another system, cylindrical canisters carry IV bags and other medications to the hospital floor (Figure 11.2).

The downside of this system is that the tube can easily get jammed. Also, fragile items, like those encased in glass, controlled substances, expensive med-

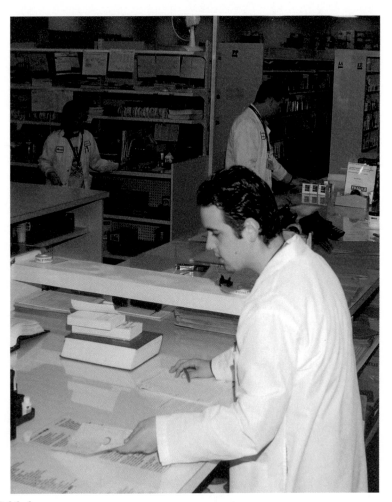

FIGURE 11.1 The flow of orders. As orders arrive, they are entered into the computer. If an order is unclear or if there is a question, the pharmacist calls the doctor.

ications, or protein-derived medications should not be sent via the pneumatic tube system because they can break during the rough ride or become lost in the system. A growing method of receiving orders is via a fax machine. Although it is a very effective way to get orders to the pharmacy quickly, often the quality of the fax can cause a delay in filling the order. Pharmacists need to verify all unreadable orders over the phone or have the order faxed again. Other methods of obtaining doctors' orders include the use of volunteers or paid staff to deliver the orders to the pharmacy.

Once the orders are received in the pharmacy, they need to be processed in the same way that a regular prescription is processed. However, instead of using the name, address, and phone number for identification, the patient's medical record number is used. Even though this method is the primary way patients are identified, all information, including name and room number, should always be verified against the order. In this way, errors are decreased, especially when two patients with the same last name are on the same floor. The pharmacy uses name alert stickers that are placed on the patients' drawer and medication when two patients have the same last name and are on the same floor. Many computer systems also have name alert functions to help distinguish between patients with similar identifying characteristics.

Most computer systems allow pharmacy technicians to enter the patient's medical record number and drug orders, although it is more common for the pharmacist to enter the order because the information, if entered by the technician, has to be checked by the pharmacist to ensure accuracy. Many pharmacists

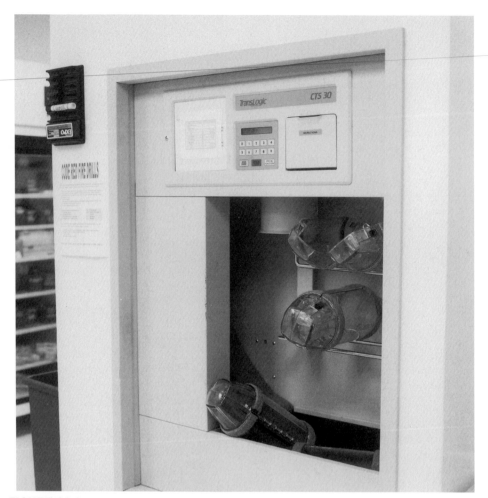

FIGURE 11.2 Pneumatic tube system. A pneumatic tube system is used to transport orders to the pharmacy and medications to hospital floors.

feel that it is double work if the technician enters the order and has to be entirely reread by the pharmacist. As the orders are entered, labels are produced from a printer that has the patient's name, medical record number, and room number along with the medication information. The name of the drug, strength, dosage form, route of administration, dose, and the dosing time are included on printed labels.

Because the labels are continually being produced, the technician usually pulls them off the printer and fills the order. Labels are placed on small zip-lock baggies so that the medication can be visibly checked against the label by the pharmacist before they are tubed or taken to the patient's floor. Some orders that are sent to pharmacy have "at once" (STAT) or "as soon as possible" (ASAP) stamped on the order. These orders need to be filled immediately because they are only ordered in this manner when an emergency situation exists.

Responsibilities of an Inpatient Technician

There are many skills that pharmacy technicians must have in today's pharmacy; because the roles of the pharmacists are ever expanding, so must the roles of the pharmacy technicians. Because pharmacists have more interaction with the

TABLE 11.2 Common Job Descriptions

Technician Responsibilities	Description
IV room	Prepares all parenteral IV preparations, including large-volume drips and parenteral nutrition
Chemotherapy	Prepares chemotherapy and other medications that may accompany these agents
Controlled substances	Gathers all controlled substance inventory sheets from all areas of the hospital; technician may also fill and deliver all controlled substances; the pharmacist is required to verify pharmacy inventory on a daily basis
Patient medication filling	Fills medication drawers on a pharmacy cart that will deliver medications to all hospital patients; may also deliver carts to all patient areas and restock any floorstock medications; if the hospital uses an automated medication dispensing system instead, the technician will need to fill this unit on all floors
Filling requisitions	Fills all requisitions sent to the pharmacy; stocks inventory; may also be responsible for checking areas containing medications for out-of-date drugs or overstocked medications that need to be returned to the pharmacy
Inventory	Orders all medications and supplies for the pharmacy; may also order specialty items for other areas of the hospital; handles all returns and recalled items that need to be sent back to the manufacturer; responsible for handling all invoices as well as putting all stock away in the appropriate bins
Discharge pharmacy	Fills prescription orders as patients are discharged from the hospital; medications are either sent to the floor for the patients or patients may come to the pharmacy window to pick them up
Satellite pharmacy	May be responsible for all tasks related to a small, isolated pharmacy such as answering phones, ordering and putting away stock, preparing parenteral medications, transcribing, pulling all medication orders, and making delivers to nursing stations

IV, Intravenous.

prescribing and implementation of formulary, the pharmacy technician completes many of the daily tasks that would otherwise require a pharmacist. The inpatient pharmacy has many different functions that depend mostly on the size of the hospital and number of pharmacies in operation. Many hospitals have 24-hour pharmacies and are open 7 days a week. Technicians need to be flexible to work all shifts, including holidays. They also need to be multifunctional because there are usually half as many technicians and pharmacists working on night and weekend shifts in most hospital pharmacies. However, the patient load may remain the same or even increase during these times. Therefore it is essential that the technician be able to perform all of the functions necessary for all shifts.

In Table 11.2, some of the more common pharmacy job descriptions are outlined. Because hospital pharmacies need to be staffed year round, it is important to have employees who can function in all areas. As a technician learns more skills throughout the pharmacy, he or she becomes more valuable.

Aseptic Technique

Aseptic technique is a method to prevent contamination of an object by microorganisms. The use of this technique is extremely important in preparing all IV medications, chemotherapy, and compounded ophthalmics. All technicians must be periodically tested on the proper guidelines of aseptic technique, which is usually done by management at the yearly evaluation. Samples are normally taken from a newly prepared parenteral medication and sent to the laboratory for testing. This is done to make sure that microbial contamination is not present in the patient's medication. To learn more about bacteria and harmful microbes see Chapter 28. Aseptic technique is discussed in more detail in Chapter 13.

Intravenous Technician

DESCRIPTION

Most IV technicians are responsible for labeling and preparing all parenteral antibiotics; large-volume drips such as heparin, aminophylline, and an assortment of potassium drips; and lactated ringer's. Some hospital pharmacies are responsible only for the large volumes of IV medications that need to be prepared; the nurses on the floor maintain a floorstock of premade, large volume bags, which can be supplied by central supply or by the pharmacy. This varies from hospital to hospital.

DUTIES

The daily routine usually includes printing all IV labels that are currently in the computer system. This IV medication information is either added or deleted as patients are admitted or discharged and as order changes occur. All changes in IV medication information are kept updated by the technician and the pharmacist who work in the IV room. Normally while the technician labels all premade IV antibiotics and other IV medications, the pharmacist answers the phones and enters new and changed orders. Pharmacists are also responsible for contacting the nurse or doctor if there is a problem with the order. For example, if an order is sent to the pharmacy for ampicillin/sulbactam (Unasyn) and the patient has an allergy to penicillin, the pharmacist calls the doctor and asks the doctor to substitute this antibiotic with one that will not cause an allergic reaction in the patient. The technician then begins to reconstitute and prepare all IV medications that must be compounded in a horizontal laminar flow hood.

Intravenous Therapy and Chemotherapy Preparation

DESCRIPTION

The hospital technician may be responsible for preparing both IV therapies and chemotherapies. However, some hospitals have separate chemotherapy centers where a technician works side-by-side with a pharmacist in preparing these medications for patients. The same aseptic techniques are used in preventing contamination when preparing any parenteral medication. However, there are a few differences between the IV and the chemotherapy settings that should be noted. One major difference involves the types of hoods used when preparing the medications. A horizontal flow hood is used for preparing IV medications. The air of a horizontal hood flows outward, away from the back of the hood, toward the technician. In this way, the environment stays bacteria free inside the hood (Figure 11.3). Chemotherapy hoods have cycled air that is sent in a vertical flow. The air is pulled down toward the tabletop filter, away from the ceiling of the hood. The chemotherapy hood does not allow the air to leave the container compartment, but gets recycled through a special filter that removes any particulate matter. The size of a chemotherapy hood is normally smaller than a horizontal laminar flow hood. In addition, technicians must wear a gown and double gloves or special chemo-safe gloves within chemotherapy hoods; it is not necessary to wear a gown or a second pair of gloves within a horizontal flow hood.

When working inside the horizontal flow hood, the orientation of the hands must not block the airflow. This means that hands cannot be moved behind the vial, needle, or IV bag. In a vertical flow hood, hands must not move over the top of any vial, needle, or IV bag. If the hands do move into these areas, then aseptic technique has been broken. Regardless of which hood is in use, it is most important that aseptic technique is always practiced. (See Chapter 13.)

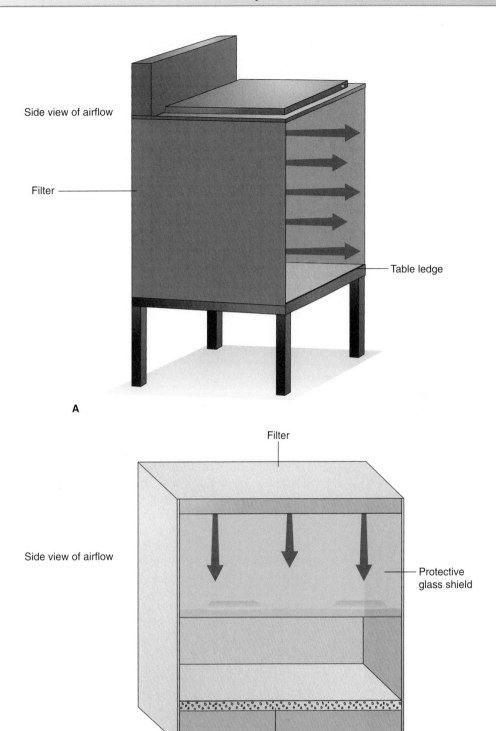

Side view of airflow

Filter

Table ledge

A

Filter

Side view of airflow

Protective glass shield

B

Filter

FIGURE 11.3 Airflow: **A,** Horizontal flow hood. **B,** Vertical flow hood.

DUTIES

Each morning at the beginning of the day shift, all IV labels representing all current orders, are printed from the computer system. Throughout the day, IV medication information is deleted or IV medications are ordered as new medication orders arrive to the pharmacy. The pharmacy technician is responsible for stocking the IV room with all of the supplies needed for the day; the supplies must also be restocked at the end of the day for the next shift. He or she must also make sure that the work area stays clean. Usually the same technician prepares all IV medications, then, at the end of the shift, he or she delivers them to the nursing floors. When the IV medications are delivered, the unused IV medications are returned to the pharmacy. If they have not expired, they are placed in the refrigerator or back into stock for future use; otherwise, they are wasted. Because each IV preparation must be accounted for, most pharmacies keep a binder or book in which information about all wasted IV preparations is written. It is important that all tasks are completed before the end of the shift and that all stock items are replaced as much as possible.

Labeling

DESCRIPTION

The proper placement of labels is important to ensure visibility of the solution and contents. The technician must initial all medications even if he or she only places a label on a premade bag. Before the IV piggybacks and drips are delivered to the appropriate floors, the pharmacist must check each one and countersign his or her initials. Labels usually contain the same type of information regardless of the facility. In addition to labeling parenteral medications, the technician must know additional information such as medications that need to be placed in light-protected bags and those requiring refrigeration. It is important for the technician to know the storage requirements and the stability of the medications he or she prepares.

DUTIES

All drugs must be labeled before they leave the pharmacy. The required parts of a label include the patient's name, patient's medical record number, room number, name of the drug, strength of the medication, the name of the solution with which the medication was mixed and the rate of infusion. This information must be checked by the pharmacy technician several times before he or she applies the label to the medication. Additional information contained on a label includes the time the dose should be given, the date, and the expiration date. Expiration dates are extremely important because all IV preparations are returned to stock if not expired. Many pharmacies use the Julian date. This is the day of the year that does not take into account the month. For instance, if the day is February 1, the Julian date is 29 because it is the 29th day of the year. It is much easier to determine the expiration date from the Julian date because it is not necessary to remember how many days are in a particular month.

All labels must be placed squarely onto the medication and should be clear and easy to read. Every drug label that is applied and initialed by the pharmacy technician must be checked and initialed by the pharmacist before leaving the pharmacy.

Controlled Substances

DESCRIPTION

The task of counting, dispensing, and tracking controlled substances is a critical job that requires perfection. Within each hospital unit that stocks controlled substances, an actual count must be conducted by two nurses at the change of every shift. Therefore all controlled substances are counted three times daily. One nurse counts the controlled substances while the other nurse confirms the count on the controlled substance sheet. At the beginning of the new day the count is moved over to a new sheet and the last day's sheet is sent to the pharmacy. Periodic automatic replenishment (PAR) levels are written at the top of the controlled substance sheets that list the amounts of medications that should be kept on the floor at all times. It is often the responsibility of the technician to retrieve these sheets daily from all units and begin assessing how many controlled substances of various sizes and strengths must be provided to keep the unit at or close to its PAR level. In the pharmacy, controlled substances are normally kept in a locked room, which may be under surveillance. All written records must be kept in pen and all inventories must be completed by a registered pharmacist.

DUTIES

After the technician has confirmed the pharmacy controlled substances count for the day, he or she must sign out each drug onto a dispensing sheet that is used to deliver the controlled substances, which is confirmed by the pharmacist. A pharmacist must do all counts and monthly inventories. Many hospitals still require pharmacists to perform the task of preparing the controlled substances for delivery; technicians are allowed to deliver them.

Each hospital has its own system of delivering controlled substances, but one of the most important aspects is to keep the controlled substances nonidentifiable. For instance, many pharmacies put controlled substances in brown paper bags that are stapled shut; most people would never know that there are controlled substances being delivered in this type of container. Even so, the pharmacy technician should never let these controlled substances out of sight when delivering them throughout the hospital. All controlled substances are signed into the department by adding them onto the controlled substances sheet. This can be done by the pharmacy technician or the nurse. All controlled substances must then be countersigned off of the pharmacy inventory sheet. The actual counting of the current levels of controlled substances should be done by both the nurse and pharmacy technician to verify all existing controlled substances before adding additional ones into stock. In addition to delivering controlled substances, the technician may be asked by the nurse to return certain ones to the pharmacy. The same validation system is used to enter onto the pharmacy inventory sheet those drugs that are to be returned to the pharmacy. Only registered nurses, not licensed practical nurses (LPNs), can sign in controlled substances.

On return to the pharmacy, all controlled substances must be signed back into the pharmacy stock. This is normally done by a pharmacist. One of the most important parts of this job is to make sure that all numbers are correct. The pharmacist must never sign in controlled substances without first visually counting the existing stock.

Additional Areas of Pharmacy

SATELLITE PHARMACIES

Description

Satellites are small specialty pharmacies that supply a clinic such as the emergency department (ED) or an entire floor of a hospital. Most are very small and minimally staffed. The satellites fill most of the daily medications for patients on their floors. Most of the floorstock used by the satellites is supplied by the hospital's large central pharmacy.

Duties

Technicians who work in the satellites are responsible for filling all medication orders and delivering them to the nurse's stations. Other duties include answering phones, keeping satellites stocked, and filling STAT orders.

DISCHARGE PHARMACY

Description

Many hospitals have a discharge pharmacy that fills prescriptions in the same manner as a community pharmacy except that it is located in the inpatient pharmacy. Doctor's orders are written on special discharge order forms that are sent down to the pharmacy with other orders via the pneumatic tube or by volunteers.

Duties

Pharmacy technicians normally process the prescription in the same fashion as in an outpatient pharmacy. After the patient information is input into the computer system, the order is filled. All auxiliary labels are attached if required and the medications must have a final check by the pharmacist. Once these medication orders are completed, they can either be sent back to the floor for the nurse to give to the patient or, if the drug is a controlled substance or a new medication for the patient, the nurse brings the patient down to receive the medications and be consulted by the pharmacist if necessary.

INVENTORY CONTROL TECHNICIAN

Description

Most hospitals have a technician who is in charge of maintaining stock levels and completing the special ordering of medications. The technician who orders the stock is responsible for the actual ordering, billing, and restocking of the pharmacy's shelves; however, it is a group effort in the pharmacy not to let stock levels drop to the point at which the stock person has to borrow items from another hospital or special order them at a higher cost. There are many methods of keeping stock at necessary levels. For instance, a hospital pharmacy may have ordering cards that are used to reorder stock when it is low. Each person is responsible for pulling the card (normally kept with the medications) and placing it in a designated area where the inventory technician can place the order. When the order arrives, the card is put back into the box along with the new stock. Another method uses bar codes that are read by a handheld device and electronically ordered. In this case, the inventory technician must visually check to see what needs to be ordered. A third alternative is when each item is tagged with a manufacturer's sticker as it arrives in the pharmacy. Stickers are provided by the manufacturer and must be adhered to each item before it is placed on the shelf. This sticker lists the stock number of the medication along with the price. When an item needs to be reordered, the sticker is taken off the container and placed on an ordering sheet. Medications may come from a warehouse or directly from the manufacturer. Either way, some medications must be ordered on an as-needed basis. This may be necessary because of short expiration dates and expense of medications.

Duties

The pharmacy runs out of drugs and supplies on a daily basis. Although pharmacies have different systems of ordering the medications, most orders normally are placed using a computer. Depending on where the warehouse or manufacturer is located, the turn-around time for the shipment may vary. For example, if a medication comes from across the country, then it must be ordered earlier than the drug that is simply sent over from the pharmacy warehouse (which usually takes less than 24 hours). Knowing the right time to order medications is a skill that pharmacy technicians must acquire; it is crucial to keep the pharmacy completely stocked with necessary medications.

When the shipment arrives, all included medications and supplies must be verified against the inventory list. It is important to initial and write *received* on each invoice. Some medications are backordered; these items are currently not in stock from the manufacturer but will be sent as soon as they are available. If the medication is one that cannot be left out of stock for any amount of time, it may be necessary to borrow from another pharmacy. This can be done by calling a pharmacist at a neighboring hospital and asking if that pharmacy has enough to share. A loan/borrow sheet is filled out and a taxi is normally sent to carry the medication from one location to the other. After the original ordered stock arrives, replacements for the borrowed items should be returned to the loaning pharmacy.

Placing stock onto the shelves is another important duty; it is the point at which the stock is rotated. Making sure that the later expiration dates are placed farthest back on the shelf ensures that the medications with the earliest expiration dates will be used first. The inventory technician is also responsible for returning damaged items and expired agents and handling recall items following the manufacturer's guidelines. Timing is probably one of the most important aspects of keeping inventory at a constant level. The technician can order appropriately if he or she learns the pharmacy's protocol for ordering and compensating for items that take longer to arrive, upcoming holidays, and patient load. In the winter and spring, there are typically more patients in the hospital. This directly relates to the types of heavily used agents as well as the overall increase in the use of medications.

Supplying Specialty Areas

There are several areas of a hospital in which the pharmacy must maintain a PAR level of medications. It is important that technicians recognize each of the abbreviations representing the units and clinics that require medication from the pharmacy; therefore a breakdown of each major area of a hospital is given in Box 11.1. The supplies kept on hand in these units are referred to as *floorstock*. The technician must be fully aware of the types of medications used in each of the following areas because each unit, ward, or clinic has its own special stock. Because of the specialty of each of the following areas, many pharmacies have special forms that are preprinted with complete descriptions of commonly used drugs. This helps to decrease the incidence of stock being sent to the wrong areas within the hospital. The pharmacy normally receives the supply ordering forms from the specialty areas daily. Although they are not a priority task, these orders should be filled before the end of the day. In addition, the technician may need to deliver the medications and check various areas of the hospital for any outdated medications. This task should be done on a monthly basis, preferably before the end of the month. Outdated medications normally can be returned to the pharmacy if they will expire within 3 months. Expired medications may be sent back to the manufacturer for credit (most manufacturers accept returned expired medications in batches of 100) or they may be taken away by an independent company and destroyed in a proper manner. This depends on the contract between the hospital and the manufacturer. Also, some hospitals contract

BOX 11.1 PRIMARY UNITS AND CLINICS THAT REQUIRE MEDICATION FROM PHARMACY

CCU	Coronary care unit
CLINICS	Patients may visit a clinic to be seen by a physician or nurse practitioner
ED	Area of hospital where patients can receive emergency care with doctors and nurses on staff 24 hours a day
ICU	Intensive care unit
L&D	Unit where mother goes through labor and delivers baby
MED	Medical unit for patients who have had surgery or who may be under observation
NICU	Neonatal intensive care unit
NSY	Nursery—unit where babies are taken for care and observation by nurses
OB/GYN	Unit that takes care of expectant mothers or those who have just had a baby
ONCOLOGY	Unit that takes care of patients with cancer
OR	Operating room
ORTHO	Orthopedics unit that takes care of patients that may need treatment or surgery on bones or joints
PACU	Postanesthesia care unit
PED	Unit for children younger than age 14 years
POST-OP	Unit where patient is kept after an operation or procedure
PRE-OP	Unit where patient is kept before an operation or procedure
UROLOGY	Unit that takes care of patients that may need treatment, surgery, or procedures on the urinary system

an outside company that specializes in drug inventory to come into the pharmacy periodically to document all expired medications before they are sent off to be destroyed.

Each department, such as the operating room (OR), postanesthesia care unit (PACU), wards, and clinics, is stocked with its own types of medications depending on what type of services it provides. Because of the many different areas throughout a hospital, the pharmacy must stock a wide variety of medications in different dosage forms. Therefore the pharmacy technician must have a good understanding of which medications are appropriate for each department. Departments such as the ED, OR, and ICU stock many drugs in injectable form and a wide variety of both oral and injectable controlled substances. Pediatrics uses many of the same medications that are used in the other departments, except in lower doses, as well as medications that are in suspension form. Labor and delivery (L&D) departments stock injectables and other drugs meant for labor, contractions, and cesarean births. The tasks of collecting and filling all floorstock medications are part of the daily routine of a technician. As always, it is necessary that all orders be verified and initialed by a pharmacist before they can be delivered to the correct departments.

Nonclinical Areas the Pharmacy Stocks

Nonclinic areas of a hospital can include areas that a patient never sees or those areas that are used as an in-and-out clinic. Some examples of these special areas of the hospital, along with the types of medications that the pharmacy may be responsible for ordering and stocking, are included in Box 11.2.

BOX 11.2 SPECIAL DEPARTMENTS STOCKED BY THE PHARMACY

Anesthesia	Doctors or nurse anesthesiologists who administer medications used before and throughout surgery
Respiratory	Therapists who administer breathing treatments to hospitalized patients
Injection clinic	Nurses administer both adult and pediatric immunizations and may also perform allergy skin tests
Radiology or imaging department	Technicians and physicians may administer dyes for imaging and may need to use a medication cart (known as crash cart) for adverse reactions or incidents

Patient Medication Filling

DESCRIPTION

One of the traditional roles of the pharmacy technician is filling the medication orders for patients. In the past, the most common way to provide a 24-hour supply of medications for the floors was to manually fill the patient medication drawer for each patient. Once the drawers were filled, the pharmacist verified them against the doctor's orders. The drawers were then taken to the floors where the patients were admitted. Nurses could then get their patients the necessary medication from this drawer. Medications were divided between routine medications, located in the front of the drawer, and as-needed (prn) medications, which were placed in the back of the drawer. Although some hospitals still use this system, more facilities are implementing automated dispensing systems. Not only do these systems speed up delivery of medication to the patient but also help to ensure accuracy. Some of the automated systems used in hospital settings include PYXIS, SUREMED, and Robot RX. Whereas the robot mechanically fills the drawers quickly and accurately, both PYXIS and SUREMED are machines that are preloaded with a variety of commonly used medications. The pharmacist needs only to type in the order and the nurse can then retrieve the medication on the patient's floor by using an access code. Although these systems seem to replace the technician, they require constant filling and updating of new medications on a daily basis. Technicians are now properly trained to use these sophisticated computer systems to fill patient prescriptions as well as to complete all other pharmacy duties.

TECH NOTE! Outpatient pharmacies have automated systems that quickly and accurately fill hundreds of prescriptions per day. Larger pharmacy distribution centers have systems that fill thousands of prescriptions per day.

DUTIES

All medications are delivered to the patient floors using two carts that are rotated daily. Before loading the patients' drawers with the next 24-hour supply, all previous medications should be emptied from the drawer. This is to decrease the possibility of errors. The front of the drawer contains the routine medications and the back contains the prn medications. Routine medications are those that have to be taken on a schedule everyday, whereas prn medications are those medications that can be taken if needed. For example, most acetaminophen (Tylenol) is ordered as a prn for headache or fever; therefore many prn medications are not used for more than one 24-hour period. All bulk items are normally sent to the floor labeled with the patient's name and room number; these items may be left in the drawer. Bulk items are those that last longer than 24 hours or medications that are not available in unit doses. For example, a bottle of medicated shampoo is a bulk item.

If the hospital uses an automated medication dispensing system, there is no need for a cart exchange. However, these systems do require regular and frequent fillings with new medications; the dispensers throughout the hospital must also be refilled. When a new medication is ordered it can be entered into the dispensing system's computer, which is located within the hospital. This is automatically prompted as the pharmacist or technician enters the order into the terminal.

A multiple-day supply is entered and delivered to the unit on the next scheduled round. For example, if a medication given once daily is ordered, a total of five or more doses may be stocked in the dispensing machine. This allows the nurses to access the medications they need without having to wait for the medication cart to arrive each day. All transactions made on a medication dispensing system are recorded and a receipt is generated. Only receipts for controlled medications are kept as records in the controlled substances room.

Controlled substances are also stocked in the dispensing machines on a daily basis. It is necessary to count the controlled substances stocked in the machine before adding additional doses. A receipt is generated by the machine after each entry and is electronically transmitted to the pharmacy computer system.

Pharmacy and Nursing Staff Relationship

The pharmacy staff probably works more with nurses than with anyone else in the hospital. Nurses depend on the pharmacy for all of their medications; they generally make more than 80% of the total calls that come into the inpatient pharmacy. The subjects of these phone calls include inquiries about the status of their patients' medications, as well as requests for information about drug interactions, dosing ranges, and pharmacy calculations. By far the most common question asked of the pharmacy is "Where are the medications that I ordered?" Any pharmacy technician can answer this question by simply checking either the computer system to see if the medication was sent or checking the orders that have not yet entered. However, for all other questions, the technician turns the phone over to the pharmacist. Good communication between the pharmacy and the nursing staff can alleviate a lot of anxiety.

TECH NOTE! Clearly identifying yourself as a technician when answering the phone immediately lets, callers know whether or not you can help them. This information prevents then from having to repeat a possibly lengthy question.

STAT and ASAP Orders

Medication orders that need to be filled within minutes are referred to as STAT orders. When the pharmacy receives a STAT order, it should take precedence over all other orders. Normally, a STAT order can be filled in 15 minutes, depending on the preparation time required for the medication. Some STAT orders can be filled quickly using stock off the shelf, whereas others may require special preparations, such as the mixing of an IV preparation. When this happens, the medication must be made as quickly as possible while using proper aseptic technique. STAT orders are those that can literally mean the difference between life and death; they must be taken seriously. If possible, a STAT order should be hand-delivered to ensure that it gets to the correct destination safely and quickly.

An ASAP order is not normally as urgent as a STAT order. However, these orders should be put in front of the new orders to ensure fast processing by the pharmacist.

Specialty Tasks

In addition to the previously outlined tasks that technicians commonly perform, there are additional duties that require the skills of a technician. These include assisting with clinical duties and anticoagulant therapy tasks. Some hospitals that have nuclear pharmacies are using technicians to handle nuclear medications. These agents may be used in diagnostic procedures. As the role of the pharmacy continues to change, so will the tasks of the pharmacy technician.

DO YOU REMEMBER THESE KEY POINTS?

- Duties of a pharmacy technician, including the areas described in this chapter
- How often medications are supplied to nursing units using a cart-filling method
- Steps in and frequency of filling automated medication dispensing systems
- The difference between a centralized pharmacy and a satellite pharmacy
- Duties involved in ordering and maintaining the pharmacy's stock levels
- Hospital areas that the pharmacy stocks
- Specialty areas of the hospital for which the pharmacy stocks or orders medication
- Abbreviations of units located within a hospital and the types of service they provide
- What PAR levels are and who is responsible for maintaining them
- Different types of hospitals, what differentiates them from one another, and how that affects the overall service that they may provide
- Which agencies monitor hospitals, including pharmacies within the hospital
- The various ways that orders are processed by the pharmacy

REVIEW QUESTIONS:

Multiple Choice

1. Policies and procedures binders contain information pertaining to all of the following except
- A. Employees' weekly schedule
- B. Emergency situations
- C. Training
- D. Daily work routines

2. JCAHO is an agency that inspects and accredits
- A. Hospitals
- B. Hospital pharmacies
- C. Pharmacists
- D. Both A and B

3. Hospital orders contain which of the following information?
- A. Laboratory orders
- B. Dietary restrictions
- C. Medications
- D. All of the above

4. All of the following information is necessary on a doctor's order except
- A. Patient's name
- B. Patient's room
- C. Patient's next of kin
- D. Patient's medical record number

5. Hospital technicians must be available to
- A. Work various shifts
- B. Work weekends
- C. Fill different jobs per operational needs
- D. All of the above

6. Technicians have all of the following responsibilities except
   A. Printing IV labels before filling them
   B. Preparing antibiotics
   C. Discontinuing IV medications per doctor's orders
   D. Calling the doctor for order clarification

7. By law, which of the following tasks cannot be done by a technician?
   A. Ordering pharmacy stock
   B. Filling chemotherapy orders
   C. Filling controlled substance orders for Schedules III-V medications
   D. Final checking and sign-off of orders

8. The following areas are stocked by the pharmacy except
   A. Respiratory therapy
   B. ED
   C. Central supply
   D. Injection clinic

9. Technicians can answer which of the following questions over the phone?
   A. Generic or trade name of drug
   B. Whether or not the drug is in stock
   C. If the drug order has been filled and sent to the floor
   D. All of the above

10. The differences between IV therapy and chemotherapy parenteral preparation include all of the following except
    A. The type of flow hood used
    B. Hand placement
    C. Size of the hood
    D. Aseptic technique

True/False

*If the statement is false, then change it to make it true.

1. Protocol is policy that is set by the pharmacist on duty.
2. Hospitals must meet both state and federal guidelines if they are to be reimbursed.
3. Orders written by doctors in a hospital setting are not the same as prescriptions.
4. Medications are normally placed in see-through zip-lock containers for security reasons only.
5. Only pharmacists can fill orders that are received from the hospital floors.
6. Technicians need to use aseptic technique only in the chemotherapy hood.
7. A PAR level refers to the pharmacy's location and capabilities within the hospital.
8. All units within a hospital have the same floorstock to treat patients.
9. Technicians cannot answer any questions that nurses direct to the pharmacy.
10. It is best to identify yourself as a technician when first answering the phone.

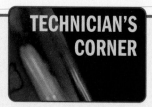

TECHNICIAN'S CORNER

While in the pharmacy, you get an order for Ms. Jen Baranowski. Only her name and her room number are written on the order. The order is for ceftriaxone 1 g q6h. This is not the appropriate dosing regimen for this medication.

What information must you have before you can process this order?

What do you do concerning the wrong dosing times for this medication?

REFERENCE

Ansel H, Allen LV, Popovich NG: *Pharmaceutical dosage forms and drug delivery systems,* ed 7, Baltimore, 1999, Lippincott Williams & Wilkins.

12

Repackaging and Compounding

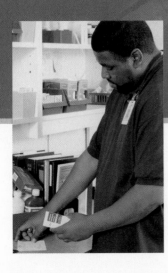

Objectives

- List the steps in repackaging medications.
- Describe the proper handling of medications when repackaging.
- Describe the way in which ointments or creams should be packed into jars.
- List the requirements for assigning expiration dates for unit dose medication.
- Explain the calculations used to determine expiration dates when repackaging.
- List the common reasons behind using unit dose medications.
- Define terms used in compounding procedures.
- Describe the equipment used in compounding drugs.
- Differentiate between types of scales used to weigh compounds.
- Explain the correct methods in preparing and clean-up of compounding areas.

Blister packs *Containers usually made of plastic that hold a single-dose tablet or capsule*

Bulk compounding *A larger quantity of medication that can fill a large order at one time or several smaller orders in the future*

Calibration *The markings on a measuring device*

Compounding *The act of mixing, reconstituting, and packaging a drug*

Cream *A hydrophilic base*

Elixir *A base solution that is a mixture of alcohol and water*

FDA *Food and Drug Administration*

Hydrophilic *Water loving; any substance that easily dissolves into water*

Hydrophobic *Water hating; any substance that does not dissolve in water*

Mortar and pestle *A bowl and rounded knob used to grind substances into fine powder*

Ointment *A hydrophobic product such as Vaseline*

Reconstitution *To mix a liquid and a powder to form a suspension or solution*

Repackaging *The act of reducing the amount of medication taken from a bulk bottle; unit dosing is a form of repackaging*

Solute *The ingredient that is dissolved into a solution*

Solution *A water base in which the ingredient(s) dissolve completely*

Solvent *The greater part of a solution*

Suspension *A solution in which solid particles do not dissolve into the base and must be shaken before using*

Syrup *A sugar-based liquid*

Tincture *A base solution of alcohol*

Unit dose *A single dose of a drug*

Introduction

Repacking medication is common in a hospital pharmacy, whereas compounding nonsterile products is more common in a community pharmacy. Because some of the same rules apply for both repackaging and compounding drug products, this chapter covers both of these skills. Repackaging, also called unit dosing, is discussed first, and nonsterile compounding is discussed in the second half of the chapter.

Repackaging

The U.S. Food and Drug Administration (FDA) is responsible for providing guidelines for all manufacturers that package medications. Expiration dates are determined based on tests run by manufacturers and the FDA; however, these rules do not apply to medications repackaged in a hospital setting for individual patient use. The expiration date for repackaging products is set by each state. Items repackaged for use within a hospital or for a specific patient's use cannot be mass-produced. Manufacturing drug companies following FDA guidelines are in the business of mass production. Following are five reasons that a pharmacy repackages a bulk drug into unit dose medications:

1. Certain drugs cannot be bought from a manufacturer prepackaged in unit dose strips. The pharmacy must make its own.
2. The cost of unit dosing certain medications may be cheaper when done by the hospital than if purchased from a manufacturer.
3. Because of the packaging, both speed and efficiency is increased.
4. Because of the label on each dose of drug, the chance of errors is decreased.
5. If unit dose medication is not used, it can be put back into stock and used for another patient at a later time.

Whatever the reason, unit dosing makes sense. By using unit dose medications, a hospital saves a substantial amount of money per patient. Although packaging guidelines are not exactly the same between hospital pharmacies and manufacturers, good manufacturing practices are used by both. Good manufacturing practices are FDA guidelines designed to guarantee safe and effective products for the consumer. Some of the guidelines that the hospital technician and pharmacist should follow are listed in Box 12.1.

DRUGS AND LABELS

The dosage forms of drugs that are normally repackaged in a pharmacy include tablets, capsules, and liquids. Tablets may be cut in half and repackaged per protocol.

Many different types of computer labeling programs are used to generate unit dose labels in the pharmacy. It is usually the responsibility of the pharmacy technician to determine not only which drugs are needed to replenish the pharmacy stock but also to calculate the correct expiration date, document the essential components of the drug, generate the labels, and load the medication (Figure 12.1). Finally, the pharmacist checks the completed work to ensure that the label, drug, and logging of the medication are correct.

BOX 12.1 EXAMPLE OF GOOD MANUFACTURING PRACTICE GUIDELINES

Item	Guidelines
Drugs and labels	All medications must be checked by a registered pharmacist
Equipment	In good condition and clean
Expiration date	6 months or $\frac{1}{4}$ of the time of the drug's manufacturing date, whichever is less (recently updated to a maximum of 1 year of the manufacturer's expiration date or, if manufacturer's date is less than 1 year, then that date may be given). The bulk container may not have been previously opened
Package	Appropriate for the drug
Preparation	Not more than one item prepared at a time
Records	All items repackaged logged for referencing

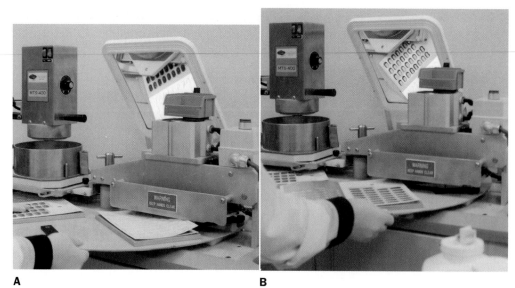

A   **B**

FIGURE 12.1 A technician is responsible for the proper preparation and labeling of all repackaged medications. **A,** The empty medication card is rotated under the hopper where the medication is placed into the card and then rotated to the heating element where the seal is made to enclose each tablet. **B,** A mirror is used by the technician to verify that each sheet is completely filled.

EQUIPMENT

Types of unit dosing equipment vary. Some packaging machines not only fill the unit dose containers but also may generate labels for the drugs as well as adhere them to the containers as they pass through. Others are much less high-tech, and the technician manually places each tablet or capsule into the individual blister pack and adheres the labels. The process of repackaging should take place in a designated area of the pharmacy, away from high-use areas. All equipment should be kept clean and in good condition. If the technician is using manual methods to load medications into blister packs, it is important that gloves are worn after washing hands. If pill counters are used to guide tablets or capsules into their containers, the tray should be washed after each use.

TECH NOTE! Cleaning counting trays after each use is for the protection of the next patient. If residue is left behind on the pill counter and the next patient is allergic to the previously counted medication, it is possible for that patient to have an allergic reaction. When chemotherapy medication is counted, a tray marked for counting chemotherapy should be used to avoid cross-contamination.

In addition to pill counters, all equipment should be cleaned after use following manufacturer's guidelines. Keeping the area clean and well-organized helps avoid contamination of drugs and reduces the chance of error when repacking.

EXPIRATION DATE

Assigning the expiration date of a repackaged medication is a simple yet extremely important process. Once a bulk bottle is opened, the manufacturer's expiration date is no longer valid. The correct length of time is determined by calculating the new expiration date from the bulk medication. One common and simple way of dating drugs is to set the expiration date at the end of the month. For example, when you are preparing a label for a drug that you have determined will expire at the end of September 2002, you would write 9/02. It is assumed that the drug is good through the month of September. Because laws change concerning appropriate expiration dating, two methods are outlined in this chapter; your specific state's requirements will determine the method used.

Method 1

The life of a repacked drug is 6 months or one fourth of the manufacturer's expiration date, whichever is less. The best way to determine this number is by determining the number of months that the drug is good for and divide by 4. This gives the exact amount of time the drug is in date. However, if that answer is more than 6 months, the expiration date is set at the least amount of time, 6 months. The examples provided shows the calculations for proper dating.

EXAMPLE 12.1 EXPIRATION DATING (6-MONTH VERSION)

Cimetidine 300 mg tablet
Expires in August 2007

Today's date: August 2003
Calculation: 4 years × 12 months = 48 months ÷ 4
= 12 months

Because the calculated time exceeds 6 months, the 6-month rule is used; the product expires in 2/04.

Method 2

The medication is given a maximum of 1 year as long as it does not exceed the safety margin given by the drug company. If the medication expires in 6 months, then 6 months is the maximum allowable expiration date. For example, a drug that expires in 5 years can be given only 1 year if the drug company's data supports its safety. The bottom line is to remember that the most important aspect of determining the proper expiration date is documentation.

EXAMPLE 12.2 EXPIRATION DATING (¼ OF THE MANUFACTURER'S TIME)

Acetaminophen 500 mg tablets
Expires in December 2004

Today's date: August 2003
Calculation: 8/03 to 12/04 = 16 months ÷ 4
= 4 months

Because the calculated date is less than 6 months, you may only give the acetaminophen 4 months, or until 12/03.

PACKAGES

The types of packages used in pharmacy include liquid cups, vials, blister packs, zip-lock bags, and light-resistant bags (Figure 12.2). Each type of container

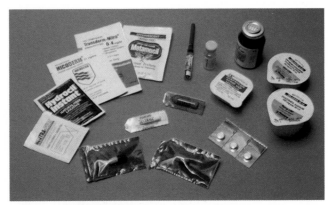

FIGURE 12.2 A sample of containers.

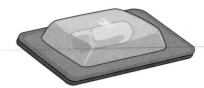

FIGURE 12.3 A sample of a blister pack container.

holds specific amounts and types of medications. Liquids are normally placed in bottles, cups, or vials. Tablets and capsules are usually placed in blister packs (Figure 12.3) or vials.

PREPARATION

The preparation required to repackage medications is relatively simple. If tablets or capsules are to be made, the main task is to have enough packages and labels ready for use. In addition to these supplies, keeping medications separate from one another is extremely important. Only one item at a time should be made because leaving multiple drugs on a countertop leads to errors. Part of the preparation of repackaging is accurate calculations for expiration dates and logging the medications to be prepared in a logbook. There are two common types of repackaged medications:

1. Unit dose: One medication per container
2. Monthly supply: Typically 30-day supply; packaged for long-term care facilities

RECORDS

Keeping track of the products that you are repackaging is one of the major steps that should not be overlooked. Just as manufacturers must know how to find drugs they have packaged, so must the hospital pharmacy. For instance, if a manufacturer recalled a drug that had been repackaged, it is important to have an accurate count of how many unit doses were made and an identifying mark on each of them. Therefore documentation for repackaged drugs must have the information shown in Box 12.2.

Compounding

Nonsterile compounding consists of compounding medications on a countertop in a pharmacy setting (Figure 12.4). Sterile compounding is discussed in Chapter 13. The most common items made in pharmacies are creams, ointments, and oral suspensions. Less common drugs that can be made include capsules, suppositories, and syringes. Only the most common compounding techniques are discussed in this chapter. Common compounding guidelines followed in pharmacies are listed in Box 12.3.

EQUIPMENT

Compounding in the pharmacy requires many different pieces of equipment. Common types of equipment are listed in Box 12.4. One of the most expensive pieces is the balance or scale used to weigh powders. Scales differ in their range of weight and style. A class A balance (Figure 12.7A) weighs lighter substances between 120 mg and 15 g, whereas a class B balance weighs heavier substances ranging from 650 mg to 120 g. Each scale has special weights that are labeled in milligrams or grams. When placing counterweights on the balance, the

BOX 12.2 EXAMPLE OF A RECORD LOG SHEET USED FOR DOCUMENTATION

Item	Description
Date	The date that the drug is made, which includes day, month, and year
Drug	Drug name, usually by generic name then brand name if indicated on log sheet
Dosage form	Tablet, capsule, spansule, troche, liquid, etc
Manufacturer	Manufacturer of the drug, usually abbreviated
Manufacturer's lot number	Control number located on the side of the label or on the bottom of the bottle
Manufacturer's expiration date	Located with the lot number; remember that if the date indicates only month and year, the drug is good through the end of the month
Pharmacy lot number	Each item repackaged in the pharmacy is given a number consecutive to the previously made batch
Pharmacy expiration date	Calculate the new expiration date, which is 6 months or ¼ of the time of the manufacturer's expiration date, whichever is less
Technician	Must initial the logbook entry
Pharmacist	Each item made must be checked off by a pharmacist

The information on the label of the unit dose item is much less than what is required in the logbook, but it is just as important. The following sample lists the components necessary on a typical unit dose label:

    Name of drug
        Generic name
        Trade name (trade name commonly given for the easy identification of the proper medication)
    Strength
    Dosage form
    Pharmacy lot number
    Pharmacy expiration date

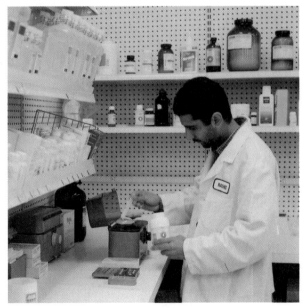

FIGURE 12.4 Technician using a class A or class III balance. Each dial must be set accurately for precise measurement.

BOX 12.3 EXAMPLE OF COMMON COMPOUNDING GUIDELINES

Item	Appropriateness
Equipment	In good condition and clean
Preparation	Not more than one item to be prepared at a time
Drugs and labels	All medications checked by a registered pharmacist
Package	All containers appropriate for each drug compounded
Expiration date	Cannot be longer than the expiration date of any of the ingredients used to prepare agent
Weighing	All ingredients must be weighed on a pharmacy balance
Meniscus	The concave upper surface of a liquid in a container. Measurement must be read at the bottom of the meniscus (see Figure 12.8)

BOX 12.4 COMMON TYPES OF EQUIPMENT USED IN COMPOUNDING

Types of Mortar and Pestles	Use
Glass	Mixing porous liquids, suspensions, or substances that may stain other containers
Porcelain	Blending powders

Other Compounding Station Equipment	Use
Filter paper	Used under compounding product to be weighed or as a filter in a funnel
Glycine paper	Used under compounding product to be weighed
Beakers/graduate	A calibrated measuring container used for liquids
Glass stir sticks	Used to stir products such as suspensions
Glass compounding slab	Smooth surface on which to mix ointments and creams
Spatulas	For mixing and filling jars
Blender	For mixing larger products or those that require high-speed or prolonged low-speed blending
Funnel	For filtering or pouring liquids into smaller bottles
Sink	For washing hands, equipment, and countertop
Solvents	For cleaning

technician must never touch the weights because the oils from his or her hands corrode the metals, which changes the correct weight. Both class A and B balances are mechanical, using independent weights for reference. Another style of balance is the electronic balance that has a digital readout of the weight. No weights are used with this balance; instead the calibrations are electronic. In either case, appropriate care and cleaning of these sensitive instruments is a must.

Graduate cylinders (Figure 12.5) come in conical and cylindrical shapes to measure liquids. When measuring liquids in a graduate, the meniscus must be read for correct measurement.

In addition to proper balances and cylinders, other pieces of equipment commonly used are a mortar and pestle, which are needed to crush tablets and other solid substances into a fine powder to be mixed with other ingredients (Figure 12.6). Mortars and pestles are made of two different substances, glass and porcelain.

If the items that need to be compounded require specialized equipment, often the pharmacy orders the product from another pharmacy that specializes in compounding products.

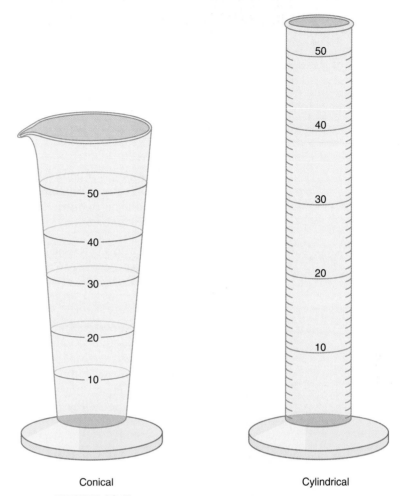

Conical   Cylindrical

FIGURE 12.5 Graduate cylinders for liquid measurement.

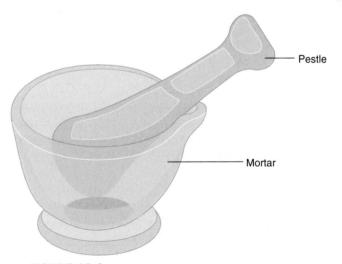

Pestle

Mortar

FIGURE 12.6 Mortar and pestle used to crush solids.

PREPARATION

Most pharmacies have a countertop station set aside for compounding products. At this station all necessary equipment for compounding is kept so it is readily available. It is the responsibility of the technician who will be preparing the compounds to make sure that all items are clean and in good working order. Before compounding, be sure your state allows compounding by a pharmacy technician. Long hair should be tied back, a lab coat should be worn, and gloves may be helpful in reducing contamination of the product. In addition to these personal considerations, a technician who is sick or has any open wounds should not make any compounding products. Only one compounding product should be made at a time to decrease the possibility of errors. For commonly compounded items, a recipe book or formula cards may be used to guide the technician, listing compounds, their weights, and step-by-step instructions.

TECH NOTE! Read all instructions before beginning to compound materials. Make sure that all the ingredients are available to avoid a delay in the product preparation. It is also important to reorder stock after ingredients are depleted so that the ingredients are available for the next time.

Additional ingredients that many pharmacies have in stock help reduce the bad taste of a drug and make them look more palatable. Sweeteners for taste, flavorings for smell, and colorings are among the main ingredients of a compounding area. In Box 12.5 is a list of the common additives.

If you have any questions on how to prepare a product, ask the pharmacist at the beginning of the compounding process, not in the middle. The only type of compounding that may be done away from the compounding area is the reconstitution of oral suspensions. These products are simple to prepare and do not need to be logged or labeled in the same manner as compounded products.

DRUGS AND LABELS

When reconstituting drugs such as amoxicillin suspension, the label is already attached to the product. All the technician must do is read the side panel and follow the directions for the proper amount of sterile water to be mixed with the powder. The expiration date is clearly marked on the side and is effective as soon as the suspension is mixed. Therefore after mixing the drug you must mark down the expiration date on the front of the label for the patient. In addition to this information, any necessary auxiliary labels must be attached. Common auxiliary labels are listed in Box 12.6.

When reconstituting a suspension, if the manufacturer calls for 110 ml of sterile water to be mixed with the powder in the bottle, you should only add one half of the water at first. This allows the powder to mix with the water, which brings down the volume within the bottle and makes it easier to mix in the remaining amount.

PACKAGING

The types of containers that are used for compounded products must be appropriate. The container must protect the contents, have a child resistant cap (if

BOX 12.5 COMMON ADDITIVES FOR TASTE AND APPEARANCE

Ingredient	Used in
Vanilla, berry	Antibiotics, antihistamines, barbiturates
Lemon	Decongestants
Grape	Electrolytes, antihistamines

BOX 12.6 COMMON AUXILIARY LABELS PLACED ON MEDICATION CONTAINERS

Dosage Form	Type of Auxiliary Label
Suspensions	Shake well
Ophthalmics	For the eye
Otics	For the ear
Ointments, creams, lotions	For topical use; for external use
Suppositories	For rectal use; for vaginal use

TABLE 12.1 Capsules Sizes

Number	Approximate Amount Contained	Example
000	1000 mg	
00	750 mg	
0	500 mg	
1	400 mg	
2	300 mg	
3	200 mg	
4	150 mg	
5	100 mg	

applicable), and have the appropriate label(s). Once mixed to the proper concentration, all products are filled into the appropriately sized container. This should be done neatly to avoid waste. Containers vary in size and in manufactured materials, depending on the use of the drug. In addition to the more traditional containers, such as bottles and jars, capsules, suppositories, and syringes are also used. Although capsules are normally acquired from the manufacturer, if a physician writes an order for a compound not available by a manufacturer, the pharmacy may have to make the capsules. There are eight sizes of capsules; each holds a different amount of drug that is measured in milligrams as shown in Table 12.1.

Syringes are sometimes used to prepare vaginal compounds. Once the drug is loaded into the barrel of the syringe, a cap is placed over the top to keep the contents inside. Suppositories are rarely made in most pharmacies because of the time required. When they are prepared, either plastic or metal molds are used to shape the suppositories. The base ingredient of a suppository is usually a combination of cocoa butter, wax and mineral oil that holds its shape until it reaches body temperature at which the drug can be released. Once the suppositories harden in the mold, they can be wrapped, packaged, and labeled for dispensing. Other containers used to package compounded products include glass and plastic bottles, dropper bottles, and jars of various sizes. Jars and syringes are the only two packages that do not have childproof caps or lids.

EXPIRATION DATES

There are several factors that affect the stability of a drug. The amount of light, air, temperature, and even pH alters the longevity of a drug. Legally, the date given to a pharmacy-prepared product cannot be longer than any of the ingredients in the product. It is up to the pharmacist or the pharmacy technician to find the appropriate expiration date from the manufacturer's literature. In addition to this reference, there are many compounding books available that contain calculations that determine appropriate expiration dates.

RECORDS

Just as in repackaging, documentation of compounded medications is extremely important. By keeping accurate records, the integrity of the product dispensed is ensured and falls within FDA guidelines under quality assurance. Although protocol varies between hospital settings, all recipe information is copied to show the step-by-step approach taken by the technician. Along with the recipe, the following information is documented:

> Date prepared
> Name of ingredients
> Manufacturer of each ingredient
> Lot number and expiration date of each ingredient (this includes sterile water container, if used)
> Amount or weight of each ingredient
> Dosage form of each ingredient
> Pharmacy lot number assigned
> Pharmacy expiration date assigned
> Technician's initials
> Pharmacist's initials
> Date dispensed
> Patient's name and medical record number

Documents are kept on the pharmacy premises for no less than 3 years from the time the medication was prepared. The following information is necessary on the label of the compounded product:

> Name of patient and medical record number
> Date
> Drug
> Doctor
> Sig: Directions
> Pharmacy lot and expiration date
> Initials of technician and pharmacist

Once the label is affixed to the container, all necessary auxiliary labels should be chosen. Many auxiliary labels, such as the following, not only tell the patient what the intended use for the product is but also indicate the appropriate storage requirements. In addition, there are labels that allow for expiration dates to be written in:

> Refrigerate
> This drug expires in ___ days
> For topical use only

WEIGHING

The components of a typical balance in a pharmacy include paper and weights. In the container that holds the weights is a pair of tweezers for grasping the metal

BOX 12.7 INSTRUCTIONS FOR USING A CLASS A BALANCE

The balance must be steadied on the counter. There are adjustable legs on every balance.

Lightweight papers are then added to both sides of the balances to protect the weighing plates and to hold the substance being weighed.

The balance must be "zeroed out" to prevent the paper being included in the weight of the drug.

At this point the counterweight can be placed on the right side of the balance.

Once the weight is in place, the balance must be set to the proper weight.

The substance to be measured can then be placed on the opposite plate until the two plates balance.

weights. This is to prevent the oils from the hands getting onto the metal. Oils corrode the metal, altering the exact weight of the metal. Each balance also has an arrest knob that is used to lock the scale in place, reducing the chance of damage to the balance. There are six steps for the proper setup of a balance; each one is critical to obtain the proper weight of a substance. The balance instrument guides are shown in Box 12.7, and a typical scale is shown in Figure 12.7.

TECH NOTE! Always place the weights on the right side of the balance. This is done to ensure continuity of measurement.

MEASURING TECHNIQUES

Pharmacy balances are very sensitive. Regardless of the substance that you are measuring, it is important to keep the air flow around the balance to a minimum. Even the motion of a person walking by can set the balance into a rocking motion, making calibration very difficult. Pharmacy balances have a glass lid that can be used to cut off air currents, but it cannot be used easily while weighing compounds. As the balance begins to come into balance, it is important to add less and less substance to the balance. One way of doing this is to use a spatula and pick up a small amount of substance, then lightly tap the side of the spatula (from behind the substance) to flick on a few granules at a time. This technique is easier with powders than with other substances. Compounding is time consuming. It is important to keep the goal of accuracy in mind at all times. Thus you must take your time. Rushing to prepare a compound is a recipe for disaster.

Measuring liquids requires a few simple steps to ensure the proper volume. Because of the water molecules clinging to the sides of a container (called capillary action), the amount of liquid appears to be more than the actual amount. When reading the calibrations of a beaker or graduate you must have the liquid at eye level. You must read the graduated cylinder at the bottom of the liquid line, also known as the meniscus as shown in Figure 12.8.

When choosing a vehicle to measure your liquids in, remember that it is best to choose the container size closer to the volume required because the calibrations are more accurate than in larger containers.

COMPOUNDING TECHNIQUES

Depending on the type of product being prepared, different techniques are required. If an ointment is prepared, a hydrophobic base such as petroleum jelly is mixed with the drug. For preparing creams, hydrophilic bases such as Eucerin or Aquaphor

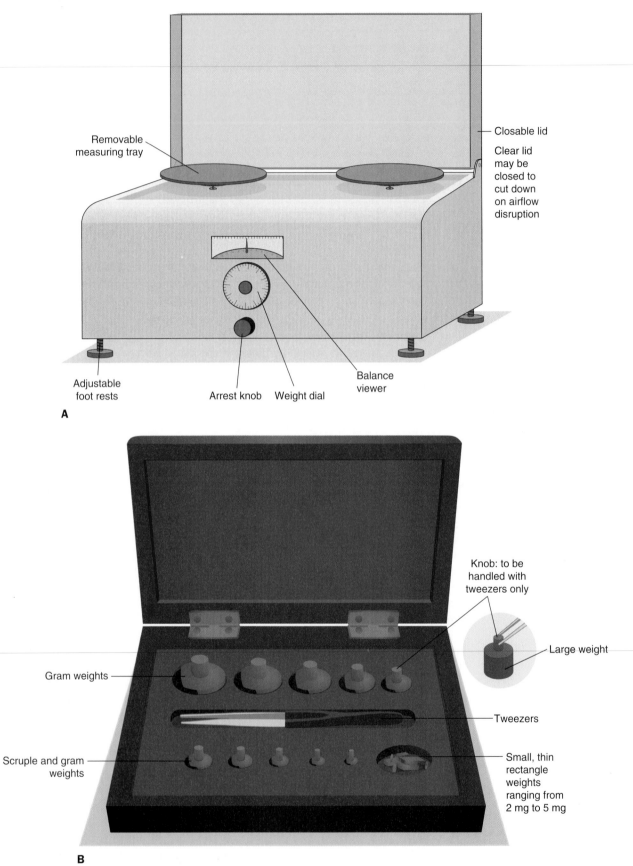

Removable
measuring tray

Closable lid

Clear lid
may be
closed to
cut down
on airflow
disruption

Adjustable
foot rests

Arrest knob   Weight dial

Balance
viewer

A

Knob: to be
handled with
tweezers only

Large weight

Gram weights

Tweezers

Scruple and gram
weights

Small, thin
rectangle
weights
ranging from
2 mg to 5 mg

B

FIGURE 12.7 A, Class A balance. **B,** Pharmaceutical weights.

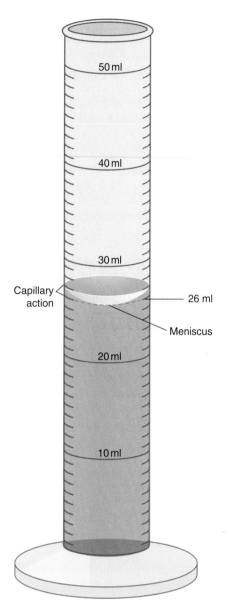

FIGURE 12.8 A 50 ml graduate showing the meniscus and proper measurement of solutions.

creams are used. To prepare a simple mixture of 2.5% hydrocortisone cream in a 50-g Dermabase, follow these steps:

1. Use a mortar and pestle to crush the tablets or coarse granules into a fine powder for mixture.
2. After both the base and drug are properly weighed, place the base on the center of a glass compounding slab. A small amount of glycerin may be added to the powder (levigated) to help it mix with the base more easily.
3. Slowly add the powdered drug to the base using a spatula to mix the two components well.
4. Once mixed thoroughly, the spatula is again used to fill the medication jar. As the jar is being filled, periodically tap the jar on the counter to compact the contents.
5. When the jar is filled, place the spatula flat across the top of the contents and slowly turn the jar to level off the top and give the final product a professional look.

When preparing capsules, the punch method is commonly used. This involves keeping the thickness of the powder in the middle of the compounding slab about one third of the length of the capsule. Then push the opened capsule into the powder, fill the entire capsule with powder, and then attach the other half of the capsule. As you can imagine, this technique is slow and arduous; therefore most pharmacies order capsules to be prepared by a compounding pharmacy. There are machines that load capsules quickly and accurately, saving the pharmacy staff hours of compounding the more difficult drugs.

When preparing solutions, you must understand the major parts of the liquid: the solvent is the larger part of the overall solution, the solute is the ingredient or agent used within the solvent, and the solution is the final dosage form that results from these two types. Most solutions are simply mixed by either adding the solute to the solvent in portions for proper mixing or by adding two solutions together. One of the most important techniques of mixing solutions is to measure carefully and mix thoroughly. Always check the final solution for any possible precipitation or discoloration that indicates a bad ingredient.

TECH NOTE! When orders indicate a solution to be a specific strength then to "qs" the solution to a final volume, this means that after the proper strength is prepared the solution is to be topped off with the additive liquid (such as sterile water) to yield a final volume as ordered by the physician.

Suspensions are different than solutions because they mix a hydrophobic (not water-soluble) ingredient into a hydrophilic (water-soluble) solution. For example, in the case of an amoxicillin suspension, the powdered ingredient is suspended in sterile water after mixing. Therefore all suspensions must be shaken well to evenly mix the powder, which can then deliver the proper amount of medication.

TECH NOTE! Most suspensions should be mixed by adding $\frac{1}{2}$ of the additive solution to the powder, mixing well, and then adding the remaining solution. This ensures thorough mixing. Remember to add the "SHAKE WELL" auxiliary label to the bottle.

DO YOU REMEMBER THESE KEY POINTS?

- The proper steps to follow when repackaging medication
- The documentation necessary for repackaged and compounded products
- The proper steps to follow when compounding a product
- The various types of scales that are used in compounding
- How expiration dates are determined when repackaging
- Why pharmacies repackage products
- The various types of equipment used in packaging medications
- The sizes of capsules used in compounding
- Common auxiliary labels used on compounded products
- The various types of containers used in compounding products

REVIEW QUESTIONS:

Multiple Choice

1. Of the reasons listed, which is not a common reason for repackaging medication?
   A. Cost effectiveness
   B. More competitive against other hospitals
   C. Reusable
   D. Reduction of errors

2. The best description of the guidelines for assigning an expiration date of a repackaged drug is
   A. Half of the manufacturer's expiration date
   B. Less than the manufacturer's date
   C. One fourth of the manufacturer's expiration date or 6 years, whichever is less
   D. One fourth of the manufacturer's expiration date or 6 months, whichever is less

3. Keeping a compounding area clean ensures
   A. Avoidance of contamination of the products
   B. Less chance of errors
   C. Ability to mix several medications at the same time
   D. Both A and B

4. Using the 6-month expiration dating method, determine the expiration date of a drug to be unit dosed that has a manufacturer's expiration date of 3/05. If today's date is 2/02, the drug will expire in
   A. 6/02   C. 3/03
   B. 8/02   D. 3/04

5. Of the information listed, which is not required to be logged into a repack logbook?
   A. The date the drug was made
   B. The patient's name
   C. The initials of the pharmacist
   D. The pharmacy lot number

6. The type of balance(s) that can accurately weigh 10 g of powder is(are)
   A. Class A   C. Both A and B
   B. Class B   D. None of the above

7. The type of mortar and pestle that is best used for grinding coarse granules into a fine powder is(are)
   A. Glass   C. China
   B. Porcelain   D. All of the above

8. A meniscus is best described as
   A. A beaker filled with a small amount of water
   B. Water molecules attaching to the sides of a container
   C. A container used to measure very small amounts of liquid
   D. The lowest level of liquid, which is the point that should be used to measure

9. The arrest knob on a balance is used to
   A. Measure the weight of a compound
   B. Balance the feet of the balance
   C. Adjust the balance's weights
   D. Lock the balance

10. A _____ base is used to prepare an ointment.
    A. Water   C. Hydrophobic
    B. Hydrophilic   D. None of the above

True/False

*If the statement is false, then change it to make it true.

1. Good manufacturing practices is a set of hospital standards on the practices of compounding medications.

2. If gloves are worn for repackaging, washing hands is not necessary.

3. A unit dose medication delivers only one dose of a drug.

4. When compounding, it is better to always place the weights on the same side of the scale.

5. Spatulas are commonly used for mixing and for loading compounds into jars.

6. Most pharmacies have recipe books for compounded products.

7. When compounding, it is not necessary to document the expiration date of water.

8. All mortar and pestles are used for the same purpose.

9. Tapping a jar of cream or ointment eliminates smoothing out the top of the compounded product.

10. A bulk bottle refers to a compounded or repackaged product made in a pharmacy.

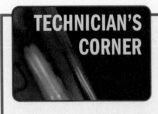

TECHNICIAN'S CORNER

You receive an order for 2.5% hydrocortisone cream in 50 g. You have 2.5% HC powder and Dermabase in stock.

What is the strength of the hydrocortisone used (in grams)?
How much Dermabase do you need to equal a total volume of 50 g?
What documentation is required for these items?
What would you place on the label (include auxiliary labels needed)?

BIBLIOGRAPHY

Allen L: *The art, science, and technology of pharmaceutical compounding,* Washington, DC, 2002, American Pharmaceutical Association.

Ansel HC, Allen LV, Popovich NG: *Pharmaceutical dosage forms and drug delivery systems,* ed 7, Baltimore, 1999, Lippincott Williams & Wilkins.

Shargel L, Mutnick A, Souney P, et al: *Comprehensive pharmacy review,* ed 4. Baltimore, 2001, Lippincott Williams & Wilkins.

CHAPTER

13
Aseptic Technique

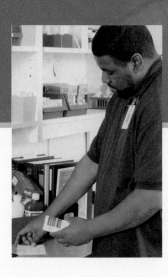

Objectives

■ List the sizes of syringes and needles used in the pharmacy setting.

■ Describe how often hoods must be inspected.

■ Describe how to properly care for laminar flow hoods.

■ Explain the use of aseptic technique within a horizontal flow hood.

■ List the types of stock used within an intravenous (IV) room.

■ Explain the differences between total parenteral nutrition (TPN) and peripheral parenteral nutrition (PPN).

■ Describe how to properly dispose of needles, vials, and cytotoxic supplies.

■ Describe how to prepare and transport medications in syringes.

■ List the medications that must be placed in glass containers.

■ Describe aseptic technique within a vertical flow hood.

■ List various containers used in the laminar flow hood.

**TERMS
AND
DEFINITIONS**

Aseptic technique *The procedures used to eliminate the possibility of a drug becoming contaminated with microbes or particles*

Gauge *The size of the needle opening*

Horizontal flow hood *Environment for the preparation of sterile products that uses air originating from the back of the hood moving forward across the hood out into the room*

Hyperalimentation *Parenteral nutrition for persons unable to eat*

Laminar flow hood *Environment for the preparation of sterile products*

Parenterals *Medications administered by injection, such as intravenously or intramuscularly*

Peripheral parenteral *Injection of a medication into the veins located on the periphery of the body system instead of a central vein or artery*

Total parenteral nutrition *Large-volume IV nutrition administered through the central vein (subclavian vein), which allows for a higher concentration of solutions*

Universal precautions *A set of standards that lowers the possibility of contamination; used to prepare medications*

Vertical flow hood *Environment for preparation of chemotherapy treatments that uses air originating from the roof of the hood moving downward that is captured in a vent located on the floor of the hood*

Introduction

One of the most crucial responsibilities a hospital pharmacy technician has is the proper preparation of parenteral medications. It is extremely important that all parenteral medications are prepared in a manner that reduces the possibility of contamination. This is possible only through the proper manipulation of materials used within the hood. All parenteral and ophthalmic medications should be prepared within a laminar flow hood. There are various sizes and types of hoods available; all are capable of keeping out bacteria and other unwanted particulates if the technician uses proper aseptic technique.

The pharmacy technician may prepare sterile products in settings such as a pharmacy as part of a home health service and pharmacies in long-term care facilities. This chapter predominantly focuses on the technician working in a hospital pharmacy. A wider variety of parenteral medications are used here than in any other setting. Within the hospital, the pharmacy technician is responsible for many daily tasks. Just as pharmacists are required to do everything from processing doctors' orders to performing clinical duties, a pharmacy technician must be versatile to complete the many tasks that will be asked of him or her. Each skill has its own set of guidelines. This chapter explores all types of parenteral medications—the terminology and the equipment commonly associated with them, as well as the various methods used in their preparation. Parenterals are prepared by pharmacies in or associated with hospitals, long-term care facilities, and home health clinics. Although these pharmacies may differ somewhat in their overall patient responsibilities, all still use the same techniques, which are outlined in this chapter. There are many important aspects of parenteral medications that must be understood before an order can be filled, including information about inventory processes, the technician's responsibilities, and the variety of abbreviations that are used in medication orders.

Terminology

When doctor's orders are written, it is important to understand the symbols and abbreviations used in filling the prescription. Box 13.1 lists some of the most common abbreviations. It is also important to pay attention to the strength, form, and timing of the dosage, as well as to the route of administration.

Supplies

Before discussing the actual techniques required to prepare intravenous (IV) drips, chemotherapy, and other sterile products, one must first learn about the types of supplies necessary for these processes. There are many different tools available, but cost can be the determining factor when pharmacies are choosing the equipment that is best suited for their purposes. For instance, there are many different types of automated pumps that automatically fill IV bags and other sterile containers (Figure 13.1). These pumps range in complexity and cost. Usually pharmacies rent the machine and purchase the tubing that is required for that specific pump. Common supplies stocked by pharmacy IV rooms are listed in Box 13.2.

Delivery Systems

There are many different types of containers used to dispense medication. Such containers are developed to be stable and easy to use. Also, because many of the medications are not premade by the manufacturer and must be made in the pharmacy, it is important to determine whether or not the medication will be wasted if the treatment is not given to the patient. Once the medication is reconstituted, it must be used within a certain time or it expires and money is lost. Sometimes, the drug may not be given to the patient for whom it was prepared; the doctor may have decided to use a medication of a different dose, type, volume, or solution. This type of waste only adds to the high costs of health care. Therefore if

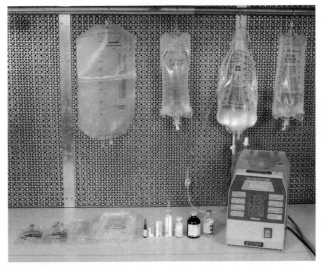

FIGURE 13.1 Supplies used with parenteral medications.

BOX 13.1 DESCRIPTIONS OF PHARMACY STOCK AND TERMINOLOGY

Types of Containers Used for Preparing Parenterals	Description of Container and/or Contents
Amp (Ampule)	1 to 50 ml glass container
Vial	0.5 to 100 ml glass or plastic container with a rubber stopper
Multi-dose vial	Holds multiple doses of medication
Single-dose vial	Holds one dose of medication
Flexible bag	Plastic container (empty or filled with various fluids ranging from 50 to 3000 ml)

Types of Solutions Used/Ordered for Parenteral Agents	
Diluent	Solution used to place medications in solution. Can be sterile water, NS, or others
D5/NS	5% dextrose in normal saline
D10NS	10% dextrose in normal saline
NS	0.9% normal saline, 0.9% sodium chloride
$\frac{1}{2}$NaCl	One-half normal saline (0.45% sodium chloride)
LR	Lactated Ringer's; isotonic solution containing sodium, potassium, calcium, and chloride
$\frac{1}{4}$NS	One-fourth normal saline (0.22$\frac{1}{2}$% sodium chloride)
D5$\frac{1}{2}$NS	5% dextrose and 0.45% normal saline contained in the same bag of solution*
SW	Sterile water, usually used to reconstitute
D5W	5% dextrose in water
D10W	10% dextrose in water

Routes of Administration for Parenteral Agents	
IV	Intravenous; into the vein
IVPush	Into the vein quickly and forcefully
IM	Intramuscular; into the muscle
ID	Intradermal; upper layers of the skin (up to 1 ml)
SQ, SC	Subcutaneous; under the skin
IT	Intrathecal; into a sheath, such as the lumbar sheath located at the base of the spine

Miscellaneous Terms Used Concerning Parenteral Medications	
On call	Doctor wants dose to be ready when he or she decides to give the medication; most anesthesiologists order preop medications as on call
NPO	Nothing by mouth
Preop	Medication ordered is to be given before surgery; usually sedative/antiemetic
Postop	Medication to be given after surgery
PRN	Medication is to be given as needed
QS	Quantity sufficient; adding enough diluent or medication to attain the correct amount needed
Drip or infusion	Usually an IV bag >500 ml that runs over a specified amount of hours

Amp, Ampule; *MDV*, multiple-dose vial; *SDV*, single-dose vial, *NS*, normal saline.
*Normal saline comes in many different combinations of dextrose to saline.

BOX 13.2 COMMONLY USED INTRAVENOUS ROOM SUPPLIES

Supplies	Common Description
70% isopropyl alcohol	Antiseptic for cleaning hood
Alcohol pads	Alcohol on pads for convenience
Amp breaker	Plastic device; one end smaller for small amps, other end for large amps; helps to prevent crushing glass or cutting oneself when opening ampules
Filter needles	A needle that includes a filter that eliminates glass from entering the final solution when drawing from an ampule
Filter straws	For pulling medication from amps
Filters	Used for specific medications to trap particles 5 microns to 0.22 microns from entering IV fluids
Male/female adapter	Universal size; fits a syringe on each end for mixing the two contents
Syringe needles	The most common bore sizes used in pharmacy are 16 G to 20 G
Syringe caps	A sterile cap used to prevent contamination of syringes during transportation out of pharmacy
Syringes	Instrument that holds between 0.3 ml to 60 ml for administration of medications
Transfer needles	A needle on both ends used to transfer a vial to a bottle
Tubing for pumps	Tubing is specific for manufacturer's machine
Tubing transfer sets	Blood transfer sets; used to transfer large containers into empty containers
Mini spike	Large spike that is pushed into vial with a syringe attachment at the other end
Forceps	Instruments that lock; used to close off tubing while transferring medications

Amp, Ampule; *G*, gauge.

methods can be devised that can decrease this waste, pharmacies will adopt these methods. Of course, sometimes methods of reducing waste are costly. However, as new innovative methods are created and adopted, the cost can decrease. The following examples show the types of containers used in the pharmacy along with some alternative containers or administration delivery systems.

PIGGYBACK CONTAINERS

Flexible bags and bottles are the two main types of piggyback containers. Containers can be purchased prefilled with solutions or empty for use in preparing a custom IV solution. The sizes and types of piggyback containers and solutions vary from 50 ml to 500 ml. Some medications, such as insulin, cannot be placed in viaflex bags and must be put into glass containers. Examples of specialized containers used for medication dispensing include large- and small-volume drips, syringe pumps, and miscellaneous systems.

Large- and Small-Volume Drips
Large-volume drips include viaflex bags in three sizes: 1-L, 2-L, and 3-L bags. The small volume containers typically hold 50 to 100 ml of fluids. These can deliver a variety of fluids, including parenteral nutrition. Parenteral nutrition is a combination of essential nutrients that are administered through a drip system over several hours or up to 24-hours. Small volume drips range from 50 ml to 500 ml.

SYRINGES

Technicians may also prepare syringes that are placed into a pump that dispenses medications over time. These pumps can be set for short or long durations, not to exceed a 24-hour period. These are often used to dispense controlled substances at a specific rate of infusion. Another type of syringe dispensing system relies on gravity for delivering the solution.

IV CHAMBERS

Another type of administration system holds a specific volume within a chamber. This system allows the nurse to administer small amounts of medication over a predetermined period. These types of volume-controlled chambers are most often used for pediatric patients.

CASSETTES

Another type of device that can be used to administer controlled substances is a controlled analgesia device, shown in Figure 13.2. Patient controlled analgesia (PCA) is a method of supplying analgesics that allows the patient to control the rate at which the drug is delivered for the relief of pain, usually using an infusion pump. These devices can be used within a hospital setting or the patient may wear the cassette home, which is one of the device's biggest advantages. Tubing is connected to a catheter plug that automatically dispenses medication. An additional bolus may be programmed into the pump. A bolus is a preset amount of drug that can be administered by the patient when his or her pain intensifies. The patient has access to a button located at the end of a cord attached to the controlled analgesia device; when depressed, the button triggers the administration of additional medication. Because the boluses are preset for amount and frequency, even if the patient presses the button many times, he or she will receive only the predetermined amount of drug. This safeguards the patient from overdosing.

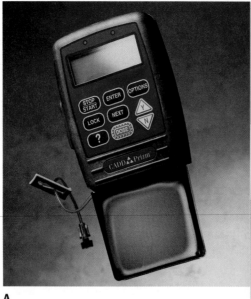

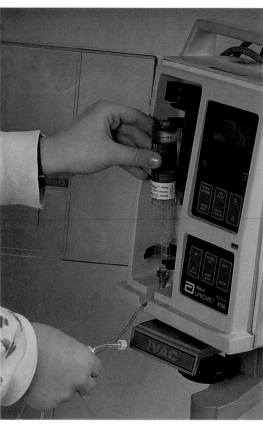

FIGURE 13.2 A, Controlled analgesia device (CAD) pump. **B,** Patient-controlled analgesia (PCA) pump.

VIALS

There are many types of vials that can be placed onto a small piggyback solution via an adapter; these are not mixed with the solution until right before it is administered. The pharmacy technician is responsible for the proper attachment of the vial to the proper solution, but the nurse is the person responsible for breaking the adapter seal between the vial and the piggyback and mixing the drug with the solution. The advantage of this system is the avoidance of wasted medication.

Controlled-release infusion system is another type of delivery system in which the vial is reconstituted (mixed) but is not added to the piggyback. At the time of administration, the vial is attached to a special port on the side of the tubing set that allows the medication to enter the piggyback, where it is then delivered into the patient's bloodstream.

SYRINGE SIZES

Syringes used in the pharmacy are available in seven basic varieties: 1, 3, 5, 10, 20, 30, and 60 ml sizes. There are two types of syringes. A tension type syringe comes in a 1-ml volume. In this case the needle is held on by friction only as seen in Figure 13.3*A* and can be used for withdrawing insulin and other medications that require volumes equal to or less than 1 ml. However, they cannot be used when preparing chemotherapy doses because of the risk of the needle coming off the syringe and causing a spill, or a possible needle stick to the technician. All other sizes of syringes hold their needles in place by a lock mechanism referred to as a Luer lock (see Figure 13.3*B*). This ensures a safe seal for the withdrawal of medication.

Most syringes are made of plastic and should be disposed of after one use. Glass syringes may be available in some facilities. Glass syringes are rarely used in the pharmacy, although they can be used when a patient has an allergy to plastics. Glass syringes, unlike plastic syringes, can be sterilized and reused.

Another type of syringe is a Tubex as seen in Figure 13.4. Tubex can hold a variety of medications and are available in 0.5-ml to 3-ml volumes. The bottom of the syringe is screwed into the Tubex holder. Tubex are reusable and are normally dispensed to the nursing units by the pharmacy on request.

As the size of the syringe increases the accuracy decreases. This is important to remember because it is necessary to obtain the exact amount of drug ordered. The anatomy of a syringe is shown in Figure 13.5.

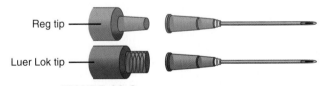

FIGURE 13.3 Two types of syringe tips.

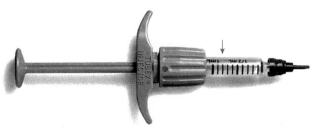

FIGURE 13.4 Tubex holder with injection cartridge inserted.

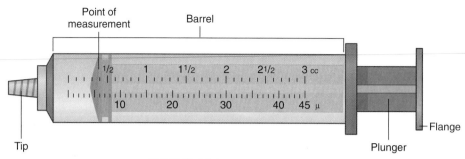

FIGURE 13.5 Parts of a syringe.

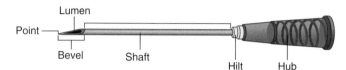

FIGURE 13.6 Parts of a needle.

NEEDLES

Needles are either made of aluminum or stainless steel. There are many different gauges (sizes) and lengths of needles, and most are used by nurses to administer injections. The nurse determines which gauge needle to use depending on the injection site. In the pharmacy, needles are used to draw solutions into a syringe, not to administer medications to patients. There are a limited number of needle gauges available in the pharmacy, and the larger gauge needles make drawing medications easier. It is more important for the pharmacist or technician to choose an appropriately sized syringe than it is to determine the correct needle gauge. The rule to remember in sizing needles is that the gauge (size) number of a needle is inversely proportional to the needle's bore size. This means that as the bore size increases the gauge decreases. For example, a 27-gauge (G) needle has a much smaller opening than a 19 G needle. In the pharmacy setting, the most common sizes used for preparing IV medications are 19 G, 18 G, and 16 G, which are used to draw medications from vials or other containers. The length of these needles is normally 1 to 1½ inches. It is important to remember that as the bore size increases, the risk of coring the vial rubber stopper is increased. When a vial is cored, a chunk of rubber is dislodged and may fall into the vial. To avoid coring, the bevel edge should face upward. If coring does occur, a filter needle must be used to prevent the piece of cored rubber from entering the IV solution.

TECH NOTE! You should not wipe needles with alcohol. If you touch the needle with alcohol or something unintended (such as the IV bag port), the needle must be discarded and replaced with a new one.

The parts of a needle are labeled in Figure 13.6 and should be memorized because it is necessary to know which areas cannot be touched when assembling needles to syringes within a laminar flow hood. No part of a needle below the hub should be touched. The point and shaft must remain sterile.

FILTERS

There are different types and sizes of filters that can be used when preparing parenteral medications. The smallest filter is the 0.22-micron filter, which removes all unwanted particles larger than 0.22 microns (thousandths of a millimeter) from the solution. Another type of filter is the filter straw. This straw-like needle can quickly take a large amount of solution, sifting it through a filter located in the hub of the needle. The filter straw is often used to remove any fine particles of glass from an ampule.

TECH NOTE! To use a filter needle, first pull the solution into the syringe using a regular needle, replace the needle with a filter needle, then push the solution through the filter into the IV container. When using a filter straw, withdraw the solution, then place a regular needle on the syringe before pushing the solution out.

STOCK LEVELS

All of the items stored in the pharmacy's IV room must be kept in stock and at their minimum levels at all times. Before and after each shift, the IV technician is responsible for reordering and restocking the IV room for the next shift. Many IV supplies can be ordered from the central supply area of the hospital and will arrive by the next shift. However, in cases in which the manufacturer or a centralized distribution center is located off site, delivery can take from 2 days to 1 week. Therefore the technician ordering stock must know how long the shipment normally takes to arrive so that the pharmacy will not run out.

Many IV antibiotics are available in premade bulk packs; 12 or 24 come frozen in boxes. Although they are very convenient, they are more expensive than having technicians make IV stock. Most of the time, technicians make extra IVs to be used throughout the week. IV medications can be frozen, but each box must be marked with the expiration date, which is determined by using the manufacturer's information. Once IV medications are thawed, they must be marked with the new expiration date, also determined by the manufacturer. Large temperature-controlled refrigerators may be used to store thawed IV medications and to recycle medications. Antibiotics and other medications that are in multiple dose vials can be stored in the refrigerator, sometimes for days, and used day-to-day.

Aseptic Technique

All parenteral medications must be prepared using aseptic technique. Normally nurses do not have the advantage of using a laminar flow hood; however, they too need to use strict aseptic technique. Aseptic technique goes hand-in-hand with universal precautions. Universal precautions are guidelines followed by all health care workers when dealing with body fluids or blood products. They are used to keep contamination from occurring by a product or to a product. Aseptic technique is a set of guidelines used by nurses when they prepare IV treatments; it must also be used by technicians who use a laminar flow hood for preparing certain agents. For technicians, the importance of using aseptic technique cannot be stressed enough. A medication that contains any microbes or unwanted debris can cause a dangerous infection, or even death, when it is administered into a patient's vein. Steps used in aseptic technique begin with washing hands as shown in Box 13.3 and follows with the proper hood cleaning and preparation of a parenteral medication.

HOOD CLEANING AND MAINTENANCE

Depending on the type of sterile product being prepared, a horizontal or vertical flow hood is used. A horizontal flow hood is used for many types of parenteral medication preparations or sterile product mixtures. For all chemotherapeutic agents, only a vertical flow hood should be used because of the direction of the airflow and the specifications of the hood. A vertical flow hood can be used to mix

BOX 13.3 TWELVE ASEPTIC TECHNIQUES FOR TECHNICIANS*

1. No jewelry should be worn in the hood. This includes artificial nails because of microbial growth around or underneath.
2. Long hair should be tied back away from the face.
3. Hands must be washed after entering the IV area and before entering the laminar flow hood (see Figure 13.7*A-D*).
4. Hands, wrists, and arms to the elbow should be washed with antimicrobial soap and hot water for at least 30 seconds; no more than 90 seconds.
5. Gloves can be worn but should be washed down with 70% isopropyl alcohol after being put on.
6. The surface of the hood should be washed down with 70% isopropyl alcohol using proper method (explained later in this chapter).
7. The hood must run at least 30 minutes before placing medications inside.
8. All vials and ports must be wiped down with alcohol. They should not be sprayed because the alcohol can make contact with the filter in the back of the hood, which breaks down the filter.
9. Hands or any object within the hood cannot block the airflow at any time.
10. Work at least 6 inches into the horizontal hood; keep pens and other objects out of the hood.
11. All needles, syringes, vials, and other byproducts must be disposed of in proper receptacles.
12. No sneezing, talking, or coughing can be directed toward the airflow in a laminar flow hood.

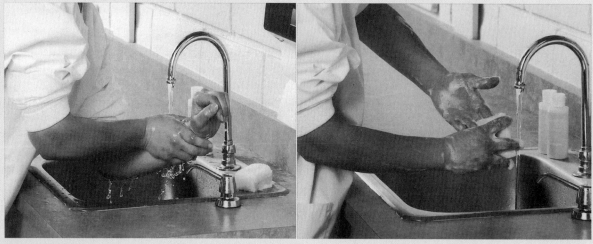
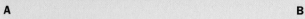
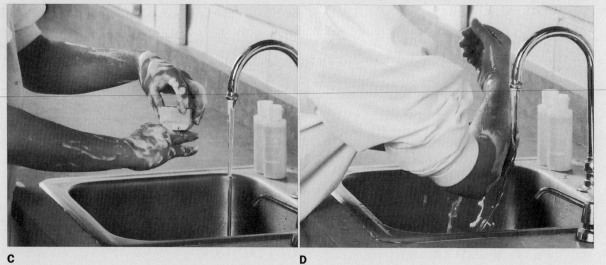

A   **B**

C   **D**

FIGURE 13.7 **A,** Wet hands and arms with warm water. **B,** Scrub top and bottom of hands. **C,** Scrub between fingers and up to the elbow. **D,** Rinse arms and hands thoroughly. Foot pedals may be used rather than handles.

IV, Intravenous.
*Sanitation of hands is found in Appendix F.

nonchemotherapeutic agents if needed; however, chemotherapeutic agents should never be mixed in a horizontal flow hood. All hoods used in the pharmacy for preparing sterile products should be inspected yearly by an authorized inspector to ensure the effectiveness of the filtering system. The direction of airflow in each type of hood is shown in Figure 11.3.

In a horizontal flow hood, the outside air flows into the back of the hood, through the hood's special filter, and out toward the opening. This special filter is a high-efficiency particulate air (HEPA) filter that traps all particles larger than 0.2 microns. The sides of the hood and items within the hood create a disruption of airflow. For this reason, the technician must work 6 inches in from the sides and front of the hood. Also, movement within the hood should be kept to a minimum to decrease disruption of airflow. An example of cleaning a horizontal flow hood is shown in Box 13.4.

In a vertical flow hood, the concept is similar, although air cannot be released back into the room. For this reason, vertical hoods have a Plexiglas shield that separates the technician from the inside work surface. The air comes into the HEPA filter and then into the workspace area. There is a grid at the front of the tabletop that draws in the air and filters it once again through a HEPA filter before it is either released out into the open or is vented to the outside, depending on the type of venting system used. The vertical flow hood should be cleaned as follows:

1. Wet a 4 × 4 inch gauze pad or other disposable cloth with 70% isopropyl alcohol and wipe down the inside of the hood. This includes the back, sides, and tabletop. Do not spray the ceiling inside the vertical hood because this is where the filtering system is located.

BOX 13.4 CLEANING THE HORIZONTAL HOOD

- It is important to be gowned up properly before cleaning the laminar flow hood. All items should be removed from the hood before cleaning.
- Moisten 4 × 4 inch gauze or other disposable cloth or gauze with 70% isopropyl alcohol and wet down the inside of the hood. This includes the sides and tabletop. Make sure you do not spray the HEPA filter at the back or the ceiling inside the hood.
- Then, starting from the top right-hand side of the hood, wipe down, across the surface, and up to the top of the left-hand side of the hood.
- Moving forward a few inches, repeat the motion in the opposite direction.
- The side-to-side, back-to-front motion must be done before using the hood each day. In addition, the hood should be cleaned periodically throughout the course of the day to ensure a sterile environment as shown below.

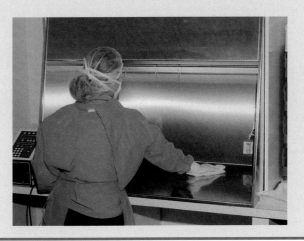

HEPA, High-efficiency particulate air.

2. Start on the (inside) back of the hood and wipe from the top right across to the left-hand side, drop down a few inches, and then back across the wall to the other side. Continue this until the back wall is completely wiped.
3. Then repeat the cleaning procedures working from the top right-hand side, across the tabletop, and up the other side until the whole hood is done.
4. In addition to the sides, tabletop, and back of the vertical flow hood, you should also wash down the inside of the Plexiglas protective shield.

HAND PLACEMENT

Regardless of which type of hood is used, the placement of the hands is one of the most important aspects to consider when preparing sterile medications. There are some simple yet important techniques that should be practiced. These decrease the possibility of both contamination and errors when preparing sterile products. The necessary steps to be taken when in the hood are outlined in Figure 13.8.

CLEAN UP

Once the technician has finished using the hood area, he or she should clean up all unused materials and discard any empty or used products. Wiping down the hood countertop should be the final step in the clean up, preparing it for the next product to be processed. In a vertical flow hood there are several steps that must be taken to maintain a sterile environment. These steps are detailed under Chemotherapy Agents later in this chapter.

PARENTERAL ANTIBIOTICS

Antibiotics have suggested guidelines for dosing regimens that most doctors follow. As shown in Table 13.1, the manufacturer's guidelines are determined by which microbe is being attacked. Pharmacies have a chart that instructs the person preparing the medication as to the type and amount of diluent needed, the normal dosing times, and expiration dates. Antibiotics also differ in how they should be prepared and how long it takes for the powder to dissolve in the diluent. Once the drug is reconstituted, the solution should be checked for color and clarity.

TECH NOTE! Each type of medication has its own unique properties. For example, ceftazidime produces gas when reconstituted. Therefore to prevent the solution from shooting out of the vial, the gas must first be released. This can be done by puncturing a needle into the vial. Erythromycin is difficult to get into solution form; therefore it is important to allow additional time when reconstituting erythromycin. Let the vial sit in the hood (shaking it every so often) until the powder turns into a solution. These are the types of details that are learned over time in the pharmacy.

Parenteral "Syringe" Medications

Intravenous push or intramuscular (IM) medications can be prepared by the nurse at the nursing station or at the patient's bedside; however, the pharmacy does prepare some IV push/IM medications. These agents are placed in a syringe and sealed with a syringe cap until it is time to administer the medication. There are

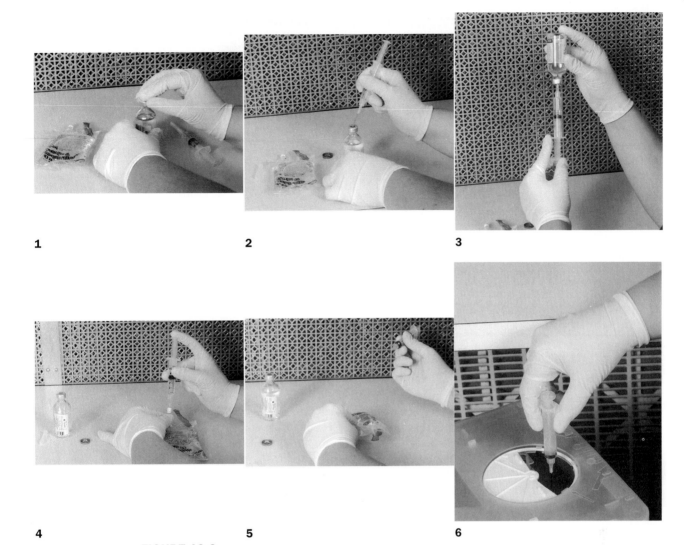

FIGURE 13.8 The six-step process of aseptic technique in the hood is as follows:

1. Using alcohol, swipe the top of the vials and the ports on the IV bags from back to front (move around the vial and bag rather than over or behind).
2. Place the needle bevel side up and push it into the vial's rubber stopper. Preload the syringe with the necessary amount of air to replace solution.
3. Invert the vial and syringe 180 degrees. Push in the air from the syringe and pull out the solution.
4. After removing the syringe from the vial, insert the needle into the IV bag and inject the medication using a steady hand.
5. After injecting the IV bag with the medication, immediately flip the bag over. This decreases the possibility of forgetting which bags have been injected and which ones have not.
6. Never recap the used needles; instead, throw away each syringe in a sharps container along with the uncapped needle after use. Syringes cannot be reused when changing from one drug to another. This decreases the chance of drug-to-drug contamination.

seven procedures to follow when preparing these syringes that are outlined in the following:

1. The liquid inside the ampule must be untrapped from the tip of the ampule by snapping, tapping, or whipping the ampule around in a half circle to force the liquid from the tip. Only then can you proceed.
2. When breaking an ampule, you can use an ampule breaker or wrap an alcohol pad around the neck of the ampule and snap at the narrowest

TABLE 13.1 Example of Suggested Dosing Times, Solutions, and Appropriate Volumes for Antibiotics

Generic Name	Trade Name	Common Dosing Regimens (in hours)	Common Solutions	Common Volumes
Ampicillin	Omnipen	q8–q6	NS	Less than 1.5g (50ml), more than 1.5g (100ml)
Cefazolin	Ancef, Kefzol	q8–q6	D5W or NS	Less than 2g (50ml), more than 2g (100ml)
Cefotaxime	Claforan	q6–q12	D5W or NS	Less than 2g (50ml), more than 2g (100ml)
Ceftazidime	Fortaz	q8–q6	D5W or NS	Less than 2g (50ml), more than 2g (100ml)
Ceftriaxone	Rocephin	q8–q24	D5W or NS	Less than 2g (50ml), more than 2g (100ml)
Doxycycline	Vibramycin	q12	D5W or NS	250ml
Erythromycin	E-mycin	q6–q24	NS	250ml[†] 10mg/20mg lidocaine
Gentamicin	Garamycin	q8–q18* based on glycosidic levels	D5W or NS	Less than 100mg (50ml), over 100mg (100ml)
Imipenem-cilastin	Primaxin	q6–q12	NS	Less than 500mg (100ml), more than 500mg (250ml)

D5NS, 5% Dextrose in normal saline; *NS*, normal saline.
*See Chapter 23 for more on antibiotics.
[†]Erythromycin stings when given intravenously; therefore it is commonly mixed with lidocaine to kill the pain.

point. This decreases the possibility of crushing the ampule or cutting your fingers.

3. If the drug is taken from an ampule, you must use a filter needle to remove all microscopic pieces of glass that can remain at the bottom of a broken ampule.
4. Syringes cannot be transported from the pharmacy with needles attached; therefore a sterile syringe cap must be adhered to the tip of the syringe.
5. Syringes must be flagged with a label. This may involve cutting the label down so that it fits the length of the barrel of the syringe.
6. When flagging a syringe, do not cover the calibrations on the side of the syringe; the nurse must be able to see how many milliliters are in the syringe.
7. Never fill a syringe to the maximum when preparing an IM or IV push syringe. The nurse must have some room to pull back the syringe before injecting the medication.

Other injectables are available premade from the manufacturer, including Tubex ampules. These are stocked in the pharmacy and dispensed by request from the nursing station or area.

ANALGESIC INTRAVENOUS PREPARATIONS

Patients who require analgesics after major surgery or those persons who are in hospice normally have their medications prepared in the pharmacy. Within the hospital setting, nursing stations stock various strengths of controlled substances aimed at relieving extreme pain. Depending on the doctor's order, the nurse can prepare IM or IV push doses from the controlled substances cabinet. For those patients who require large volumes of morphine sulfate or patients who are sent home on strong analgesics, medications are prepared by the pharmacy technician. As mentioned previously in the section on containers, syringe pumps and controlled analgesic devices are two common types of devices that can be used to load controlled substances. Many controlled substances are also prepared in viaflex bags and dispensed to the nursing floor after being documented on the controlled substances board.

TECH NOTE! All dosage forms of controlled substances that are delivered to nursing floors must be signed out of the pharmacy stock and into the floorstock of the receiving station. These documents are maintained and all controlled substances should be counted at the end of every shift to account for all narcotic use or waste.

CHEMOTHERAPEUTIC AGENTS

A ~~horizontal~~ Vertical flow hood and additional supplies are needed to prepare chemotherapy medications. Many facilities do not require a technician to wear a gown when preparing parenteral medications. However, when preparing chemotherapy agents you must wear a gown and gloves. Also, the chemotherapy supplies must be disposed of in appropriate containers. There are specially marked plastic pails clearly identified as "Hazardous Waste" containers kept inside the hood. After thoroughly washing hands and arms to the elbows, the technician should put on the first pair of gloves, followed by a full gown. The gowns typically have Velcro tabs or ties to secure them. Once the gown is on, a second pair of gloves should be placed over the cuff of the chemotherapy gown. This is to prevent any contamination of chemotherapy agents, if they should come into contact with the gloves. This also protects the technician from contamination. If contamination should occur, the outside pair should be removed and discarded appropriately. Goggles normally are not worn by technicians working with a chemotherapy hood because there is the added protection of the Plexiglas shield that does not allow any solution to come out of the hood toward the face or eyes.

TECH NOTE! Keep a sterile 4 × 4-inch gauze pad inside the chemotherapy hood just in case you have a minor spill. You can cover the spill with the gauze pad, decreasing the aerosolization of vapors and isolating the spill until you clean it up. Remember that all products discarded from the chemotherapy hood must be placed in an appropriate container.

Proper Disposal of Chemotherapeutic Agents and Supplies

When the chemotherapeutic agent preparation is done, it is important to discard the wrappings, needles, syringes, and the gown and gloves in appropriate containers. Most chemotherapy hoods contain a small sharps container in which all needles, syringes, and the remains of chemotherapy agents should be discarded. When these receptacles are two thirds full, they should be discarded following the pharmacy protocol. Many hospital pharmacies have environmental services collect the receptacle when it is full.

TECH NOTE! Always check your pharmacy's protocol regarding the disposal of sharps containers. This information can be found in the policies and procedures handbook.

When preparation is complete, the gloves, gown, and all paper products, such as the outside wrappings of alcohol prep pads, should be placed within a plastic ziplock bag identified as hazardous waste. The bag is then disposed of inside a large waste receptacle that is marked "hazard chemicals, dispose of properly." This too should be taken away by environmental services or per protocol when two-thirds full.

TECH NOTE! You should always know the location of the clean-up kit for hazard waste spills and review the policies and procedures in case of a chemotherapy spill.

HYPERALIMENTATION

Hyperalimentation (also known as hyperals) are large volumes of parenteral medications normally made for persons who cannot take in nutrition orally (they cannot eat). Reasons for this inability to eat can range from a recent stomach or intestinal surgery to various conditions that affect the gastrointestinal system. There are two main types of hyperalimentation that are prepared in the pharmacy, total parenteral nutrition (TPN) and peripheral parenteral nutrition (PPN). In a hospital setting, after the initial hyperal is prepared and hung, daily laboratory tests of electrolyte levels are drawn from the patient to determine necessary changes. For example, if a patient's potassium levels begin to drop, then the next hyperal will be altered to compensate for the decrease. In this way, the patient gets exactly what nutrients are needed on a daily basis. Home health clinics and some hospitals prepare a week's worth of hyperals; electrolyte levels are tested weekly instead of daily. Some patients may remain on this type of nutrition for many months.

There are many different protocols used to prepare parenteral nutrition; following is an example of a hospital pharmacy's solutions. These large volumes are premixed and ordered in cases from the manufacturer. Added to these solutions are the various electrolytes and other medications requested by the patient's attending physician.

TPN   Normally contain 50% dextrose, 10% amino acids, and 20% fat
PPN   Normally contain 25% dextrose, 10% amino acids, and 10% fat

These two preparations are administered differently because of their different concentrations. TPNs are given intravenously via the subclavian vein and superior vena cava because of the higher concentration of nutrients. Patients must have a surgically inserted catheter. PPNs are given via a large peripheral vein located in the back of the hand or in another peripheral area located in the upper extremity and therefore are less complicated. Most facilities have a standard order to start a patient on hyperal. The volume of a hyperal can typically range from 2 L to 3 L. The doctor determines the rate of infusion over the course of 24 hours. Regardless of how many milliliters run per hour, the hyperal must be changed at least every 24 hours to ensure the sterility of the solution. A standard rate of infusion is 100 ml per hour; therefore 2400 ml may be used over the course of a day. If a 3-L TPN is hung at 1700 hours, then the following day at 1700 hours a new bag is hung and the remaining 600 ml of TPN are discarded down the drain. Most hyperals are tailor-made for each patient. An example of a protocol order is given in Figure 13.9.

TECH NOTE! Some chemicals can precipitate other chemicals, creating solid flakes in the IV solution. Always check your IV bag for clarity after you finish preparing the solution.

ELECTROLYTES AND ADDITIVES

All TPNs contain dextrose and amino acids; both help to nourish the body. Dextrose (sugar) allows quick energy for the body, whereas amino acids are the essential parts that the body uses to build needed enzymes and other important molecules. In addition, lipids are commonly added to give the body the necessary fat needed to metabolize important cell components such as cell walls. The rest of the additives are additional electrolyte ions such as those listed in Table 13.2. These components can be determined on a daily basis if the patient is in a hospital setting. Other medications, such as ranitidine, cimetidine, or famotidine

TPN ORDER SHEET

HOME HEALTH	DATE
PATIENT	ADDRESS

TPN FORMULA:

AMINO ACIDS: ☐ 5.5% ☐ 8.5% ☑ 10% ☐ WITH STANDARD ELECTROLYTES	425 ml
DEXTROSE: ☐ 10% ☐ 20% ☐ 40% ☐ 50% ☑ 70% (check one)	357 ml
LIPIDS: ☐ 10% ☑ 20% FOR ALL-IN-ONE FORMULA	125 ml

FINAL VOLUME qsad STERILE WATER FOR INJECTION 400mL	1307 ml

Calcium Gluconate	0.465m Eq/ml	5 mEq
Magnesium Sulfate	4m Eq/ml	5 mEq
Potassium Acetate	2m Eq/ml	mEq
Potassium Chloride	2m Eq/ml	mEq
Potassium Phosphate	3m M/ml	22 mM
Sodium Acetate	2m Eq/ml	mEq
Sodium Chloride	4m Eq/ml	35 mEq
Sodium Phosphate	3m M/ml	mM
TRACE ELEMENTS CONCENTRATE	☐ 4 ☐ 5 ☐ 6	ml

Patient Additives:

☐ MVC 9 + 3 10 ml Daily

☐ HUMULIN-R 10 u Daily

☐ FOLIC ACID ______ mg
______ times weekly

☐ VITAMIN K ______ mg
______ times weekly

☐ OTHER: MVI 12 1.5mL/daily

☐ OTHER: ______

Directions:

INFUSE: ☑ DAILY
☐ ____ TIMES WEEKLY

OTHER DIRECTIONS:

______

______

______

______

Rate: ☐ CYCLIC INFUSION: OVER ______ HOURS (TAPER UP AND DOWN) " ☐ CONTINUOUS INFUSION: AT ______ ml PER HOUR " ☑ STANDARD RATE: AT 110 ml PER HOUR FOR 12 HOURS

LAB ORDERS:

☐ STANDARD LAB ORDERS
SMAC-20, CO2, Mg+2 TWICE WEEKLY
CBC WITH AUTO DIFF WEEKLY
UNTIL STABLE, THEN:
SMAC-20, CO2, Mg+2 WEEKLY
CBC WITH AUTO DIFF MONTHLY

☐ OTHER: ______

______

______

VALIDATION:

______
DOCTOR'S SIGNATURE

Print Name: ______

Office Address: ______

______

Phone: ______

WHITE: Home Health CANARY: Physician

FIGURE 13.9 Example of a total parenteral nutrition (TPN) order.

TABLE 13.2 Types of Parenteral Additives

Abbreviation	Electrolyte Ions	Concentration	Notes
KCL	Potassium chloride	2 mEq/ml	
KPO$_4$	Potassium phosphate	K$^+$ 2 mEq/ml, phosphate 3 mEq/ml	Always work out phosphate first
CaGluconate	Calcium gluconate	0.465 mEq/ml	
MgSO$_4$	Magnesium sulfate	1 mg/ml	
K Ac	Potassium acetate	2 mEq/ml	*Used to balance
NaAcetate	Sodium acetate	2 mEq/ml	*Used to balance
NaPO$_4$	Sodium phosphate	2 mEq/ml	
NaCL	Sodium chloride	2 mEq/ml	*Used to balance

Miscellaneous Additives

MVI	Multivitamin		Comes in PEDI dosing
MTE	Multiple trace elements		Comes in PEDI dosing
Zn	Zinc		
Se	Selenium		
Regular insulin	Insulin		Can be added to TPNs and PPNs

Other Nonsupplements Added to TPN or PPN Solutions

Generic	Brand	Concentration
Ranitidine	Zantac	40 mg/ml
Famotidine	Pepcid	20 mg/ml
Cimetidine	Tagamet	150 mg/ml

PEDI, Pediatrics; *PPN*, peripheral parenteral nutrition; *TPN*, total parenteral nutrition.
*To *balance* means the pharmacist determines the amount to be added.

(all histamine-2 [H$_2$] antagonists), which help patients with stomach problems can also be added to a hyperal. In addition to stomach medications, insulin is often added in quantities up to 100 units per bag. Only regular insulin is added to hyperals.

Compatibility Considerations of Parenteral Medications

There are many different types of medications that are prepared in an IV room. Some medications must be protected from light, whereas others must be kept in bottles (as discussed earlier). Refer to Table 13.3 for additional considerations in the preparation of parenteral drugs. All IV rooms have reference books that can be used to find special instructions for all types of parenteral medications. The IV technician must become familiar with the idiosyncrasies of medications to ensure that all solutions he or she makes are effective and safe.

TABLE 13.3 Additional Considerations for the Preparation of Drugs

Medication	Special Instructions
Insulin	NS or $\frac{1}{2}$ NS
Amiodarone	D5/NS
Nitroglycerin	D5/NS or NS
Ciprofloxacin	Protect from light
Lorazepam	Protect from light; stable longer in glass than in plastic

NS, Normal saline; *D5/NS*, 5% dextrose in normal saline.

```
                    HOME INFUSION PHARMACY

          Patient A
          RX#37856


          Amino*Acids 10%=425 ml  Dextrose*70%=357 ml
          Ster*Water=400 ml  Lipids*20%=125 ml
          MVI=10 ml/day  *Additives per liter*
          Sod*Chlor=35 mEq  Pot*Phos=15 mM  Calcium=
          5 mEq  Magnesium=5 mEq


          Qty#      TPN 40–51GM Protein+Lipids
          Infuse nightly 8pm to 8am thru IV PICC line via sigma
          pump.  *****Add 10 units Humulin-R to each bag just
          prior to infusion***** **Note: contains TPN soln+lipids:
          rate adjusted** Settings: rate=104 ml/hr
          volume=1248 ml


                        ***REFRIGERATE***

          Expiration date: 04/01/1999
```

FIGURE 13.10 Example of an intravenous (IV) label.

All labels produced for parenteral medications must be initialed by the technician who prepares them. Labels get their final check from a registered pharmacist. Many pharmacy labels rely on the Julian date for determining the expiration date of the medication. If the medication does not get used, perhaps because of a discontinued order, it is recycled for use on another patient. The Julian date is the actual consecutive day of the year. For example, January 1 is day 1, whereas after January 30 February begins and the days continue in sequence with 31, 32, 33, and so on until day 365, which is December 31. It is easier to determine an expiration date when using the Julian date instead of a traditional month/day/year system. However, if a computer system is used that relies on the calendar date, it should indicate the expiration date as well.

Components of an Intravenous Label

The final step in preparing parenteral medications is the application of the label. The label should first be checked against the medication and the doctor's orders to make sure that the right medication is being given to the patient. Although each pharmacy prepares its own label, all labels require the same minimum information. An example of an IV label is shown in Figure 13.10. After the label has been applied, the IV preparations are set out for the pharmacist to check along with the vial or container of medication used to make the IV preparation. Once this is done, the IV preparations are loaded onto a cart or delivery vehicle that delivers them to their destinations. In a home-health setting, a delivery service may be used to transport the medications to the patient's home. Within a hospital, this task normally is done by the technician. When the IV preparations are placed in the correct nursing unit, all unused IV preparations are obtained and are returned to the pharmacy for recycling. As long as the IV preparations are within their expiration dates and are kept at proper temperature, they can be used to fill new orders.

DO YOU REMEMBER THESE KEY POINTS?

- The major responsibilities of a hospital technician
- The types and sizes of syringes available in an IV room
- The parts of a syringe and needle
- The important aspects of aseptic technique and when they should be used
- How to determine the Julian date
- Different types of parenteral medications and when they are used
- Different equipment and supplies used in an IV area
- The types of solutions used to mix various antibiotics and parenterals
- The main routes of administration

REVIEW QUESTIONS:

Multiple Choice

1. Which of the skills listed is the *most* important aspect of preparing sterile products?
   A. Aseptic technique
   B. Working in a horizontal flow hood
   C. Using 70% isopropyl alcohol to wipe down the hood
   D. Filter needles

2. A male/female adapter is used for which of the following reasons?
   A. To attach a needle to a syringe
   B. To attach syringes to tubing
   C. To attach syringes to syringes
   D. To attach two IV bags together

3. The smallest filter that can be used is a
   A. Filter straw
   B. Filter needle
   C. Micron 5 filter
   D. Micron 0.22 filter

4. Which of the following sizes of syringes is not commonly found in an IV room?
   A. 3 ml
   B. 4 ml
   C. 5 ml
   D. 10 ml

5. Which of the following sizes of needles is not commonly used in an IV room?
   A. 16 G
   B. 18 G
   C. 19 G
   D. 25 G

6. Hands should always be washed or sanitized when
   A. Entering the IV room
   B. Before working in the horizontal flow hood
   C. Before working in a vertical flow hood
   D. All of the above

7. Laminar flow hoods should be cleaned
   A. With 70% isopropyl alcohol
   B. At least 30 minutes before using
   C. At least once a day
   D. All of the above

8. Chemotherapeutic agents should be disposed of
   A. In a plastic chemotherapy bag
   B. In a sharps container
   C. Only at the end of a shift
   D. By a biohazard team of professionals

9. HEPA stands for _____ and traps particles larger than _____
   A. Heated environmental parenteral air filter; 2 microns
   B. High-environmental particulate air filter; 0.2 microns
   C. Horizontal-efficiency particulate air filter; 0.2 microns
   D. High-efficiency particulate air filter; 0.2 microns

10. You may find all of the following medications in a hyperal except
    A. Heparin   C. Ranitidine
    B. Insulin   D. Ampicillin

True/False

*If the statement is false, then change it to make it true.

1. IV stock ordering should be done on a weekly basis.
2. NPO means nothing by mouth.
3. Vials and IV bag ports should be wiped from front to back.
4. Syringes are normally made of glass.
5. Needles are made of aluminum or stainless steel.
6. As the syringes increase in size, the calibration is less accurate.
7. Laminar flow hoods should be checked monthly.
8. You may recap syringes if they have been used only once.
9. You must wear goggles when preparing chemotherapy agents.
10. A sharps container must be replaced when it is full.

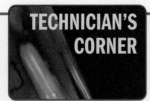

TECHNICIAN'S CORNER

The pharmacy receives an order for patient R. Jones.
Allergies: PCN, sulfa, morphine
Dx: Sepsis, diabetes
Transcribe the following order into lay terms and determine if any of the orders should be brought to the attention of a pharmacist; if so, explain why.

#1 Unasyn 3 g q6h in 100 ml NS
#2 Vancomycin 1 g in 100 ml D5NS
#3 NPH insulin "rainbow coverage" or "sliding scale"

BIBLIOGRAPHY

American Society of Health-Systems Pharmacists: *Manual for pharmacy technicians,* Bethesda, MD, 1993, ASHP.

Ballington D: *Pharmacy practice for technicians,* St Paul, MN, 1999, Paradigm.

Potter P, Perry AG: *Fundamentals of nursing,* ed 5, St Louis, 2001, Mosby.

14

Pharmacy Stock and Billing

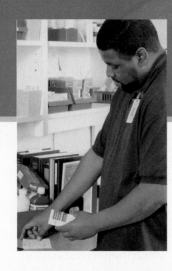

Objectives

- Explain the function of a drug formulary.

- List the primary types of insurance companies and how they manage drug coverages.

- Describe the differences between generic and trade drugs and how they affect cost to the patient and pharmacy.

- Differentiate between Medicaid and Medicare programs and who is eligible.

- Explain the purpose of worker's compensation.

- Describe three main ordering systems available in a pharmacy to keep stock levels constant.

- List the types of automated dispensing systems.

Adjudication *Electronic insurance billing for medication payment*

Formulary *A list of preferred drugs to be stocked by the pharmacy; also a list of drugs covered by an insurance company*

Generic name *Non-proprietary name of a drug*

POS *Point of sale*

Recall *When a drug or device must be returned to the manufacturer due to failure to meet FDA standards*

Trade name *Brand name drug; the company that first applies for a patent on the chemical structure of a medication or generic name is allowed to name the product with a patented name*

TYPES OF INSURANCE

Government *Medicaid and Medicare*

HMO *Health maintenance organization*

PPO *Preferred Provider Organization*

Worker's compensation *A government-required and enforced coverage for workers injured on the job*

Introduction

Everyone working in the pharmacy is responsible for maintaining the inventory stock. It is an essential part of the daily tasks of pharmacy staff. As stocks are depleted it is important that replacement inventories be ordered. Although there are many different systems available for ordering stock, the task of ordering can be delegated to a specific person within the pharmacy. It then falls on the rest of the staff to inform the inventory control person of falling stock levels.

Along with ordering stock, pharmacy technicians are often placed in charge of the billing process. Proper knowledge of billing procedures is a skill that is normally learned over time as one works in the pharmacy. Because each pharmacy may accept different insurance claims, the technician must become acquainted with the normal billing procedures of that pharmacy. However, there are common types of billing practices that are covered in this chapter that may help you understand the proper information needed to file a claim for reimbursement.

In addition, there is basic information on the major types of insurance coverage of which every technician should be aware. A firm knowledge of formulary must be in place for the proper ordering and billing practices. This chapter begins with the formulary and the necessary knowledge needed concerning insurance companies. Then pharmacy inventory, some major types of devices used to keep track of inventory, and how to handle special obstacles as they occur are discussed.

Formulary

A formulary is analogous to a backbone. It is a list that describes all the medications covered under insurance plans. It also offers alternative medications if the first choice is not covered. For medications to become part of a formulary they must meet certain requirements such as effectiveness and cost.

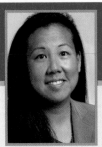

Pharmacist's Perspective
BY SUSAN WONG, PHARM.D.

Drug Utilization and Formulary Selection Process

Today's healthcare is in crisis. Health insurance companies and plans come and go. Ownership and management of hospitals and pharmacy benefits are in a state of flux. One of the greatest contributors to this instability is rising drug costs. The last few years have seen double digit increases in annual drug costs. As medicine evolves and progresses, the average lifespan of Americans becomes longer and longer. But as we live longer, we need more medicines to treat our ills and keep us alive. Drug companies spend a great deal of time and money to develop and market their new drugs. They must recoup these investments during a drug's patent life.

During the time in which a drug is under patent, its rights and exclusivity are under the sole ownership of usually one, sometimes more than one, drug company. They have the right to price these new medicines in relation to its use, its costs over time, and what the market will bear. Not until the patent expires and all efforts to lengthen a drug's patent life are exhausted will drug company competitors be allowed to manufacture a generic version, thereby lowering the retail cost through open competition.

In the past decade there has also been an explosion of "me-too" drugs. These drugs are in the same or a similar chemical class, have the same or very similar action, but have very slight modifications in their chemical structures. These slight differences might affect a drug's side effect profile or its half-life (length of activity), or the different chemical structures may not have any variations in action at all. The slight variation in chemical structure allows the different drugs to be registered and licensed as separate drug entities within a drug class. Many of the drugs commonly used today for heart disease, hypertension, diabetes, hyperlipidemia, and others have brother or sister drugs that are in the same class (or family) and have the same action—hence the name "me-too" drugs.

All of these factors have necessitated the use of the formulary system for many organizations such as insurance companies, health maintenance organizations, and others. A formulary is a list of medicines that are preferred agents that provides a way of managing the utilization of drugs so that they are the most cost effective for a given organization. The goal for any health care organization is to use the right medicine in the right amount at the right time to achieve a favorable outcome (i.e., health). The formulary system employs a team of professionals to review all the possible medicines for a given use and their costs to an organization for an average patient, and then to encourage or regulate the use of a preferred agent or agents for a given class or type of drug. The formulary review process also includes periodic reevaluations of medicines as new drugs come to market, or as problems arise with old drugs.

The next time you go to the supermarket and go down the laundry soap aisle, look at how many types, sizes, colors, additives, and so on there are on the shelves for laundry soap. Now I would be willing to guess that they all clean your clothes pretty well. Some have fresh scents, some have no scent, some have bleach alternatives, and some claim to save the colors in your clothes. Some may cost $5, some may cost $15. But they all clean your clothes. You might buy the brand that cleans your clothes for the most economical price. Some folks may need certain brands or formulations because of allergies. Most will buy the bigger sizes (because they get more for their hard-earned cash). Choosing a preferred medicine for a formulary is a similar process (but a bit more scientific). If a patient has an allergy to, or has failed therapy with the preferred agent, the patient may need to use a nonformulary medicine. In this instance, the pharmacy may have to specially order a nonpreferred medicine for the patient.

As a pharmacy technician you may be involved with the recording or billing of medicine that a patient has received. Or you may be involved with procuring a medicine that is not on the formulary and is used infrequently. Accuracy is the key here because the misrecording of a medicine can affect both what a patient must pay for their medicines and what your employer is reimbursed from the patient's insurance plan. Accuracy can also affect your employer if you are involved in supply chain management or inventory/stocking of your supplies. It is crucial for all involved to use the medicines that do the job and are most cost-effective. This helps patients spend their health care dollars wisely. ■

Many formulary drugs are generic. These drugs are as effective as the brand name drugs but are less expensive. A committee composed of pharmacists, physicians, and other healthcare administrators review drugs that have been approved by the Food and Drug Administration (FDA) and that are cost effective. In addition, consideration may be given to drug companies that bid or give rebates when their drug is chosen. This decrease in price to the pharmacy ultimately saves money for the insurance company and the patient. Although most insurance companies cover most of the cost of a generic drug, some do allow the patient to choose the brand name drug. However, if the patient selects the brand name drug, the patient must pay the difference between the generic and brand name drug and may also be responsible for any copay required. For example, if the normal copay is $5 per prescription and the patient chooses a brand name medication that costs $10 more than the generic equivalent, then the patient must pay $15. Finally, formularies are not permanent by any means. If and when new generics come into the market, cost and other factors are again reviewed. Typically the types of drugs not included on a formulary are new drugs, uncommon drugs, and extremely expensive drugs. Also, if a nonformulary drug can be justified as a medically necessary substitution by the physician, it may be approved.

Generic Versus Trade Drugs

The terms *trade*, *brand*, and *proprietary* are used interchangeably to refer to the name of the drug that was first patented and marketed by the owner or manufacturer. After a certain amount of time passes the patent runs out. Eventually other drug companies can apply for the right to produce the same drug. These drugs produced by other companies are considered "generic." Although the FDA approves generic drugs as equivalent to the trade drug, they may have different appearances because of different manufacturing procedures.

Third-Party Billing

The term *third-party billing* refers to the third part of the three parties—patient, pharmacy, and insurance company—involved in the overall payment process, the insurance company. After the patient has paid his or her portion of the drug cost, the pharmacy must submit an invoice for the remaining cost for payment to the insurance company. This chapter begins by listing the primary types of insurance, followed by their common traits and the problems that may arise when processing medication claims.

TYPES OF INSURANCE

It is important for the technician to know the type of insurance, if any, each patient has for billing purposes. Learning about all of the different insurance policies is nearly impossible, especially because their guidelines change regularly. Therefore this chapter covers the most basic information that can be applied to the major types of billing. The four types of insurance plans in use today are the following:

Health maintenance organization (HMO)
Preferred Provider Organization
Government programs–Medicare and Medicaid
Worker's compensation

HEALTH MAINTENANCE ORGANIZATION

An HMO has specific features that set it apart from traditional insurance programs. An HMO is an effective method of controlling health care costs. Blue Cross, United Healthcare, Pacificare, Champus Tricare Program, and Kaiser are some of the many insurance companies that offer HMO coverage. Special features of HMOs include the following:

1. Primary care physician (PCP): The insurance company allows the patient to choose a main physician rather than having to be seen by the physician on duty.
2. Independent physician association (IPA): The provider offers a discounted rate to the patient through the contract made with the insurance company. In return, the doctor accepts a lesser amount than is normally charged for the procedure performed. These are considered contracted providers; examples of contracted providers are certain hospitals, clinics, and medical groups.
3. Copay: The insurance company requires a predetermined amount to be paid by the patient for office visits, emergency room visits, and drugs, regardless of the final cost. The rate varies depending on the type of coverage the patient has. The insurance company is responsible for the remainder of the cost.

What If Your Patient Has HMO Insurance?

If a patient has HMO insurance, the technician must obtain information from the patient such as address, date of birth (DOB), insurance number, and full name. If the pharmacy accepts the patient's insurance, the technician charges the patient the copay per medication filled. The pharmacy in turn bills the insurance company for the remaining balance of the medication. The patient is responsible for the entire cost only if the insurance company denies coverage based on eligibility or authorization not received before service. An HMO may require prior authorization on certain medications per their formulary guidelines. State regulations regarding the types of forms used to approve such medications may vary.

PREFERRED PROVIDER ORGANIZATION

The difference between HMOs and PPOs is that the patient usually pays more out-of-pocket expenses for PPOs. The benefit is that the patient can choose a physician from the insurance plan's list of contracted providers or may choose any physician a patient wants. There are no requirements for a PCP.

PPOs are offered by Blue Shield, Blue Cross, United Healthcare, State Farm Insurance, and others. As you can see, some insurance companies offer both PPOs and HMOs. This is why it is important for the patient to choose the right insurance plan.

Patients choosing a PPO may have a copay for their visits, the copay tends to be higher, and PPOs may have a deductible (the amount that the patient must pay before the insurance company pays). The insurance then pays a certain percentage of the medical expenses and medication bills if the patient's claims meet the criteria (i.e., charges were incurred by a contracted provider and the service provided was within the PPO's allowed amount). This helps control the cost to the insurance because the patient pays everything that the insurance company does not pay.

What If Your Patient Has PPO Insurance?

You must find out whether the patient has medication coverage through the PPO plan. In addition, you must find out whether the patient pays upfront for the medication or has a copay. This information is determined from the information on the patient's health insurance card. After the information is transmitted to the provider, an approval code is sent to the pharmacy. If the claim is rejected, the technician must call the help desk to find out why. Unless it is a minor error such as the patient's last name was spelled wrong or the wrong DOB was given, the technician may instruct the patient to call the provider to rectify major problems.

GOVERNMENT-RUN INSURANCE PROGRAMS

Programs such as Medicare and Medicaid are examples of state and federal medical insurance plans. Each person who works pays the government a percentage of his or her income toward Medicare. A percentage of each state's budget is applied toward Medicaid. Each plan has specific guidelines that must be followed to the letter for patients to qualify for reimbursement.

Medicare

Medicare is a federally run program for seniors, the disabled, and dialysis patients. It works much like an HMO and a PPO. The patient must go to a provider that accepts Medicare, but the patient has a yearly deductible and a percentage share of cost. The share of cost is similar to a deductible and copay put together. The patient is responsible for paying up to a certain amount in a hospital setting. At present, Medicare pays outpatient costs with the exception of some diabetic supplies and equipment. In addition, Medicare offers no prescription drug coverage.

Some major drug companies offer drug programs to the elderly and the disabled that will provide medications to those who use specific products.

Medicaid

Each state has its own Medicaid program for low-income residents. This also includes uninsured pregnant women and those with certain disabilities. Federal funding accounts for only a small portion of the revenue. Medicaid can be used in conjunction with Medicare if the person qualifies. In addition, each state may have many different programs that help defer the cost of health care and medication. The following are the three major levels of coverage within the Medicaid system:

1. The patients may not be responsible for any cost.
2. Share of cost. In the share of cost level, the patient's plan requires that the patient pay a deductible (i.e., a specific dollar amount must be met before the insurance company pays). For instance, the patient may be responsible for the first $1000, but any remaining amount is paid by Medicaid.
3. Geographical managed care program. A geographical managed care plan allows patients to belong to a medical group with which Medicaid has a contract agreement. This includes HMOs, thus allowing patients to have benefits similar to benefits offered by HMOs. (Each state's regulation may vary.)

What If Your Patient Has Medicaid Insurance?

You must know whether the patient has medication benefits. If so, you need a copy of the insurance card. This card identifies the program under which the patient is covered. These plans include county-run programs as well. Each differs in the patient's coverage.

WORKER'S COMPENSATION

Worker's compensation is a type of insurance paid by employers to fully cover injuries suffered by employees while on the job. The federal government requires employers with a certain number of employees to offer worker's compensation. Insurance coverage is paid to private insurance carriers.

Anyone who works for a company that pays into worker's compensation may be eligible to use this insurance if he or she has a work-related injury. The patient does not have to pay anything. Instead, claims are filed either electronically or in hard copy to the insurance companies. However, pre-authorization must be given to the pharmacy before medications are dispensed.

BILLING THE INSURANCE COMPANY

The information that insurance companies must know to process a claim from the pharmacy or to reimburse the patient is the same as the requirements on a pharmacy label plus date of birth, insurance group, and identification numbers. All information must be verified before the medication is dispensed. Once the patient's information is in the pharmacy's computer system, it is important to keep that information updated for both the pharmacy and the insurance company.

Minimum information required by the insurance company includes the following:

Required by the Insurance Company	Reason
Patient's name	To verify the insurance coverage
Date medication is filled	May be important to process claim
Pharmacy name and address	The insurance company must pay the pharmacy
Medication prescribed	To verify whether the drug is on the formulary
Dosage	Determines the cost of the medication
Date of birth	
Identification number	

Each plan has its own formulary, limitations, and exclusions. In addition to these variances, each pharmacy has certain insurance that they accept or reject. This means, if the pharmacy accepts the copayment as payment in full, they will bill the insurance company for the cost of the medication. Otherwise, the pharmacy may not accept the insurance based on their limits of payment.

Patient Profiles

Each pharmacy has its own specific computer system, which details each patient's profile. This profile must be kept updated for proper billing. Basic information that can be viewed on this computer system includes the following:

- Patient's name
- DOB
- Address
- Phone number
- Gender
- Allergies
- Insurance provider's information, including provider's phone number and insurance number

If the information contains a mistake, the insurance claim may be rejected.

If the patient does not have insurance, he or she must pay full price for prescriptions. The cost of a prescription can vary greatly. Many pharmacies offer coupons on new prescriptions. The use of generics can greatly reduce the price of a medication.

If the patient has insurance, determining the guidelines of the program is of primary importance if the pharmacy is to receive reimbursement. The process by which all claims are processed over a computerized system is referred to as adjudication. The insurance determines the amount of coverage per medication based on various criteria such as the following:

1. Average wholesale price (AWP): The AWP can be found in *Drug Topics Red Book*. Use *Red Book* or *Blue Book* to determine the price of a medication based on the manufacturer's price.
2. Copay: The insurance company pays a certain amount based on the patient's copay. This also depends on whether the patient has an HMO, PPO, or a government-run program.

Processors, companies that work for insurance companies, are responsible for the approval of drug coverage, collecting and processing claims, and payment.

Processing Claims

When handling a patient's medication claim, the pharmacy is responsible for relaying the necessary information about each patient. Because each insurance company needs specific information, the technician must know each insurance company's specific needs. The general types of information required may include the following:

- Processor, typically the insurance company
- Member's identification (ID) number, usually the Social Security number, or an assigned number of the policy owner
- Group number (if applicable)
- Plan code (if applicable)
- Insurance carrier

Claim Problems

There are many reasons why a prescription may not be covered for the insured patient. This can be a frustrating time for the patient and the technician who is trying to get a prescription covered as well as for the insurance company's representative. The most common reasons that a prescription may not be covered are as follows:

- Coverage has expired
- Coverage limits exceeded
- National drug code (NDC) is not covered
- Patient is trying to refill a prescription too soon
- The cardholder's information does not match the processor's information
- Doctor is not the Primary Care Physician

Coverage Expiration Policy for Drugs. If the patient has lost his or her coverage, the claim is rejected. Following HIPAA regulations in 2003, the pharmacy does not have access to information regarding reason for rejection, and is only disclosed a termination date. Patients often are unaware of why this has happened and may want the pharmacy to investigate. Pharmacy personnel are not allowed to call the patient's insurance carrier regarding these types of inquiries. Patient confidentiality would be breached and legal action could result. The only recourse is to explain to the patient that he or she must contact the insurance company to resolve the issue. In the meantime, the patient must pay full price for the medications. If there has been an error, reimbursement is made after the insurance company corrects the problem.

Limitation of Plan Exceeded. This problem can arise for several reasons. One reason is that the drug is not covered in the insurance plan's formulary (i.e., non-formulary). In this case, a special authorization form must be submitted to the insurance company from the physician explaining why the patient must have a specific (nonformulary) medication. Another reason is that the prescription calls for a greater amount of the drug than is allowed by the insurance plan. For example, some government insurance plans limit the number of prescriptions that can be filled per month or per year. If the prescription calls for a specific quantity of medication that exceeds the maximum amount to be filled per day, the prescription is rejected and the patient can contact the insurance company for special permission to obtain the drug.

Some patients are exempt from these types of limitations because of their illness. These include people who suffer from diabetes or those who have been diagnosed with human immunodeficiency virus (HIV) or acquired immune deficiency syndrome (AIDS). Those persons suffering from diabetes require a continuing refill of lancets and blood-testing strips to monitor their blood glucose. In addition, they must refill their insulin syringes monthly. In the case of persons being treated for HIV or AIDS, the medication is very expensive and they usually have to take many medications simultaneously. When a claim is rejected because limits are exceeded, the technician must explain the problem and adhere to the maximum limit permitted by the insurance company. The patient is ultimately responsible for contacting the insurance company to dispute the problem.

Handling Nonformulary Drugs or Non-Covered NDC Numbers. Formularies tend to be very specific. This includes the decision of which drug manufacturers' products are included on the member's plan. These drug products are identified by their NDC, a code assigned to every drug in the United States. If the code submitted is not in the formulary, the claim is rejected by the insurance company. In pharmacy, these types of medications are referred to as nonformulary drugs. In this case two options can be explored. First, the pharmacist can contact the doctor and request that the prescription be changed to a drug that is covered under the patient's insurance plan.

TECH NOTE! The NDC was developed by the FDA for the drug industry for identification purposes. It is composed of three sections, each with a different meaning. The first set of numbers refers to the manufacturer; the second, the drug product; and the third, the trade package identification.

TECH NOTE! Only a pharmacist can call the doctor to change a medication.

The other option is to submit a prior authorization form to the insurance company indicating why the patient must take the nonformulary drug. The type of prior authorization forms vary depending on the insurance company's guidelines. Physicians normally fill out and submit the prior authorization forms for approval. This approval process can take up to 2 weeks. The patient must pay upfront for the medication, or he or she can wait to have the prescription filled after the approval or rejection is given by the insurance company. If the patient pays upfront and the medication is approved, the patient is reimbursed by the insurance company after the pharmacist fills out a reimbursement form for the patient. The form is sent to the insurance company to reimburse the patient for the covered drug cost.

Filling a Prescription Too Soon. There are several reasons why patients attempt to get their prescription refilled before they run out. Prescriptions are usually filled for a 30-day supply, or more rarely a 60-day or 90-day supply. The amount of medication supplied may be directly related to safety issues that surround a medication because many medications are extremely dangerous. Many insurance plans allow additional savings if refills are ordered via mail-order pharmacies that are on their list of participating pharmacies. Most of the time it is not a problem to call in for a refill on the last week of the drug's supply; however, there are instances in which the patient may call in as early as only 1 week after receiving the prescription. The patient may be leaving the country for an extended time and wants to make sure that he or she has enough medication to last until return. In this case, the pharmacist can decide to fill a prescription depending on the type of medication. If the patient's insurance will not pay, the patient is responsible for the cost of the medication.

TECH NOTE! If the patient received 2–30-day supply, then reimbursement may not be sent until $^3/_4$ of the prescription has been taken.

Sometimes a physician instructs the patient to increase the dosage, thus forcing the refill process before its allotted time. In this case a new prescription order must be submitted to the insurance company. In some cases the technician must call the insurance company's help desk to explain the circumstances of the prescription change. However, some insurance companies may require a direct response from the patient's physician before approval is given.

Non-ID Match. Probably one of the most common problems is when the cardholder's information does not match up to the processor's information, thus resulting in a claim rejection. To determine whether this is the case, the technician should always recheck the information submitted to the insurance company. Items to double-check include the following:

- Health plan card number, ID number, insurance number, and so forth
- Patient's name, DOB, and relationship to the insured person

The relationship of the patient to the cardholder is important because he or she may be a new spouse or adopted child, or other changes may have been made. In this case, the technician may be able to ask for a new insurance card for the member through the insurance's help desk.

TECH NOTE! More insurance companies are now hiring pharmacy technicians because of their in-depth knowledge of drugs.

Inventory Control

Each pharmacy orders drugs that include formulary drugs and some nonformulary drugs. The established level of medication stock kept on hand at any given time is referred to as the periodic automatic replenishment level. This is the minimum amount of medication that should be maintained in the pharmacy at any given time. Just as insurance billing has become a common task of pharmacy technicians, so has the responsibility of ordering medications. Different systems are available that can keep a running inventory of medications as well as order them. This can be done several ways, such as at the point of sale (POS), by order cards, or by handheld inventory computers. Because there are so many different types of systems in use today, this chapter explores the main idea behind these various systems as well as looking into when and how stock arrives to the pharmacy. This also includes proper storage of all drugs. In addition, this chapter discusses how recalls are handled and how returns are processed.

Although some pharmacies may contract out the job of writing up returns and sending them back to the manufacturer, this is usually done by a pharmacy technician who is an employee of the pharmacy. This technician typically is in charge of all aspects of ordering, restocking, and returning stock within the pharmacy.

SYSTEMS

It is very important to maintain a periodic automatic replenishment level in the pharmacy for several reasons. Many manufacturers do not fill orders on the weekend or holidays. This means the pharmacy could run out of stock during the weekend. The pharmacy may have to wait until the following delivery day to receive the necessary stock. This is extremely serious if a patient cannot obtain an essential medication because the pharmacy is out of stock. Patients visiting a community pharmacy may be able to go elsewhere to have prescriptions filled, but hospitalized patients rely on the hospital pharmacy to stock medications.

In cases when stock is not going to arrive until the following Monday or Tuesday, the only recourse is to express deliver the medication or borrow it from another pharmacy. Express delivery can range from a courier delivering the medication to having the medication flown in from a long distance. Of course this is used only in case of an emergency when all other options will not work. It is also very expensive and in many cases unnecessary if the pharmacy staff understands when to reorder a specific drug. Shipping time varies depending on the type of drug ordered. This is when pharmacy personnel must show their teamwork. It is not proper or appropriate to assume it is someone else's job.

More pharmacies rely on computerized systems that know when to order medications. This is by far one of the best ways to maintain appropriate stock levels, although not all pharmacies have this system. Three main systems are discussed in this chapter, although there are many more types. All systems are somewhat similar to those discussed in the following sections.

BAR CODING

Most manufacturers identify their products with bar codes that can be scanned. This process speeds up the input of information because one pass of the bar code device identifies the drug, strength, dosage form, quantity, cost, package size, and any other information. Pharmacies can use these bar codes as well. The medication is scanned at the register, called the POS, and is electronically taken off the computerized inventory list. When the in-stock quantity drops to a certain level (PAR), it is reordered automatically. Other devices used to scan drugs are handheld components that identify the necessary drug information. The operator (the technician) only needs to put in the quantity to be ordered. The information from this handheld set is then transferred to the main computer ordering system.

AUTOMATED DISPENSING SYSTEMS

For the pharmacy to determine the necessary stock levels, there has to be a way to inventory the stock that is not on the stock shelves but is in use or in a different location. For example, community pharmacies' computerized dispensing units keep track of the inventory as tablets and capsules are dispensed into a drug vial. As the pills pass a beam of light, they are automatically taken off the inventory. An example of this type of system is a Baker Cell System. Systems of this type are being developed constantly, and they all work similarly.

In a hospital, the pharmacy is responsible for supplying various clinics and nursing units with stock. To avoid everyone needing stock at the same time and having a shortage of stock on hand to fill the orders, dispensing systems that link the nursing units to the pharmacy's computer system allow the stock levels to be viewed at any time. Each time the nurse indicates the type and amount of drug taken from these drug cabinets, it is deducted from the current stock levels in the cabinet and this information is then transferred electronically to the pharmacy's unit. Various reports can be run from this centralized unit, which can give an overall stock inventory for a specific drug. In addition to the inventory status, such units also monitor controlled substance use and inventory. All persons adding drugs to or taking drugs from the unit are identified and a log is kept of all users. This also ensures the proper use of controlled substances and detects any discrepancies. Examples of this type of automated dispensing systems are PYXIS and OMNICELL.

TECH NOTE! Automated systems used in hospitals are switching from nurses and pharmacy personnel having to enter personal codes to using fingerprint ID, therefore making it more difficult to misuse the system.

MANUAL ORDERING

Although manual ordering is slowly being eliminated as the main ordering technique, it is still important in the continued monitoring of stock levels. Many pharmacies visually note that stock is getting low or use ordering cards that stay inside the medication box. These cards list the drug information, including the ordering number and the necessary periodic automatic replenishment levels to aid the technician in ordering the proper amount. The card system or simply writing down the right amount of stock to be ordered depends on the technician knowing which drugs fall into which of the following categories:

- Formulary: Nonformulary drugs normally are kept at a low level because they are not ordered often. They may not be kept at all, depending on the preferences of management.

- Fast mover: These drugs are typically kept in a separate area from the normal stock because of the high volume of use. These must be ordered in larger quantities, keeping the overstock nearby, or must be ordered more often.
- Slow mover: These drugs are prescribed on a regular basis by a few doctors, but are not commonly prescribed. These must be checked before ordering and periodically to ensure that the drugs are not close to expiring.
- Special orders: These typically are drugs that are used by only a few patients, but they may be extremely important for proper treatment. It is easy to forget to order these drugs because of their infrequent use. Usually they are ordered at the time of use.
- Time of year: The drugs that fall into this category vary depending on the time of year. Many medications that are fast movers during a particular time of year may need their periodic automatic replacement levels raised during that period. For example, albuterol inhalers are normally fast movers in the spring, when allergies increase. At this time of year there may be many more people diagnosed with asthma or respiratory problems, which may double normal periodic automatic replacement levels. All pharmacy staff must be aware of the types of medications used during different times of the year and how they fluctuate.

Responding early when a trend is seen is a skill that takes time and experience. When stock begins to run low, it is everyone's responsibility to make sure that the stock is ordered.

NEW STOCK

Stock may arrive daily to the pharmacy. It is important for billing purposes that all stock be checked completely against the invoice when first received. The following is a step-by-step approach that should be used when receiving stock:

1. Retrieve the manufacturer or warehouse invoice.
2. All boxes should be accounted for. For example, if the invoice indicates there are five boxes, your first task is to verify that there are five boxes.
3. If any box is marked refrigerate or freeze, you must comply with the instructions immediately to avoid product damage.
4. All information must be checked against the invoice. For example, check the following:
   Name of drug
   Strength or dosage
   Dosage form
   Quantity
   Expiration date of product*
5. The invoice should be compared with the order form to make sure that only what was ordered was sent.
6. The invoice is then signed and dated by the technician and sent for processing per pharmacy protocol.
7. Once the received order has been confirmed as correct, the technician may put the stock away. Rotating stock is another important priority. New stock typically has later expiration dates and should be placed behind the existing stock that expires sooner. All stock should be rotated in this manner to avoid accumulation of expired drugs, which may be used accidentally.
8. Finally, it is important to return inventory cards to the medication box for future use.

---

*Checking the expiration date is extremely important. Drugs that are used rarely and have short expiration dates sit on the shelf and expire before use.

TECH NOTE! One of the best ways to learn drug names and to know where they are located in your pharmacy is to put new stock away.

Inventory may not sound difficult. However, marking stock shelves clearly ultimately affects the probability of drug errors. For example, if a drug is accidentally put in a box intended for a different drug with a similar-sounding name, it may be used to fill a prescription for the sound-alike drug and make its way into the patient's possession.

TECH NOTE! You should not allow any medication into the pharmacy unless it has good dating on it. "Good dating" means that the expiration date is long enough to make it likely that the drug will be used before expiration. Most pharmacies use a 3-month expiration time. This means that a drug that expires in 3 months or less may expire before use unless it is a fast mover, and may be sent back to the manufacturer for a refund.

RETURNS

There are three main reasons that medication is sent back to the warehouse or manufacturer. Depending on the reason, certain paperwork must accompany the medication. Except for schedule drugs that fall under the jurisdiction of the Drug Enforcement Agency, most medications can be sent back by the technician without a pharmacist's signature. The three reasons for returning drugs to the manufacturer are as follows:

1. Drug recalls
2. Damaged drugs
3. Expired drugs

Drug Recalls

Manufacturers are required by law to recall any product that has been found to violate any of the following guidelines:

1. Labeling is wrong.
2. Product was not packaged or produced properly.
3. Drug batch was contaminated.
4. Any other change occurs that causes the drug to fall outside the FDA or manufacturer's guidelines.

Recall notices may arrive by mail or fax and identify the necessary information about the drug or device in question and how to handle the recall procedure. This information includes the drug's name and why it is being recalled. One of the most important pieces of information given is the drug's lot number. This is the key to identifying the recalled medication. Technicians are responsible for checking all of the drug stock throughout the pharmacy and facility to make sure that the recalled drug is not in stock. If this is the case, the recall form is initialed to indicate that the item is not in stock. If pharmacy stock does include a drug with the recalled lot number, the pharmacist must be notified in case a patient has been issued one of these products. Any patient who may have been issued a recalled item should be notified by phone so that he or she may check the lot number of the drug or device. All recalled items must be sent back to the manufacturer as indicated. If all of a pharmacy's stock of a particular drug is recalled, more stock must be reordered immediately, possibly from another manufacturer. All of these tasks may be performed by the pharmacy technician.

Damaged Stock

If you notice that some drugs were damaged en route to the pharmacy but you did not catch it at the time of delivery, it is still not too late to send the damaged stock back to the manufacturer. It may be necessary to call first and get an approval code to send back the damaged goods.

Expired Stock

Many pharmacies have a policy to pull any medication that will expire in 3 months or less. This ensures that there are no drugs on the shelves close to their expiration date. Depending on the contract between the pharmacy and the manufacturer, it may be allowable to send back items as long as they can be bundled into a minimum package size rather than partials. For instance, if the stock of cimetidine expires within 3 months, the manufacturer may allow it to be returned for full or partial credit if a box of 100 tablets can be returned at one time. Following manufacturer's guidelines for returns is important. Hazardous chemicals, including cytotoxic agents, must be repackaged carefully to avoid breakage during transport.

NONRETURNABLE DRUGS AND THEIR DISPOSAL

There are many examples of items that are not taken back by manufacturers. Any drug that is reconstituted or compounded within the pharmacy may not be returned to the manufacturer. Partially used bottles of medication are not normally taken back, nor are any drugs that have been repackaged by the pharmacy. These drugs, including most reconstituted agents such as amoxicillin suspension, can be dumped in the pharmacy garbage, but in most cases, especially in chain pharmacies, the drugs are sent to a central location for destruction or return to manufacturer for credit. Many agents must be disposed of carefully. Cytotoxic agents must be disposed of in a sharps container marked "hazardous waste." Nontoxic intravenous agents should be disposed of in a regular sharps container marked for proper disposal. Controlled substances must be counted and cosigned by a pharmacist before they are destroyed. Before any scheduled medications are destroyed, the DEA must be contacted for specific instructions for destruction. Controlled substances disposal is the only task for which the pharmacist must be present, must cosign the disposal of the drug, and must return information required by the DEA. The DEA issues a receipt for Schedule II merchandise destroyed. This receipt must be kept for 5 years with the Schedule II inventory.

SUPPLIERS

When ordering stock for the pharmacy, the technician orders from a centralized warehouse that the pharmacy owns, from a wholesaler, or directly from the manufacturer.

There are pros and cons to each of these suppliers. As seen in Table 14.1, the benefits of using wholesalers compared with dealing directly with the manufacturer differ mostly in the amount of stock that must be ordered and kept as overstock and the difference in cost. The final column describes a warehouse situation in which a company orders extremely high volumes of drugs from the manufacturer and may repackage the medications into more suitable sizes for the ordering physician. This serves several purposes, such as easier handling, increased productivity, and lower cost. Large-quantity bottles are hard to handle. They are more likely to be dropped, spilling the contents. Medications may be prepacked in smaller, easy-to-handle containers to eliminate the bulkiness of the larger bottles. If the pharmacy warehouse prepackages common dosages, it speeds up the labeling process. For example, sulfamethoxazole/trimethoprim (Septra) is normally ordered to be taken twice daily for 10 days or twice daily for 15 days. These tablets are prepackaged in bottles of 20 and 30, eliminating the time it takes to count out the proper amount at the pharmacy counter. The technician must check the label against the prescription to determine the appropriate drug and quantity, and the prescription is ready to be checked by the pharmacist and dispensed. Finally, because the volume of drugs is much higher than what a normal pharmacy can stock, pharmacies have contracts with these warehouses that save the pharmacy a substantial amount of money. This ultimately keeps the cost lower for the consumer.

TABLE 14.1 Difference in Ordering From Manufacturers, Wholesalers, and Warehouse Repackaging Plant

Factors to Consider	Manufacturer	Wholesaler/Vendor Warehouse	Warehouse Repackaging Plant
Supplier cost	No shipping fees	Lower per contract	Lowest cost
Supplier has electronic inventory control mechanism	No	Yes	Yes
Supplier able to stock large supplies when ordering	Yes	No	No
Supplier provides special delivery service	Varies by manufacturer	Yes	Yes
Supplier handles special orders	Yes	Some special orders must be done through the manufacturer	Some special orders must be done through the manufacturer

SPECIAL ORDERING CONSIDERATIONS

Special considerations must be given to a host of drugs ordered by pharmacy. Some of these include controlled substances, investigational drugs, cytotoxic drugs, and hazardous substances. Each of these types of medications require special ordering, inventory, handling, and return paperwork. The FDA requires special forms to be completed for ordering controlled substances with a CII schedule as well as for returning them (see Chapter 2). In addition, controlled substances need to be inventoried daily by a trained pharmacy staff person. Usually, the ordering technician does not have this additional task.

Investigational drugs typically come with paperwork that must be completed and returned to the manufacturer each time a medication is given. Cytotoxic drugs do not need special paperwork, but they should be handled with great care and placed in a safety cabinet under the guidelines of the manufacturer. Some cytotoxic agents must be refrigerated and should be well marked to separate them from other agents. Most pharmacies stock certain chemicals that are considered hazardous. It is important to know where your pharmacy's material safety data sheets (MSDSs) are located in case of a spill. Agents such as phenol should be kept behind cabinet doors to protect people from accidentally knocking the bottle off a shelf and inhaling the toxic fumes.

DO YOU REMEMBER THESE KEY POINTS?

- Why pharmacy formularies are important
- The difference between a generic name and a trade name
- The major types of insurance and the differences between them
- The differences between government insurance programs
- The necessary information that patients must provide to the pharmacy for billing prescriptions to third parties
- The types of problems that often arise associated with insurance claims
- The importance of the NDC code and how to decipher it
- The responsibilities of a pharmacy technician concerning stock levels and ordering stock for the pharmacy
- Common types of automated dispensing systems and where they are used
- The set of steps that should be used when receiving stock

REVIEW QUESTIONS:

Multiple Choice

1. All of the following are types of insurance except
   A. HMO
   B. PPO
   C. Medicaid
   D. FDA

2. Medicare is a government-run insurance program that covers all of the following except
   A. Senior citizens
   B. Patients using dialysis
   C. Children
   D. Persons who are disabled

3. Medicaid covers all of the following people except
   A. Persons who are disabled
   B. People with low income
   C. Women who are pregnant
   D. Single working people with above-average income

4. Geographical managed care can be best described as
   A. A medical group that is covered under Medicare and works much like an HMO
   B. A program that belongs to a medical group covered by Medicare and works much like an HMO
   C. A program that belongs to a medical group covered by Medicaid and works much like an HMO
   D. An HMO program that covers general medical groups

5. Information required by insurance companies does not include
   A. Date medication is filled
   B. Name of pharmacy filing the prescription
   C. Name and dosage form of drug
   D. Name of technician

6. Insurance claims that are electronically transmitted to the insurance provider are called
   A. E-mail
   B. NDC claims
   C. Adjudication
   D. Copay

7. Of the automated systems listed, which is most commonly used to manage controlled substances levels?
   A. PYXIS
   B. Baker Cell Systems
   C. Bar coding
   D. Both A and C

8. Various types of drugs ordered for a pharmacy may include
   A. Formulary drugs
   B. Hazardous substances
   C. Cytotoxic drugs
   D. All of the above

9. One of the most important aspects of keeping stock in date is
   A. Sending back expired drugs
   B. Throwing away drugs that are close to expiring
   C. Rotating stock
   D. None of the above

10. An inventory system that automatically orders stock as it is used is called
    A. PYXIS
    B. POS
    C. MSDS
    D. Inventory cards

True/False

*If a statement is false, then change it to make it true.

1. Both trade and generic drugs cost the pharmacy the same price.

2. If a patient's drug claim is rejected by the insurance company, the technician may call the help desk and attempt to reactivate it.

3. Periodic automatic replacement levels are levels of drugs that should be kept at a predetermined level in the pharmacy.

4. All drug recall notifications must be initiated by the FDA.

5. It is the sole responsibility of the pharmacy inventory technician to keep all drugs and pharmacy supplies in stock.

6. Drug companies never allow pharmacies to return drugs.

7. The only drug return that requires a pharmacist's signature is controlled substances return.

8. All hazardous substances should be kept behind cabinet doors for safety purposes.

9. MSDS stands for medication safety drug sheets and gives descriptions of drugs.

10. Drugs that expire within 3 months may (in many cases) be pulled and returned to the manufacturer.

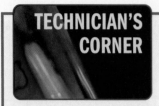
TECHNICIAN'S CORNER

The pharmacy technician accidentally fills the quinine stock box with quinidine. What is the difference between these two medicines? As a technician, what can you do to avoid confusion between these two drugs?

15
Psychopharmacology

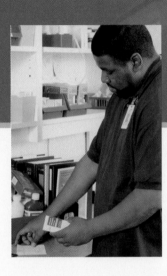

Objectives

- List the major medications used for each of the conditions described in this chapter.

- List the most common side effects of each of the drugs discussed.

- Describe the main emotional conditions affecting the brain.

- Differentiate between a normal depression and a severe depression.

- List the types of insomnia that can occur and why.

- Differentiate between older and newer treatments for the mentally disabled.

- Distinguish the capabilities of a psychologist versus a psychiatrist.

- List the differences between the uses of monoamine oxidase inhibitors (MAOIs), tricyclic antidepressants (TCAs), and selective serotonin reuptake inhibitors (SSRIs).

- Explain the reasons for the use of SSRIs over MAOI and TCA agents.

- Describe the differences between the uses of phenothiazines and thioxanthenes.

- Describe the types of nondrug therapy available for patients suffering from various mental disorders.

TERMS AND DEFINITIONS

Anxiety *Feelings of apprehension, dread, and fear, with characteristics including tension, restlessness, tachycardia, dyspnea, and a sense of hopelessness*

Bipolar disorder *Depressive psychosis, alternating between excessive phases of mania and depression; Formerly known as manic-depressive*

Depression *A mental state characterized by sadness, feelings of loss and grief, loss of appetite, and may include suicidal thoughts*

Dystonia *Symptoms that include twisting, repeated jerking movements, and/or abnormal posture*

Extrapyramidal *Symptoms of taking antipsychotic medications that include parkinsonism, dystonia, and tremors*

Insomnia *Difficulty falling or staying asleep*

Mania *A form of psychosis characterized by excessive excitement, elevated mood, and exalted feelings*

Neurosis *Mental illness arising from stress or anxiety in the patient's environment without loss of contact with reality; phobias can be listed in this category*

Pruritis *Severe itching that can be caused by an allergic reaction*

Psychosis *A mental illness characterized by loss of contact with reality*

Schizophrenia *A group of mental disorders characterized by inappropriate emotions and unrealistic thinking*

Tardive dyskinesia *Unwanted side effects of taking phenothiazines that include slow, rhythmical, involuntary movements that are either generalized or specific to a muscle group*

Tourette's syndrome *A disorder characterized by multiple motor tics, lack of muscle coordination, and involuntary purposeless movements that are accompanied by grunts and barks*

PSYCHOTHERAPEUTIC MEDICATIONS

Trade Name	Generic Name	Pronunciation	Trade Name	Generic Name	Pronunciation
Antipsychotic Agents			Norpramin	desipramine	deh-sip-**rah**-meen
			Pamelor	nortriptyline	nor-**trip**-tah-leen
Compazine	prochlorperazine	**pro**-klor-pear-ah-zeen	Paxil	paroxetine	par-**ox**-eh-teen
Eskalith	lithium	**lith**-e-um	Prozac	fluoxetine	flew-**ox**-eh-teen
Haldol	haloperidol	ha-low-**pear**-i-doll	Sinequan	doxepin	**dock**-seh-pin
Loxitane	loxapine	**lock**-sah-peen	Tofranil	imipramine	ih-**mip**-rah-meen
Mellaril	thioridazine	thy-oh-**rid**-ah-zeen	Wellbutrin	bupropion	bew-**pro**-peon
Navane	thiothixene	thy-oh-**thick**-seen	Zoloft	sertraline	**sir**-tra-leen
Orap	pimozide	**pim**-oh-zyde			
Prolixin	fluphenazine	flew-**fen**-ah-zeen			
Risperdal	risperidone	ris-**pear**-ih-doan	**Antianxiety Agents**		
Stelazine	trifluoperazine	try-flew-**pear**-ah-zeen	Atarax	hydroxyzine HCl	high-**drok**-seh-zeen
Thorazine	chlorpromazine	klor-**pro**-ma-zeen	Ativan	lorazepam	lor-**az**-ah-pam
Trilafon	perphenazine	per-**fen**-ah-zeen	Buspar	buspirone	bew-**spear**-on
Zyprexa	olanzapine	oh-**lan**-zah-peen	Equanil	meprobamate	meh-**pro**-bah-mate
			Librium	chlordiazepoxide	klor-dye-az-eh-**pox**-ide
Antidepressants			Serax	oxazepam	ox-**az**-eh-pam
Asendin	amoxapine	ah-**mox**-ah-peen	Tranxene	clorazepate	klor-**az**-eh-pate
Celexa	citalopram	cit a **lo** pram	Valium	diazepam	dye-**az**-eh-pam
Desyrel	trazodone	**trah**-zoe-doan	Vistaril	hydroxyzine pamoate	high-**drok**-seh-zeen
Effexor	venlafaxine	ven-**la**-facks-een	Xanax	alprazolam	al-**pra**-zoe-lam
Elavil	amitriptyline	am-eh-**trip**-tah-leen			

Introduction

Over the course of history, one of the most difficult studies of medicine has been the study of the brain, because of its complexities. Specifically, what makes people behave they way they do? Historically, a person suffering from mental illness who did not "fit" into "normal" society easily could have been institutionalized for life. Families would try to forget or hide their knowledge of a mentally ill relative. The traditional treatments used ranged from electric shocks, straight jackets, isolation and even to physical punishment. There were few medications known to help a mental disease. Even after some medications were discovered, most of them treated the illness by sedating the patient so that he or she could not "act out." It was not until the 1960s that advancements were made in psychopharmacology.

There are many different specialists trained in the study of human emotions, feelings, and behavior, such as psychiatrists, psychologists, and counselors. Psychiatrists are medical doctors who have completed a residency in the field of psychiatry. A psychologist has a doctorate degree in psychology. Unlike psychiatrists, psychologists cannot write prescriptions, but they are trained extensively in the treatment of mental illness through counseling. In addition to psychiatrists and psychologists, there are other professionals available to treat individuals with emotional problems, such as family counselors and clergy. For many people, this type of therapy may be adequate for help through difficult times. A person suffering from a severe emotional, behavioral, or biological instability involving the emotional portion of the brain may need to be seen by a psychiatrist for proper diagnosis and treatment. Depending on the diagnosis, a patient may also need to see a neurologist, a specialist of the nervous system. Many mental illnesses are caused by neuronal disturbances within the nervous system, such as twitching, or emotional problems stemming from a brain tumor or other physical problem.

Emotional Health

Emotional and behavioral instability can often be linked to functions of the body. A physician must evaluate the central nervous system (CNS) as well as the environment a person lives in. The CNS can be divided into two main functions, autonomic and somatic. The autonomic system works without conscious control, whereas the somatic system is under conscious control (see Chapter 17). The nervous system is an intricate network of chemical reactions that causes specific responses when activated. If any chemicals within the nervous system are out of balance or cease to produce, symptoms can appear as inappropriate behavior.

Nondrug Treatments

Because of the wide range of mental health conditions that exist, there are many alternative nondrug treatments available. In the case of disorders that involve addictions or behavior disorders, there are many group therapies available through nonprofit groups, such as Alcoholics Anonymous, or for-profit groups, such as Weight Watchers. Both give the patient a safe place where he or she can speak freely and not feel guilty. For more serious conditions or in cases in which the person does not feel comfortable speaking in front of others, a person can see a psychologist or counselor. For conditions that affect the whole family or a child, there are many family counselors that specialize in group therapy within the family unit. For persons suffering from more severe crises, there are psychiatrists who are able to meet one-on-one to discuss problems. If the psychiatrist feels that medication is appropriate, he or she can write prescriptions, unlike psychologists or family

TABLE 15.1 Conditions and Available Treatments

Examples of Conditions	Specialist	Special Notes
Mild depression, anxiety	Psychologist	Cannot prescribe drugs
Mild family problems, stress, child-rearing problems	Psychologist, family counselor, or support group	Cannot prescribe drugs
Psychosis, schizophrenia, manic depressive disorders, major phobias	Psychiatrist (medical doctor)	Can prescribe drugs if necessary

counselors. Mental health professionals and their scopes of practice are listed in Table 15.1.

Medication Therapy

Schizophrenia, mania, or psychotic depression are often treated with antipsychotic drugs and/or tranquilizers. These agents reduce the symptoms that often accompany these conditions. Mania, schizophrenia, and even psychotic depression tend to induce high-stress states in the patient. Antipsychotic agents and tranquilizers sedate the patient and produce a calming effect, lessening anxiety and depression.

ANTIPSYCHOTIC AGENTS

The two main classifications of antipsychotic drugs are phenothiazines and thioxanthenes. They differ in their lengths of effectiveness. Long-acting medications are called decanoates and are dosed monthly. In addition to the decanoates, there are the short-acting daily doses of the same type of drug. For instance, haloperidol can be dosed daily or on an as needed (prn) basis. In addition to this type of dosing, the patient may be given a monthly dose of injectable haloperidol decanoate. The following medications are available as long-term decanoates.

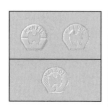

Ortho-McNeil

CLASSIFICATION: LONG-ACTING DECANOATES
GENERIC NAME: haloperidol decanoate
TRADE NAME: Haldol
INDICATIONS: psychoses; Tourette's disorder
STRENGTH: 50 mg injectable, 100 mg injectable; 0.5 to 5 mg tablets
ROUTE OF ADMINISTRATION: injectable, po
COMMON DOSAGE: 10 to 15 times the normal daily dose every (q) month (maximum dose should not exceed 100 mg). Most daily oral (po) doses range between 5 mg to 20 mg per day individed doses
AUXILIARY LABELS:
- Do not drink alcohol.
- May cause dizziness and drowsiness.

GENERIC: fluphenazine decanoate
TRADE NAME: Prolixin
INDICATION: Psychotic disorders
STRENGTH: 25 mg/ml
ROUTE OF ADMINISTRATION: injectable
COMMON DOSAGE: 10 to 15 times the normal daily dose q month
AUXILIARY LABELS:
- Do not drink alcohol.
- May cause dizziness and drowsiness.

Side effects of decanoates include respiratory depression, tardive dyskinesia, drowsiness, orthostatic hypotension, and dry mouth.

Drug Action of Phenothiazines and Thioxanthenes

The drug action as it relates to the mechanism of action for the agents within two common classes of antipsychotics (phenothiazine and thioxanthene) is the inhibition of dopamine within the CNS. This antianxiety effect is caused by the effects on the brainstem area. These agents can cause blood pressure to drop but also (as a side effect) can decrease nausea and vomiting via their antiemetic effects. It can take up to 6 weeks or longer before the desired effects of these agents are obtained. If a change in medication is necessary, doses must be tapered slowly.

The main indications for these agents are psychosis, nausea, and vomiting. They can be given orally (po) or parenterally (intravenously or intramuscularly). Side effects of these agents include drowsiness, confusion, insomnia, hypotension, and dry mouth. Alcohol and monoamine oxidase inhibitors (MAOIs) may potentiate (increase) CNS depression, whereas antacids and antidiarrheals can reduce the absorption rate of both phenothiazines and thioxanthenes. One adverse reaction that can occur while taking these types of agents is tardive dyskinesia. The symptoms include involuntary movement of the facial muscles, tongue, jaw, and head. If these symptoms appear, the medication must be stopped immediately, because these effects can be irreversible. Another type of adverse effect that is related to overdosing is extrapyramidal effects that mimic Parkinson's disease, causing both the hands and head to shake. Drooling and a shuffling gait are present as well. These symptoms usually disappear if the medication strength is lowered or medication is stopped. Following are the shorter acting agents listed under their perspective classifications:

CLASSIFICATION: PHENOTHIAZINES

> **GENERIC NAME:** prochlorperazine
> **TRADE NAME:** Compazine
> **INDICATION:** psychotic disorders; nausea and vomiting
> **ROUTE OF ADMINISTRATION:** po, injectable, rectal
> **COMMON DOSAGE (po):** 5–10 mg (for nausea) 1 q6 or 8h prn
> **AUXILIARY LABELS:**
> - May cause dizziness and drowsiness.
> - Do not take if you become pregnant.
> - Do not drink alcohol.

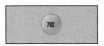

Sandoz

> **GENERIC NAME:** thioridazine
> **TRADE NAME:** Mellaril
> **INDICATIONS:** psychotic disorders; anxiety, agitation, depression, sleep disturbances
> **ROUTE OF ADMINISTRATION:** po
> **COMMON DOSAGE:** 10 mg twice a day (bid) or three times a day (tid)
> **AUXILIARY LABELS:**
> - May cause dizziness and drowsiness.
> - Do not take if you become pregnant.
> - Do not drink alcohol.

> **GENERIC NAME:** perphenazine
> **TRADE NAME:** Trilafon
> **INDICATIONS:** psychotic disorders, nausea, and vomiting, hiccoughs
> **ROUTE OF ADMINISTRATION:** po, injectable
> **COMMON DOSAGE:** 4 mg to 8 mg tid
> **AUXILIARY LABELS:**
> - May cause dizziness and drowsiness.
> - Do not take if you become pregnant.
> - Do not drink alcohol.

SmithKline
Beecham

GENERIC NAME: chlorpromazine
TRADE NAME: Thorazine
INDICATION: manic depressive reactions, hyperactivity in children
ROUTE OF ADMINISTRATION: po, injectable, rectal
COMMON DOSAGE: 25 mg tid up to 400 mg every day (qd)
AUXILIARY LABELS:
- May cause dizziness and drowsiness.
- Do not take if you become pregnant.
- Do not drink alcohol.

GENERIC NAME: trifluoperazine
TRADE NAME: Stelazine
INDICATION: psychotic disorders, anxiety
ROUTE OF ADMINISTRATION: po, injectable
COMMON DOSAGE: 1 mg to 5 mg qd or bid
AUXILIARY LABELS:
- May cause dizziness and drowsiness.
- Do not take if you become pregnant.
- Do not drink alcohol.

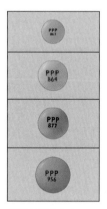

Bristol-Myers
Squibb

GENERIC NAME: fluphenazine
TRADE NAME: Prolixin
INDICATION: psychotic disorders, emesis
ROUTE OF ADMINISTRATION: po, injection
COMMON DOSAGE: 0.5 mg to 10 mg qd
AUXILIARY LABELS:
- May cause dizziness and drowsiness.
- Do not take if you become pregnant.
- Do not drink alcohol.

The side effects of phenotiazines are drowsiness, dizziness, extrapyramidal symptoms, dry mouth, and tardive dyskinesia.

CLASSIFICATION: ANTIPSYCHOTIC
GENERIC NAME: thiothixene
TRADE NAME: Navane
INDICATION: psychotic disorders
ROUTE OF ADMINISTRATION: po, injectable
COMMON DOSAGE: 2 mg tid to 15 mg qd
AUXILIARY LABELS:
- May cause dizziness and drowsiness.
- Avoid alcohol.

The side effects of thioxanthes are extrapyramidal symptoms, dry mouth, akathisia, dystonia, and tardive dyskinesia.

Alternative Antipsychotic Agents

Alternative antipsychotic agents are used to treat psychotic patients that do not respond well to phenothiazines or thioxanthenes, or who have adverse reactions to them. Many of these agents are new on the market and their drug actions are not entirely understood. A list of the most common agents are given in the following.

CLASSIFICATION: DIBENZAPINE DERIVATIVES

GENERIC NAME: loxapine

TRADE NAME: Loxitane

INDICATION: psychotic disorders

ROUTE OF ADMINISTRATION: po, injection (IM)

COMMON DOSAGE: 10 mg bid up to 50 mg qd (in divided doses)

AUXILIARY LABELS:

- May cause dizziness and drowsiness.
- Do not drink alcohol.
- Do not take if you become pregnant.

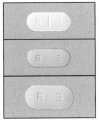

Janssen

CLASSIFICATION: BENZISOXAZOLE DERIVATIVES

GENERIC NAME: risperidone

TRADE NAME: Risperdal

INDICATION: psychotic disorders and agitation in elderly people

ROUTE OF ADMINISTRATION: po

COMMON DOSAGE: 1 mg up to 3 mg bid

AUXILIARY LABELS: none

The side effects of dibenzapines are drowsiness, hyperactivity, seizures, and tardive dyskinesia.

GENERIC NAME: olanzapine

TRADE NAME: Zyprexa

INDICATION: psychotic disorders

ROUTE OF ADMINISTRATION: po

COMMON DOSAGE: 5 mg to 10 mg qd

AUXILIARY LABELS: none

The side effects are headache, agitation, insomnia, and constipation.

CLASSIFICATION: BUTYROPHENONE

GENERIC NAME: pimozide

TRADE NAME: Orap

INDICATION: Tourette's syndrome; psychosis

ROUTE OF ADMINISTRATION: po

COMMON DOSAGE: 1 mg to 2 mg qd

AUXILIARY LABEL:

- Avoid grapefruit juice.

ANTIMANICS

The word *mania* is derived from the word *manic*. This form of psychosis is characterized by excessive mood swings that range from manic (high) to depressive (low) states, which is also known as bipolar behavior, indicating the extreme mood swings. Lithium is used to treat the mania phase. Although the complete mechanism for lithium is not fully understood, it is believed to alter behavior by enhancing nerve cells' uptake of serotonin and norepinephrine (see Chapter 17). This sets it apart from all the other psychiatric drugs, because it does not cause any major CNS changes such as sedation, feelings of euphoria, or depression. Lithium's effects are more powerful in older adults; therefore it is important that their lithium levels are monitored more closely. It may take several weeks to see the desired effect of this agent.

TECH NOTE! All patients taking lithium must have their blood levels monitored on a regular basis to monitor for toxicity.

CLASSIFICATION: ANTIMANIC
   GENERIC NAME: lithium
   TRADE NAME: Eskalith
   INDICATION: mania, depression
   ROUTE OF ADMINISTRATION: po
   COMMON DOSAGE: for acute mania; 600 mg tid or 900 mg bid. Doses vary based on laboratory results of serum lithium levels
   AUXILIARY LABELS:
- Do not drink alcohol.
- May cause dizziness and drowsiness.
- Take with food or milk.
- Drink plenty of water.

The side effects include dizziness, drowsiness, ataxia, hypotension, slurred speech, and weight gain.

ANTIDEPRESSANTS

Everyone is depressed at one time or another during their lifetime. Most persons who experience depression do not seek medical help and recover within a short period. However, for those persons in whom the depression does not subside within a few weeks, professional attention may be necessary.

There are many drugs used for depression. This mental state can range from prolonged feelings of extreme sadness to thoughts of suicide. Patients with manic-depression fluctuate between the two extremes. There are three closely related agents that are commonly used to treat depression. These are the tricyclic antidepressants (TCAs), monoamine oxidase inhibitors (MAOIs), and selective serotonin reuptake inhibitors (SSRIs). Each of these agents increases the norepinephrine, serotonin, and dopamine chemicals of the brain, which elevates the mood of the patient. However, each type of agent accomplishes this by a different drug action.

Tricyclic Antidepressants

TCAs are used for depression, obsessive-compulsive disorders, and, in some cases, chronic pain. These agents inhibit (stop) the reuptake (the cells taking back excess amounts) of norepinephrine and serotonin. There is a wide range of concerns with TCAs in general. One of the main concerns with taking TCAs is the possibility of tardive dyskinesia. Worsening of symptoms in patients with heart disease, schizophrenia, seizure disorders, and renal or hepatic problems are also a concern. Because of these problems, TCAs are not the first line of treatment for depression. However, for some people, they work well when all other medications fail. Side effects range between the various types of TCAs and are described in the following.

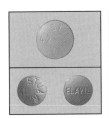

Astra Zeneca

CLASSIFICATION: TRICYCLIC ANTIDEPRESSANT
  GENERIC NAME: amitriptyline
  TRADE NAME: Elavil
  INDICATION: depression
  ROUTE OF ADMINISTRATION: po, injectable
  COMMON DOSAGE: 75 mg to 100 mg qd (divided doses) up to 300 mg qd
  AUXILIARY LABELS:
  - May cause dizziness and drowsiness.
  - Take with food.

GENERIC NAME: doxepin
  TRADE NAME: Sinequan
  INDICATION: depression, anxiety
  ROUTE OF ADMINISTRATION: po, cream*
  COMMON DOSAGE: 50 mg to 150 mg qd
  AUXILIARY LABELS:
  - May cause dizziness and drowsiness.
  - May cause sensitivity to sun light.

*Cream is indicated for dermatological pruritus, alopecia, or rashes

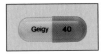

Navortis

GENERIC NAME: imipramine
  TRADE NAME: Tofranil
  INDICATION: depression, enuresis (bedwetting)
  ROUTE OF ADMINISTRATION: po (pamoate + HCL), injectable (HCL only)
  COMMON DOSAGE: po 75 mg to 150 mg qd*
  AUXILIARY LABELS:
  - May cause dizziness and drowsiness.
  - Do not drink alcohol.

*In children dosage is determined by the child's weight.

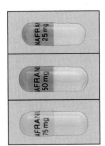

Basel

GENERIC NAME: clomipramine
  TRADE NAME: Anafranil
  INDICATION: obsessive compulsive disorder, depression
  ROUTE OF ADMINISTRATION: po
  COMMON DOSAGE: 25 mg qd, up to 100 mg qd (divided doses)
  AUXILIARY LABELS:
  - May cause dizziness and drowsiness.
  - Do not drink alcohol.

The side effects of tricyclic antidepressants include drowsiness, dry mouth, blurred vision, orthostatic hypotension, dizziness, and headache.

Monoamine Oxidase Inhibitors

MAOIs mostly differ from TCAs and SSRIs by their side effects. Patients taking MAOIs can exhibit hypertension. There are many food interactions with MAOIs as well. Certain foods containing tyramine, such as wine, can be extremely dangerous to a patient taking MAOIs. In addition to wine, in general, foods that use bacteria or other microbes in their processing cause interactions. Produce such as raisins, bananas, avocados, and papaya can cause adverse reactions also. A sample list of foods with microbial ingredients are listed in Table 15.2.

Because of the many food interactions with MAOI agents, they are reserved for use in patients who do not respond to TCAs or SSRIs or who have a reaction to them. The following drugs are MAOIs.

TABLE 15.2 Foods That Contain Tyramine

Foods	Additive
Cheese	Bacteria and fungi
Sour cream	Bacteria
Beer	Yeast
Wine	Yeast
Avocados	Bacteria
Soy sauce	Fungi
Yogurt	Bacteria
Chocolate	Caffeine
Tea	Caffeine
Coffee	Caffeine

CLASSIFICATION: MONOAMINE OXIDASE INHIBITORS
GENERIC NAME: tranylcypromine
TRADE NAME: Parnate
INDICATION: depression
ROUTE OF ADMINISTRATION: po
COMMON DOSAGE: 30 mg qd (divided doses) up to 60 mg qd
AUXILIARY LABELS:
- Take with food.
- Do not drink alcohol.

GENERIC NAME: phenelzine
TRADE NAME: Nardil
INDICATION: depression
ROUTE OF ADMINISTRATION: po
COMMON DOSAGE: 15 mg tid up to 60 mg qd
AUXILIARY LABEL:
- Do not drink alcohol.

The side effects of MAOIs include GI upset, insomnia, drowsiness, hypotension, dry mouth, and anorexia.

Selective Serotonin Reuptake Inhibitors

SSRIs act specifically on keeping higher levels of serotonin in the brain. When serotonin is increased, mood is elevated. These agents work differently than the MAOIs and TCAs. Because they have fewer side effects, they are preferable to treat depression and obsessive compulsive disorders. The doses that follow are the maximum doses. Patients may be started at a lower dose initially, and the dose may be gradually increased to the maximum dosage. It is important to note that patients cannot take MAOIs and SSRIs concurrently. There have been reports of death caused by this dangerous combination. Typically these medications can take up to 6 weeks to work at their full potential.

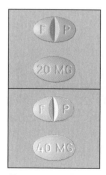

Forest

CLASSIFICATION: SELECTIVE SEROTONIN REUPTAKE INHIBITORS
GENERIC NAME: citalopram
TRADE NAME: Celexa
INDICATION: antidepressant
ROUTE OF ADMINISTRATION: po
STRENGTH: tablet 20 mg, 40 mg, 60 mg; solution 10 mg/5 ml
COMMON DOSAGE: po 20 mg qd
AUXILIARY LABEL:
- May cause dizziness and drowsiness.

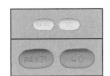

SmithKline
Beecham

GENERIC NAME: paroxetine
TRADE NAME: Paxil
INDICATION: depression, obsessive compulsive disorder
ROUTE OF ADMINISTRATION: po
COMMON DOSAGE: depression, 10 mg qd; OCD, 40 mg qd
AUXILIARY LABELS:
- Take with food.
- Do not drink alcohol.

GENERIC NAME: fluoxetine
TRADE NAME: Prozac
INDICATION: depression, obsessive compulsive disorder
ROUTE OF ADMINISTRATION: po
COMMON DOSAGE: 60 mg qd maximum; usually 10–20 mg daily
AUXILIARY LABELS:
- Take with food.
- Do not drink alcohol.
NOTE: May increase suicidal tendencies.

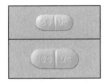

Roerig

GENERIC NAME: sertraline
TRADE NAME: Zoloft
INDICATION: depression, obsessive compulsive disorder
ROUTE OF ADMINISTRATION: po
COMMON DOSAGE: 50 mg qd up to 200 mg qd
AUXILIARY LABEL:
- Do not drink alcohol.

The side effects of SSRIs include insomnia, nausea, dizziness, drowsiness, sexual dysfunction, headache, constipation, dry mouth, and anorexia.

Additional Antidepressants

The antidepressants discussed here do not fit into the previous categories because they do not have the same drug actions as the other antidepressants. In some cases, the exact drug action is not known; however, they work well for some patients.

CLASSIFICATION: OTHER ANTIDEPRESSANTS
GENERIC NAME: trazodone
TRADE NAME: Desyrel
INDICATION: depression
ROUTE OF ADMINISTRATION: po
DRUG ACTION: inhibits serotonin uptake mechanism
COMMON DOSAGE: 150 mg up to 600 mg qd (divided doses)
SIDE EFFECTS: dizziness, drowsiness, SOB, chest pain, tachycardia
AUXILIARY LABELS:
- Take with food.
- May cause dizziness and drowsiness.
- Do not drink alcohol.

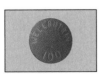

Glaxo-Wellcome

GENERIC NAME: bupropion*
TRADE NAME: Wellbutrin, Zyban (Either can be used for smoking cessation)
INDICATION: depression
ROUTE OF ADMINISTRATION: po
DRUG ACTION: a weak blocker of the uptake mechanism of serotonin and norepinephrine, and dopamine to an extent
COMMON DOSAGE: 100 mg tid or 150 mg bid
SIDE EFFECTS: dizziness, drowsiness, hallucinations, blurred vision
AUXILIARY LABELS:
- Do not drink alcohol.
- May cause dizziness and drowsiness.

*Has been known to cause seizures when dosage is over 450 mg per day

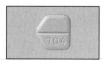

Wyeth-Ayerst

GENERIC NAME: venlafaxine
TRADE NAME: Effexor
INDICATION: depression
COMMON DOSAGE: 75–225 mg/day in split dosages given bid or tid
ROUTE OF ADMINISTRATION: po
DRUG ACTION: this agent inhibits the dopamine inhibitors, thus increasing dopamine levels in the brain
SIDE EFFECTS: dry mouth, elevated BP, dizziness, drowsiness, sweating, sexual dysfunction
AUXILIARY LABELS:

- Do not drink alcohol.
- May cause dizziness and drowsiness.

SEDATIVE AND HYPNOTIC AGENTS

Sedative and hypnotic agents affect the CNS. The difference between the two types of agents is the degree to which they affect the CNS. Because sedatives affect the CNS to a lesser degree than do hypnotics, they are used to relax and ease a nervous or irritated person by producing a soothing effect. For example, they are sometimes given to relax patients before a procedure, such as a magnetic resonance imaging or computed tomography (CT) scan. Hypnotics affect the CNS to a higher degree than sedatives, causing sleepiness. Examples of their use include inducing sleep before surgery or inducing sleepiness for those who suffer from insomnia. Insomnia can occur for many reasons, including side effects of drugs, whether they are over-the-counter (OTC) or prescriptions. It is common for older persons to suffer from insomnia because of pain or physiological changes. Another major cause of insomnia is stress. Listed in Table 15.3 are three types of insomnia and their specific descriptions.

For persons suffering from mild cases of insomnia there are many OTC drugs available. Some of the most popular agents are listed in Table 15.4.

The main ingredient in OTC sedative and hypnotic agents is diphenhydramine. Diphenhydramine (Benadryl) is classified as an antihistamine. The main side effect of this agent is sleepiness, which, in the case of insomnia, is the desired effect. Acetaminophen or magnesium salicylate are additive analgesics used to

TABLE 15.3 Types and Description of Insomnia

Types	Description
Initial insomnia	Difficulty falling asleep
Intermittent insomnia	Difficulty staying asleep
Terminal insomnia	Waking early and unable to fall back to sleep

TABLE 15.4 Over-the-Counter Agents to Treat Insomnia

OTC Trade Name	Generic Name	Common Dosage
Nytol	Diphenhydramine	25 mg
Excedrin PM	Diphenhydramine/acetaminophen	38 mg/500 mg
Sominex Caps	Diphenhydramine	50 mg
Nighttime Pamprin	Diphenhydramine/acetaminophen	50 mg/650 mg
Extra Strength Doans PM	Diphenhydramine/magnesium salicylate	25 mg/500 mg

treat insomnia caused by pain resulting from injury or illness. OTC sedatives are meant to treat short-term insomnia and work well. However, if the insomnia continues over a longer period, a stronger medication may be needed, such as a prescription sedative-hypnotic agent.

The first two classes of drugs that are discussed are the barbiturates and benzodiazepines. These two drug classes are not considered a permanent solution to insomnia. One negative effect of using certain hypnotics is the hangover effect the following morning. Because both agents are controlled substances (C-IV) they have an ability to become addictive; therefore, they are normally used for short-term treatment. Each class of drug has different indications, drug actions, dosing, and side effects that are discussed next.

Barbiturates

Barbiturates are controlled substances that have been used for many years as sedation for persons suffering from different conditions such as seizures and insomnia and as a hypnotic before surgery. Barbiturates are differentiated by the time it takes them to work. They range from short- to long-acting and are listed in Table 15.5.

Drug Action. Barbiturates act on the brainstem area reducing nerve impulses to the cerebral cortex. Because they affect the respiratory system, nerves, and smooth muscles, their effects cause relaxation and sleep. If a low dose is given, they produce a mild sedative effect, whereas a high dose causes anesthesia. Examples of these agents include thiopental and methohexital, which are used in surgery to keep the patient under general anesthesia.

Side Effects. There are several side effects associated with the use of barbiturates such as drowsiness, dizziness, nausea, vomiting, constipation, and a hangover effect after the drug wears off. Because of the effect barbiturates have on the CNS and the respiratory system, they can cause death if the patient takes an overdose. Because of the many side effects produced by barbiturates, benzodiazepines are more often prescribed.

Benzodiazepines

Benzodiazepines have several effects on the body system. They are known to affect parts of the brain, decreasing convulsions and affecting emotional stability. Effects

TABLE 15.5 Common Barbiturates

Schedule	Generic Name	Trade Name	Common Dosage	Length of Action	ROA
C-IV	phenobarbital	Luminal	Sedative: 30 mg–120 mg qd Seizures: 60 mg–120 mg qd	Long acting	po, IV, IM
C-IV	mephobarbital	Mebaral	Sedative: 32 mg–100 mg tid/qid Seizures: 400 mg–600 mg qd	Long acting	po
C-III	butabarbital	Butisol	Sedation: 15 mg–30 mg tid/qid Sleep: 50 mg–100 mg Preop: 50 mg–100 mg	Intermediate	po, IV
C-II	secobarbital	Seconal	Sleep: 100 mg Preop: 200 mg–300 mg	Short acting	po, IV IM
C-II	pentobarbital	Nembutal	Sedation: 20 mg tid/qid Insomnia: 100 mg qhs Preop: 1–3 mg/kg	Short acting	po, IV, po, IM, IV, supp

ROA, Route of administration; *qd,* every day; *po,* oral; *IV,* intravenous; *IM,* intramuscular; *tid,* three times a day; *qid,* four times a day; *qhs,* at bedtime; *preop,* preoperative; *supp,* suppository.

within the spinal cord cause muscle relaxation, and benzodiazepines can cause sedation. Because these agents affect the CNS, they can decrease breathing rate. Their main use is as hypnotic agents to induce sleep. Other common uses include seizure control and as muscle relaxants.

The benzodiazepines are lipid (fat) soluble. This means that they can enter into and through cells and areas within the body system that are made of lipids or are protected by a lipid barrier. The brain is a delicate and extremely important area that must be protected from foreign bodies. It is protected by a blood-brain barrier that stops many chemicals from passing into the brain. Drugs that are lipid soluble can pass through the blood-brain barrier, which is why mental function is changed after taking the medication. Excretion is through the urine. All the benzodiazepines are legend (prescription) drugs and are labeled controlled substances C-IV. A list of commonly prescribed benzodiazepines follow.

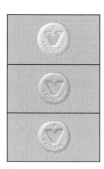

Roche

CLASSIFICATION: BENZODIAZEPINES
  GENERIC NAME: diazepam
  TRADE NAME: Valium
  INDICATION: anxiety, acute alcohol withdrawal, muscle relaxant, anticonvulsant
  ROUTE OF ADMINISTRATION: po, injection
  COMMON DOSAGE: anxiety, 2 mg to 10 mg; alcohol withdrawal 10 mg tid or four times a day (qid); muscle spasms, 15 mg to 30 mg qd
  AUXILIARY LABELS:
  ■ May cause dizziness and drowsiness.
  ■ Do not drink alcohol.

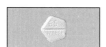

Wyeth-Ayerst

GENERIC NAME: lorazepam
  TRADE NAME: Ativan
  INDICATION: anxiety, insomnia
  ROUTE OF ADMINISTRATION: po, injection
  COMMON DOSAGE: anxiety, 2 mg to 6 mg qd; insomnia, 2 mg to 4 mg at bedtime (qhs)
  AUXILIARY LABELS:
  ■ May cause dizziness and drowsiness.
  ■ Do not drink alcohol.

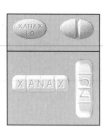

Pharmacia &
UpJohn

GENERIC NAME: alprazolam
  TRADE NAME: Xanax
  INDICATION: anxiety, panic disorders
  ROUTE OF ADMINISTRATION: po
  COMMON DOSAGE: 0.25 mg to 0.5 mg tid
  AUXILIARY LABELS:
  ■ May cause dizziness and drowsiness.
  ■ Do not drink alcohol.

GENERIC NAME: oxazepam
  TRADE NAME: Serax
  INDICATION: anxiety, tension, alcohol withdrawal
  ROUTE OF ADMINISTRATION: po
  COMMON DOSAGE: anxiety, 10 mg to 15 mg tid or qid; alcohol withdrawal, 15 mg to 30 mg tid or qid
  AUXILIARY LABELS:
  ■ May cause dizziness and drowsiness.
  ■ Do not drink alcohol.

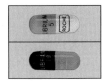

Roche

GENERIC NAME: chlordiazepoxide
TRADE NAME: Librium
INDICATION: anxiety, acute alcohol withdrawal
ROUTE OF ADMINISTRATION: po, injection
COMMON DOSAGE: 5 mg to 10 mg tid or qid
AUXILIARY LABELS:
- May cause dizziness and drowsiness.
- Do not drink alcohol.

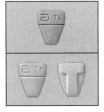

Abbott

GENERIC NAME: clorazepate
TRADE NAME: Tranxene
INDICATION: anxiety, alcohol withdrawal
ROUTE OF ADMINISTRATION: po
COMMON DOSAGES: anxiety, 30 mg qd (divided doses); alcohol withdrawal, 1 mg up to 30 mg qd
AUXILIARY LABELS:
- May cause dizziness and drowsiness.
- Do not drink alcohol.

CLASSIFICATION: benzodiazepine-like
GENERIC NAME: zolpidem
TRADE NAME: Ambien
INDICATION: insomnia
DRUG ACTION: non-benzodiazepine hypnotic—does not have muscle relaxant or anticonvulsant
ROUTE OF ADMINISTRATION: po
COMMON DOSAGE: 5–10 mg hs x 5–7 days
AUXILIARY LABELS:
- May cause dizziness and drowsiness.

The side effects of benzodiazepines include drowsiness, dizziness, blurred vision, dry mouth, and fatigue.

MISCELLANEOUS ANTIANXIETY AGENTS

Each of the antianxiety agents listed in the following have a different drug action. Most, if not all, of the agents that affect certain parts of the CNS produce anticholinergic effects. This includes the drying out of secretions throughout the body, which can involve dry mouth, dry eyes, and constipation. Each type of agent causes these side effects to one degree or another.

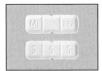

Bristol-Myers
Squibb

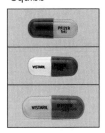

Roerig

CLASSIFICATION: ANTIANXIETY
GENERIC NAME: buspirone
TRADE NAME: Buspar
INDICATION: anxiety
ROUTE OF ADMINISTRATION: po
COMMON DOSAGE: 15 mg per day
DRUG ACTION: unknown
SIDE EFFECTS: none
AUXILIARY LABEL:
- Take as directed.

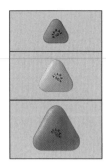

Pfizer

CLASSIFICATION: ANTIHISTAMINE
GENERIC NAME: hydroxyzine HCl; hydroxyzine pamoate
TRADE NAME: Atarax; Vistaril
INDICATION: anxiety, pruritus resulting from allergic reactions, preoperative sedation
ROUTE OF ADMINISTRATION: po; injectable form
DRUG ACTION: affects the CNS, producing muscle relaxation, analgesic, and anticholinergic effects
COMMON DOSAGE: anxiety or nausea 25 mg to 100 mg tid/qid; pruritus 25 mg tid or qid
SIDE EFFECTS: drowsiness, dry mouth
AUXILIARY LABELS:
■ May cause dizziness and drowsiness. Alcohol intensifies these effects.

CLASSIFICATION: ANTIANXIETY
GENERIC NAME: meprobamate
TRADE NAME: Equanil, Miltown
INDICATION: anxiety, muscle relaxant, and for insomnia
ROUTE OF ADMINISTRATION: po
DRUG ACTION: affects the CNS and also inhibits spinal reflexes causing overall relaxation
COMMON DOSAGE: 400 mg tid to qid
SIDE EFFECTS: drowsiness, dizziness, dry mouth
AUXILIARY LABELS:
■ May cause dizziness and drowsiness.
■ Do not drink alcohol.
NOTE: Antianxiety/antipsychotic medications are C-IV medications

TECH NOTE! Pharmacy technicians have the knowledge of classifications of drugs and personal patient information, and it is important to remember that all medical information should be kept private. If patient confidentiality is broken, the consequences can possibly be devastating to the patient. Never disclose to anyone what medication the patient is taking or condition the patient has.

DO YOU REMEMBER THESE KEY POINTS?
■ The main causes of insomnia
■ Various treatments for depression, including the types of agents used
■ The differences between MAOIs, TCAs, and SSRIs
■ Under what circumstances might a decanoate agent be used
■ The method of action of phenothiazines
■ The major side effects of TCAs
■ How long most antidepressants must be taken before they are effective
■ What foods contain tyramine and what importance they have when taking MAOIs
■ Why MAOIs are normally less popular than SSRIs and TCAs for treating depression
■ What major OTCs are available for treating insomnia
■ What barbiturates are prescribed for and their schedules
■ What benzodiazepines are prescribed for and their schedules

REVIEW QUESTIONS:

Multiple Choice

1. The blood-brain barrier protects the brain from
A. Toxins
B. Drugs
C. Large molecules
D. All of the above

2. A prescription can be written by
  A. A psychiatrist   C. A family counselor
  B. A psychologist   D. All of the above

3. A type of nondrug therapy for emotional problems may include
  A. Family counseling   C. Visiting a psychologist
  B. Group therapy   D. All of the above

4. The illness that is marked by extremes in elevated and depressed moods is defined as
  A. Schizophrenia   D. All of the above
  B. Bipolar disorder   D. Depression

5. Long-acting decanoates are given
  A. Every other day   C. Every month
  B. Every week   D. In any of these combinations

6. The main neurotransmitters of the brain that are affected by benzodiazepines are
  A. Dopamine   C. Epinephrine
  B. Norepinephrine   D. All of the above

7. Extrapyramidal effects that include shaky hands and head are mainly caused by
  A. Overdosing MAOIs   C. Overdosing SSRIs
  B. Overdosing TCAs   D. All of the above

8. _____ is (are) the main drug(s) used for the treatment of mania phases of people with bipolar disorder.
  A. TCAs   C. Lithium
  B. SSRIs   D. Diphenhydramine

9. The antidepressant class that has the mildest side effects and is used for depression is
  A. SSRIs   C. TCAs
  B. MAOIs   D. Benzodiazepines

10. SSRIs inhibit the reuptake inhibitors within the neuronal transmission, which increases the levels of _____.
  A. Norepinephrine   C. Serotonin
  B. Epinephrine   D. Dopamine

True/False

*If the statement is false, then change it to make it true.

1. Tardive dyskinesia is a mental illness.

2. Short-acting phenothiazines include oral fluphenazine (Prolixin), thioridazine (Mellaril), chlorpromazine (Thorazine), and trifluoperazine (Stelazine).

3. Decanoate dosage forms include po and parenteral.

4. Persons taking SSRIs should avoid foods that contain tyramine.

5. MAOIs are used less than SSRIs and TCAs because of their side effects.

6. Most antidepressants must be taken for up to 1 week before the desired effects can be seen.

7. Two of the most common auxiliary labels for benzodiazepines are "Take with plenty of water" and "Take with food."

8. TCAs, MAOIs, and SSRIs can be used to treat bipolar behavior.

9. Bipolar behavior is also referred to as a manic-depressive disorder.

10. Hypnotic agents are often used to relax patients before procedures such as CT scans.

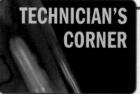
TECHNICIAN'S CORNER

The doctor has ordered Tofranil for a child who is 5 years old and weighs 45 lbs. He orders 1.5 mg/kg/day to be given tid.

Is this dosage safe according to the *Mosby's Drug Consult* recommendations?

How much drug per day would this child be given based on the dose ordered?

How much drug per dose would be given based on the dose ordered?

Is there a generic equivalent to Tofranil; if so, what other companies manufacture this drug?

Body Systems

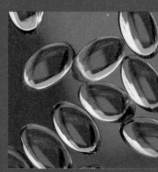

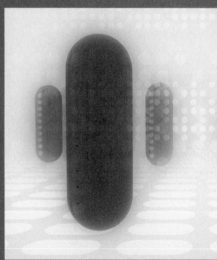

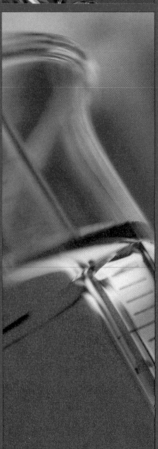

16 Endocrine System

17 Nervous System

18 Respiratory System

19 Visual and Auditory Systems

20 Gastrointestinal System

21 Urinary System

22 Cardiovascular System

23 Reproductive System

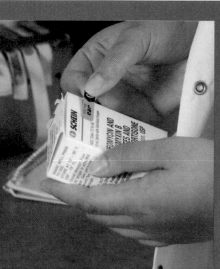

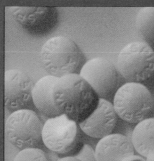

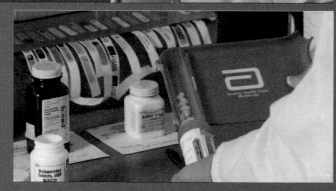

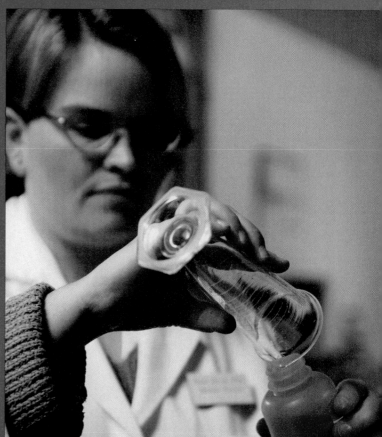

16 Endocrine System

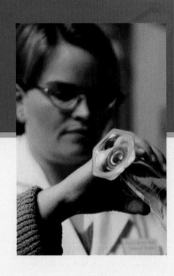

Objectives

■ Write the generic and trade names for all drugs discussed in this chapter.

■ List both classifications and indications of each drug discussed.

■ Name the major glands of the body.

■ Write the location and function for the glands discussed.

■ Differentiate between the endocrine and exocrine glands.

■ Explain the role of iodine in the metabolism of hormones of the thyroid gland.

■ Explain the role of calcium in bones.

■ Describe the causes and symptoms of osteoporosis.

■ Describe the conditions caused by improper gland functioning.

■ List the main hormones that are produced in women and men.

■ Explain the uses of androgens in both men and women.

■ List the causes of diabetes mellitus.

■ Describe the differences between insulin dependent diabetes mellitus (IDDM) and non-insulin dependent diabetes mellitus (NIDDM).

■ Explain the relationship between the central nervous system and the release of hormones from the adrenal gland.

■ List the primary side effects of the medications discussed in the chapter.

■ List the auxiliary labels required when filling prescriptions for hormones.

Addison's disease *Condition resulting in a decrease in adrenal cortical hormones, such as mineralocorticoids and glucocorticoids, that causes symptoms including muscle weakness and weight loss*

Autoimmune disease *Condition in which a person's tissues are attacked by his/her immune system; abnormal antigen-antibody reaction*

Cretinism *Condition in which the development of the brain and body is inhibited by congenital lack of thyroid secretion*

Cushing's disease *Syndrome causing an increase in secretion of the adrenal cortex with excessive production of gluco-corticoids that includes symptoms such as a moon face and deposits of fat (buffalo hump)*

Euthyroid *Normal functioning thyroid gland*

Exophthalmos *Prominence of the eyeball due to increased thyroid hormone*

Glucose *Simple sugar*

Goiter *Condition in which the thyroid is enlarged because of a lack of iodine, known as simple goiter, or because of a tumor, known as toxic goiter*

Graves' disease *Condition caused by hypersecretion of thyroid with diffuse goiter, exophthalmos, and skin changes*

Homeostasis *Equilibrium of the body by feedback and body regulation processes*

Hormone *Chemical substances produced and secreted by an endocrine duct into the bloodstream or duct that result in a physiological response at a specific target tissue*

Hypercalcemia *Unusually high concentration of calcium in the blood*

Hyperglycemia *Abnormally high glucose content circulating in the bloodstream*

Hypocalcemia *Low concentration of calcium in the blood*

Hypoglycemia *Abnormally low glucose content circulating in the bloodstream*

Myxedema *Condition associated with a decrease in overall thyroid function in adults; also known as hypothyroidism*

Osteoporosis *Condition associated with the decrease of bone mass and softening of bones, resulting in the increased possibility of bone fractures*

Paget's disease *Condition that affects older adults in which the density of the bones decreases, resulting in softening and weakening*

Thyroxine *Known as T_4; contains four ions of iodine*

Triiodothyronine *Known as T_3; contains three ions of iodine*

DRUGS

Trade Name	Generic	Pronunciation	Trade Name	Generic	Pronunciation
Thyroid Replacement			**Hyperthyroidism**		
Armour Thyroid	desiccated thyroid	**des**-eh-kate-ed **thigh**-roid	Propylthiouracil	propylthiouracil	pro-pull-thigh-oh-**your**-ah-sill
Synthroid, Levoxyl	levothyroid	lee-vo-**thigh**-roid	Tapazole	methimazol	meth-**em**-ah-zoll
Cytomel	liothyronine	lie-oh-**thigh**-row-neen	Thyro-block	potassium iodide	poh-tas-ee-um **eye**-oh-dyed
Thyrolar	liotrix	**low**-tricks			

263

DRUGS—cont'd

Trade Name	Generic	Pronunciation	Trade Name	Generic	Pronunciation
Calcium Regulator			**Estrogens**		
Calcimar	calcitonin	**cal**-sit-toe-nen	Estrace	estradiol	ess-tra-**dye**-ole
Didronel	etidronate disodium	eh-tea-**droh**-nate dy-sew-dee-um	Premarin	conjugated estrogens	**kon**-juh-gated **ess**-troe-gens
			Estinyl	ethinyl estradiol	**eth**-in-ill ess-tra-**dye**-ole
Biphosphonates			Estrovis	quinestrol	kwye-**ness**-troll
Fosamax	alendronate	al-den-drone-ate	Diethylstilbestrol	diethylstilbestrol	dye-eth-ill-still-**best**-roll
Aredia	pamidronate	pa-mi-**droe**-nate	Prempro	combined estrogen/progestin	**ess**-troe-jen/pro-**jess**-tin
Calcium					
Oscal	calcium carbonate	**kal**-see-um **car**-bone-ate	**Progestins**		
			Progesterone	progesterone	pro-**jess**-tur-own
Calcium gluconate	calcium gluconate	**kal**-see-um **glue**-ko-nate	Megace	megestrol acetate	me-**jess**-trall
			Provera	medroxyprogesterone	me-drock-see-pro-**jess**-tur-own
Phos Lo	calcium acetate	**kal**-see-um **as**-see-tate			
			Aygestin	norethindrone acetate	nor-**eth**-in-drone
Calcium lactate	calcium lactate	**kal**-see-um **lack**-tate	**Insulin**		
Adrenal Corticosteroids			Humulin N	normal insulin	**in**-su-lin
Acthar	corticotropin	**kore**-tye-co-troe-pin	Humulin R	regular insulin	
Cortrosyn	cosyntropin	koe-sin-**troe**-pin	Humalog	lispro	**lis** pro
Mineralocorticoids			**Oral Antidiabetic Drugs**		
Florinef	fludrocortisone acetate	floo-droe-**kor**-ti-sone **as**-e-tate	Orinase	tolbutamide	toll-**butte**-tah-myde
			Diabinese	chlorpropamide	klor-**pro**-pah-myde
			Tolinase	tolazamide	toll-**laze**-ah-myde
			Micronase, Diabeta	glyburide	**glye**-burr-eyed
Glucocorticoids			Glucotrol	glipizide	**glip**-eh-zyed
Cortef	hydrocortisone	hye-droe-**kor**-ti-sone	Glucophage	metformin	met-**four**-men
Solu-Medrol	methylprednisolone	meth-il-pred-**nis**-oh-lone	Precose	acarbose	**ay**-car-bose
			Actos	pioglitazone	pye-oh-**gli**-ta-zone

Introduction

The endocrine system encompasses the production and secretion of hormones from the glands. The Greek word *orme* means "to excite." This is exactly what hormones do. They activate specific target cells, causing a response. There are many different types of hormones that are produced in different glands. Doctors who specialize in the study of glands and hormones of the body are endocrinologists. In this chapter we look at the location and function of the major glands of the body. Major conditions affecting the endocrine system are discussed along with the types of agents used to treat them.

Endocrine Anatomy

Three glands are located in the head—the pituitary, hypothalamus, and pineal gland. These glands play an important role in hormone production. The pituitary gland produces hormones that affect other glands and specific organs of the body as shown in Figure 16.1. The hypothalamus, located above the pituitary gland, is a bridge between the nervous system and hormone system. It secretes hormones

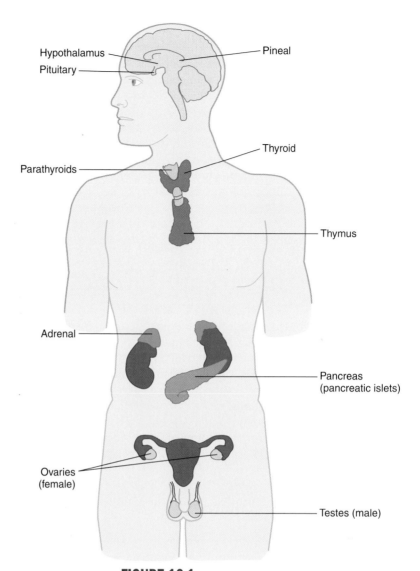

FIGURE 16.1 Endocrine anatomy.

that affect the pituitary gland. The pineal gland, located behind and below the hypothalamus, is responsible for controlling the circadian rhythms, sexual growth, and other body functions, which are discussed later in this chapter.

Located at the base of the neck, the thyroid gland is responsible for hormones that participate in metabolism. The parathyroid glands, positioned slightly behind and above the thyroid gland, secrete hormones that help the body keep the calcium levels adequate. Located lower in the chest is the thymus gland, which secrets hormones that play an important role in the body's defense system. The adrenal glands are located in the abdominal area right above the kidneys and secrete specific hormones linked to the body's stress level.

The largest gland is the pancreas, located behind the left kidney at the back of the abdominal wall. It is responsible for the production and secretion of different types of hormones and digestive juices. Two major hormones produced are insulin and glucagon. Glands that are specific to reproduction are the ovaries in women and the testes in men. In women, the ovaries secrete hormones, such as progesterone and estrogen. In men, the main hormone secreted is testosterone. Each of these hormones is also responsible for gender characteristics.

Description of Hormones

Hormones are responsible for many different human functions, including emotions, in both women and men. Hormones are classified by the distance they travel. Autocrine hormones act on the same cell from which they are secreted, such as interleukin-2, which stimulates T cells (part of the immune system). The paracrine hormones act on cells that are in proximity to the target cells such as prostaglandins, and the endocrine hormones act on cells that are located further away. These endocrine hormones are the focus of this chapter. Glands have two mechanisms of action, either endocrine or exocrine. Hormones produced within endocrine glands enter into the bloodstream to reach their target site, whereas those produced in the exocrine glands are sent to the target organ or tissue via a tube or duct. An example of a tube or duct that secretes outwardly to the surface of the skin is the duct of the sweat glands.

Structure and Function of Hormones

The regulation of hormones throughout the body is constantly kept in balance within a normal range through a feedback system similar to your home thermostat. However, hormones, in general, can be thought of as specialized keys that unlock only one door. When the key enters the lock, a reaction takes place. As the hormone travels through the body it does not react with any keyhole other than the one it was made to fit. It is not good for homeostasis if glands secrete too many hormones; rather a delicate balance must be kept to produce the right amount of response. When a gland either stops producing or secretes too much hormone, various conditions of the endocrine system may result.

There are two different types of hormones within the endocrine system; as shown in Figure 16.2; one type is composed of proteins and the other is composed of steroids.

Hormones perform many functions throughout the body, including the following:

Maintain homeostasis—keep the body within normal physiological limits through the use of increasing and decreasing blood glucose levels for energy use.

Prepare the body for an emergency situation—"fight or flight" reaction.

Participate in the human body's development and reproductive system—sexual maturity and reproductive functions, such as menstruation and pregnancy.

Mechanism of Action

Receptor sites are located inside and outside of cells. Protein hormones fit into receptor sites outside cells, whereas steroid hormones enter into and attach to receptor sites inside the cell. Both mechanisms cause a reaction. The following are the three systems that influence the endocrine system:

1. Negative feedback is the first way in which hormones are produced and secreted. For example, if the level of sugar drops below a certain point in the body, it triggers the secretion of the specific gland. The gland secretes hormones (the key) that target organs (the door lock) to bring the glucose level back up to the necessary level.
2. The second response system is by hormonal chemicals that may also participate in a chain reaction. For example, a chemical response may initiate the first set of hormones to be released from the pituitary gland that interact with the receptors on the adrenal glands; in turn this response releases hormones into the bloodstream.

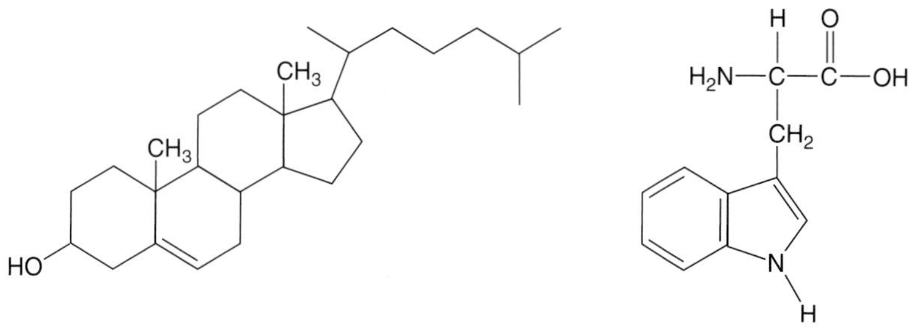

Cholesterol—a steroid   Tryptophan—a protein

FIGURE 16.2 Anatomy of a steroid and protein.

3. The third response system is via the nervous system. Stressful situations can alter the production and secretion of specific hormones that, when released, prepare the body for the situation. For example if a person is in an emergency situation, the body requires more energy; therefore chemicals such as epinephrine may be released, giving the body an extra boost of energy.

Functions of the Endocrine Glands

HYPOTHALAMUS

Located in the brain below the thalamus gland, the hypothalamus is a very small organ that links the nervous system to the endocrine system. The hypothalamus plays a key role in the regulation of several functions such as water balance, metabolism of fat and carbohydrates, body temperature, appetite, and emotions. This organ also produces hormones that regulate the anterior pituitary gland to various degrees. Although the hypothalamus is responsible for the production of two hormones, oxytocin and antidiuretic hormone (ADH), they are stored in the posterior section of the pituitary gland. The hypothalamus stimulates the pituitary gland by neuronal impulses. The pituitary glands then release oxytocin, which stimulates the ovaries, or ADH (also known as vasopressin), which affects the kidneys. The hypothalamus also produces and secretes two substances known as releasing or inhibiting hormones. Their target organ is the anterior lobe of the pituitary gland, where they either stimulate or inhibit the release of other hormones.

PINEAL GLAND

This gland is responsible for the production and secretion of melatonin. Melatonin is a chemical substance that helps to regulate the sleep-wake cycle. Its target tissue is the hypothalamus. Although this gland is small in adults, it is larger in small children. As a person ages, it becomes smaller in relation to other structures and also begins to function less. It is affected by light and secretes melatonin more during the night and less during the daytime. The effects of melatonin have been linked to the beginning of puberty and the menstrual cycle.

PITUITARY GLAND

The pituitary gland is like the control tower of the endocrine system. It is commonly called the master gland of the body system. It is composed of two portions, the anterior and posterior lobes. Although small, the anterior lobe makes the hormones that stimulate many different organs as listed in Table 16.1. The posterior lobe also contains hormones that regulate the kidneys via reabsorption (ADH), and oxytocin is responsible for uterine contractions initiating labor and milk production (lactation) in postpartum women. This entire system is regulated via negative feedback control from the nervous system (specifically the hypothalamus) and other hormone glands. It is no surprise that the pituitary gland is referred to as the "master" gland.

THYROID GLAND

The thyroid gland is located at the base of the neck. It is the gland responsible for producing and secreting three hormones, thyroxine (T_4), triiodothyronine (T_3), and calcitonin. Iodine is necessary within the thyroid gland to synthesize both T_4 and T_3; each is named to indicate the number of atoms of iodine contained. Both T_4 and T_3 are transported via the bloodstream along with plasma proteins; the hormones pass through target cells into the interior of the cell where they bind to a specific protein. This ultimate reaction helps trigger the rate of metabolism of proteins, fats (lipids), and sugars (carbohydrates) throughout the body; therefore they play an important role in the growth and homeostasis of the body. Calcitonin plays an active role in the regulation of calcium. Calcium is the major mineral found in bones. It is also important for the proper functioning of muscle contractions, nerve impulses, and blood clotting. A constant level is maintained by three different hormones, including calcitonin. Its function is to inhibit the resorption of calcium from the bone and kidney. Vitamin D and parathyroid hormone (PTH) are the two other hormones that help regulate calcium and are discussed in other sections of the chapter.

PARATHYROID GLANDS

Located behind the thyroid gland are the parathyroids (*para* meaning "across"). The parathyroid organ is composed of two sets of secreting glands. They are the

TABLE 16.1 Hormonal Production of Anterior and Posterior Pituitary Gland

Abbreviation	Hormone	Target Tissue	Result
Anterior Pituitary Gland			
ACTH	Adrenocorticotropic hormone	Adrenal glands	Secretes glucocorticoids and adrenocortical hormones
FSH	Follicle-stimulating hormone	Ovaries in women; testes in men	Estrogen secretion in women, sperm production in men
GH	Growth hormone	Tissues and bones throughout the body	Growth throughout childhood
LH	Luteinizing hormone	Ovaries in women; testes in men	Progesterone production in women, testosterone production in men
Prolactin	Prolactin	Mammary glands in women	Produces milk for lactation
TSH	Thyroid-stimulating hormone	Thyroid gland	Causes the thyroid gland to produce thyroid hormones
Posterior Pituitary Gland			
ADH	Antidiuretic hormone	Kidneys	Resorbs water back into the bloodstream
Oxytocin	Oxytocin	Uterus	Causes contraction of the smooth muscle; also stimulates anterior pituitary lobe to produce prolactin

main regulators of calcium levels in the blood through the release of PTH. The glands can draw calcium out of the bone when needed to increase the concentration of calcium in the body's extracellular fluid. Along with the calcium increase, they affect the concentration of phosphate by lowering it, thus allowing more calcium to be used.

ADRENAL GLANDS

Located directly on top of each of the two kidneys, the adrenal glands participate in the activities of the kidneys. The adrenal glands secrete steroids and catecholamines. If the adrenal glands are dissected in a cross section, two layers of tissue can be seen: the medulla (located in the center) and the cortex (outer portion) of the gland. Each of the two layers within the adrenal gland is specific to its function.

The adrenal medulla synthesizes and secretes catecholamines, norepinephrine and epinephrine. They are stored in the adrenal medulla until activated by the sympathetic nervous system. As mentioned previously, one of the functions of the endocrine system is to stimulate the "fight or flight" reaction. For instance, when one comes into contact with a stressful situation such as when one is scared, the body prepares itself for either fighting or running, depending on the situation. The heart rate increases and the veins dilate to allow more blood to reach all muscles and to increase blood flow to the brain. Stored glucose is released into the bloodstream to fuel the body. The secretion of epinephrine accounts for approximately 70% to 80% and norepinephrine is 20% to 30%.

The cortex of the adrenal glands produces three types of hormones: the glucocorticoids, mineralocorticoids, and the sex hormones (androgens or estrogens). The adrenal hormones and their effects are listed in Table 16.2.

Glucocorticoids affect the metabolism of lipids (fats), carbohydrates (sugars), and proteins (meats). Glucocorticoids produce a reaction opposite to the effect of insulin produced by the pancreas. They increase glucose levels. They also reduce inflammation and increase the capacity to cope with stressful situations. Mineralocorticoids are also produced within the cortex but within a different layer than the glucocorticoids. Their function is to regulate the secretion of both water and salt by the kidney.

PANCREAS

The pancreas is the largest organ of the endocrine system. Its function is to maintain energy homeostasis throughout the body. It does this by secreting glucagon and insulin, inhibiting the release of somatostatin. Glucagon is secreted in response

TABLE 16.2 Adrenal Hormones and Their Effects on the Body

Class of Hormones	Specific Hormone	Produced and Secreted	Effects
Glucocorticoids	Cortisol	Adrenal cortex	Increases blood sugar concentration; also has antiinflammatory and antiallergy effects
Mineralocorticoids	Aldosterone	Adrenal cortex	Increases urinary output, including potassium and hydrogen while retaining sodium; keeps blood volume at par
Sex hormones	Androgens in men	Adrenal cortex	Affects male and female characteristics such as hair growth and sex drive
	Estrogens in women	Adrenal cortex	Affects female sex drive, fat deposition, and bone formation

to low blood glucose. This hormone triggers the liver to release stored glucose for use by the body when levels are low. It also triggers fatty acids to be released by adipose (fat) tissue for energy use. When blood glucose is high, insulin is released into the bloodstream. This hormone targets tissues such as the liver, muscle, and adipose tissues to take up excess glucose from the bloodstream, where it can be stored for later use. Somatostatin, secreted by the hypothalamus, inhibits the release of insulin and glucagon.

OVARIES

The two ovaries in women are responsible for production (oogenesis) and secretion of one or, rarely, two eggs or more (ovulation) on a monthly basis. Located on either side of the uterus, the ovaries sit above the uterus and are attached to the fallopian tubes, which connect the two organs. Although the ovulation of eggs begins at puberty, it is not possible to become pregnant until the menstrual cycle begins. The ability to have children ends as the hormones responsible, such as estrogen, decline until the ovarian cycle stops. The ovaries also secrete the hormones estrogen and progesterone. The function of estrogen is the development of breasts and genitals and the menstrual cycle, which prepares the female for pregnancy. The anterior pituitary gland releases follicle-stimulating hormone (FSH) that triggers estrogen levels to increase, which causes luteinizing hormone (LH) (another pituitary hormone) to be secreted. The combination of these two hormones causes ovulation.

TESTES

The two testes in men are responsible for the production and secretion of sperm (spermatogenesis). They are located within the scrotum. Sperm production begins before the age of puberty and decreases with age, although most men produce sperm throughout their lifetime. FSH is released as puberty begins and causes the stored sperm to divide. Each sperm contains one half of the genetic material that will be contributed to a new life. The production of testosterone (also from the testes) is responsible for the growth of adjacent organs: prostate gland, seminal vesicles, vas deferens, and others. It is also responsible for changes in the voice pitch as a boy enters puberty and for muscle development. This hormone also affects the differences in the physiques of men and women.

Conditions of the Endocrine System and Their Treatments

There are many different types of conditions and illnesses that can affect the endocrine system. Causes can range from the effects of aging and genetic factors to those that are the result of a condition affecting another part of the body. The failure of the endocrine system to perform correctly affects other areas of the body such as heart, brain, and kidney function. Table 16.3 lists the common conditions that affect the endocrine system.

CONDITIONS OF THE PITUITARY AND HYPOTHALAMUS GLAND AND THEIR TREATMENTS

Hyperfunction of the pituitary gland can be caused by various tumor growths. Giantism and acromegaly are two conditions that involve an increase in growth hormone (GH). If this condition is present in children, it is referred to as giantism.

TABLE 16.3 Endocrine Conditions with Corresponding Glands and Hormones

Glands/Hormones	Condition/Disease	Possible Treatments
Thyroid/T_3, T_4, Calcitonin	Hyperthyroidism (Grave's disease)	Medication, surgery
	Hypothyroidism (myxedema, cretinism)	Medication
Parathyroid	Hyperparathyroidism	Reduce Ca intake, diuresis
	Hypoparathyroidism	Ca and Vitamin D replacements
Pituitary		
Anterior Pituitary		
	Deficiency	
TSH, ACTH, FSH, LH	Sexual dysfunction, metabolism imbalance, sterility	Hormone replacement therapy
GH	Dwarfism	Growth hormone replacement
	Overproduction	
TSH	Giantism (child)	Radiation, surgical intervention
	Acromegaly (adult)	
Posterior Pituitary		
	Deficiency	
Vasopressin (antidiuretic hormone)	Diabetes insipidus	Medication (DDAVP)
Oxytocin	Reduce uter	
Adrenal		
	Deficiency	
Mineralocorticoids (Aldosterone)	Body chemical imbalance	Medication for hormone replacement
Glucocorticoids (Cortisol)	Addison's disease	Hormone replacement
Gonadocordticoids (Androgens/Estrogens/Progestins)	Sexual immaturity/dysfunction	Hormone replacement
	Overproduction	
Mineralcorticoids/Glucocorticoids	Cushing's syndrome	Surgery, medication
Pancreas		
Insulin		
	Deficiency	
	Diabetes mellitus, IDDM	Insulin, diet
	NIDDM (Insulin resistance)	Oral medication, diet, insulin
	Gestational diabetes	Insulin during pregnancy
	Overproduction	
	Hypoglycemia	Diet, lifestyle changes
Testes		
Testosterone		
	Deficiency	
	Stunted sexual growth, sexual dysfunction	Hormone replacement therapy
	Overproduction	
	Precocious puberty	Female hormones, treatment of cause
Ovaries		
Estrogen/Progesterone		
	Deficiency	
	Stunted sexual growth	Hormone replacement therapy
	Menopause	Hormone replacement therapy
	Overproduction	
	Precocious puberty	Male hormones, treatment of cause

The bones elongate, resulting in heights that have reached 8 feet. If this condition arises in adulthood, it is called acromegaly and symptoms involve increased size of the head, tongue, nose, hands, feet, and toes. This excess of GH can also cause more serious conditions such as hyperglycemia and hypercalcemia. Treatment involves removal of the tumor, although any bone growth preceding removal cannot be reversed. These tumors tend to be benign.

Hypofunction of the pituitary gland causes a decrease of hormones to secondary target organs. A congenital defect of the pituitary gland can cause dwarfism.

Tumors can also disturb the functioning of both the pituitary and hypothalamus. Simmonds' disease affects adults, causing a lack of menstruation in women and impotence in men. Oxytocin is a hormone released by the posterior pituitary gland that has a direct affect on the uterus and is responsible for the beginning stages of labor. Oxytocin is commonly used as a medication in hospitals to help induce labor or to abort a fetus. It is administered parenterally only.

Diabetes insipidus can be caused by a lack of ADH resulting from lesions, tumors, or an infection in or on the hypothalamus or posterior pituitary gland. Treatment for this type of diabetes and diabetes mellitus is discussed later.

CONDITIONS OF THE THYROID AND THEIR TREATMENT

The two main conditions of the thyroid are hyperthyroidism and hypothyroidism. Hyperthyroidism is due to an excess of thyroid hormones. This can be caused by autoimmunity, as in Graves' disease. An autoimmune disease is one in which the body attacks itself; in Graves' disease the body produces antibodies to thyroid-stimulating hormone (TSH) receptors. When this happens, the thyroid is triggered to produce more hormones, which results in the enlargement of the glands behind the eye, known as exophthalmos. Other symptoms of Graves' disease include restlessness, nervousness, sweating, weight loss, and tachycardia.

A goiter is caused by the lack of iodine, which is needed for thyroid hormone production, and by tumors that can cause overproduction of hormone. Goiters are also due to excessive amounts of T_3 and T_4, causing enlargement of the thyroid gland. This gives the appearance of an enlarged neck and is usually caused by a tumor. It is not commonly found in developed countries because of the addition of iodine to salt.

Treatment of hyperthyroidism includes removal of the tumor, if that is the cause. Antithyroid agents can be used in Graves' disease, and radioactive iodine is used to decrease nodules in goiters. Radiation may also be used to destroy part of the thyroid gland.

CLASSIFICATION: AGENTS USED TO TREAT HYPERTHYROIDISM
GENERIC NAME: propylthiouracil (PTU)
TRADE NAME: Propylthiouracil (PTU)
INDICATION: hyperthyroidism
COMMON DOSAGE: 300 mg to 450 mg every day (qd)
SIDE EFFECTS: nausea, headache (HA), urticaria
AUXILIARY LABEL: Take as directed

GENERIC NAME: methimazole
TRADE NAME: Tapazole
INDICATION: hyperthyroidism
COMMON DOSAGE: 5 mg to 15 mg qd
SIDE EFFECTS: fever, rash, itching
AUXILIARY LABEL: Take as directed

Hypothyroidism occurs when the thyroid is unable to secrete enough T_3 and T_4. This can be caused by congenital deficiencies referred to as thyroid aplasia. A lack of iodine in the diet can cause a deficiency because iodine is necessary for the synthesis of T_3 and T_4. Inflammation of the thyroid, known as thyroiditis, can also be caused by an autoimmune effect. Thyroid aplasia affects children that are not born with a thyroid gland. The lack of the thyroid gland affects the growth of the child's body and nervous system. If the condition is not discovered early, the child's growth will be stunted (dwarfism) and the child will develop mental retardation (cretinism). Once diagnosed, thyroid medication is given for life, although any retardation that has occurred cannot be reversed.

Hypothyroidism in adults causes the condition myxedema. Symptoms include skin that appears puffy. The overall deficiency of thyroid hormones has a dramatic effect on all the organs of the body. This results in an overall decrease in energy and mental alertness. Tumors that affect the thyroid are usually benign (adenomas) and rarely are malignant (carcinoma). The main treatment for these types of tumors is removal. Thyroid hormone replacement agents need to be taken for life (one dose a day), because there are no other available treatments. Because the body's metabolism is at its highest in the morning, doctors advise patients to take their thyroid medications in the morning at the same time daily.

CLASSIFICATION: AGENTS USED TO TREAT HYPOTHYROIDISM
GENERIC NAME: thyroid desiccated
TRADE NAME: Armour Thyroid
INDICATIONS: hypothyroidism, thyroid cancer
COMMON DOSAGE: 60 mg to 120 mg qd
SIDE EFFECTS: no major effects if correct dosage taken
AUXILIARY LABEL: Take as directed

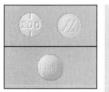

Kroll

GENERIC NAME: levothyroxine sodium
TRADE NAME: Synthroid, Levothroid
INDICATION: hypothyroidism
COMMON DOSAGE: 0.2 mg qd*
SIDE EFFECTS: no major effects if correct dosage taken
AUXILIARY LABEL: Take as directed

GENERIC NAME: liothyronine sodium
TRADE NAME: Cytomel
INDICATION: hypothyroidism
COMMON DOSAGE: 0.25 mg to 0.1 mg qd
SIDE EFFECTS: no major effects if correct dosage taken
AUXILIARY LABEL: Take as directed

GENERIC NAME: liotrix
TRADE NAME: Thyrolar, Euthroid
INDICATION: hypothyroidism
COMMON DOSAGE: 60 mg to 120 mg qd
SIDE EFFECTS: no major effects if correct dosage taken
AUXILIARY LABEL: Take as directed

*Dosage may vary depending on weight of patient and extent of illness

CONDITIONS OF THE PARATHYROID GLANDS AND THEIR TREATMENT

There are two parathyroid glands on each side of the thyroid gland. Hyperparathyroidism is a condition in which there is an increase of parathyroid hormone (PTH) secreted into the bloodstream; it can arise from just one of the four glands. The most common cause of this condition is benign tumors. Another condition closely related is secondary parathyroid hyperplasia in which all four glands are enlarged; this is linked to chronic renal disease.

Symptoms of these two conditions are similar; this includes increase of calcium because the increased levels of PTH promote the release of calcium into the bloodstream, which leads to bone weakening with an increase in possibility of fractures. This softening of the bones resulting from the loss of calcium may lead to Paget's disease, and commonly causes osteoporosis in postmenopausal women. Also, the increase of calcium in the blood causes a buildup of the calcium salts in the kidneys, which can cause kidney stones. Other side effects of hypercalcemia include muscle weakness, lethargy, and heart conduction changes.

Treatment depends on the underlying cause. If the hyperparathyroidism is due to improper kidney function, then transplantation may be necessary to stop the problem. If transplantation does not work, removal of the glands may be necessary. Following are the common drugs used for replacement therapy for hyperparathyroidism.

CLASSIFICATION: BONE METABOLISM REGULATOR
GENERIC NAME: calcitonin-salmon
TRADE NAME: Calcimar
INDICATIONS: Paget's disease, hypercalcemia, postmenopausal osteoporosis
COMMON DOSAGE: Paget's disease 50 units qd; hypercalcemia 4 units/kg q12h; osteoporosis 100 units qd 200 units qd intranasal for osteoporosis (all injected intramuscularly or subcutaneously)
SIDE EFFECTS: nausea, vomiting, diarrhea, facial flushing
AUXILIARY LABEL: None

CLASSIFICATION: BISPHOSPHONATES
GENERIC NAME: etidronate sodium
TRADE NAME: Didronel
INDICATION: Paget's disease
COMMON DOSAGE: 5 mg to 10 mg/kg/day (may be given orally for 6 mo or intravenously for 3 to 7 days)
SIDE EFFECTS: Headache, gastrointestinal (GI) upset
AUXILIARY LABELS: Oral (po): Take as directed (Intravenous [IV] form is administered in hospital)

GENERIC NAME: alendronate
TRADE NAME: Fosamax
INDICATIONS: Paget's disease, postmenopausal osteoporosis
COMMON DOSAGE: Paget's disease 40 mg qd po; osteoporosis 10 mg qd; 70 mg q week
SIDE EFFECTS: Headache, GI upset
AUXILIARY LABEL: Take 30 min before breakfast
Take with full glass of water

GENERIC NAME: pamidronate
TRADE NAME: Aredia
INDICATIONS: hypercalcemia, Paget's disease, osteolytic bone lesions resulting from myelomas
COMMON DOSAGE: hypercalcemia 60 mg to 90 mg IV over 24 hour; Paget's 30 mg qd IV ×3 days; osteolytic lesions 90 mg over 2 hours q 3 to 4 weeks
SIDE EFFECTS: HA, GI upset
AUXILIARY LABEL: None, administered in hospital as medicine is IV only

Hypoparathyroidism

Hypoparathyroidism involves the malfunctioning of the parathyroid glands and can occur after removal of the parathyroid glands; in very rare cases it may be congenital or an autoimmune disease. The result is hypocalcemia, which is the decrease or lack of calcium. Symptoms include muscle spasms, irregular heart contractions, and alteration of normal nerve conduction. Treatment is limited to replacement therapy with calcium supplements listed as follows.

Generic Name	Trade Name	Normal Dosage for Replacement
Calcium acetate	PhosLo	250 mg–1 g po qd
Calcium carbonate	Tums, Os-cal	500 mg–1.5 g po qd
Calcium chloride	Calcium Chloride	10% IV
Calcium citrate	Citracal	950 mg PO qd
Calcium gluconate	Calcium Gluconate	500 mg–1 g qd; 10% IV

CONDITIONS OF THE ADRENAL GLANDS AND THEIR TREATMENT

The adrenal glands are divided into the cortex and the medulla. Diseases of the adrenal cortex range from either an overproduction or underproduction of steroids. The cortex can be subdivided into three separate areas, each with their own specialized functions. Conditions affecting the cortex can be within one or more of the three areas. The three types of steroids include mineralocorticoids, glucocorticoids, and sex steroids. A decrease in secretion of any of these steroids can affect the levels of sodium, potassium, and chloride within the body (Table 16.4). Carbohydrate metabolism may be affected or sexual problems may result.

The most common syndrome of those listed in Table 16.4 is Cushing's syndrome. Most cases of Cushing's syndrome are caused by the oversecretion of glucocorticoids. This overproduction of adrenocorticotropic hormone (ACTH) often results from tumors of the pituitary glands. The remaining conditions occur from other tumors located either in the lungs or tumors of the adrenal cortex. Cushing's syndrome can also be caused by overmedication with steroids. The adrenal glands enlarge and symptoms are developed that can include obesity, flushing of the face, hypertension, and thick, scaling skin. Other symptoms include overall weakness and fatigue. Treatment may include the use of aminoglutethimide, or surgery may be used to remove tumors.

Hypofunction of the adrenal cortex can be caused by autoimmune disease, infections, or tumors that cause the destruction of the gland. In approximately 70% of persons suffering from Addison's disease, the condition is due to an autoimmune disease. Addison's disease results in the total necrosis of the adrenal cortex. Symptoms include fatigue, weight loss, nausea, and syncope. Treatment consists of replacement therapy of glucocorticoids and mineralocorticoids.

CLASSIFICATION: MINERALOCORTICOID

   GENERIC NAME: fludrocortisone acetate
   TRADE NAME: Florinef
   INDICATION: Addison's disease
   COMMON DOSAGE: 0.1 mg qd
   SIDE EFFECTS: GI upset
   AUXILIARY LABEL: Take as directed

An overexuberant, inflammatory response can result in more serious conditions. Under certain conditions, glucocorticoids can help the healing process of an inflamed, injured area. Following are glucocorticoid agents used for Addison's disease and for inflammation.

TABLE 16.4 Hyperfunction of Three Types of Adrenal Hormones

Condition	Common Name	Increased Secretion	Specific Steroid
Hyperaldosteronism	Conn's syndrome	Mineralocorticoids	Aldosterone
Hypercortisolism	Cushing's syndrome	Glucocorticoids	Cortisol
Adrenogenital syndrome	Adrenogenital syndrome	Sex steroids	Androgens

CLASSIFICATION: GLUCOCORTICOIDS
GENERIC NAME: hydrocortisone
TRADE NAME: Cortef
INDICATIONS: adrenal deficiency, inflammation
COMMON DOSAGE: 20 mg to 240 mg qd
SIDE EFFECTS: GI upset
AUXILIARY LABEL: Take as directed
           Take with food

GENERIC NAME: methylprednisolone sodium succinate
TRADE NAME: Solu-Medrol, Depo-Medrol
INDICATIONS: Addison's disease, inflammation
COMMON DOSAGE: 10 mg to 40 mg IV or intramuscular (maximum 3 days)
SIDE EFFECTS: GI upset
AUXILIARY LABEL: None

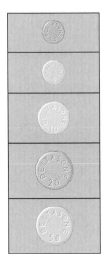

Forest

GENERIC NAME: prednisone
TRADE NAME: Deltasone
INDICATION: inflammation
COMMON DOSAGE: 5 mg to 60 mg qd
SIDE EFFECTS: GI upset
AUXILIARY LABELS: Take as directed.
           Do not stop taking abruptly
           Take with food or milk

GENERIC NAME: triamcinolone (#1), triamcinolone hexacetonide (#2), triamcinolone acetonide (#3)
TRADE NAME: Aristocort (po), Aristospan (IV), Kenalog-40 (IV)
INDICATIONS: adrenocortical deficiency, respiratory diseases
COMMON DOSAGE: adrenal 4 mg to 12 mg qd; respiratory 16 mg to 48 mg
SIDE EFFECT: GI upset
AUXILIARY LABEL: Take as directed
           Take with food

Pharmacia &
Upjohn

GENERIC NAME: dexamethasone
TRADE NAME: Decadron
INDICATION: allergic disorders
COMMON DOSAGE: 0.7 5 mg to 9 mg qd
SIDE EFFECTS: GI upset
AUXILIARY LABEL: Take as directed
           Take with food

Adrenal Medulla

Most of the conditions that affect the adrenal medulla result from tumor growths. The two main tumors are neuroblastomas and pheochromocytomas. Although neuroblastomas are known to grow rapidly and metastasize, they can be treated with chemotherapy, radiation, and surgical removal. Pheochromocytomas are usually benign and can cause hypertension. With surgical removal, the hypertension is relieved and the patient's prognosis is good.

CONDITIONS OF THE PANCREAS GLAND AND THEIR TREATMENT

One of the most well known conditions that can affect the pancreas is diabetes mellitus. There are two categories: insulin-dependent diabetes mellitus (IDDM) and non-insulin-dependent diabetes mellitus (NIDDM). The main difference between the two is the age of onset and the type of treatment normally given. Most people with IDDM are affected during childhood and require subcutaneous injections of insulin for the rest of their lives (hence the name insulin-dependent). NIDDM diabetes affects people older than 40 years and is referred to as non–insulin-dependent diabetes because oral medications usually can be used if lifestyle changes are not effective. NIDDM is more common.

TECH NOTE! The terms *rainbow coverage* and *sliding scale* refer to the varying doses of insulin that should be given depending on the reading of the blood glucose meter.

The cause of diabetes is the inability of the pancreas to secrete insulin or a resistance to insulin that affects the levels of glucose. The result is hyperglycemia. Diabetes mellitus can lead to renal disease, blindness, and even gangrene, which can lead to amputations of extremities. There are two main types of insulin that are used for IDDM: natural insulin, which is taken from animals such as pigs or cows, and synthesized human insulin, which is made in a laboratory and is chemically identical to human insulin. Persons who are newly diagnosed with insulin-dependent diabetes are given the newer DNA recombinant human insulin, but some persons remain on insulin derived from animals. Injected insulin helps maintain the glucose levels of the blood. There are short- and long-acting insulins used to keep the body's metabolism in homeostasis. Typical insulins prescribed are listed in Table 16.5.

The first line of treatment for patients with NIDDM is a change of lifestyle. Incorporating diet, exercise, and oral medications may take care of the problem. In more severe cases, insulin may be necessary. The drugs listed in Table 16.6 are a sample of hypoglycemic agents used to treat NIDDM.

TABLE 16.5 Commonly Prescribed Insulins for IDDM

Generic	Trade	Human/Animal	Length of Action
Insulin injection	Regular Iletin I	Beef or pork	Rapid
	Regular Iletin II	Purified pork	Rapid
	Novolin R	Human	Rapid
Isophane insulin	NPH Iletin I	Beef or pork	Intermediate
	Humulin N	Human	Intermediate
Isophane insulin suspension and insulin injection	Humulin 70/30	Human	Intermediate
Isophane insulin suspension and insulin injection	Humulin 50/50	Human	Intermediate
Insulin zinc suspension	Lente L	Purified pork	Intermediate
	Humulin L	Human	Intermediate
Insulin zinc suspension; extended lente	Humulin Ultralente	Human	Long Acting
Insulin analog injection	Humalog	Human	Rapid
Insulin glargine	Lantus	Human	Long Acting

TABLE 16.6 Oral Antidiabetic Agents for NIDDM

Generic	Trade	Normal Dosage
Oral Antidiabetic Agents		
Biguanides		
Metformin	Glucophage	500–1000 mg qd
Sulfonylureas		
Acetohexamide	Dymelor	250–500 mg qd
Chlorpropamide	Diabinese	100–250 mg bid
Glimepiride	Amaryl	1–4 mg qd
Glipizide	Glucotrol	5–10 mg qd
Glyburide	Micronase	1.5–20 mg qd
Tolazamide	Tolinase	100–500 mg qd
Tolbutamide	Orinase	500 mg qd
Antidote for Antidiabetic Agents or to Treat Hypoglycemia		
Glucagon	Glucagon	1 mg oral–10 ml by injection

Newer oral agents in use to treat NIDDM include the following agents. Because so many new agents are making their way into the pharmacy, it is important for technicians to always stay abreast of the new agents being used.

CLASSIFICATION: ORAL HYPOGLYCEMICS
 GENERIC NAME: pioglitazone
 TRADE NAME: Actos
 COMMON DOSAGE: 15 mg to 30 mg qd

GENERIC NAME: acarbose
 TRADE NAME: Precose
 COMMON DOSAGE: 50 mg to 100 mg three times daily (tid) maintenance dose*

GENERIC NAME: repaglinide
 TRADE NAME: Prandin
 COMMON DOSAGE: 0.5 mg to 4 mg twice daily (bid), tid, or four times daily (qid) maintenance dose*

GENERIC NAME: rosiglitazone
 TRADE NAME: Avandia
 COMMON DOSAGE: 4 mg qd or 2 mg bid maintenance dose*

*These doses are recommended after initial doses are given; initial doses vary.

Blood Glucose Meters

Patients with diabetes must monitor their blood glucose levels by blood draw, often several times daily. Small needles called lancets are placed into a device that is used to collect a drop of blood, which is then compared with a color-coded strip of paper. Reading the amount of glucose by checking the glucose content of urine is another commonly used method. When the strip comes into contact with glucose in the urine, the strip changes color. The resulting color is compared with the chart provided, which indicates the amount of glucose in the blood or urine and the amount of insulin necessary. From the determination made, the patient can take the proper amount of insulin necessary to balance his or her system. See

TABLE 16.7 Common Diagnostic Devices Used for Monitoring Glucose Levels in NIDDM Patients

Name	Type	Sizes Available
Urinalysis		
Chemstrip bG	Strips	100/bottle
Clinistix	Strips	50/bottle
Diastix	Strips	50 and 100/bottle
Clinitest	Tablets	36 and 100/bottle
Blood Analysis		
Glucostix	Strips	50, 100 /bottle
One Touch	Strips	25, 50,100/bottle*
First Choice	Strips	25, 50, 100/bottle†

*Used with One Touch brand meter.
†Used with First Choice brand meter.

Table 16.7 for a list of common diagnostic devices used for monitoring glucose levels.

HORMONES SECRETED BY THE OVARIES AND THEIR USES

There are many important hormones that regulate the female reproductive system. Within the ovaries, many hormones are produced that are responsible for the secondary sex characteristics of the female body and for reproduction. The two main hormones produced are estrogen and progesterone. Estrogen is primarily responsible for the development of female organs, breasts, and female body contours caused by fat distribution. Estrogen also stimulates growth of epithelial cells that line the uterus. Progesterone is secreted toward the halfway mark in the menstrual cycle and is responsible for changes in the uterus that prepare it for normal menstrual periods.

Treatment with estrogen is indicated for the following:

- To correct estrogen deficiency; estrogen deficiency results in abnormal uterine bleeding, hypogonadism, decreased ovarian functioning, and post-menopausal osteoporosis
- For cancer therapy in the breast or advanced prostatic carcinomas

Treatment with progesterones is indicated for the following:

- To correct female hormonal imbalance that may cause amenorrhea, dysmenorrhea, endometriosis
- To prevent pregnancy

See Chapter 23 for drugs found with these hormones.

CONDITIONS OF THE TESTES AND THEIR TREATMENT

For men, the main hormone secreted is androgen; testosterone is one of the main androgens. Testosterone regulates the secondary development of the male gender. It also provides protein development to the musculoskeletal system and to the development of sperm.

Treatment with testosterone is indicated for the following:

- Testosterone deficiency resulting from a formation of a cyst or removal of the testicles
- Treatment of delayed onset of puberty
- Certain types of breast carcinoma in women
- Certain types of anemia

See Chapter 23 for drugs with this hormone.

DO YOU REMEMBER THESE KEY POINTS?

- The main glands of the endocrine system
- The main function of the thyroid, pituitary, hypothalamus, adrenal, and pancreas
- The common diseases associated with the organs of the endocrine system
- The affect melatonin has on the body and what gland produces it
- How hormones regulate the reproductive system
- Types of replacement therapies available to treat conditions of the reproductive system
- Where the main regulators of calcium are located and where secretion takes place
- The cause and types of diabetes
- The treatments of diabetes
- The differences between types of insulin

REVIEW QUESTIONS:

Multiple Choice

1. Three glands located in the head are the
   A. Pineal, pituitary, and pancreas
   B. Hypothalamus, pituitary, and pineal
   C. Pituitary, exocrine, and endocrine
   D. None of the above

2. _____ hormones act on the same cell they are secreted from, whereas _____ hormones must travel to their target organ in the blood.
   A. Endocrine; autocrine   C. Paracrine; endocrine
   B. Autocrine; paracrine   D. Autocrine; endocrine

3. T_4 and T_3 are secreted from the
   A. Thymus gland   C. Thyroid gland
   B. Adrenal gland   D. Pituitary gland

4. The endocrine system keeps the body in balance by a mechanism known as
   A. Endocrine mechanism   C. Homeostasis mechanism
   B. Exocrine mechanism   D. Negative feedback mechanism

5. The hormones TSH, FSH, and ACTH are all secreted from the
   A. Hypothalamus   C. Posterior pituitary gland
   B. Anterior pituitary gland   D. Thyroid

6. The essential ions necessary for both T_3 and T_4 production are
   A. Proteins   C. Fatty acids
   B. Carbohydrates   D. Iodines

7. The endocrine gland(s) that help regulate the kidneys and secrete epinephrine and norepinephrine is(are)
   A. Parathyroid glands   C. Pancreas
   B. Pituitary glands   D. Adrenal glands

8. The most common causes of conditions affecting the endocrine system are
   A. Tumors   C. Congenital factors
   B. Cancer   D. Smoking

9. The condition that affects children suffering from hypothyroidism is known as
   A. Aphasia   C. Myxedema
   B. Cretinism   D. None of the above

10. The cause of diabetes is
    A. The inability of the pancreas to secrete enough insulin to regulate glucose
    B. A resistance to insulin that can affect the metabolism of glucose
    C. Other factors such as blindness or renal failure
    D. Both A and B

True/False

*If the statement is false, then change it to make it true.

1. Acromegaly is a childhood disease caused by a deficiency of growth hormone.
2. The hypothalamus links the central nervous system to the endocrine system.
3. Hormones are produced in the primary gland and secreted from the target gland.
4. Graves' disease is marked by the enlargement of the neck region.
5. Types of insulin can be long- or short-acting.
6. Aphasia is another term for hyperthyroidism.
7. Persons with NIDDM usually need to make lifestyle changes, whereas those with IDDM need insulin injections for life.
8. Insulin helps maintain glucose levels in the pancreas.
9. The two main hormones secreted by the ovaries are estrogen and progesterone.
10. The hormone androgen is responsible for the secondary development of the male, and also affects women's sex drives.

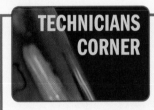

TECHNICIANS CORNER

Using *Mosby's Drug Consult,* find out whether there are any drug interactions between the following drugs:

Calcium carbonate (Oscal) 500 mg qd
Levothyroid (Synthroid) 0.1 mg qd
Aspirin enteric-coated 325 mg qd
Glipizide (Glucotrol) 5 mg qd

BIBLIOGRAPHY

Damjanov I: *Pathology for the health-related professions,* ed 2. Philadelphia, 2000, Saunders.
Facts and comparisons, St Louis, 1999, Wolters Kluwer.
Mosby's Drug Consult, St Louis, 2004, Elsevier.
Salerno E: *Pharmacology for health professionals*, St Louis, 1999, Mosby.
Thibodeu GA, Patton KT: *Structure & function of the body,* ed 11, St Louis, 2000, Mosby.
Voet D: *Biochemistry*, Indianapolis, 1990, Wiley & Sons.

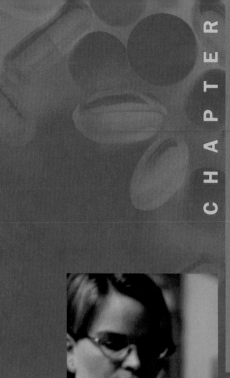

CHAPTER 17

Nervous System

Objectives

- Describe the main functions of the nervous system.

- Identify the main parts of a neuron.

- Describe how nerves function in transmitting impulses.

- List the main neurotransmitters of the nervous system.

- Describe the differences between the central nervous system (CNS) and the peripheral nervous system (PNS).

- Explain how the efferent system functions as opposed to the afferent system.

- Describe the main neurotransmitters of the PNS and the CNS.

- Identify the types of drugs affecting the nervous system.

- Identify the differences between cholinergics, adrenergics, and their blocking agents.

- Give examples of conditions that affect the nervous system and how they are treated.

- List the drugs that affect the nervous system, their methods of action, and normal dosing.

- Identify the auxiliary labels for the drugs discussed.

Afferent *The direction of neuronal impulse from the body toward the central nervous system (CNS)*

Autonomic *Self-controlling or involuntary*

Autonomic nervous system (ANS) *Division of the nervous system that controls the involuntary body functions; consists of sympathetic and parasympathetic divisions*

Axon *The part of a nerve cell that conducts impulses away from a cell body*

Blood-brain barrier *A barrier formed by special characteristics of capillaries to prevent certain chemicals from moving to the brain*

Cell body *The main part of a neuron from which axons and dendrites extend*

Central nervous system (CNS) *Brain and spinal cord*

Cerebrospinal fluid (CSF) *A fluid that fills the ventricles of the brain and also lies in the space between the arachnoid layer of the meninges and the brain or spinal cord*

Cervical *The neck region*

Dendrites *The part of a neuron that branches out to bring impulses to the cell body*

Efferent *The conduction of electrical impulses away from the CNS to the body*

Homeostasis *The equilibrium pertaining to the balance of the body with respect to fluid levels, pH level, and chemicals*

Lumbar *The region of the back that includes the area between the ribs and the pelvis: the area around the waist*

Monoamine oxidase (MAO) *An enzyme (includes MAO-A and MAO-B) found in the nerve terminals, the neurons, and liver cells; inactivates chemicals such as tyramine, catecholamines, serotonin, and certain medications*

Nerve terminal *The end portion of the neuron where nerve impulses cause chemical to be released; these cross a small space, called a synaptic cleft, to carry the impulse to another neuron*

Neuron *The functional unit of the nervous system, which includes the cell body, dendrites, axon, and terminals*

Parasympathetic nervous system *Division of the autonomic nervous system that functions during restful situations; "breed or feed" part of ANS*

Peripheral nervous system (PNS) *The division of the nervous system outside the brain and spinal cord*

Somatic *The motor neurons that control voluntary actions of the skeletal muscles*

Sympathetic nervous system *Division of the autonomic nervous system that functions during stressful situations; "fight or flight" part of ANC*

Thoracic *Relates to the thorax area or the chest*

CENTRAL NERVOUS SYSTEM DRUGS

Trade Name	Generic Name	Pronunciation	Trade Name	Generic Name	Pronunciation
Muscle Relaxants			Robaxin	Methocarbamol	meth-o-**kar**-ba-mol
Lioresal	Baclofen	**back**-low-fen	Norflex	Orphenadrine	or-**fen**-ah-dreen
Soma	Carisoprodol	kar-isoe-**proe**-dole			
Paraflon	Chlorzoxazone	klor-**socks**-ah-zone	**Neuromuscular Blocking Agents**		
Flexeril	Cyclobenzaprine	sigh-klo-**benz**-ah-preen	Pavulon	Pancuronium	pan-kur-**roe**-nee-um
Dantrium	Dantrolene	**dan**-tro-lean	Zemuron	Rocuronium	row-kur-**oh**-nee-um

CENTRAL NERVOUS SYSTEM DRUGS—cont'd

Trade Name	Generic Name	Pronunciation	Trade Name	Generic Name	Pronunciation
Anectine	Succinylcholine	sucks-in-ill-**koe**-leen	**Multiple Sclerosis Agents**		
			Avonex	Interferon Beta 1a	in-tur-**fear**-on bay-ta 1
Anticonvulsants			Betaseron	Interferon Beta 1b	in-tur-**fear**-on bay-ta 1
Tegretol	Carbamazepine	kar-ba-**maz**-e-peen			
Klonopin	Clonazepam (C-IV)	kloe-**naz**-e-pam	**Amyotrophic Lateral Sclerosis**		
Valium	Diazepam (C-IV)	die-**az**-e-pam	Rilutek	Riluzole	**ril**-you-zole
Cerebyx	Fosphenytoin	fos-**fen**-i-toyn			
Neurontin	Gabapentin	gab-a-**pen**-tin	**Alzheimer's Disease Agents**		
Mebaral	Mephobarbital (C-IV)	mep-oh-**bar**-bi-tall	Aricept	Donepezil	don-**nay**-pa-zil
Luminal	Phenobarbital (C-IV)	fee-no-**bar**-bi-tall	Cognex	Tacrine	**tac**-kreen
Mysoline	Primidone	**prim**-i-don			
Depakene	Valproic acid	val-**pro**-ic acid	**Myasthenia Gravis Agents**		
			Eserine	Neostigmine	knee-o-**stig**-meen
Parkinson's Disease Agents			Mestinon	Pyridostigmine	pie-rid-o-**stig**-meen
Symmetrel	Amantadine	ah-**man**-tie-deen			
Cogentin	Benztropine	benz-**tro**-peen	**Alpha and Beta Adrenergics**		
Parlodel	Bromocriptine	bro-mo-**krip**-teen	Levophed	Norepinephrine	nor-epi-**nef**-rin
Sinemet	Carbidopa/levodopa	car-bih-**doe**-pa/lee-vo-**doe**-pa	Yutopar	Ritodrine	**rye**-toe-dreen
Dopamine	Dopamine	do-**pa**-meen	**Alpha and Beta Adrenergic Blocking Agents**		
Larodopa	Levodopa	lee-vo-**doe**-pa	Cardura	Doxazosin	doks-ah-**zo**-sin
Permax	Pergolide	pur-go-**lide**	Regitine	Phentolamine	fen-**toll**-ah-meen
Mirapex	Pramipexole	pra-mi-**pex**-ole	Minipress	Prazosin	**pra**-zoe-sin
Requip	Ropinirole	row-**pin**-ah-roll	Hytrin	Terazosin	tur-**az**-oh-sin
Eldepryl	Selegiline	sel-eh-geh-**leen**	Brevibloc	Esmolol	**es**-mo-lol
Artane	Trihexyphenidyl	try-heks-ah-**fen**-a-dill	Normodyne	Labetalol	la-**bay**-ta-lol

Introduction

The nervous system is a complex system controlling and coordinating the movements and many functions of the body. This includes activities that we do not usually consciously think about, such as walking or running. Nerves also enable the body to perform internal functions involuntarily, such as the heart beating, the digestive system breaking down a meal, or the brain interpreting visual awareness. We take much for granted when it comes to the nervous system; however, if we lost a simple function, such as moving our eyes along a page of a book, it would be a devastating event in our lives. The nervous system is better understood when broken down into divisions and specific functions of those divisions. I begin with a generalized overview of the nervous system and its main branches, working through some of the basic functions of each. It is important to understand the nervous system and how drugs affect the various levels. Some conditions that affect the nervous system are discussed along with the medications that treat those conditions.

Nervous System

There are four main functions of the nervous system. One function consists of impulses sent to the central nervous system (CNS); a second function sends impulses from the CNS. A third function coordinates activities of all parts of the nervous system (those functions that rely on outside stimulation), and finally, there is a sensory function that detects various changes of the body. The many functions of the nervous system serve to keep the body in a balanced mode, which is referred to as homeostasis. The nervous system can be described as a complex mainframe computer system with its network of nerves connected to the body much like the Internet is connected to millions of homes. The mainframe (CNS) is connected to computers (target sites) that interpret the signals; likewise, the computer extensions can send messages to the mainframe computer (CNS) where it can be interpreted, and a response is then sent back (Figure 17.1).

The nervous system (the mainframe) is composed of the CNS (brain and the spinal cord) and the peripheral nervous system (PNS). The PNS has four distinct functions composed of two efferent and two afferent nerve tracts. The two efferent functions serve as the highways for motor impulses traveling from the CNS to the body's muscles and two sensory afferent functions that travel from the body to the CNS. The two efferent branches are called the somatic and the autonomic branches. Each efferent branch reaches out to specific areas of the body and relays motor messages from the CNS. The somatic branches make contact with skeletal muscles throughout the body, whereas the autonomic branches makes contact with the cardiac (heart) and smooth muscles such as those in the blood vessels, stomach, and other large organs. The branches that represent the afferent system carry impulses from the soft tissue areas and involuntary muscles of the body and other organs back to the CNS via visceral branches and the somatic branches. The various branches of the PNS allow the CNS to work at an optimal level because each area of the nervous system is in charge of a specific type of motor action or sensory response (Figure 17.2).

Recall that all the components of the nervous system are considered one system. We begin with the smallest functional part of the CNS, the neuron.

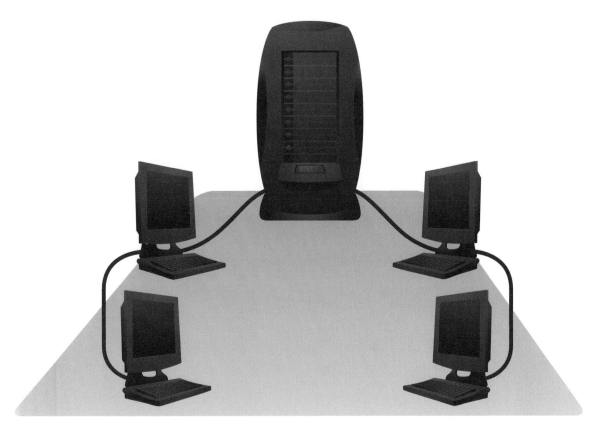

FIGURE 17.1 Computer mainframe with extensions to other computers.

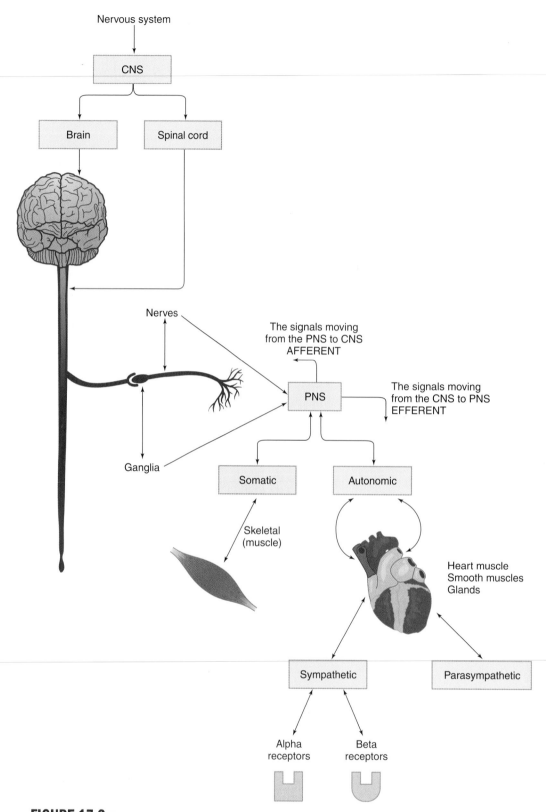

FIGURE 17.2 The nervous system: the divisions include the somatic and autonomic branches.

TECH NOTE! The nervous system is composed of the CNS and the PNS. The CNS comprises the brain and spinal cord. The PNS comprises the branches of nerves that travel between the CNS and the body systems. The PNS can be divided into the somatic and autonomic systems.

The Neuron

The smallest unit of the nervous system is the neuron. Billions of neurons make up the nervous system. This highly sophisticated circuitry is somewhat analogous to a computer chip that is responsible for relaying information within a computer system. The computer chip is very small and carries a massive amount of information; similarly millions of nerves run throughout our bodies and carry messages back and forth from the CNS.

The cell body, dendrites, axon, and the nerve terminal compose the four main sections of a neuron. As neurons branch out, forming a network of relay stations, they allow nerve impulses to travel from one neuron to another. The dendrites are extensions that receive electrical impulses. The cell body processes the electrical message before it enters the axon. There is a specialized insulation called a myelin sheath that wraps around the axon. The myelin sheath is composed of the same fatty material that is found in the white matter of the brain. It helps with impulse conduction (Figure 17.3).

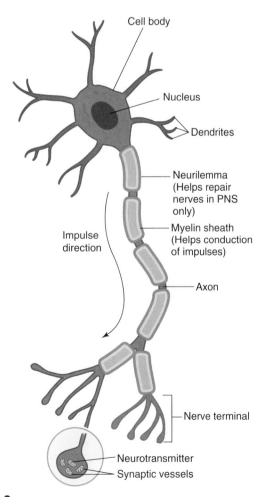

FIGURE 17.3 Complete neuron and cell membrane of efferent (motor) nerve.

TABLE 17.1 Neuronal Transmitters, Their Most Important Clinical Locations, and Some of Their Actions

Neurotransmitter	Type of Response
Acetylcholine (PNS)	Excitatory (skeletal muscles, GI muscles); inhibitory (heart)
Norepinephrine (PNS)	Excitatory (increases heart rate)
Epinephrine (PNS)	Inhibitory (bronchodilator); excitatory (increases heart rate)
Dopamine (CNS)	Helps to inhibit involuntary movement
Serotonin (CNS)	Helps to inhibit pain perception

PNS, Peripheral nervous system; *GI,* gastrointestinal; *CNS,* central nervous system.

Nerves are not separate from one another in the PNS, but form bundles made of axons. Bundles of cell bodies are called ganglions. However, within the CNS the terminology differs—the axons are called tracts and the cell bodies are called either nuclei or ganglia. The electrical nerve impulses are transmitted from one neuron to another by various chemicals called neurotransmitters. There are many different neurotransmitters, each responsible for a different message. The most common neurotransmitters are listed in Table 17.1, along with their type of response. When the impulse is activated by an neurotransmitter, a series of actions take place to transmit the nerve impulse.

Nerve Transmission

There are three main states of a neuron. These are polarized, depolarized, and repolarized. When the cell is in a resting state there is an overall negative charge inside the neuron that is made up of potassium (K^+—positive) and chloride ions (Cl^-—negative). The outside of the neuron is more positive, with sodium (Na^+) as the positive charge. At this point the cell is considered polarized and waiting to be excited. When a neurotransmitter activates the cell membrane, an influx of outside sodium ions rushes through channels, changing the negative charge inside to a positive charge, as shown in Figure 17.4. This is called depolarization. The cell restores the resting state by allowing the inside positive charges (K^+) to escape. As the transition back to the resting state is made, the cell actively transports the sodium back to the outside and allows the potassium to reenter the cell. This repolarizes the cell, bringing the cell full circle and back to the resting stage again.

TECH NOTE! Nerves are made of millions of axons. Each neuron is made of a cell body, dendrites, axon, and nerve endings. Electrical impulses travel along the nerves to and from the CNS via afferent and efferent branches. Impulses are made by the change in polarity of the axon, which moves the impulse very rapidly. This electrical conduction is helped by the myelin sheath. The impulse is started by neurotransmitters. There are many different types of neurotransmitters.

Central Nervous System

THE BRAIN

The brain is composed of two types of matter. Gray matter is made up of neuron cell bodies and dendrites, and the white matter is made up of bundles of nerve fibers (myelinated axons). These fibers are woven in a pattern, making up the contents of the brain. There are several sections of the brain that serve specific

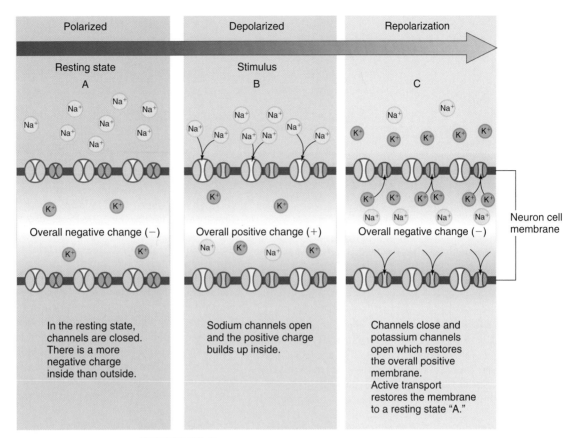

FIGURE 17.4 Neuronal impulse transfer.

functions of the body. The largest area of the brain is the cerebrum. This area deals with the ability to reason, remember, speak a language, and create. The cerebrum is divided into two hemispheres: The right hemisphere controls logical thinking processes and the left hemisphere controls creativity. Each of the two hemispheres can be further divided into four different lobes, each having their own function. These functions cover the six senses—hearing, vision, balance, taste, touch, and smell—as well as motor functions to muscles. The next largest segment is the cerebellum, located at the base of the brain, which helps control most of the muscle functions and precise movements of the body. This includes balance, posture, and overall coordination. The brainstem connects the brain to the spinal cord and consists of three main areas: the midbrain, pons, and medulla oblongata. These three areas are linked to many of the nerves within the brain. Each area serves as a control center with specific functions (Figure 17.5).

The midbrain and pons are a collection of nerves that branch off into other areas and serve as an intersection, whereas the medulla oblongata controls breathing or respiration, cardiac rate, the force of the heart's contraction, and dilation of blood vessels. Wedged between the midbrain and the cerebrum are two other parts of the brain, the thalamus and hypothalamus. When activated, these structures produce chemical reactions throughout the body, linking the nervous system to the endocrine system. The hypothalamus is a built-in thermostat and appetite center; it also relays messages to the thalamus. The thalamus is in charge of most of our sensory stimuli and is responsible for interpreting messages sent via the nervous system and for relaying them to other areas It is also responsible for initiating motor impulses from the cortex (see Chapter 16).

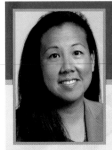

Pharmacist's Perspective

SUSAN WONG

What's New In Headache Management?

Many people say "I've got a migraine." What is a migraine headache? Migraines are a distinct type of headache with the following features: episodic, not continuous or daily, usually on one side of the head, may or may not be associated with aura, autonomic dysfunction (nausea, vomiting, photophobia, etc.), strong family history, and may be significantly disabling—not "just a headache." Daily throbbing headaches are more likely to be rebound headaches than migraines. Daily or near-daily throbbing headaches coupled with daily analgesic use are likely analgesic rebound headaches. Rebound headaches typically occur in patients who have been initially diagnosed with migraine and get caught up in a cycle of frequent and excessive analgesic use. Management includes educating the patient about the cause of analgesic rebound, initiating preventive therapy, and tapering the patient off analgesics over several weeks.

The primary goal of management of migraine headaches is prevention. This involves identifying and eliminating risks or triggers for headaches such as fatigue, noise, bright lights, certain foods, and other lifestyle factors. Simple analgesics (aspirin, nonsteroidal antiinflammatory drugs [NSAIDs]) work well for acute attacks, especially in patients with mild to moderate pain in whom risks and trigger factors are under control. Antiemetics, such as metoclopropamide or prochlorperazine, are useful additions if nausea is a prominent symptom. Analgesic combinations (e.g., Fiorinal, Midrin) and ergots (e.g., Ergostat, Cafergot) are usually effective for more severe migraines. Dihydroergotamine (DHE) injectable and more recently DHE nasal spray (Migranal) has been a mainstay of migraine treatment.

The "triptans": sumatriptan (Imitrex), rizatriptan (Maxalt MLT), zolmitriptan (Zomig), and naratriptan (Amerge), are useful for patients whose migraines do not respond to or who are intolerant of other classes of agents. Compared with sumatriptan (Imitrex), the new triptans are more selective 5-HT (serotonin) agonists and offer greater oral bioavailability, a potentially improved risk-to-benefit ratio, and a potentially greater therapeutic benefit through a combination of both peripheral and central effects.

Preventive drug therapy is indicated when a patient has frequent (two or more) headaches per month that create significant disability at home, school, or work (cancelled plans, etc.), causing significant emotional distress, or when a patient requires large quantities of medications to acutely stop the pain. Prevention should be part of a treatment plan that emphasizes behavioral changes and should be given an adequate trial to assess effectiveness (usually 2 to 3 months unless side effects are intolerable). Prescribing inadequate doses of preventive medications for brief periods is a major cause of therapeutic failure. Beta-blockers and tricyclic antidepressants remain the drugs of choice for prevention. Propranolol is found to be the most effective agent but may cause a slow heart rate; it should be used with caution in patients with asthma. Failure of one beta-blocker does not preclude success with another. A number of over-the-counter (OTC) alternatives may be effective; they include riboflavin (400 mg/day), or magnesium (500 to 700 mg/day for adults and 7 mg/kg for children). Magnesium supplementation may also improve the efficacy of triptan medications. Diarrhea and intestinal cramping are rare side effects at these doses; caution is necessary in renal impairment or disease.

Your role as a technician is to be aware of what a patient tells you or asks for. If it seems like the same patient is asking for OTC pain or headache medicine either in a large quantity or on a regular basis, it should be a red flag, causing you to ask: how often do you need to take this type of medicine? Are you using it for headaches or other pain? Does it help? If any of the answers are more than just on an occasional basis, tell the pharmacist. Sometimes chronic use of OTC medicines can be a problem because they can interfere with some of the prescription medicines, they can worsen or cause other problems, and, in the case of headaches, they can actually contribute to having them (hence the description of analgesic rebound). A patient may ask you for single-agent supplements such as riboflavin or magnesium. Make sure he or she speaks with the pharmacist to prevent drug interactions or adverse effects from too much of a certain substance. ■

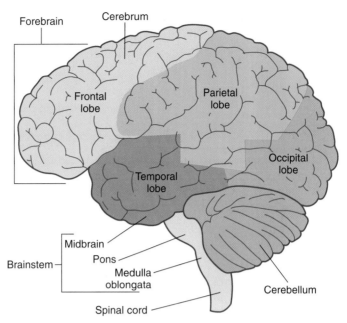

FIGURE 17.5 Anatomy of the brain.

TECH NOTE! The nerves of the brain crisscross so that the left side of the brain controls the right side of the body. Thus persons suffering from a stroke (blocked blood flow) on one side of the brain can lose the ability to move parts of the body located on the opposite side.

THE SPINAL CORD

The spinal cord is composed of an inner gray matter that houses many nerve cells and an outside white matter containing nerve fibers. The meninges, a thin covering lining the inside of the bones, separates and protects the brain and the spinal cord from the bony structure of the skull and spinal column. The brain and spinal cord are also cushioned by a watery liquid called the cerebrospinal fluid (CSF). This combination of the meninges and fluid serves to protect and cushion the CNS.

The brain and spinal cord are protected by a barrier called the blood-brain barrier. This barrier is another protectant that allows only certain types of very small molecules to pass into the brain. This includes some drugs. Most drugs that can pass through the blood-brain barrier are lipid soluble (i.e., they dissolve in fat).

The spinal cord is divided into sections, each identified by its attachment location along the spinal cord. The five main areas of the spinal cord include the cervical (neck), thoracic (chest), lumbar (lower back), sacral (below lower back), and coccygeal areas (Figure 17.6).

AFFERENT (SENSORY) NEURONS

The afferent branch's main functions include transferring information via electrical impulse from the peripheral area (outside the CNS) back to the CNS. The afferent, or sensory, branch is composed of neurons that have long axons (the dendrites at the ends of the axon going to the cell body) and a short axon. The cell body is located within the PNS axon that enters the CNS.

EFFERENT (MOTOR) NEURONS

After the CNS receives a message, a response via nerve impulse is sent through the efferent branch to a target muscle. The neurons, which compose the efferent

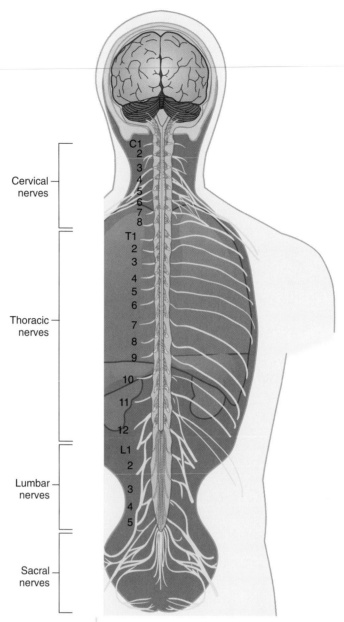

FIGURE 17.6 Segments of the spinal cord.

branch, have short dendrites and a long axon. The dendrites and cell body of these efferent neurons are located within the CNS, and the axon becomes part of the PNS (Figure 17.7).

TECH NOTE! The brain and spinal cord make up the CNS. The brain has three main areas: the cerebrum, cerebellum, and brainstem. The brain is composed of both gray and white matters that contain neurons. The meninges, CSF, and the blood-brain barrier protect the brain and spinal cord. The afferent nerves bring messages from our body to the CNS, and the efferent nerves send messages back to the muscles of the skeleton, organs, and other tissues in response to the stimulus. The axon synapses are located in the CNS in the afferent system, whereas the axon synapses are located in the CNS and PNS in the efferent system.

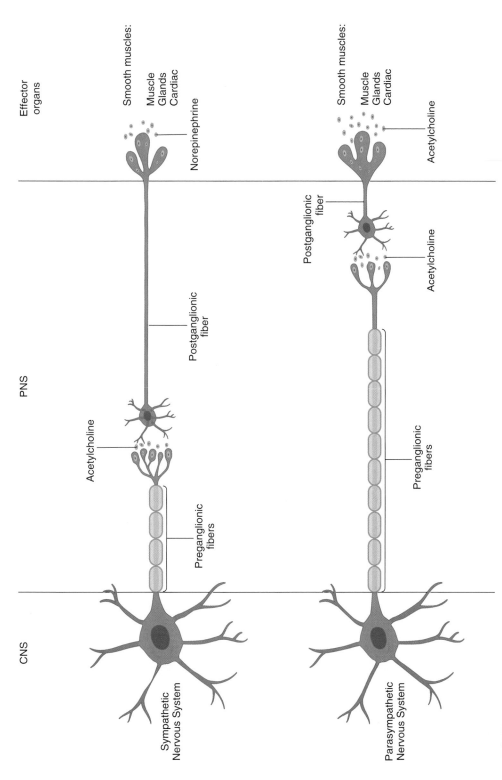

FIGURE 17.7 The afferent and efferent nerves and the areas attached by the sympathetic and parasympathetic systems. Preganglionic and postganglionic nerves and cell bodies with the axon for both are shown. Efferent and afferent neurons are also included.

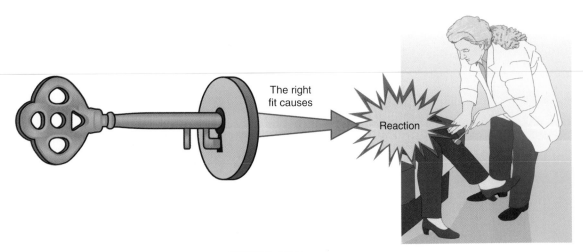

FIGURE 17.8 Lock and key mechanism.

Peripheral Nervous System

THE SOMATIC SYSTEM

The somatic system is a network of nerves that relay messages to the CNS from the outside world and return messages back to the body. It is part of the PNS and regulates the motor nerves that control voluntary actions of the skeletal muscles as well as impulses from sensory receptors. Receptor sites are sensitive to a stimulus and include smell, taste, touch, and hearing.

THE AUTONOMIC SYSTEM

A subdivision of the PNS, the autonomic branch is called the autonomic system because it controls automatic functions. These are the functions that you do not have to consciously think about, such as heart beat. It is called the involuntary nervous system and is further subdivided into two branches of the PNS called the sympathetic and parasympathetic nervous systems. Both of these systems serve to regulate organs, tissues, and blood vessels. They can perform this function in response to outside and inside stimuli with the use of specific neurotransmitters. Both sympathetic and parasympathetic systems are made of nerves and ganglia. Both systems have neurons of approximately the same length that carry impulses from the CNS to target tissue. The ganglia is the area where the synapse (relay) is located. The nerve fibers are considered to be either preganglionic or postganglionic, depending on whether the nerve fibers come before or after the ganglia. Each neurotransmitter has its own specific receptor that it contacts opposite the synapse (the lock and key mechanism) (Figure 17.8).

SYMPATHETIC SYSTEM

The areas of the CNS where the sympathetic nerves emerge are the thoracic and lumbar regions of the spinal cord. The function of the sympathetic division is to respond to stressful situations, such as the "fight or flight" response. During the fight or flight stress response, the sympathetic system shuts down the nonessential systems of the body. This redirects energy to other areas such as the muscular system. The nerves that are responsible for this type of behavior are composed of preganglionic neurons imbedded into the gray matter of the spinal cord. As the impulses travel through this gray matter, they synapse with postganglionic neurons that go out into the body systems. The sympathetic preganglionic neurons synapse and affect many postganglionic neurons. This massive transfer to many areas of the body allows humans to respond quickly and powerfully to a situation. The sympathetic system also sends impulses to various organs and tissues for other emotional situations such as anxiety, hate, and even stress. When you go for an interview and your palms get sweaty, your heart rate increases, and breathing becomes quick and shallow, you are experiencing a sympathetic reaction but to a lesser degree than a person having a panic attack or who is in fear for his or her life. Whether you are in a life-threatening situation or in minor stress, the sympathetic nervous system keeps the body in homeostasis through its "fight or flight" responses. Table 17.2 shows the response of each major organ when affected by the sympathetic system. All of the nonessential energy-consuming functions, such as urination or digestion, are placed on hold while blood flow to large muscles, the release of glucose from the liver, the heart rate, and other functions are increased. This sympathetic response is one that is not mentally activated, but is an instinctive or autonomic reaction.

TECH NOTE! Drugs that mimic the sympathetic system are called adrenergic drugs; those that block the actions of the sympathetic system are called adrenergic blockers. Drugs that mimic the parasympathetic system are called cholinergic drugs; those that block the actions of the parasympathetic system are called anticholinergics. Monoamine oxidase (MAO) enzymes are responsible for destroying excess neurotransmitters. Activators like adrenergics and cholinergics either increase the amount of neurotransmitters or stop the MAOs from destroying the neurotransmitters. When blockers are used, they block the receptor sites of the neurotransmitters so that they cannot connect and cause a response.

Adrenergic Agents and Adrenergic Blockers

The main neurotransmitters of the sympathetic system are norepinephrine and epinephrine. Dopamine is a precursor for norepinephrine and is found as a neurotransmitter within the CNS, specifically the basal ganglia. Persons suffering from Parkinson's disease have low levels of dopamine, causing tremors and other physiological problems.

Within the nerve ending there are enzymes that destroy excess norepinephrine, or they are taken up to be reused. One of the enzymes responsible for this action is called monoamine oxidase (MAO). It is important that excessive amounts of norepinephrine are destroyed, or overexcitement can cause unwanted effects.

There are four types of receptors found opposite the sympathetic postganglionic fiber endings. α-1 receptors are located in peripheral blood vessels, the

TABLE 17.2 Major Organ Response When Sympathetic System is Activated

Organ/Tissue	Sympathetic Response
Heart	Increases force of contraction, speed of conduction within the heart, and rate
Lung	Bronchi and bronchioles become dilated, secretions are suppressed
Blood vessels	Constricts all surface areas so person looks pale; increases to areas where blood is most needed, such as the GI system, muscles, heart, brain
Digestive system	Inhibition—decreases GI motility, and GI secretions are suppressed
Urinary system	Bladder wall relaxes; sphincter contracts
Liver	Increases release of glucose
Eyes	Pupils dilate for better vision; ciliary muscle relaxes for far vision
Adrenal medulla	Epinephrine is released into the blood
Sweat glands	Increases secretion

GI, Gastrointestinal.

heart, and the eyes. α-receptors are located on the smooth muscle; β-1 receptors are located on the heart muscle; and β-2 receptors are located in the respiratory system and elsewhere. Drugs that mimic natural sympathetic neurotransmitters are referred to as sympathomimetics or adrenergics, and the drugs used to block them are called sympatholytics or are named after the specific receptor they block. The adrenergic agents that mimic the sympathetic nervous system are epinephrine and norepinephrine. Some uses for α- and β-sympathomimetics are listed in Table 17.3 with their effects.

CLASSIFICATION: SYMPATHOMIMETICS OR ADRENERGIC AGENTS
GENERIC NAME: epinephrine
TRADE NAME: Adrenalin
DRUG ACTION: activates α-1 and β-1 sites, causing vasoconstriction and increasing the heart rate
INDICATION: low blood pressure; used to treat heart attacks and shock
ROUTE OF ADMINISTRATION: injectable
COMMON DOSAGE: 1 mg/mL
SIDE EFFECTS: headache (HA), tachycardia, and high blood pressure

GENERIC NAME: dopamine
TRADE NAME: Intropin
DRUG ACTION: stimulates both α-1 (but only at high rates of infusion) and β-1 receptors
INDICATIONS: in low dosages it causes vasodilation and increased urine output; in moderate doses it releases norepinephrine, which affects β-1 receptors, increasing heart contractions; in high doses it is used for patients suffering from shock
ROUTE OF ADMINISTRATION: injectable
COMMON DOSAGE: 1 to 5 μg/kg/min up to 50 mg/kg/min
SIDE EFFECTS: tachycardia, HA, vomiting

GENERIC NAME: ritodrine
TRADE NAME: Yutopar
MOA: activates β-2 receptors that inhibit contraction of the uterine muscles
INDICATION: premature labor
ROUTE OF ADMINISTRATION: injectable
COMMON DOSAGE: 50 to 100 μg/min
SIDE EFFECTS: bradycardia, nausea, and vomiting

PARASYMPATHETIC SYSTEM

There are many differences between the sympathetic and parasympathetic systems. The parasympathetic system can be thought of as the opposite or counterbalance to the sympathetic system. In the parasympathetic system, nerves emerge from the brainstem and the sacral part of the cord. Another important difference is the location of the preganglionic nerves. In the parasympathetic system these are

TABLE 17.3 α- and β-Receptors and Their Effects on the Body Systems

Receptors	Effects
α-1	Heart contraction increases
	Eye dilation
	Peripheral vasoconstriction
α-2	Smooth muscles contract
β-1	Heart rate increases
β-2	Bronchial muscles dilate
	Uterus relaxes

located in the gray matter of the brainstem or spinal cord. They exit the CNS and have a long preganglionic fiber. The impulse moves to the target organ creating a response. One of the main functions of the parasympathetic system is activation of the digestive system. This function includes secreting acidic juices, increasing peristalsis, and inducing hormonal secretion of insulin. The parasympathetic system also slows the heart rate. The parasympathetic system works while we rest and is inhibited only when the sympathetic system takes over during periods of intense stress. Table 17.4 describes the organs and effects of the parasympathetic system.

TECH NOTE! The autonomic system is an involuntary branch of the PNS. It is divided into sympathetic and parasympathetic systems. The sympathetic system releases the neurotransmitter norepinephrine when we are stressed, and the parasympathetic system releases acetylcholine (ACh) when we are at rest. Sympathetic ganglions synapse with many postganglionic fibers for a widespread effect, whereas parasympathetic preganglionic fibers synapse with fewer postganglionic fibers.

Cholinergic Agents and Cholinergic Blockers

The main neurotransmitter of the parasympathetic system is ACh. ACh is important in the CNS and PNS. It works quickly and has a short duration of action. There are two types of cholinergic agents, those that mimic ACh, and those that stop the destruction of ACh by the enzyme acetylcholinesterase. Because these cholinergic drugs mimic the parasympathetic system, they are referred to as parasympathomimetics, whereas drugs that inhibit the cholinergic reaction by blocking the receptor are most commonly called anticholinergics. The main side effects of anticholinergics are dry mouth and an inhibition of urine output.

Parasympathetic receptors, which respond to the neurotransmitter ACh, are located on smooth and cardiac muscle cells. Cholinergic blockers stop the response. They prevent ACh from combining with the receptor, causing the nerve impulse to stop. This is useful when patients must be sedated or when their eyes have to be dilated by the optometrist. There are many uses for anticholinergic drugs, including many of the conditions that are discussed later.

Conditions of the Nervous System and Their Treatments

Many disorders involve inappropriate or excessive muscle contractions. Some muscular disorders involve the wasting away of the muscles. Many of the following conditions are still without cures, and researchers are still trying to find the causes.

TABLE 17.4 Response of the Body Systems to Parasympathetic Stimulation

Organ/Tissue	Parasympathetic Response
Heart	Slows
Lungs	Dilates bronchi
Blood vessels	None
Digestive system	Increased motility; digestion takes place
Urinary system	Urinary bladder muscle contracts; sphincter relaxes
Liver	None
Eyes	Pupils constrict; ciliary muscle contraction for near vision
Adrenal medulla	None
Sweat glands	None

Some are hereditary, whereas others may be random genetic mutations. Other disorders are being investigated to determine whether environmental conditions may increase the incidence of their occurrence.

GENERAL NERVOUS SYSTEM DISORDERS

Skeletal Muscle Pain

Pain in the muscles is a warning signal from the body. Although everyone experiences some pain at one time or another, severe injury or chronic pain may need additional care. Treatments include surgery followed by physical therapy or drug therapy. Other causes of pain related to the nervous system include headaches, migraines, and various bone conditions affecting the skeletal system. Analgesics and nonsteroidal antiinflammatory drugs used to treat head pain are discussed in Chapter 24. For chronic muscle pain that cannot be identified, the patient may be treated only with skeletal muscle relaxants. There are two main types of these drugs used—centrally acting and direct acting.

Actions of Central-Acting Medications

Although the drug actions of central-acting medications are not well known, the result of the medications is well documented. One of most important effects of these agents is the depression of the CNS. They affect the brainstem, thalamus, basal ganglia, and the spinal cord. Side effects include dizziness, drowsiness, blurred vision, and headaches. These agents are not meant for long-term use. These drugs are classified as smooth muscle relaxants. The main drugs used as smooth muscle relaxants follow, along with their primary indication, drug action, and necessary auxiliary labels. In several instances the specific drug action is not currently known; therefore a general drug action is supplied. Auxiliary labels are placed on certain prescription bottles and contain brief information about the drug for the patient's reference. The information usually refers to side effects. For instance, if an auxiliary label states, "Take with food," the medication can cause stomach upset.

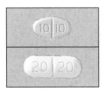

Novartis

CLASSIFICATION: SMOOTH MUSCLE RELAXANTS
  GENERIC NAME: baclofen
  TRADE NAME: Lioresal
  DRUG ACTION: inhibits synaptic reflexes at CNS level
  INDICATION: spasticity associated with multiple sclerosis (MS) or spinal cord injury
  ROUTE OF ADMINISTRATION: oral, injectable
  COMMON DOSAGE: oral dosage ranges from 5 mg tid to 80 mg maximum per day
  AUXILIARY LABELS:
  - Take with food or milk
  - May cause dizziness or drowsiness

Wallace

  GENERIC NAME: carisoprodol
  TRADE NAME: Soma
  DRUG ACTION: blocks neuron activity at CNS level
  INDICATION: acute muscle pain
  ROUTE OF ADMINISTRATION: oral
  COMMON DOSAGE: 350 mg tid or qid
  SIDE EFFECTS: dizziness, drowsiness, vertigo, upset stomach, HA
  AUXILIARY LABELS:
  - May cause dizziness or drowsiness
  - Take with food

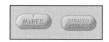

Ortho-McNeil

GENERIC NAME: chlorzoxazone
TRADE NAME: Parafon Forte DSC
DRUG ACTION: reduces multisynaptic impulses at CNS level
INDICATION: discomfort caused by muscle pain and spasms
ROUTE OF ADMINISTRATION: oral
COMMON DOSAGE: ranges from 250 mg tid to qid to 750 mg tid to qid, tapering off dose as pain decreases
SIDE EFFECTS: dizziness, drowsiness, and stomach upset
AUXILIARY LABELS:

- May cause dizziness or drowsiness
- Take with food

GENERIC NAME: cyclobenzaprine
TRADE NAME: Flexeril
DRUG ACTION: decreases muscle spasms without loss of muscle function
INDICATION: acute muscle pain
ROUTE OF ADMINISTRATION: oral
COMMON DOSAGE: 10 mg tid; maximum length 3 weeks
SIDE EFFECTS: dizziness, drowsiness, blurred vision, dry mouth
AUXILIARY LABELS:

- May cause dizziness or drowsiness
- Avoid alcohol

GENERIC NAME: methocarbamol
TRADE NAME: Robaxin
DRUG ACTION: general CNS depression
INDICATION: acute muscle pain and muscle pain associated with tetanus
ROUTE OF ADMINISTRATION: oral, injectable
COMMON DOSAGE: oral dosage, 1.5 g qid up to 8 g per day in severe cases
SIDE EFFECTS: drowsiness, dizziness; urine may change color to black, brown, or green
AUXILIARY LABELS:

- May cause dizziness or drowsiness
- Avoid alcohol
- Urine may change color

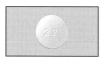

3M

GENERIC NAME: orphenadrine
TRADE NAME: Norflex
DRUG ACTION: acts at the brainstem using analgesia
INDICATION: acute muscle pain and bedtime leg cramps
ROUTE OF ADMINISTRATION: oral, injectable
COMMON DOSAGE: oral dosage 100 mg bid
SIDE EFFECTS: dizziness, drowsiness, blurred vision, fainting, dry mouth
AUXILIARY LABELS:

- May cause dizziness or drowsiness
- Avoid alcohol

Direct-Acting Agents

Direct-acting agents work directly on the muscles by inhibiting calcium release, which results in decreased muscle response. Side effects include fatigue, dizziness, drowsiness, diarrhea, and respiratory depression. (The medication dantrolene is listed under multiple sclerosis.) Commonly used oral agents are listed in the following. These are samples of combinations of agents that include a variety of popular analgesics and antiinflammatories.

CLASSIFICATION: MUSCLE EXLAXANTS WITH ANALGESICS/ANTIINFLAMMATORIES
GENERIC NAME: carisoprodol/aspirin
TRADE NAME: Soma Compound
COMMON DOSAGE: 200 mg, 1 to 2 tablets qid

GENERIC NAME: carisoprodol/aspirin/codeine
TRADE NAME: Soma Compound with codeine
COMMON DOSAGE: 16 mg codeine, 1 to 2 tablets qid

GENERIC NAME: orphenadrine/aspirin/caffeine
TRADE NAME: Norgesic
COMMON DOSAGE: 25 mg/385 mg/30 mg, 1 to 2 tablets q6-8 h

Conditions Affecting the Peripheral Nervous System

MYASTHENIA GRAVIS

Myasthenia gravis is a rare autoimmune disorder in which electrical messages from the CNS to muscles throughout the body, especially the muscles of the throat and eyes, are affected. The body's immune system attacks and destroys the receptors that normally receive neuronal impulses. A tumor within the thymus may sometimes be the cause. Although the muscles in the face, eyes, and mouth areas are affected, other areas can be affected as well. Both vocal and vision difficulties often occur, and drooping of the eyelids is a common side effect seen in persons suffering from this autoimmune disease. Muscles tire easily and take a much longer time to recover. This is a chronic disease that worsens over time. Eventually the respiratory system is affected and death results. Myasthenia gravis affects more women than men; only 3 : 100,000 persons are affected in the United States. Drugs that block the destruction of ACh, called anticholinesterases, are most often used for treatment. Surgery is performed to remove the thymus if a thymic tumor is found. Of people with myasthenia gravis, 8 out of 10 can be helped; only rare cases result in death when the respiratory system fails. There is no cure for myasthenia gravis, except in those cases in which the cause is a tumor in the thymus (15% of cases).

Drug Treatments

The class of drugs used for treating myasthenia gravis is cholinergics. The drug action is to block the destruction of the neurotransmitter ACh by the enzyme acetylcholinesterase. Side effects of the medications may occur because of overstimulation that can result in nausea, vomiting, diarrhea, and severe abdominal pain.

CLASSIFICATION: CHOLINERGIC AGENTS
GENERIC NAME: neostigmine
TRADE NAME: Prostigmin
INDICATION: Myasthenia gravis
ROUTE OF ADMINISTRATION: oral, injectable
COMMON DOSAGE: oral dosage ranges from 15 mg to 375 mg qd

GENERIC NAME: pyridostigmine
TRADE NAME: Mestinon
INDICATION: Myasthenia gravis
ROUTE OF ADMINISTRATION: oral, injectable
COMMON DOSAGE: oral dosage ranges anywhere from 70 mg to 1.5 g per day

Disorders of the Brain and Spinal Cord

EPILEPSY

Epilepsy is a seizure disorder in which there is a hyperexcitability in some of the nerve cells in the brain. Diagnosis is normally based on an electroencephalogram (EEG). For an EEG, electrodes are attached to the head of the patient and the electrical impulses corresponding to brain waves are transferred onto paper strips that can be read by a physician. There are two types of seizures, partial or generalized. Partial seizures affect only one hemisphere of the brain and may result in only a twitching of a limb without any loss of consciousness. Generalized seizures affect both hemispheres and have different levels of intensity ranging from petit mal (the least violent) to grand mal seizures that are longer and more intense. Children often have petit mal seizures, causing them to stare off into space for a time. In grand mal seizures, also known as tonic-clonic seizures, the person loses consciousness and falls to the ground; there are widespread muscle spasms (tonic phase) followed by muscle relaxation (clonic phase). The person can be injured depending on where and when he or she has the seizure. The person having the seizure does not remember the episode. Other causes for seizure include skull fracture or tumor, although often no cause is found. Treatment can range from drugs to surgery in the case of an operable tumor. Anticonvulsants are the types of drugs used for epilepsy. Often the dosage or type of medicine must be adjusted to help the patient become seizure-free. It is extremely important for the patient to take the medication on time every day to avoid the possibility of seizures.

Drug Treatment

Anticonvulsants inhibit abnormal impulses within the CNS by inhibiting one or more of the ions such as sodium, calcium, or potassium within the nervous system. When dosed correctly, these agents stop seizures from occurring. The various agents used for treatment of seizures—hydantoins, barbiturates, succinimides, and benzodiazepines—and their maintenance dosing is discussed.

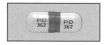

Parke-Davis

CLASSIFICATION: HYDANTOIN ANTICONVULSANT
GENERIC NAME: phenytoin
TRADE NAME: Dilantin
DRUG ACTION: inhibits seizure activity at the motor cortex; decreases sodium ion gradient
INDICATION: most often tonic-clonic seizures and partial seizures
ROUTE OF ADMINISTRATION: oral, injectable
COMMON DOSAGE: oral dosage is 100 mg tid, although the dosage can range widely
AUXILIARY LABELS:
■ May cause dizziness or drowsiness
■ Avoid alcohol

GENERIC NAME: fosphenytoin
TRADE NAME: Cerebyx (intravenous [IV] only—because phenytoin given IV irritates and burns the vein, fosphenytoin, a different form of phenytoin, is given instead; after it enters the body, it converts into phenytoin). Note: The drug action and trade name are the same as phenytoin.

CLASSIFICATION: SUCCINIMIDE ANTICONVULSANT
GENERIC NAME: ethosuximide
TRADE NAME: Zarontin
INDICATION: absence (petit mal) seizures
ROUTE OF ADMINISTRATION: oral
COMMON DOSAGE: 250 mg qd
AUXILIARY LABEL:
- May cause dizziness or drowsiness

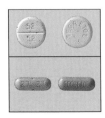

Wyeth-Ayerst

CLASSIFICATION: CNS ANTICONVULSANT
GENERIC NAME: carbamazepine
TRADE NAME: Tegretol; Tegretol XR
INDICATION: all types of seizures
ROUTE OF ADMINISTRATION: oral
COMMON DOSAGE: 200 mg to 1200 mg; 200 mg bid for XR
AUXILIARY LABELS:
- May cause dizziness or drowsiness
- Avoid alcohol
- Take with food

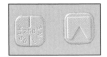

Roche

CLASSIFICATION: BARBITUATE ANTICONVULSANT
GENERIC NAME: primidone
TRADE NAME: Mysoline
INDICATION: all types of seizures
ROUTE OF ADMINISTRATION: oral
COMMON DOSAGE: 250 mg tid or qid
AUXILIARY LABELS:
- May cause dizziness or drowsiness
- Take with food

CLASSIFICATION: CNS ANTICONVULSANT
GENERIC NAME: valproic acid
TRADE NAME: Depakene, Depakote, Depacon
INDICATION: all types of seizures
ROUTE OF ADMINISTRATION: oral, injectable
COMMON DOSAGE: oral dosing 30 to 60 mg/kg/day tid or qid
AUXILIARY LABELS:
- Take with food or milk
- Do not crush or chew
- May cause dizziness or drowsiness

CLASSIFICATION: CNS ANTICONVULSANT
GENERIC NAME: gabapentin
TRADE NAME: Neurontin
INDICATION: all types of seizures
ROUTE OF ADMINISTRATION: oral
COMMON DOSAGE: 900 mg to 1.8 g tid
AUXILIARY LABEL:
- May cause dizziness or drowsiness

CLASSIFICATION: BARBITURATES (CONTROLLED SUBSTANCES)
GENERIC NAME: phenobarbital
TRADE NAME: Luminal
DRUG ACTION: depress the sensory cortex
INDICATION: partial and generalized seizures; also used for sedation and other effects
SIDE EFFECTS: nausea and vomiting; also can cause respiratory depression if overdosed
ROUTE OF ADMINISTRATION: oral, injectable
COMMON DOSAGE: oral dosage varies from 60 mg to 100 mg qd

GENERIC NAME: mephobarbital
TRADE NAME: Mebaral
ROUTE OF ADMINISTRATION: oral
COMMON DOSAGE: 400 mg to 600 mg qd
Drug action, indication, and side effects same as phenobarbital

TECH NOTE! It usually takes days to weeks for these medications to work. For instance, mephobarbital can take several days and phenobarbital can take up to 3 to 5 weeks to become effective. Blood levels should be monitored when taking barbiturates.

CLASSIFICATION: BENZODIAZEPINES (CONTROLLED SUBSTANCES)
　　DRUG ACTION: stop seizures by affecting areas of the brain such as the thalamus, cortex, and limbic areas
　　INDICATIONS: anxiety and insomnia (diazepam and clonazepam are indicated additionally for seizures)

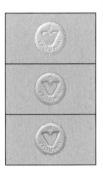

Roche

GENERIC NAME: diazepam
TRADE NAME: Valium
INDICATIONS: seizures,* antianxiety
ROUTE OF ADMINISTRATION: oral, injectable
COMMON DOSAGE: oral dosage 2 mg to 10 mg bid to qid
SIDE EFFECTS: drowsiness
AUXILIARY LABEL:
■ Do not drink alcohol

*Not to be used as sole treatment for seizures. Parenteral dose is for control of acute seizures.

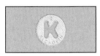

Roerig

GENERIC NAME: clonazepam
TRADE NAME: Klonopin
INDICATIONS: seizures, antianxiety
ROUTE OF ADMINISTRATION: oral
COMMON DOSAGE: ranges from 1.5 mg tid up to a maximum of 20 mg qd to control seizures
Indications and side effects same as diazepam

TECH NOTE! All benzodiazepines are controlled substances. Although these agents can work well, they are all C-IV controlled substances and are not usually used for long-term treatment but instead are used with other anticonvulsants or in emergency situations. The main side effect of these drugs is CNS depression

ALZHEIMER'S DISEASE

Alzheimer's disease affects millions of elderly people, including some famous people such as former President Ronald Reagan and actor Charlton Heston. It is a degenerative brain condition that progresses as one ages but can occur in younger people. Because of the loss of neuronal synapses, the transfer of electrical stimuli that holds the memory banks cannot process information and memory loss occurs. Brain cells are replaced with deposits of protein that can be described as tangles and knots. The brain begins to shrink in size and memory is affected.

Most people lose some memory as they age; however, an abnormal loss of memory and basic mental function is called dementia. Other symptoms include inability to perform normally familiar tasks, difficulty talking, and disorientation in familiar surroundings. Alzheimer's disease affects approximately 7% of people younger than 65 years; incidence rises to 30% for people older than 85. Researches are getting closer to the possible causes of this condition, and it is now known that most people suffering from Alzheimer's disease lack the neurotransmitter ACh, which is needed to transmit impulses properly. There have been many hypotheses for the cause of Alzheimer's disease, including viruses, immunizations, and tainted water. It has been shown to run in families as well. In addition to the use of drugs to help slow the advancing progression of this disease, patients usually need 24-hour care in skilled nursing facilities if their families cannot take on the responsibility.

Drug Treatment

Although the main therapy for Alzheimer's disease tends to be cholinesterase inhibitors, other agents such as nimodipine and physostigmine may help delay the progressive disease.

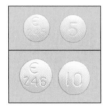

Parke-Davis

CLASSIFICATION: CHOLINESTERASE INHIBITOR
　　GENERIC NAME: donepezil
　　TRADE NAME: Aricept
　　DRUG ACTION: inhibits acetylcholinesterase, which is responsible for destroying ACh; therefore it allows a higher concentration of ACh to activate receptors
　　INDICATION: mild to moderate Alzheimer's disease
　　ROUTE OF ADMINISTRATION: oral
　　COMMON DOSAGE: 5 mg to 10 mg qd
　　SIDE EFFECTS: nausea, vomiting, and diarrhea with initial dosing

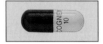

Novartis

CLASSIFICATION: CHOLINESTERASE INHIBITOR
　　GENERIC NAME: tacrine
　　TRADE NAME: Cognex
　　DRUG ACTION: elevates ACh concentrations in the cerebral cortex
　　INDICATION: mild to moderate Alzheimer's disease
　　ROUTE OF ADMINISTRATION: oral
　　COMMON DOSAGE: varies depending on status of disease; initial dose 10 mg qid
　　SIDE EFFECTS: most effects are due to high dosage, nausea, vomiting, and diarrhea

TECH NOTE! Tacrine is associated with liver damage and is dosed four times daily rather than once, as is donepezil. Therefore it is not used as often.

MULTIPLE SCLEROSIS

Multiple sclerosis involves deterioration of the myelin sheath as shown in Figure 17.10.

The insulating myelin sheaths that surround neurons help in the conduction of electrical current as the impulses travel. With multiple sclerosis, the body begins to attack the myelin sheaths, destroying this important material. The sheaths are replaced by plaques of sclerotic (hard) tissue. When this happens, the electrical impulses cannot pass from one neuron to another and the person fails to complete the movement he or she wishes to make. The average age of onset is in the early 30s. Some symptoms include muscle weakness, abnormal sensations such as numbness or tingling over any part of the body, vision change, and loss of coordination. Many people experience a period of remission followed by attacks of loss of function. The cause is considered an autoimmune response to some unknown stimulus.

Drug Treatment

Currently only autoimmune stimulants (interferons) are used to treat multiple sclerosis specifically, although other medications are used to treat the symptoms.

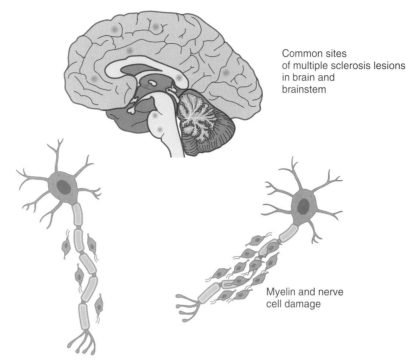

Common sites of multiple sclerosis lesions in brain and brainstem

Myelin and nerve cell damage

FIGURE 17.10 Normal versus nonnormal basal ganglia.

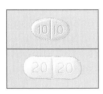

Somerset

CLASSIFICATION: ANTISPASMODIC MEDICATIONS
GENERIC NAME: baclofen
TRADE NAME: Lioresal
DRUG ACTION: inhibits synaptic reflexes at CNS level
INDICATION: spasticity in multiple sclerosis and some spinal cord injuries
ROUTE OF ADMINISTRATION: oral
COMMON DOSAGE: increasing dosage over several weeks from 5 mg tid to 20 mg qid
AUXILIARY LABEL:
■ May cause dizziness or drowsiness

CLASSIFICATION: CENTRAL-ACTING SMOOTH MUSCLE RELAXANTS; ANTISPASMODICS
GENERIC NAME: dantrolene
TRADE NAME: Dantrium
INDICATION NAME: (antispastic) multiple sclerosis, cerebral palsy, and cerebrovascular accident
ROUTE OF ADMINISTRATION: oral
COMMON DOSAGE: 25 mg qd

CLASSIFICATION: INTERFERON
GENERIC NAME: interferon β-1a
TRADE NAME: Avonex
INDICATION: Multiple sclerosis
ROUTE OF ADMINISTRATION: injectable
COMMON DOSAGE: 30 µg intramuscular q week
AUXILIARY:
■ Avoid sunlight

CLASSIFICATION: INTERFERON
GENERIC NAME: interferon β-1b
TRADE NAME: Betaseron
INDICATION: Multiple sclerosis
ROUTE OF ADMINISTRATION: injectable
COMMON DOSAGE: 0.25 mg subcutaneously qod
AUXILIARY LABEL:
■ Avoid sunlight

PARKINSON'S DISEASE

Parkinson's disease is a condition that has affected famous persons such as Michael J. Fox and Mohammed Ali. This condition is another progressive disease that is a disorder of the basal ganglia and is associated with the loss or deficiency of dopamine. The basal ganglia is a group of cells (gray matter) located in the medulla (white matter) of the cerebrum. The function of the basal ganglia is to regulate skeletal muscle tone and overall body movement. Dopamine is a natural chemical produced in the brain that inhibits movement. ACh activates the neurons and dopamine inactivates them. If dopamine is lacking, then there is movement without ending. The overall degeneration of dopamine-producing neurons brings about the symptoms of Parkinson's disease (Figure 17.11).

The severity of symptoms increases over months to years. The most common symptoms include tremors, muscle rigidity, loss of balance, and hypokinesia and bradykinesia. Hypokinesia results in a decrease in the range of motion, and bradykinesia involves an overall slowing of motion and performing simple tasks such as buttoning a shirt or eating. As this disease progresses, the patient's movement slows and eventually stops; the person becomes wheelchair bound. Swallowing may become difficult, and speech may be slurred. Signs of Parkinson's disease develop at approximately 60 years of age. The cause is unknown; although researches have found a genetic defect in some cases, it is still unclear whether the disease is genetic or environmental or a combination of both. Diagnosis is difficult because the disease can progress very slowly; doctors usually order computed tomography scans or magnetic resonance imaging to rule out other possibilities. Often, administration of anti-Parkinson's agents is used to make the correct diagnosis of Parkinson's disease. Treatments include surgery, physical therapy, and drugs. Various drugs increase the dopamine and ACh levels in the brain, which are responsible for fine motor movements, and improve balance. However, these drugs have major side effects. Following is a list of some of the most common drugs.

Drug Treatment

The following drugs are all classified as anti-Parkinson's agents. Most of these agents increase the neurotransmitter dopamine in one way or another.

CLASSIFICATION: ANTI-PARKINSONISM DRUGS; ANTICHOLINERGICS
  GENERIC NAME: amantadine
  TRADE NAME: Symmetrel
  DRUG ACTION: stimulates dopamine receptors, relieving tremors and rigidity
  INDICATION: Parkinson's disease
  ROUTE OF ADMINISTRATION: oral
  COMMON DOSING: 10 mg to 40 mg per day
  SIDE EFFECTS: may cause insomnia if taken late in the day

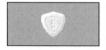

Merck

  GENERIC NAME: selegiline
  TRADE NAME: Eldepryl
  DRUG ACTION: inactivates monoamine oxidase, which is responsible for destroying dopamine; therefore it increases the amount and duration of dopamine
  INDICATION: Parkinson's disease
  ROUTE OF ADMINISTRATION: oral
  COMMON DOSING: 5 mg bid along with other anti-Parkinson agents such as levodopa/carbidopa (Sinemet)
  SIDE EFFECTS: most adverse effects happen only when an overdose is given

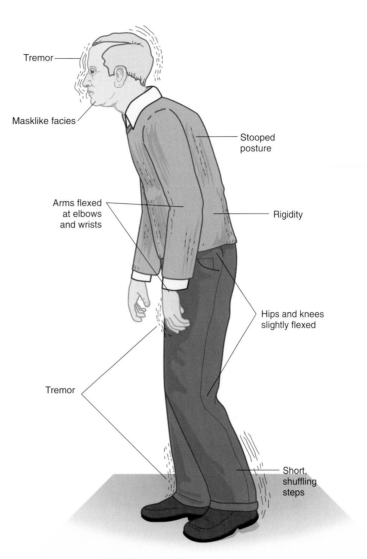

Tremor

Masklike facies

Stooped posture

Arms flexed at elbows and wrists

Rigidity

Hips and knees slightly flexed

Tremor

Short, shuffling steps

FIGURE 17.11 Parkinson's disease.

GENERIC NAME: levodopa/carbidopa

TRADE NAME: Sinemet

DRUG ACTION: levodopa is a precursor of dopamine (which is decreased in Parkinson's disease); in this form it can cross the blood-brain barrier where it is converted into dopamine; carbidopa is only given with levodopa to extend the life and transport of dopamine by inhibiting the transformation into dopamine outside of the blood-brain barrier; because carbidopa cannot cross the BBB, once inside levodopa can easily convert to dopamine

INDICATION: Parkinson's disease

ROUTE OF ADMINISTRATION: oral

COMMON DOSING: doses range from 25 mg/100 mg tid to 25 mg/250 mg tid

SIDE EFFECTS: dystonic movements, anorexia, nausea and vomiting, dry mouth, dizziness, headache, weakness, fatigue

AUXILIARY LABELS:

May cause dizziness or drowsiness.

- Do not crush tablet
- Take with food

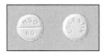
Rhone-Poulene

CLASSIFICATION: ANTICHOLINERGIC
  GENERIC NAME: benztropine
  TRADE NAME: Cogentin
  DRUG ACTION: prolongs the effects of dopamine by inhibiting the reuptake mechanism
  INDICATION: Parkinson's disease, normally used in conjunction with other anti-Parkinson agents
  ROUTE OF ADMINISTRATION: oral, injectable
  COMMON DOSING: oral dosages ranges from 0.5 mg to 6 mg per day
  AUXILIARY LABELS:
  - May cause dizziness or drowsiness
  - Take with food
  - No alcohol

CLASSIFICATION: ANTICHOLINERGIC
  GENERIC NAME: trihexyphenidyl
  TRADE NAME: Artane
  DRUG ACTION: prolongs the effects of dopamine by inhibiting the reuptake mechanism
  INDICATION: Parkinson's disease, normally used in conjunction with other anti-Parkinson agents
  ROUTE OF ADMINISTRATION: oral
  COMMON DOSING: 2 mg to 5 mg bid to tid
  AUXILIARY LABELS:
  - May cause dizziness or drowsiness
  - Take with food
  - No alcohol

AMYOTROPHIC LATERAL SCLEROSIS

Amyotrophic lateral sclerosis (ALS) stands for *without* (a) *spinal cord* (myo) *degeneration* (trophic) *sides* (lateral) and *hardening* (sclerosis). Although this disease was first discovered in the mid 1800s, it is known in the United States as Lou Gehrig's disease, after the famous baseball player who contracted ALS. It is a progressive degeneration of the motor tract in the spinal cord. One theory is that it may be caused by the excitatory neurotransmitter glutamate at the synapse and that this causes cell death.

Although the motor functions of the body decrease, the mind is left unaffected Those who suffer from this fatal disease describe it as being trapped inside a dying body. The cause for this disease is unknown, but it affects more men than women and usually begins between the ages of 50 and 60 years. Only 10% of patients can be expected to live 10 years or more, and approximately 50% of persons die within 18 months of diagnosis. Initially, the symptoms include weakness in the skeletal muscles and, toward the end, difficulty swallowing and talking. The respiratory muscles become affected and dyspnea (shortness of breath) occurs. The patient is eventually wheelchair bound and ultimately dies by choking because he or she can no longer swallow. Treatment is limited to a few agents, such as muscle relaxants, to help the side effects, which include muscle spasm, depression, muscle cramping, and excessive salivation.

Drug Treatment
Only riluzole has been developed specifically for treating ALS, and it only slows the progression of the disease. There is no cure.

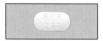
Rorer

CLASSIFICATION: ANTISPASMODICS
  GENERIC NAME: riluzole
  TRADE NAME: Rilutek
  DRUG ACTION: inhibits glutamine release and decreases the influx of sodium
  INDICATION: ALS
  ROUTE OF ADMINISTRATION: oral
  COMMON DOSAGE: 50 mg q12h
  SIDE EFFECTS: nausea, dizziness, diarrhea, and abdominal pain

MISCELLANEOUS MUSCLE AGENTS

Neuromuscular Blockers

Neuromuscular blocking agents are used in conjunction with anesthetics when a patient is having surgery. They are not used outside of the hospital setting. Many hospitals prepare "conscious sedation packs" of various medications, including neuromuscular blocking agents. The reason for this terminology is that although these agents will almost instantly paralyze a patient, they do not sedate or affect any pain levels. The pharmacy technician is responsible for preparing, delivering, and refilling these packs.

Polarizing Agents

Polarizing agents are used as adjunctive agents with anesthetics. The result is a complete loss of muscle skeletal function. Most of the agents are short acting and are useful when intubating a patient. Intubation is necessary when a person is placed on a ventilator; these types of agents keep patients stationary so they do not fight the breathing rhythm of the ventilator.

TABLE 17.5 Agents Used for Various Conditions of the Nervous System

Disease	Generic Name	Trade Name	Effect
Myasthenia gravis	Pyridostigmine	Regonol	Cholinergic
Multiple sclerosis	Baclofen	Lioresal	Steletal muscle relaxant
	Interferon	Avonex β-1a	Immune modulator
	Interferon	Betaseron β-1b	Immune modulator
	Dantrolene	Dantrium	Skeletal muscle relaxant
	Riluzole	Rilutek	Benzathiazol
Parkinson's disease	Amantadine	Symmetrel 1	Dopaminergic
	Benztropine	Cogentin	Anticholinergic
	Bromocriptine	Parlodel	Dopaminergic
	Carbidopa/levodopa	Sinemet	Dopaminergic
	Ropinirole	Requip	Dopaminergic
	Diphenhydramine	Benadryl	Anticholinergic
	Dopamine	Dopamine	Dopaminergic
	Levodopa	Larodopa	Dopaminergic
	Pergolide	Permax	Dopaminergic
	Pramipexole	Mirapex	Dopaminergic
	Trihexyphenidyl	Artane	Anticholinergic
	Selegiline	Eldepryl	Dopaminergic
Alzheimer's disease	Donepezil	Aricept	Cholinesterase inhibitor
	Tacrine	Cognex	Cholinesterase inhibitor
Epilepsy	Carbamazepine	Tegretol	Anticonvulsant
	Fosphenytoin	Cerebyx	Anticonvulsant
	Gabapentin	Neurontin	Anticonvulsant
	Mephobarbital	Mebaral C-IV	Anticonvulsant
	Phenobarbital	Luminal C-IV	Anticonvulsant
	Phenytoin	Dilantin	Anticonvulsant
	Primidone	Mysoline	Anticonvulsant
	Valproate	Di-Valproic	Anticonvulsant

> **GENERIC NAME:** pancuronium
> **TRADE NAME:** Pavulon
> **INDICATION:** muscle rigidity; patient should be under anesthesia before use because pancuronium has no effect on pain levels
> **ROUTE OF ADMINISTRATION:** IV only
> **DOSAGE FORMS:** 1 mg/mL, 2 mg/mL, in volumes of 2 mL, 5 mL, and 10 mL vials and 2 mL and 5 mL amps and syringes

> **GENERIC NAME:** rocuronium
> **TRADE NAME:** Zemuron
> **INDICATION:** muscle contractions during procedures; patient should be under anesthesia before use because rocuronium has no effect on pain levels
> **ROUTE OF ADMINISTRATION:** IV only
> **DOSAGE FORMS:** 10 mg/mL, 5 mL vials

Depolarizing Agents

> **GENERIC NAME:** succinylcholine
> **TRADE NAME:** Anectine
> **INDICATION:** intubation and during surgical procedures (currently the only depolarizing agent)
> **ROUTE OF ADMINISTRATION:** IV only
> **DOSAGE FORMS:** 20 mg/mL vials, 50 mg/mL amps, 100 mg/mL 5 mL and 10 mL vials

Table 17.5 lists some of the conditions affecting the nervous system and the agents used in treating those specific diseases. Other drugs that affect the CNS are listed in Table 17.6. These are discussed under their respective chapters within this textbook.

TABLE 17.6 Miscellaneous Agents That Affect the Central Nervous System

Treatment	Class of Drug	Effect
Analgesics	Controlled substances	Reduce pain
Antiemetics/antivertigo	Anticholinergics	Decrease secretions
Antianxiety	MAOIs	Antidepressant
Sedatives/hypnotics	Benzodiazepines	Antianxiety, antiinsomnia
Anesthetics	Barbiturates	Inhibits pain perception
Diet aids	Stimulants	Reduces hunger

MAOIs, Monoamine oxidase inhibitors.

DO YOU REMEMBER THESE KEY POINTS?

- Both generic and trade names of drugs covered in this chapter
- The divisions of the nervous system (nervous system tree)
- The major divisions of the brain covered in this chapter and their primary functions
- Conditions in which the sympathetic or parasympathetic systems are stimulated
- Medications that directly affect the sympathetic or parasympathetic system
- Composition of a neuron
- The anatomy of the ganglionic neuronal system with respect to the CNS
- The importance of the blood-brain barrier with respect to medications
- The major classifications of medications used on the sympathetic system and their side effects

- The major classifications of medications used on the parasympathetic system and their side effects
- Major conditions that affect the CNS
- Commonly used medications to treat conditions covered in this chapter

REVIEW QUESTIONS:

Multiple Choice

1. Cholinergic agents are stimulants of which system?
   - A. Nervous system
   - B. Sympathetic system
   - C. Parasympathetic system
   - D. None of the above

2. Afferent and efferent fibers have the function of
   - A. Relaying messages to and from the CNS
   - B. Running the CNS
   - C. Stimulation
   - D. Inhibiting NTs

3. Neurons are made of the following components except
   - A. Dendrites
   - B. Cell body
   - C. Nerve terminals
   - D. Amino acids

4. The area where an neurotransmitter crosses over to another neuron is called
   - A. The nerve ending
   - B. The axon
   - C. The cell body
   - D. The synapse

5. All of the following are neurotransmitters except
   - A. Dopamine
   - B. Norepinephrine
   - C. Serotonin
   - D. Succinylcholine

6. Which of the following drugs is not a used as a smooth muscle relaxant?
   - A. Baclofen
   - B. Cyclobenzaprine
   - C. Cerebyx
   - D. Soma

7. Which of the following systems activities is not increased during a sympathetic response?
   - A. Digestive system
   - B. Heart
   - C. Lung
   - D. Liver

8. The part of the brain that controls memory, reason, and language skills is the
   - A. Medulla oblongata
   - B. Cerebellum
   - C. Cerebrum
   - D. Brainstem

9. The area that controls breathing and cardiac functions is the
   - A. Medulla oblongata
   - B. Right hemisphere
   - C. Left hemisphere
   - D. Thoracic spinal cord

10. The hypothalamus functions as the body's
    - A. Thermostat
    - B. Appetite relay center
    - C. Memory
    - D. Both A and B

11. Which of the following medications used for Parkinson's disease can pass the blood-brain barrier?
    - A. Dopamine
    - B. Levodopa
    - C. Carbidopa
    - D. Both A and B

12. Which of the statements describing dopamine is inaccurate?
    - A. Dopamine is a naturally occurring substance within the body.
    - B. Dopamine allows for smooth movements of the muscle system.
    - C. Dopamine can be injected to replace low levels within the basal ganglia.
    - D. Dopamine is a precursor to norepinephrine.

13. Which of the following classes of drugs is used most often for epileptic seizures?
    - A. Barbiturates
    - B. Benzodiazepines
    - C. Hydantoins
    - D. All of the above may be used

14. Which of the types of seizures listed is normally due to not taking medications?
    - A. Tonic-clonic
    - B. Absence seizures
    - C. Atonic type seizures
    - D. All of the above

15. The most common reason neuromuscular blocking agents are used is to
    - A. Keep the patient asleep during an operation
    - B. Keep the patient from fighting a respirator (ventilator)
    - C. Stop all pain and movement while being intubated
    - D. Both B and C

16. _____ is converted into norepinephrine within the _____ system.
    A. ACh, sympathetic
    B. Epinephrine, sympathetic
    C. ACh, parasympathetic
    D. Dopamine, CNS

17. Which of the following statements is not true concerning the sympathetic system?
    A. When activated, glucose is released from the liver.
    B. All parasympathetic system functions stop.
    C. It is responsible for the fight or flight reaction.
    D. Drugs that activate this system are called cholinergics.

18. Of the components listed, which one is not housed in the brainstem?
    A. Hypothalamus and thalamus
    B. Pons
    C. Midbrain
    D. Medulla oblongata

19. The name of the enzyme that is responsible for destroying norepinephrine is
    A. Anticholinergic
    B. Antiadrenergic
    C. ACh
    D. Acetylcholinesterase

20. _____ affect the sympathetic system, whereas _____ affect the parasympathetic system.
    A. Cholinergics, anticholinergics
    B. Cholinergics, adrenergics
    C. Adrenergics, antiadrenergics
    D. Adrenergics, cholinergics

True/False

*If a statement is false, then change it to make it true.

1. Gray matter makes up the brain and white matter makes up the spinal cord.
2. Homeostasis is when the body is in a sympathetic response mode.
3. The PNS can be divided into two divisions.
4. The thalamus and hypothalamus link the nervous system to the endocrine system.
5. The blood-brain barrier serves to prevent large molecules (such as toxins) from passing into the CNS.
6. Carbidopa is an ingredient added to Sinemet to extend the life of the drug.
7. ALS is a degenerative disease of the motor cells of the CNS that affects the myelin sheaths surrounding the neuronal axon.
8. Tonic seizures involve stiffening of the muscles, whereas clonic is rapid jerking.
9. Neuromuscular blocking agents block both pain perception and muscle movement.
10. Drugs that mimic the cholinergic neurotransmitters of the sympathetic system are also called sympathomimetics.

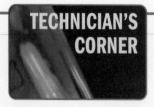

TECHNICIAN'S CORNER

Mr. Perkins was just diagnosed with Parkinson's disease. He comes into the pharmacy with a new prescription for levodopa. What auxiliary labels are necessary? (Use *Mosby's Drug Consult* for reference.)

BIBLIOGRAPHY

Facts and comparisons. St Louis, 1999, Wolters Kluwer.

Gutierrez K, McCuistion LE: *Real-world nursing survival guide: pharmacology.* Philadelphia, 2002, WB Saunders.

Mosby's Drug Consult, St Louis, 2004, Elsevier.

Potter PA, Perry AG: *Fundamentals of nursing,* ed 5. St Louis, 2001, Mosby.

Thibodeau GA, Patton KT: *Structure and function of the body,* ed 11. St Louis, 2000, Mosby.

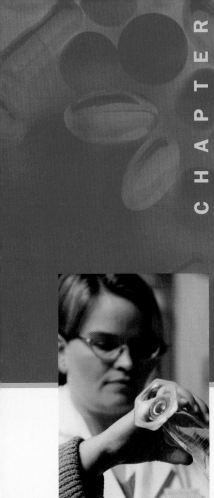

18 Respiratory System

Objectives

- Define all terms used in this chapter as they pertain to the respiratory system.

- List the functions of the respiratory system.

- Describe the act of respiration in transferring oxygen for carbon dioxide.

- Identify the components of the respiratory system outlined in this chapter.

- Differentiate between emphysema, asthma, and bronchitis.

- List the most common conditions that affect the lungs and the types of medications used to treat them.

- List the drugs' generic and trade names.

- List the classification and indication for each of the drugs described in this chapter.

- Choose the appropriate auxiliary labels when filling prescriptions for respiratory conditions.

- List the most common side effects for medications discussed in this chapter.

Antitussives *Medication that prevents or relieves coughing*

Asthma *A condition in which narrowing of the airways impedes breathing*

Chronic obstructive pulmonary disease (COPD) *a disease process where the lungs have decreased capacity for gas exchange; also known as emphysema and chronic bronchitis*

Cough reflex *Response of the body to clear air passages of foreign substances and mucus by a forceful expiration*

Cystic fibrosis *An inherited disorder that causes production of very thick mucus in the respiratory tract and affects the pancreas and sweat glands; patient experiences difficulty breathing and has frequent respiratory infections*

Decongestant *Drugs that reduce swelling of the mucous membranes by constricting dilated blood vessels, reduces blood flow to nasal tissues, thus reducing nasal congestion*

Expectorant *Chemical that cause the removal of mucous secretions from the respiratory system; loosens and thins sputum and bronchial secretions*

Influenza *A respiratory tract infection caused by an influenza virus*

Metered dose inhaler (MDI) *a method of supplying medication to the lungs through inhalation*

Nonproductive cough *Cough that does not produce mucous secretions (dry cough)*

Productive cough *Cough that expectorates mucous secretions from respiratory tract*

Prophylaxis *Preventative treatment*

Sputum *Fluid coughed up from the lungs and bronchial tissues*

Viscosity *The thickness of a solution or fluid (e.g., corn syrup is very viscous)*

RESPIRATORY MEDICATIONS

Trade Name	Generic Name	Pronunciation	Trade Name	Generic Name	Pronunciation
Antitussives			Adrenalin	epinephrine	epi-**nef**-rin
Benylin	dextromethorphan/	dex-troh-meh-**thor**-fan	Isuprel	isoproterenol	eye-so-pro-**tear**-in-all
Tessalon perles	guaifenesin	gwi-**fen**-ah-sin	Alupent	metaproterenol	meta-pro-**tear**-in-all
	benzonatate	**ben**-zoe-na-tate	Serevent	salmeterol	sal-**met**-er-ol
Expectorant			**Xanthines**		
Robitussin	guaifenesin	gwi-**fen**-ah-sin	Aminophylline	aminophylline	am-in-**off**-eh-lin
			Theo-Dur	theophylline	thee-**off**-ah-lin
Antihistamines					
Benadryl	diphenhydramine	dye-**fen**-hi-dra-meen	**Leukotriene Receptor Antagonists**		
Chlor-Trimeton	chlorpheniramine	klor-**fen**-air-ra-meen	Singulair	montelukast	mon-**tea**-lu-cast
Claritin	loratadine	lor-at-ah-**dean**	Accolate	zafirlukast	zay-**fur**-lu-cast
Mucolytic					
Mucomyst	acetylcysteine	a-sea-**till**-sis-teen	**Corticosteroids**		
			Beclovent	beclomethasone	**beck**-low-meth-the-sewn
Decogestants			Azmacort	triamcinolone	try-am-**sin**-oh-lone
Sudafed	pseudoephedrine	sue-doe-e-**fed**-dren	AeroBid	flunisolide	**flew**-nis-oh-lide
Neo-Synephrine	phenylephrine	**fen**-ill-ehf-rin			
Afrin	oxymetazoline	ox-e-met-**taz**-o-leen	**Anticholinergics**		
			Atrovent	ipratropium bromide	ih-prah-**trow**-pea-um
Bronchiolar Dilators			Intal, NasalCrom	cromolyn	**krom**-oh-lin
Proventil, Ventolin	albuterol	al-**bu**-ter-all			

Introduction

The respiratory system plays an important role in the body's overall system, working to keep us alive and well. It is one function that we become acutely aware of when it is not working properly. As seen in Figure 18.1, the respiratory system is composed of many organs, each having specific functions. For example, the lungs enable the body to extract oxygen from the atmosphere when inhaling and remove carbon dioxide (CO_2) from the body when exhaling. The respiratory system also works to remove unwanted particles from the air before they enter the body system through fine hairs of the nose and the mucosal lining of the bronchi. In addition, the nose helps to heat and humidify cold, dry air so that it is more compatible with our body temperature. This chapter discusses respiration, form and function, and the conditions that affect the respiratory system, including medications to treat them. The drug action, normal dosages, and any auxiliary labels that need to be affixed to prescriptions are also listed in this chapter.

TECH NOTE! The average respiration rate for adults is 12 to 18 breaths per minute, whereas a child's rate is 40 breaths per minute.

Structure of the Respiratory System

Imagine a large tree with many branches, hollow it out, and invert it, and you have an idea of what the respiratory system looks like. The large trunk is analo-

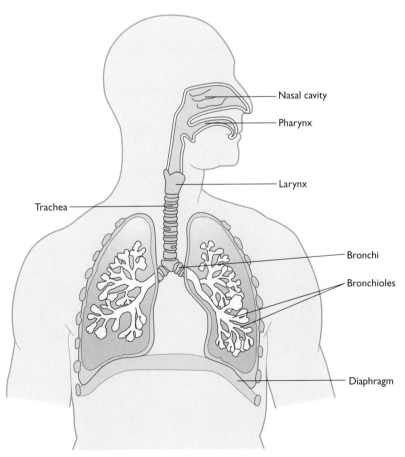

FIGURE 18.1 Diagram of respiratory system.

gous to the trachea, and the two main branches represent the bronchi. The smaller branches are the bronchioles, and the leaves are the alveolar sacs where gas exchange takes place (Figure 18.2). Let's begin to take a more in-depth look at the respiratory tract, starting with the upper respiratory system.

THE UPPER RESPIRATORY SYSTEM

The upper respiratory system is composed of the nose, pharynx, larynx, and nasal cavities. A mucosal lining covers the inside of the respiratory tract. More than 125 mL (approximately $1/2$ cupful) of mucus is produced each day by the body, which forms a protective mucous blanket over much of the respiratory tree. The mucus also serves as an air purification mechanism by trapping inhaled irritants such as dust and pollens. The nasal septum separates the interior of the nose into two distinct cavities. The cavities are also lined by a mucous membrane with small microscopic hairlike structures called cilia. The function of the mucous membrane is to warm and moisten inhaled air. The cilia catch small dust particles in the air that we breathe. Other functions of the nose include the sense of smell and a drain system for tears from the eye. The pharynx is a tube approximately 5 inches long that is shared with the digestive system. Food goes into the esophagus and air goes to the trachea, also known as the windpipe. The tonsils, composed of lymphatic tissue, are located in the pharynx.

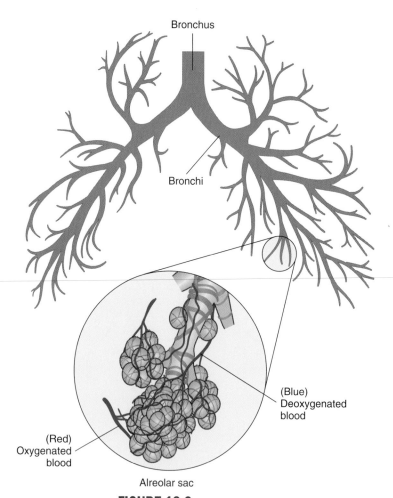

FIGURE 18.2 Bronchial tree.

THE LOWER RESPIRATORY SYSTEM

The lower respiratory system is composed of the trachea, bronchial tree, and lungs. The trachea is lined with a mucous membrane that traps airborne particles, and cilia (fine microscopic hairlike structures) that move the particles upward where they are swallowed. The trachea branches off into the right and left bronchi. In turn, each bronchus branches off into smaller and smaller bronchi and into smaller and smaller bronchioles. The function of the bronchioles is to provide oxygen distribution and a passageway for air to reach the alveoli. The bronchioles end in millions of clusters of microscopic alveolar sacs deep in the lungs.

The pleural cavity is composed of moist, smooth, slippery membranes that line the chest cavity and cover the outer surface of the lungs. This lining is called the pleura and serves to reduce friction between the lungs and the chest wall during breathing. The larynx is also known as the voice box, because it is responsible for the sounds that we produce. The epiglottis, a thin leaf-shaped structure, is located at the entrance of the larynx. Its function is to close off the trachea automatically when swallowing takes place to keep food, liquid, and saliva from going down the airway. If food enters the trachea rather than the esophagus, choking occurs.

The epiglottis is formed by one piece of cartilage. Both men and women have a larynx, although it is much smaller in women and does not protrude from the neck as it does in men. This cartilage (usually only visible in men) is referred to as the "Adam's apple." The vocal cords are in the larynx. They provide air distribution and voice production.

The trachea (windpipe) is approximately 4.5 inches long and also has a mucosal lining. At the lower end it branches off into two tubes called bronchi that lead to the right and left lungs, respectively. The right bronchus is bigger than the left because the heart displaces some of the left side of the chest. The trachea has incomplete rings of cartilage reinforcing it so that it will not collapse when the neck is bent.

At the base of the chest cavity is a muscle called the diaphragm. This large muscle layer separates the chest cavity from the abdominal area. In the chest cavity, within the alveoli sacs that are surrounded by tiny capillaries, oxygen is picked up and CO_2 is released and exhaled. The lungs fill the chest cavity, except for the space occupied by the heart and large vessels. The lungs are divided into lobes: three in the right lung and two in the left. The right lung has a greater volume capacity, whereas the left lung is longer and has less capacity. The lungs' consistency is like that of a sponge because of the millions of alveolar sacs and connective tissue surrounding them. The lungs are separated from each other by the mediastinum, which is where the heart is located. The left lung has a notch, called the cardiac notch, where the left side of the heart is located. The main function of the lungs is breathing, also known as pulmonary ventilation.

Respiration

The act of respiration can be broken down into two distinct phases: inspiration, the movement of air into the lungs, followed by expiration, the movement of air out of the lungs. The thorax is another name for the chest cavity. The changes in the size and shape of the thorax during respiration cause a change in air pressure. This change in pressure, resulting from expansion and contraction of the chest wall caused by the raising and lowering of the diaphragm (breathing), causes air to move into and out of the lungs. As a person actively inhales (inspiration), air moves into the lungs causing the muscles of the diaphragm and intercostal areas to change. Specifically, the diaphragm flattens while the intercostals expand and increase the size of the thoracic cavity. This increase in the size of the chest cavity reduces pressure inside so that air can enter the lungs. Expiration is a passive response because, unlike inspiration, it does not use any energy to perform. As the chest relaxes during expiration, the thorax returns to its resting size and shape. The reduction in the size of the thoracic cavity causes the pressure within the thorax to increase, and air leaves the lungs (Figure 18.2).

Exchange of Gases

The air we breathe is composed of approximately 21% oxygen, 79% nitrogen, and less than 0.5% CO_2. As we breathe, the lungs exchange inspired oxygen for CO_2 (waste) carried by the blood to the lungs. This waste is then expelled from our lungs. An average adult inhales approximately 250 mL of oxygen and produces approximately 200 mL of CO_2 per minute at rest, using a type of diffusion (transfer) to accomplish this function.

After air travels through the bronchioles, it enters more narrow corridors (the alveolar sacs). In the alveolus, each oxygen molecule is able to move across the thin membrane into the waiting blood cells that are passing closely by on the other side of the membrane. The moving blood cells drop off the CO_2 before picking up the oxygen molecule. The CO_2 molecule then moves out of the lung capillary blood supply into the alveolar sacs and out of the body via expired air. The fully saturated blood moves into larger veins where it returns to the left atrium of the heart via four pulmonary veins. From the left atrium it moves into the left ventricle where it is pumped back out through the body via the arteries, replenishing oxygen to all tissues and organs.

The regulation of respiration permits the body to adjust to varying demands for oxygen supply and CO_2 removal. This is done efficiently with the help from the respiratory center within the medulla. The medulla is situated in the brainstem and is influenced by various inputs or receptors located in other body areas. The exchange of oxygen and CO_2 also helps keep our blood pH balanced. The body uses some of the CO_2 to make bicarbonate, which maintains the blood pH either by reducing the amount of hydrogen in the blood, causing the pH to become more alkaline, or by increasing the hydrogen, making the blood more acidic. The blood pH must remain close to 7.4 to sustain life (Figure 18.3).

TECH NOTE! Our body takes in 79% nitrogen but does not use it. Nitrogen is sent back into the air along with the CO_2 and leftover oxygen molecules.

Breathing

Breathing is an involuntary mechanism. This means you do not have to think about it; the body automatically exhales and inhales when needed. This response is partly due to the respiratory control center located in the medulla in the brain. As the lungs fill with air, nerve impulses originating in the stretch receptors of the lungs are transferred to the respiratory center, which begins a series of neuronal impulses to the respiratory muscles to relax them, resulting in expiration. Impulses are then sent via the respiratory center in the brain that cause the muscles to contract, causing inspiration.

Depending on the size of the person, breathing rates will vary—the smaller the size, the faster the breathing. The breathing rates of small children can be

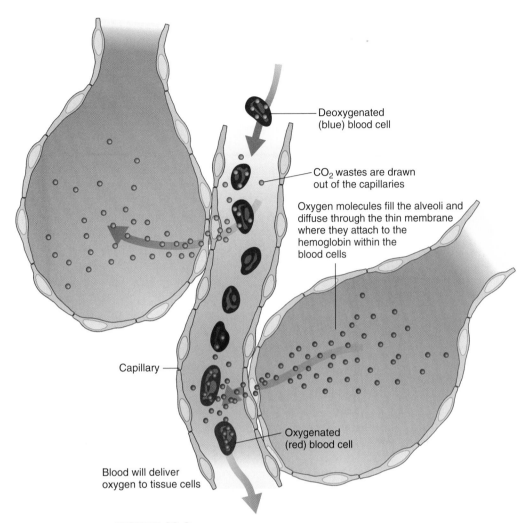

FIGURE 18.3 Inhalation/exhalation for exchange of O$_2$ and CO$_2$.

twice as fast as those of adults. The normal amount of air expelled from the lungs in a typical exhale is approximately 500 mL or 0.5 L for an average adult, although the total lung capacity is more than 5 L of air. When a person is running, the body needs more oxygen than when sitting or sleeping. The elasticity of the lungs allows for the capacity to vary widely depending on the need for oxygen. Table 18.1 lists common breathing problems.

SNEEZING

A common reflex action that occurs is sneezing. The result of breathing irritating materials, such as dust or dander, into the respiratory passageway causes the body to expel the foreign substance. There are three mechanisms that cause someone to sneeze: (1) ciliary action, (2) peristaltic motion of the bronchioles, and (3) cough reflex. When a foreign particle comes into contact with the sensory receptors of the ciliary hairs, they trigger the reflex of deep inspiration, which is then followed by closure of the vocal cords. The vocal cords remain closed until the actual sneeze is underway, at which point the outward push of air expels the foreign material from the passageways, usually accompanied by a loud noise. Other examples of air movement include coughing, yawning, hiccoughing, sighing, crying, and laughing.

TABLE 18.1 Types of Breathing Dysfunctions

Condition	Symptoms
Apnea	Respiration stops as in heart failure
Cyanosis	Lack of oxygen causes skin to turn blue-gray
Dyspnea	Labored or difficult breathing
Hyperventilation	Deep and rapid breathing
Hyponea	Shallow, inadequate breathing
Orthopnea	Labored or difficult breathing while lying down
Tachypnea	Rapid breathing
Bradypnea	Slow breathing

Disorders of the Upper Respiratory System

There are many conditions of the respiratory system. Some may be genetic, and others may be contracted because of other factors, such as contagious infections, habits such as smoking, and other environmental factors. One common condition that affects the respiratory system periodically is respiratory colds. Colds are caused by viruses. Because there are more than 140 cold viruses, the common cold has remained an untreatable illness; although recently there have been breakthroughs in the research for finding a cure. Symptoms include coughing, congestion, and sometimes wheezing within the upper respiratory system. Common treatments include decongestants and antihistamines. Other symptoms that accompany colds are rhinitis (inflammation of the lining of the nose), pharyngitis (sore throat), or rhinorrhea (a runny nose).

Hoarseness is another problem that affects the vocal cords and may be due to several conditions that cause a loss of voice. Laryngitis is the temporary loss of speech resulting from an inflammation, irritation, or infection of the larynx. A more severe type of cold, also caused by viruses, is commonly known as the flu or influenza. This is a viral illness that strikes millions of people each year; each strain of virus is usually named after the region where it was first detected. Influenza is responsible for millions of dollars of lost wages and health care costs annually. Influenza can be deadly, especially to those who are older or those with weakened immune systems. Influenza vaccines are normally given each winter season to those at high risk of infection, especially older adults and health care workers.

Another infection common to the upper respiratory tract is rhinitis. Colds, influenza, or allergies produce this nasal inflammatory condition. Allergies are one of the most common types of respiratory problems and are experienced by millions of people. Most allergy remedies can be obtained without a prescription. The most common remedies include oral and nasal decongestants and antihistamines.

Common Cold and Sore Throat Remedies

CLASSIFICATION: MINERAL
ENERIC NAME: zinc combinations
TRADE NAME: Halls Zinc Defense
ROUTE OF ADMINISTRATION: Oral
INDICATION: To decrease the duration of the common cold and sore throat
DRUG ACTION: Unknown
COMMON DOSAGE: 5-mg lozenges as needed
SIDE EFFECTS: Vomiting

CLASSIFICATION: LOCAL ANESTHETICS FOR THROAT
GENERIC NAME: benzocaine/menthol
TRADE NAME: Vicks Chloraseptic Sore Throat
ROUTE OF ADMINISTRATION: Oral
INDICATION: For the relief of sore throats
DRUG ACTION: Deadens nerve endings
COMMON DOSAGE: As needed
SIDE EFFECTS: Vomiting

GENERIC NAME: benzocaine, cetylpyridium chloride
TRADE NAME: Cepacol
ROUTE OF ADMINISTRATION: Oral
INDICATION: For the relief of sore throats
DRUG ACTION: Deadens nerve endings
COMMON DOSAGE: As needed
SIDE EFFECTS: Vomiting

GENERIC NAME: phenol
TRADE NAME: Vicks Chloraseptic mouth rinse
ROUTE OF ADMINISTRATION: Oral
INDICATION: For the relief of sore throat
DRUG ACTION: Deadens nerve endings
COMMON DOSAGE: As needed
SIDE EFFECTS: Vomiting

Disorders of the Lower Respiratory Tract

Pneumonia is an infection that causes acute inflammation in lung airways that become blocked with thick mucus. The cause for this infection can be bacterial, viral, fungal, chemical, or, in rare cases, parasitic. Older adults are at high risk, especially after an injury that requires them to remain in bed. Viral pneumonia is not preventable because there are no vaccines available that can be used as a prophylactic. There is a vaccine available, Pneumovax, that gives immunity for 14 common bacterial pneumonia infections. This injection is given only once in a lifetime. Persons with a weakened immune system are at a higher risk than most, but pneumonia can strike anyone.

ACUTE AND CHRONIC CONDITIONS

Acute bronchitis is an inflammation of the bronchi and the trachea caused by infection. In some individuals it can become chronic. When this happens, the repeated inflammation of the bronchioles causes them to become narrow. Smokers commonly contract chronic bronchitis. Chronic bronchitis can progress to emphysema. Either disorder is considered a chronic obstructive pulmonary disease (COPD).

There are three types of COPD: chronic bronchitis, emphysema, and bronchiectasis. Emphysema is a condition that causes the destruction of the alveolar walls that eventually leads to a loss of elasticity of the lungs and heart failure. This can be caused by smoking, environmental hazards such as asbestos and fiberglass, or, in rare cases, by a genetic predisposition. Because normal exhalation requires elastic recoil of the lungs, the affected lungs allow air to get in but cannot expel all the air. The condition worsens as the surface area of the lungs becomes further reduced because of destruction of the alveolar walls. Bronchiectasis is less common than chronic bronchitis or emphysema and is not discussed.

Asthma

Millions of people suffer from asthma. It is a major childhood respiratory problem. Asthma is an obstructive airway disease that can be caused by genetic defects or a chronic allergic reaction to irritating substances in the environment. It is classified as an inflammatory disease. The muscles around the bronchioles contract, narrowing the air passages so air cannot be inhaled properly. In addition to this increase of resistance to airflow, the condition is worsened by edema and secretion of mucus of the airway. This causes the crackling sound heard during an asthma attack. In severe cases, the end result is equivalent to suffocation as the brain is deprived of oxygen. Although there are many medications that can prevent or reverse asthma attacks, there are deaths reported from asthma. Usually these deaths occur because many asthmatic persons do not have their medication available when an attack occurs or they delay going to an emergency room for treatment. Treatments for bronchitis, emphysema, and asthma include bronchodilators, corticosteroids, xanthenes, and leukotriene receptor antagonists.

Tuberculosis

Worldwide, tuberculosis (TB) is the most common bacterial disease affecting the pulmonary system. This highly contagious lung infection is characterized by an infection within the lining of the lungs by a bacterium that needs oxygen to survive. The lungs provide an environment that is extremely oxygenated where the causative bacteria, *Mycobacterium tuberculosis,* may reside for an extended time with few or no symptoms. When the immune system becomes weakened, the bacteria multiply and symptoms appear. TB has been on the rise for several years because of the emergence of drug-resistant strains. This occurs partly because many persons with TB do not complete their course of treatment once they feel better, allowing the bacterium to not only return but also mutate, making it resistant to traditional drugs. Persons at high risk are those in a confined living space, such as a prison.

Emergency Disorders of the Lungs

The following conditions affect the lungs and its lining, usually requiring hospitalization: pneumothorax, pulmonary embolism, and hemothorax. Pneumothorax can be caused by COPD, TB, and chest wounds. It is characterized by a collapse of the alveoli resulting from air escaping into the pleural space. A pulmonary embolism results when an embolus (small blood clot that breaks away from origin) blocks a branch of the pulmonary artery that goes from the heart to the lungs. Pneumothorax is the collapse of a lung resulting from blood leaking into the pleural space. All of these examples are very serious conditions that need to be treated immediately, or death may result. Cancer of the respiratory tract can occur in any part of the respiratory system. Persistent hoarseness is one of the first signs of laryngeal cancer. Persons who smoke pipes, cigars, cigarettes, or those who have inhaled chemicals that contain hazardous particles are at higher risk than most. Treatments may include surgery, chemotherapy, radiation, or a combination of these. Other conditions that can affect the respiratory system are listed in Table 18.2.

Cardiopulmonary Resuscitation. If cardiopulmonary resuscitation (CPR) is started immediately when someone stops breathing, there is a good chance of reviving him or her. People collapsing from cardiac arrest or respiratory arrest, or children who have accidentally fallen into water and are not breathing are some of the types of victims that have been saved from death through the use of CPR. Most hospitals train pharmacy staff to learn CPR, free of charge. It is in the best

TABLE 18.2 Conditions of the Respiratory System

Condition	Definition
Pleurisy	Inflammation of the lining of the lungs and lung cavities
Croup	A childhood condition that causes obstruction of the larynx, a barking cough, and noisy breathing
Whooping cough	Also known as pertussis, this bacterial infection is contagious. It affects the larynx and trachea, and produces coughing spasms.
Pulmonary edema	Caused by fluid filling the respiratory air sacs (alveoli) and bronchioles

interest of all pharmacy technicians to take a CPR class because they are in contact with the sick and with older adults on a daily basis.

Treatment of Respiratory Disorders

The following drugs are listed in order of their indication with a brief description that includes their drug action, normal adult dosage, common side effects, and auxiliary labels most commonly used.

TREATMENT OF COLDS AND ALLERGIES

Cough Suppressants: Antitussives

Antitussives are agents that suppress coughing. Types of medications include controlled substances such as codeine and hydrocodone. Usually each is prescribed as a liquid combination with other agents to treat coughing. For instance, codeine with acetaminophen or codeine with promethazine are found in fixed combinations for coughs. Common over-the-counter (OTC) agents include guaifenesin and dextromethorphan. Common side effects may include nausea, vomiting, drowsiness, and constipation. All normal dosing regimens are based on the average adult dose.

CLASSIFICATION: NARCOTIC ANTITUSSIVES (C-II may be classified as C-IV if the C-II drug concentration is reduced)

    GENERIC NAME: codeine*

    TRADE NAME: codeine (codeine technically has no trade name)

    DRUG ACTION: decreases the cough reflex by binding to opiate receptor sites located in the central nervous system (CNS)

    ROUTE OF ADMINISTRATION: oral

    INDICATION: nonproductive cough (dry cough) and mild to moderate pain

    SIDE EFFECTS: drowsiness, constipation, nausea and vomiting

    COMMON DOSAGE: 10 mg to 20 mg every 4 to 6 hours

    AUXILIARY LABELS:

- Do not drink alcohol.
- Alcohol intensifies the effects.
- Take with food.
- Take with plenty of water.

*Codeine is usually given for coughing in a combination form with dextromethorphan or promethazine.

CLASSIFICATION: OPIOID ANALGESIC, C-III
    GENERIC NAME: hydrocodone/phenylpropanolamine, hydrocodone/chlorpheniramine
    TRADE NAME: Hycomine, Tussionex
    DRUG ACTION: decreases the cough reflex by binding to opiate receptors sites located in the CNS
    INDICATION: pain and coughing
    ROUTE OF ADMINISTRATION: oral
    SIDE EFFECTS: drowsiness, constipation, nausea and vomiting
    COMMON DOSAGE: 5 mg to 10 mg every 4 to 6 hours
    AUXILIARY LABELS:
- Do not drink alcohol.
- Alcohol will intensify the effects.
- Take with food.
- Take with plenty of water.

CLASSIFICATION: NONNARCOTIC ANTITUSSIVE
    GENERIC NAME: dextromethorphan/guaifenesin
    TRADE NAME: Benylin
    DRUG ACTION: acts on the medulla (cough center) of the brain, decreasing the urge to cough
    INDICATION: nonproductive coughs
    ROUTE OF ADMINISTRATION: oral
    COMMON DOSAGE: 10 mg to 30 mg every 4 to 8 hours
    AUXILIARY LABEL:
- Drink plenty of water.

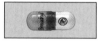

Parke-Davis

CLASSIFICATION: ANTIHISTAMINE
    GENERIC NAME: diphenhydramine
    TRADE NAME: Benadryl
    DRUG ACTION: inhibits CNS, as well as binding to histamine receptor sites for the control of allergies
    INDICATION: coughs caused by colds or allergies
    ROUTE OF ADMINISTRATION: oral, topical, injectable
    COMMON DOSAGE: 12.5 mg to 25 mg every 4 hours (not to exceed 150 mg every 24 hr)
    SIDE EFFECT: drowsiness
    AUXILIARY LABEL:
- May cause dizziness or drowsiness.

Expectorants. Expectorants are agents that break up thick mucous secretions of the lungs or bronchi so that they can be expelled from the system through coughing. The main example of an expectorant is guaifenesin. Following administration of expectorants, the patient should be told to increase fluid intake to assist with thinning of mucus secretions.

CLASSIFICATION: EXPECTORANT
    GENERIC NAME: guaifenesin
    TRADE NAME: Robitussin
    DRUG ACTION: increases respiratory tract fluid, allowing for the removal of excess mucus; dry coughs become productive and there is an overall decrease in the amount of coughing
    INDICATION: dry, nonproductive coughs
    ROUTE OF ADMINISTRATION: oral
    COMMON DOSAGE: 200 mg to 400 mg every 4 hours
    SIDE EFFECTS: dizziness, headache, nausea and vomiting
    AUXILIARY LABELS:
- May cause drowsiness.
- Drink plenty of water.

Mucolytics. Mucolytics are agents that break up mucus in patients suffering from COPD and cystic fibrosis; this type of medication is limited to acetylcysteine.

CLASSIFICATION: MUCOLYTIC
GENERIC NAME: acetylcysteine
TRADE NAME: Mucomyst
DRUG ACTION: breaks the bonds between proteins responsible for mucus buildup; this decreases the viscosity of the mucus, allowing it to be expelled
INDICATION: COPD and cystic fibrosis; also overdoses of acetaminophen
ROUTE OF ADMINISTRATION: inhalation
COMMON DOSAGE: inhalant: 10% (3 to 5 mL) to 20% (6 to 10 mL) tid to qid
SIDE EFFECTS: nausea, vomiting, runny nose
AUXILIARY LABELS: none (most treatments are given in the hospital, although family members can be taught how to give treatments at home)

Decongestants. Decongestants also help to clear respiratory passages but work more on the swollen nasal passages that usually accompany common colds or allergies. Most cold remedies are available OTC and consist of oral liquids, tablets or capsules, or nasal inhalants. Examples of these agents include pseudoephedrine, phenylephrine, and oxymetazoline. Persons suffering from hypertension (high blood pressure) should not take decongestants because they raise blood pressure. This is the type of information about which a physician or pharmacist will notify the patient.

CLASSIFICATION: SYMPATHOMIMETIC, NASAL DECONGESTANT
GENERIC NAME: pseudoephedrine
TRADE NAME: Sudafed
DRUG ACTION: affects the adrenergic receptors of the vascular smooth muscle, causing vasoconstriction and a decrease in mucus
INDICATION: nasal congestion
ROUTE OF ADMINISTRATION: oral, nasal
COMMON DOSAGE: 60 mg every 4 to 6 hours
SIDE EFFECTS: insomnia, restlessness
AUXILIARY LABELS: none

GENERIC NAME: phenylephrine
TRADE NAME: Neo-synephrine
DRUG ACTION: affects the adrenergic receptors of the vascular smooth muscle, causing vasoconstriction of nasal arterioles
INDICATION: nasal secretions
ROUTE OF ADMINISTRATION: oral, nasal, injection, ophthalmic
COMMON DOSAGE: 1 to 2 sprays every 4 hours as needed
SIDE EFFECTS: nasal congestion, if used longer than a few days (rebound congestion)
AUXILIARY LABEL:
■ For nasal use.

GENERIC NAME: oxymetazoline
TRADE NAME: Afrin
DRUG ACTION: affects the adrenergic receptors of the vascular smooth muscle, causing vasoconstriction of nasal arterioles
INDICATION: nasal congestion; allergic rhinitis
ROUTE OF ADMINISTRATION: nasal spray
COMMON DOSAGE: 2 or 3 sprays every 10 to 12 hours
SIDE EFFECTS: nasal congestion, if used longer than a few days (rebound congestion)
AUXILIARY LABEL:
■ For nasal use.

TREATMENT OF CHRONIC OBSTRUCTIVE PULMONARY DISEASE

COPD includes conditions such as emphysema and chronic bronchitis that can progress to the point at which there is irreversible damage to the lung. The dosage forms used to treat COPD include liquids, syrups, inhalants, and, in some instances, parenterals. Examples of the types of agents used are bronchodilators, corticosteroids, xanthines, and sympathomimetics. In the following drug monographs, when several classifications have the same indications and side effects, these are outlined before the monographs.

Drug Action

For the following bronchodilator medications, the drug action is sympathomimetic. These agents produce bronchodilation by relaxing the smooth muscle of the bronchioles. Common side effects for this class of drugs are headache, nervousness, and shakiness.

CLASSIFICATION: SYMPATHOMIMETIC, BRONCHODILATOR
GENERIC NAME: salmeterol
TRADE NAME: Serevent
INDICATION: asthma
ROUTE OF ADMINISTRATION: inhalant disc
COMMON DOSAGE: 2 puffs bid (not meant for acute attacks)

GENERIC NAME: metaproterenol
TRADE NAME: Alupent
INDICATIONS: asthma, bronchitis, emphysema
ROUTE OF ADMINISTRATION: inhalant, oral
COMMON DOSAGE: Liquid: 10 mg every 6 to 8 hours; MDI: 2 to 3 puffs every 3 to 4 hours
SIDE EFFECTS: tremors, shakiness, nausea and vomiting
AUXILIARY LABEL:
■ Shake well.

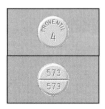

Schering

CLASSIFICATION: SYMPATHOMIMETIC
GENERIC NAME: albuterol
TRADE NAME: Proventil, Ventolin
INDICATION: COPD
ROUTE OF ADMINISTRATION: inhalant, oral, liquid for nebulizer
COMMON DOSAGE: syrup: 2 mg to 4 mg tid to qid; MDI: 2 puffs every 4 to 6 hours; tablets: 4 mg tid to qid
AUXILIARY LABEL:
■ (MDI: inhalants) Shake well.
■ Can cause dizziness.

GENERIC NAME: epinephrine
TRADE NAME: Adrenalin
INDICATIONS: asthma, bronchitis, emphysema
ROUTE OF ADMINISTRATION: inhalant, injectable
COMMON DOSAGE: MDI: 2 puffs waiting between 1 to 10 minutes between doses
AUXILIARY LABELS:
■ (Inhalants) Shake well.
■ Rinse mouth with water after inhalation.

Xanthine Bronchodilator Agents

Xanthine bronchodilator agents relax the smooth muscle of the bronchi and pulmonary blood vessels. Drugs under this heading include theophylline and aminophylline and dosage forms include tablets, capsules, liquids, syrup, and injectable forms. Indications for these agents include asthma and emphysema. Side effects include shakiness, restlessness, and trembling.

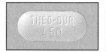

Schering

CLASSIFICATION: XANTHINE BRONCHODILATOR

    GENERIC NAME: theophylline, aminophylline

    TRADE NAME: Theo-Dur, Slo-Bid, Uni-Dur

    ROUTE OF ADMINISTRATION: oral, inhalant, injectable, rectal

    COMMON DOSAGE: oral forms: 16 mg/kg or approximately 400 mg every 6 to 12 hours; dose varies depending on whether it is sustained release; injectable: dose varies based on weight and age of patient*

    AUXILIARY LABEL:

    ■ Drink plenty of water.

    *Note that theophylline IV 400 mg/500 mL is equivalent to 500 mg/500 mL

Leukotriene Receptor Antagonist Agents

Leukotriene receptor antagonist agents' drug action is to inhibit the mechanisms that produce symptoms including edema and smooth muscle constriction that lead to asthma attacks. These agents are used for both prophylaxis and chronic treatment of asthma. Side effects include headache.

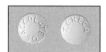

Astra Zenaca

CLASSIFICATION: LEUKOTRINE RECEPTOR ANTAGONISTS

    GENERIC NAME: zafirlukast

    TRADE NAME: Accolate

    ROUTE OF ADMINISTRATION: oral

    COMMON DOSAGE: 20 mg 2 times daily

    AUXILIARY LABEL: none

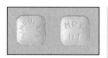

Merck

    GENERIC NAME: montelukast

    TRADE NAME: Singulair

    ROUTE OF ADMINISTRATION: oral

    COMMON DOSAGE: 10 mg once daily in the evening (qd in PM); 2 mg, 4 mg, 5 mg chewable tablet for pediatric use

    SIDE EFFECTS: Headache

    AUXILIARY LABEL:

    ■ Do not take aspirin.

Corticosteroid Agents

Corticosteroids are steroids. Their drug action includes acting as an antiinflammatory, thus lessening the constriction of the bronchial tubes. They produce smooth muscle relaxation. These medications are indicated for chronic asthma and as a prophylactic agent.

CLASSIFICATION: CORTICOSTEROID AGENTS

    GENERIC NAME: beclomethasone

    TRADE NAME: oral—Beclovent, Vanceril; nasal—Beconase AQ, Vancenase AQ

    ROUTE OF ADMINISTRATION: oral, nasal

    COMMON DOSAGE: oral inhalant: 2 puffs tid to qid; nasal inhalant: 1 spray into each nostril tid to qid

    AUXILIARY LABELS:

    ■ Shake well.

    ■ Take as directed.

GENERIC NAME: triamcinolone acetonide*
TRADE NAME: Azmacort
ROUTE OF ADMINISTRATION: inhalation
COMMON DOSAGE: 2 puffs tid to pid
AUXILIARY LABELS:

■ Shake well.
■ Take as directed.

*Other triamcinolone agents differ by their additive ingredient: triamcinolone diacetate, triamcinolone hexacetonide, and plain triamcinolone.

GENERIC NAME: flunisolide
TRADE NAME: AeroBid, Nasalide
ROUTE OF ADMINISTRATION: inhalation, oral and nasal
COMMON DOSAGE: oral inhalant (Aero Bid): 2 puffs bid; nasal inhalant (Nasalide): 2 sprays into each nostril, bid
AUXILIARY LABELS:

■ Shake well.
■ Take as directed.

GENERIC NAME: fluticasone
TRADE NAME: Flovent, Flonase, Cutivate
ROUTE OF ADMINISTRATION: Nasal and oral inhalant, topical
COMMON DOSAGE: oral inhalation (Flovent): 2 to 4 puffs bid; nasal inhalation (Flonase): 2 sprays per nostril qd
SIDE EFFECTS: Headache
AUXILIARY LABELS:

■ Shake well.
■ Take as directed.

Anticholinergic Agents

Anticholinergics inhibit the action of acetylcholine thus relaxing smooth muscle of the bronchioles. They are indicated for bronchospasms resulting from COPD. Side effects include dryness of airway membranes.

CLASSIFICATION: ANTICHOLINERGIC AGENTS
GENERIC NAME: ipratropium bromide
TRADE NAME: Atrovent*
ROUTE OF ADMINISTRATION: inhalant, oral and nasal
COMMON DOSAGE: oral inhalent: 2 puffs qid; nasal inhalation: 2 sprays into each nostril bid to tid
AUXILIARY LABEL:

■ Shake well.

*Also available in combination with albuterol (Combivent)

CLASSIFICATION: ANTIASTHMATIC, MAST CELL STABILIZER
GENERIC NAME: cromolyn
TRADE NAME: Intal, NasalCrom, Crolom
ROUTE OF ADMINISTRATION: inhalant, oral, nasal, and ophthalmic
COMMON DOSAGE: oral solution (Intal): 20 mg qid; nasal inhalent (Nasal Crom): one spray into each nostril tid to qid
AUXILIARY LABELS: none (available as an OTC medication)

TREATMENT FOR TUBERCULOSIS

Most of the primary antituberculin agents are bactericidal. This means that they kill the bacterium that causes TB. They are used in combination for a course of treatment lasting many months. Although the medication used to treat TB is very effective, many patients do not continue to take the medication once they are feeling better because they are unaware that the TB will return. Also, one of the many side effects is nausea, which can complicate the lengthy treatment. For this reason, patients must be educated by their physician about the importance of finishing their medication regimen to fully eradicate the bacteria from their system. The commonly used multiple medication treatment plans include isoniazid and rifampin given together as a daily dose. Another regimen includes isoniazid, streptomycin, and ethambutol. Another commonly used agent is pyrazinamide. Examples of the types of combination therapy are given in Table 18.3. These therapies can be given as a short or long course depending on the diagnosis. In the monographs that follow, specific side effects for each agent are listed along with the auxiliary labels and other drug information pertaining to that specific agent. To determine whether TB is entirely gone, sputum tests are required before treatment can stop.

CLASSIFICATION: ANTITUBERCULOSIS AGENTS

GENERIC NAME: isoniazid

TRADE NAME: Laniazid, Nydrazid

ROUTE OF ADMINISTRATION: oral, injectable

SIDE EFFECTS: Gastrointestinal upset

COMMON DOSAGE: 300 mg qd 1 to 2 hours before or after meals (oral Laniazid)

AUXILIARY LABELS:

- Take on an empty stomach.
- Take as directed.
- Do not drink alcohol.
- Special instructions: Avoid alcohol because of risk of hepatitis. Avoid certain foods such as fish or those containing tyramine such as aged foods. Must not discontinue unless instructed to do so by physician.

TABLE 18.3 Tuberculosis Regimens

Regimen 1		
Drug 1	Isoniazid	300 mg
Drug 2	Rifampin	600 mg
Regimen 2		
Drug 1	Isoniazid	500 mg
Drug 2	Ethambutol	800–1600 mg
Drug 3	Streptomycin	750 mg to 1 g
Regimen 3		
Drug 1	Isoniazid	500 mg
Drug 2	Rifampin	600 mg
Drug 3	Pyrazinamide	1–2 g

GENERIC NAME: rifampin
TRADE NAME: Rifadin
ROUTE OF ADMINISTRATION: oral
SIDE EFFECTS: orange to reddish urine and other secretions
COMMON DOSAGE: 600 mg qd 1 to 2 hours before or after meals
AUXILIARY LABELS:

- Take on an empty stomach.
- Take as directed.
- Special instructions: Must not discontinue unless instructed to do so by physician. Treatment normally lasts 6 to 9 months or 6 months if sputum culture is negative.

GENERIC NAME: ethambutol
TRADE NAME: Myambutol
ROUTE OF ADMINISTRATION: oral
COMMON DOSAGE: 100 mg to 300 mg qd
SIDE EFFECTS: gastrointestinal upset, nausea, vomiting, fever, or decrease in visual acuity
AUXILIARY LABELS:

- Take with food.

GENERIC NAME: pyrazinamide
TRADE NAME: pyrazinamide (no trade name)
ROUTE OF ADMINISTRATION: oral
SIDE EFFECTS: nausea, vomiting, anorexia, myalgia, gout
NORMAL DOSAGE: 500 mg qd for 2 months
AUXILIARY LABEL:

- Take as directed.

DO YOU REMEMBER THESE KEY POINTS?

- The main functions of the respiratory system
- The major organs of the respiratory system
- Common upper respiratory conditions
- Common lower respiratory conditions
- Medications used to treat respiratory conditions
- Main side effects of the drugs discussed in this chapter
- Major auxiliary labels that should be affixed to the container
- Differences between emphysema, bronchitis, and asthma
- Special instructions given for patients that are taking antituberculin agents
- Types of contributing factors that can influence respiratory conditions

REVIEW QUESTIONS:

Multiple Choice

1. Which of the following statements is not true?
   A. Respiration is an involuntary response.
   B. Expiration is an active response.
   C. The diaphragm flattens while the intercostal muscles contract, increasing the thoracic cavity and allowing for inspiration.
   D. There are two phases that describe respiration: expiration and inspiration.

2. The act of gas exchange within the lungs takes place specifically in the
   A. Brainstem
   B. Brain
   C. Medulla
   D. Alveoli

3. The main function(s) of the cilia within the upper respiratory tract is
   A. To smell
   B. To catch foreign material
   C. To warm and moisten air molecules
   D. Both A and C

4. The normal exhalation of air in an adult is

A. 0.25 L

B. 0.5 L

C. 1 L

D. More than 5 L

5. Which of the following symptoms are not common in a typical cold?

A. Laryngitis

B. Congestion

C. Wheezing

D. Coughing

6. Pneumonia can be described as

A. Viral or bacterial in origin

B. An upper respiratory tract infection

C. Contagious

D. Both A and C

7. A patient diagnosed with asthma might receive which of the following drugs as a prophylaxis

A. Narcotic antitussive

B. Bronchodilator

C. Xanthines

D. Leukotriene receptor antagonist

8. Persons who smoke are more likely to suffer from

A. Bronchitis and emphysema

B. Emphysema and asthma

C. Bronchitis and asthma

D. All of the above

9. Tuberculosis is on the rise mostly because of

A. Noncompliance with drug regimen

B. Lack of money to buy medication

C. Living in close quarters

D. Both A and C

10. The function of gas exchange includes all of the following except

A. Balancing the pH of the body

B. Oxygenation of the bloodstream

C. Discarding unused carbon dioxide

D. Exchanging nitrogen for carbon dioxide

True/False

*If the statement is false, then change it to make it true.

1. The highest percentage of gas in the air that we breathe is oxygen.

2. The larynx is also known as the voice box.

3. Colds can be caused by viruses, bacteria, or both.

4. Influenza only strikes older adults.

5. Allergies are due to genetics traits.

6. The main function of the epiglottis is to protect the vocal cords.

7. People who smoke are not any more at risk of getting COPD than nonsmokers.

8. The overall effect of bronchodilators is vasodilation.

9. Tuberculosis is caused by a bacterium and is not contagious.

10. Asthma is caused by rupture of the alveolar sacs.

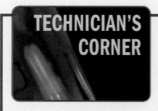

TECHNICIAN'S CORNER

A 37 lb 4-year-old was admitted into the hospital, and the doctor wants the pharmacy to calculate enough doses of metaproterenol to medicate the child for a 3-day hospital stay based on the recommended dose. If the recommended dose is 1.3 to 2.6 mg/kg/day and you have metaproterenol sulfate syrup 10 mg/5 mL in stock, how many milliliters will you need to fill the dose for one day? How much for the whole course of treatment?

BIBLIOGRAPHY

Facts and comparisons. Wolters Kluwer, 1999, St Louis.

Grollman S: *The human body: it's structure and physiology,* New York, 1965, Collier-Macmillan Limited.

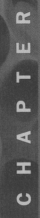

19 Visual and Auditory Systems

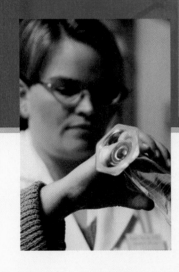

Objectives

- List the agents used on the eyes and ears, including their trade and generic names.

- Describe the functions of the eyes and ears.

- List the major components of the eyes and ears.

- Explain the drug action of the medications listed.

- Describe what causes glaucoma.

- Describe the different types of conjunctivitis and their treatments.

- List the various infections that affect the eyes and ears.

- Explain how medications work to relieve glaucoma.

Accommodation *The change that occurs in the ocular lens when it focuses at various distances*

Aqueous humor *The fluid that is found in the anterior and posterior chambers of the eye*

Cataract *Loss of transparency of the lens of the eye*

Cones *Photoreceptors responsible for color (daylight vision)*

Cornea *The transparent tissue covering the anterior portion of the eye*

Cycloplegia *Paralysis of the ciliary muscle in the eye*

Miosis *Contraction of the pupil*

Mydriasis *Dilation of the pupil*

Myopia *Nearsightedness*

Ophthalmic *Pertaining to the eye*

Rods *Photoreceptors responsible for black and white color (night vision) that respond to dim light*

Acoustic nerve *The cranial nerve that controls the senses of hearing and equilibrium which eventually leads to the cerebellum and medulla*

Auditory canal *A 1-inch segment of tube that runs from the external ear to the middle ear*

Auditory ossicles *The set of three small bony structures in the ear: malleus, incus, and stapes*

Eustachian tube *A tubular structure within the middle ear that runs to the nasopharynx (throat)*

Labyrinth *A bony maze composed of the vestibule, cochlea, and semicircular canals of the inner ear*

Otic *Pertaining to the ear*

Tympanic membrane *A membranous skin that separates the external ear from the middle ear*

DRUGS USED FOR THE EYE

Trade Name	Generic Name	Pronunciation	Trade Name	Generic Name	Pronunciation
Beta-Adrenergic Blocking Agents			**Prostaglandin Agonist**		
Betoptic	betaxolol	be-**tax**-oh-lol	Xalantan	latanoprost	la-**tan**-o-prost
Timoptic	timolol	**tye**-moe-lol			
Optipranolol	metipranolol	me-ti-**pran**-oh-lol	**Sympathomimetics**		
Ocupress	carteolol	**car**-tee-oh-lol	Glaucon, Epifrin	epinephrine	ep-i-**nef**-rin
Betagan	levobunolol	lee-voe-**byoo**-noe-lol			
			Anticholinergics		
Carbonic Anhydrase Inhibitors			Isopto Atropine	atropine	**a**-troe-peen
Neptazane	methazolamide	meth-a-**zoe**-la-mide	Cyclogyl	cyclopentolate	sye-kloe-**pen**-toe-late
Miostat	carbachol	**kar**-ba-kol	Isopto Homatropine	homatropine	hoe-**ma**-troe-peen
Trusopt	dorzolamide HCL	dor-**zoe**-la-mide	Mydriacyl	tropicamide	troe-**pik**-a-mide
Azopt	brinzolamide	brin-**zoh**-la-mide	Isopto Hyoscine	scopolamine	skoe-**poll**-a-meen
			Adrenergic Agonists		
Cholinergics (miotics)					
Pilocar, Ocusert	pilocarpine	pye-low-**kar**-peen	Vasocon, Allerest	naphazoline	naf-**az**-oh-leen

DRUGS USED FOR THE EYE—cont'd

Trade Name	Generic Name	Pronunciation	Trade Name	Generic Name	Pronunciation
Ocuclear	oxymetazoline	oxy-met-**tah**-zoe-leen	**Aminoglycosides**		
Visine	tetrahydrozoline	tet-ra-hye-**droz**-oh-leen	Genoptic	gentamicin	jen-tah-**my**-sin
Propine	dipivefrin	dye-**pihv**-eh-frin	Tobrex	tobramycin	toe-bra-**my**-sin
Corticosteroids			**Antivirals**		
Betnesol	betamethasone	beh-tah-**meth**-ah-zone	Herplex	idoxuridine	eye-docks-**yur**-eh-dean
Maxidex	dexamethasone	dex-a-**meth**-ah-zone	Viroptic	trifluridine	try-**floor**-eh-dean
FML	fluorometholone	floor-**oh**-meth-oh-lone	Vira-A	vidarabine	vi-**dar**-ah-bean

DRUGS USED FOR THE EAR

Trade Name	Generic Name	Pronunciation	Trade Name	Generic Name	Pronunciation
Domeboro	acetic acid	a-**see**-tic acid	Cerumenex	triethanolamine,	tri-eth-ah-**noll**-am-in
Americaine	benzocaine	**ben**-zoe-kane		polypeptide,	poly-**pep**-tide
Chloromycetin Otic	chloramphenicol	klor-am-**fen**-eye-chole		oleate-condensate	**oh**-lee-ate
Tridelsilon	desonide, acetic acid	**deh**-so-nide	Cortisporin Otic	hydrocortisone	hi-drow-**core**-tah-zone
				neomycin,	knee-oh-**my**-sin
				polymyxin	poll-ee-**mix**-in

Introduction

We rely on our senses from the moment we are born until we die. Although there are six main senses of the body system—sight, hearing, touch, smell, taste and equilibrium—the two senses that can change a life the most dramatically are seeing and hearing. Every day from the moment we wake until the time we fall asleep our senses are taking in new information, and our memory relies on the past memories of sights and sounds. The ability to see enables us to navigate, whereas the ability to hear can prevent walking into an area where we might be harmed. The conditions that can affect the eyes and ears may not seem as important as other conditions; however, the ramifications of neglecting these conditions can be earth-shattering. In this chapter, we cover the major components of the eyes and ears, as well as major conditions that can affect these two senses and their common treatments.

The Eyes

As one of the five main sensors of the body, the eyes link the outside world and the mind. As images are perceived, they are translated into impulses that create lasting memories in the mind. There are three different levels or categories of persons that work in the field of eye care—opticians, optometrists, and ophthalmologists. Opticians are skilled in making lenses that compensate vision loss. Optometrists are trained to perform eye examinations. Ophthalmologists are medical doctors who treat major conditions affecting the eye, including performing surgery.

ANATOMY OF THE EYE

The eye has several structures working in unison to help protect it, maintain its shape, and enhance vision. Box 19.1 lists the major structures of the eye that are

BOX 19.1 MAJOR STRUCTURES OF THE EYE

Structures	Eyebrows, eyelashes, orbit
Eyelid	Major structures such as the skin, muscle, connective tissue, and conjunctiva
Outer eye	Cornea, sclera
Middle eye	Ciliary body or muscle, iris, aqueous humor, pupil
Inner eye	Retina, optic disc
Chemicals	Rods, cones, rhodopsin
Glands	Lacrimal
Secretions	Vitreous humor, vitreous body
Nerves	Optic nerve
Muscles	Superior and inferior oblique; superior, inferior, medial, and lateral rectus

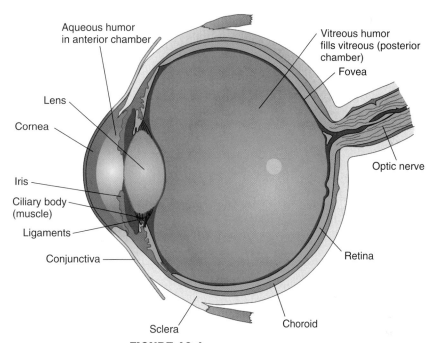

FIGURE 19.1 Anatomy of the eye.

defined in this chapter. The eyebrows shade the eyes from light. There are more than 2000 eyelashes that work to catch debris, help keep the eyes moist, and help shade the eyes. The eye sits in a bony socket called the orbit. The position of the eyes allows for peripheral vision up to approximately 100 degrees. Covering the eyes are the eyelids, which are composed of four individual layers—the outer skin, the muscles, connective tissue, and the conjunctiva. The muscles and the fibers of connective tissues are under the skin within the lid. They allow the eyelid to open and close. The natural reaction of blinking serves to protect the eye from foreign objects and allows lacrimal fluid to cleanse the eye. The conjunctiva is a thin transparent layer that is composed of a mucous membrane that covers the anterior eye, the eyelids, and the sclera. The lacrimal gland is located within the orbit, secretes tears into the eye, and has ducts that lead into the nasal cavity. Tears contain an enzyme called lysozyme that has antimicrobial properties. An overview of the anatomy of the eye is shown in Figure 19.1.

TECH NOTE! When we cry, the lacrimal glands are directly activated by the parasympathetic nervous system.

The cornea is a bulged transparent cover that allows light into the eye for visual acuity. It is composed of connective tissue and covered in a thin coating of epithelium. The cornea does not contain blood vessels to provide nourishment; instead it is nourished by being bathed in a solution called the aqueous humor and from oxygen from the air. The aqueous humor is the tissue found within the anterior eye. There are many nerve fibers within the cornea that are sensitive to pain. The sclera is attached to the cornea but wraps around to the back of the eyeball. Unlike the cornea, however, it is not transparent. It is the protective white portion of the eye and it also contains many fibers and muscles. The optic nerves extend from the back of the eye through the sclera. They send images from the eye to the brain for interpretation.

The layer just inside the sclera is the choroid coat, followed by the innermost layer the fovea. The fovea is the area where the sharpest vision occurs. From the front of the eye the sclera joins with the iris and the ciliary body. The iris is responsible for the color of the eye. Its function is to filter light. The largest space of the eye is an area called the posterior cavity, which is surrounded by the lens, ciliary body, and retina. The ciliary body forms a ring around the front of the eye. It is responsible for holding the lens in place. When certain fibers in the eye contract, the choroid coat is pulled forward, shortening the ciliary body. This in turn thickens the lens, allowing for up-close focusing. The area between the lens and the retina is filled with a jelly-like substance called the vitreous humor. A function of the vitreous body is to hold the shape and form of the eye. The retina is a thin layer that contains layers of neurons, nerves, pigmented epithelium, and membranous tissues. Receptor cells (known as photoreceptors) of the retina are responsible for vision and the neurons provide a path to the brain.

Six major muscles of the eye extend from the skeletal bone. These muscles are responsible for the movement of the eye. The direction of movements is shown in Figure 19.2. Other important muscles include those that close and open the eye and dilate and constrict pupils.

When focusing on a distant figure or in the dark, the pupil of the eye dilates (mydriasis), allowing more light in. When the eye is in extreme light, the pupil constricts (miosis). Through complicated connections, visual information is trans-

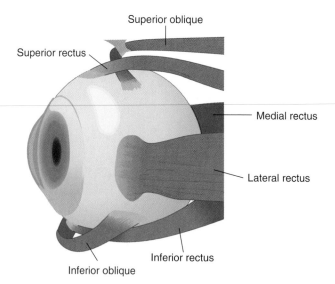

FIGURE 19.2 Eye muscles and direction of movement. Superior rectus rotates upward and inward; inferior rectus rotates downward and inward; medial rectus rotates inward; lateral rectus rotates outward; superior oblique rotates downward and outward; inferior oblique rotates upward and outward.

ferred to the nerve endings located at the back of the eye, which then send information to the brain, causing the necessary change in the lens to accommodate the incoming image. Aqueous humor is the watery fluid that plays an important function within the eye by keeping the eye moist so it maintains its shape. The aqueous humor provides the nutrients and oxygen to maintain the lens and cornea. As aqueous humor is formed it must be released to maintain the pressure within the anterior chamber. It does this by the use of built-in ducts called the canals of Schlemm. After the aqueous humor moves across the lens through the pupil and into the anterior chamber, it drains out of the eye through small openings located near the sclera and cornea. The retina contains the nerve endings that transmit electrical impulses to the brain. The retina also contains the components, rods and cones, that are responsible for color vision and for distinguishing the shapes of objects as well as darkness and light.

VISION

Each area of the eye has a specific function. As an image passes through the lens it reaches the back of the eye, the retina. It is here that the rods and cones are located. Rods are responsible for sight in dim light. They can only produce an image in black and white, whereas in bright light, cones detect color. As the rods and cones synapse (connect) with nerve endings, the signals are sent through the optic nerve to the brain. The occipital lobe is responsible for visual interpretation.

CONDITIONS THAT AFFECT THE EYE

There are a variety of conditions that can affect the eye. Depending on the cause, treatment can range from medication to surgery. Over the past decade there have been many new developments made in corrective lens treatment. Laser surgery is becoming an alternative to wearing glasses. For certain persons who are blind, there is a new surgical technique that implants new lenses allowing some individuals to see. As new techniques become available, many more eye conditions will be able to be treated and even cured. In this section, we cover commonly used medications for examinations and current treatments for the following common conditions of the eye:

- Glaucoma
- Conjunctivitis
- Congestion of the eye
- Viral infections
- Bacterial infections

Glaucoma

Glaucoma is a condition of the eye in which the pressure within the eye is higher than normal. This is referred to as increased intraocular pressure. There are two main causes for this condition: Either aqueous humor is overproduced, or the ducts that drain excess aqueous humor are blocked. Although glaucoma is easily treated, if left untreated it can cause blindness. There are three types or levels of glaucoma as listed in Box 19.2. Depending on the degree of severity, there are a wide range of medications and treatments that are available.

Conjunctivitis

This condition is very common in daycare centers and is contagious. Also known as "pink eye," it is an acute inflammation of the conjunctiva. The cause can be viral, bacterial, fungal infections, or allergies. Major symptoms include inflammation, itching, burning, and a production of white mucus in the eye.

BOX 19.2 TYPES OF GLAUCOMA*

Primary (Includes Angle-Closure or Open-Angle Conditions)
Acute congestive: Termed angle-closure, this refers to the closure of the anterior chamber possibly resulting from genetic defects.
Chronic simple: Termed open-angle, refers to the increase in IOP rather than a closed duct. About 90% of persons suffering from glaucoma have this type of condition.
Treatment: Corrected by medication or surgery (laser).

Secondary
This condition may result from an existing eye condition or may happen following cataract extraction.
Treatment: Corrected or controlled by medication.

Congenital
Exists because of genetic predisposition.
Treatment: Corrected by surgery.

IOP, Intraocular pressure.
See Table 19.1 for agents used to treat glaucoma.

Color Blindness

As previously discussed, the cones are responsible for color perception. The cones produce three photopigments, each responsible for the identification of a different color—green, blue, and red. If a pigment is missing or abnormal, then detection of individual colors becomes difficult or impossible. There is no treatment for this condition.

Blindness

Depending on the cause of blindness, there are new treatments available to possibly reverse the effects. For many persons, a corneal transplant may correct blindness. Another type of treatment for certain damaged corneal linings is stem cell transplant. This may reverse blindness through regeneration of a new membrane lining.

OPHTHALMIC AGENTS

Most ophthalmic medications are aimed at controlling glaucoma, controlling infection or inflammation, or manipulating dilation. For an overview of some of the more common agents used in treating the eyes for glaucoma refer to Table 19.1.

Dosage forms used in treating the eyes include drops, suspensions, ointments, and, in some cases, medicated disks or corrective lenses. Dosage forms and their method of action are discussed in the following section under each type of medication used in treatment.

Antiglaucoma Agents

There are five classifications of drugs that can be used topically to treat glaucoma—beta-adrenergic blockers, carbonic anhydrase inhibitors (CAIs), miotics, sympathomimetics, and prostaglandin agonists. It is important that the right diagnosis is made in order to prescribe the right medication because these are very specific in their actions. In many cases more than one medication is used.

Beta-Adrenergic Blockers. The beta-adrenergic blockers are referred to as beta-blockers. These medications lower the intraocular pressure in open-angle glaucoma. These medications are used topically as drops. Side effects of these ophthalmic drops are decreased vision after application and alteration of night or distance vision.

TABLE 19.1 Commonly Used Agents for the Treatment of Glaucoma

Classification of Drug	Generic	Trade	Indication	Side Effects
Beta-adrenergic blocking agents	Betaxolol	Betoptic	Open-angle glaucoma	Burning, stinging, eye irritation
	Carteolol	Ocupress	Open-angle glaucoma	
	Levobunolol	Betagan	Open-angle glaucoma	
	Metipranolol	OptiPranolol	Open-angle glaucoma	
	Timolol	Timoptic	Open-angle glaucoma	
Carbonic anhydrase inhibitors	Dorzolamide methazolamide	Trusopt, Kaptazane	Lower IOP open-angle angel-closure	
	Brinzolamide dorzolamide	Azopt	Lower IOP open-angle angel-closure	
Miotics, cholinergic	Carbachol intraocular	Miostat	open-angle angel-closure	Blurred vision, irritation, myopia, headache
Cholinergic	Pilocarpine	Isopto Carpine	Glaucoma	
Adrenergic agonist	Dipivefrin	Propine	Elevated IOP	Burning, stinging, eye irritation
Sympathomimetics Adrenergic agonists	Epinephrine	Glaucon, Epifrin	Open-angle glaucoma	
	Dipivefrin HCL	Propine	Open-angle glaucoma	
Anticholinergics	Atropine	Isopto Atropine	Glaucoma	Stinging, increased IOP
	Cyclopentolate	Cyclogyl	Glaucoma	
	Homatropine	Isopto Homatropine	Glaucoma	
	Scopolamine	Isopto, Hyoscine	Glaucoma	
Midriacyl	Tropicamide	Tropicamide	Glaucoma	
Prostaglandin agonist	Latanoprost	Xalatan	Elevated IOP	

IOP, Intraocular pressure.

Drug Action. These agents affect a specific site within the adrenergic system also known as the sympathetic system. The site they lock onto is the beta-receptor. Because there are two different beta sites available and it is not specified, it can be assumed that this medication will affect both beta sites. When beta sites are activated (agonistic effect), the response in many of the areas of the body is altered (see Chapter 17) including the constriction of the vessels in the eyes. This worsens glaucoma by increasing the intraocular pressure; therefore if the beta response can be blocked, then the vessels relax and the eyes can drain properly, decreasing the intraocular pressure.

CLASSIFICATION: BETA-ADRENERGIC BLOCKING AGENTS
 GENERIC NAME: betaxolol
 TRADE NAME: Betoptic, Betoptic S*
 ROUTE OF ADMINISTRATION: Opthalmic
 COMMON DOSAGE: 1 drop into eye(s) twice daily (1 gtt bid)
 AUXILIARY LABELS:
■ For the eye

*If suspension is used, apply: "Shake well before using"

GENERIC NAME: caretolol
TRADE NAME: Occupress
ROUTE OF ADMINISTRATION: Opthalmic
COMMON DOSAGE: 1 drop into eye(s) twice daily (1 gtt bid)
AUXILIARY LABEL:
- For the eye

GENERIC NAME: levobunolol
TRADE NAME: Betagan
ROUTE OF ADMINISTRATION: Opthalmic
COMMON DOSAGE: 1 drop into affected eye once or twice daily (1 gtt qd or bid)
AUXILIARY LABEL:
- For the eye

GENERIC NAME: metripranolol
TRADE NAME: OptiPranolol
ROUTE OF ADMINISTRATION: Opthalmic
COMMON DOSAGE: 1 drop into the affected eye once or twice daily (1 gtt qd or bid)
AUXILIARY LABEL:
- For the eye

GENERIC NAME: timolol
TRADE NAME: Timoptic, Timoptic XE*
ROUTE OF ADMINISTRATION: Opthalmic
COMMON DOSAGE: 1 drop into the affected eye once or twice daily (1 gtt qd or bid)
AUXILIARY LABEL: For the eye
***SPECIAL NOTE:** Patient must be instructed to shake Timoptic XE once only before application. This is done by a pharmacist at the time of consultation.

Carbonic Anhydrase Inhibitors. Carbonic anhydrase inhibitors are medications used for open-angle glaucoma or preoperatively for procedures to treat angle-closure glaucoma. These medications are sometimes given along with other miotic and osmotic ophthalmic agents. Side effects include eye irritation, such as blurring, and a stinging sensation.

Drug Action. These agents inhibit a specific enzyme, carbonic anhydrase, from increasing formation of the aqueous humor in the eye. By directly applying these medications to the eye, the intraocular pressure is reduced in persons suffering from chronic simple open-angle glaucoma. In persons suffering from secondary (angle-closure) glaucoma it can only be used for a short duration to lower the intraocular pressure in order to perform surgery.

CLASSIFICATION: CARBONIC ANHYDRASE INHIBITORS
GENERIC NAME: dorzolamide
TRADE NAME: Trusopt
ROUTE OF ADMINISTRATION: Opthalmic
COMMON DOSAGE: 1 drop into the affected eye three times daily (1 gtt tid)
AUXILIARY LABEL:
- For the eye

GENERIC NAME: brinzolamide
TRADE NAME: Azopt
ROUTE OF ADMINISTRATION: Opthalmic
COMMON DOSAGE: 1 drop into the affected eye three times daily (1 gtt tid)
AUXILIARY LABELS:
- For the eye
- Shake well before using

GENERIC NAME: methazolamide
TRADE NAME: Neptuzane
ROUTE OF ADMINISTRATION: Oral
COMMON DOSAGE: 50-100 mg bid or tid
AUXILIARY LABEL:
- May cause drowziness

Miotics. Miotics are similar to carbonic anhydrase inhibitors with regard to the types of glaucoma that they treat. Carbonic anhydrase inhibitors are used as a long-term treatment for open-angle glaucoma, whereas miotics are used only preoperatively for persons with angle-closure glaucoma. The side effects of these types of medications include headaches and decreased night vision.

Drug Action. These medications reduce the intraocular pressure by increasing the outflow of aqueous humor from the eye. Within the classification of miotics, there are direct-acting agents and indirect-acting agents. Direct-acting agents lower the intraocular pressure by contracting the ciliary muscle around the eye increasing the outflow of aqueous humor. Certain ophthalmics are injectable and are used in eye surgery. Indirect agents inhibit an enzyme (cholinesterase) that brings about muscle contraction, reducing the resistance of the aqueous humor outflow. The result is the same in either case.

Direct-Acting Agents

CLASSIFICATION: MIOTICS
GENERIC NAME: acetylcholine HCL
TRADE NAME: Miochol-E
ROUTE OF ADMINISTRATION: Opthalmic
COMMON DOSAGE: 15 to 20 mg injection before or after suture is in place
SPECIAL NOTE: Used for eye surgery

GENERIC NAME: carbachol
TRADE NAME: Miostat
ROUTE OF ADMINISTRATION: Opthalmic
COMMON DOSAGE: 1 to 2 drops into affected eye up to three times daily (1 to 2 gtts max tid)
AUXILIARY LABEL:
- For the eye

GENERIC NAME: pilocarpine
TRADE NAME: Pilocar, Isopto Carpine
ROUTE OF ADMINISTRATION: Opthalmic
COMMON DOSAGE: 1 or 2 drops into affected eye three to four times daily (1 to 2 gtts tid to qid)
AUXILIARY LABEL: For the eye
SPECIAL NOTE: Pilocarpine has an ocular insert (Ocusert), which is a disk that is placed onto the eye to release the medication over 7 days.

Indirect-Acting Agents

CLASSIFICATION: MIOTICS
GENERIC NAME: physostigmine
TRADE NAME: Eserine sulfate
ROUTE OF ADMINISTRATION: Opthalmic
COMMON DOSAGE: Apply small amount (ointment) to inside of lower eyelid up to three times daily (tid)
AUXILIARY LABEL:
- For the eye

GENERIC NAME: demecarium bromide
TRADE NAME: Humorsol
ROUTE OF ADMINISTRATION: Opthalmic
COMMON DOSAGE: 1 to 2 drops into affected eye twice per week (1 to 2 gtt biw)
AUXILIARY LABEL:
- For the eye

GENERIC NAME: echothiophate iodide
TRADE NAME: Phospholide Iodide
ROUTE OF ADMINISTRATION: Opthalmic
COMMON DOSAGE: For glaucoma, 1 drop into affected eye two times daily
AUXILIARY LABELS:
- For the eye
- Keep refrigerated

SPECIAL NOTE: This medication must be prepared by reconstitution and is stable only 1 month if kept at room temperature. It is good for 6 months if refrigerated.

Sympathomimetics. The name sympathomimetics refers to mimicking or "acting like" the sympathetic system. The primary agent, phenylephrine, is commonly used along with miotics to treat glaucoma. Other uses include dilating the eye for examination and, in lower concentrations, as a decongestant for eye irritation. Most of the agents in this class are meant specifically for persons suffering from allergies and congestion in the eyes.

Drug Action. When the sympathetic system is activated (among the changes in the body system) the vessels in the eyes contract, pupils dilate, and the ciliary muscle relaxes. The result is an increase in drainage and, with certain agents, a decrease in aqueous humor. These medications are used to treat open-angle glaucoma in addition to other antiglaucoma agents, reducing intraocular pressure. Common side effects include blurriness and, if overused, redness of the eyes.

CLASSIFICATION: SYMPATHOMIMETICS, OPTHALMIC
GENERIC NAME: epinephrine
TRADE NAME: Glaucon, Epifrin
ROUTE OF ADMINISTRATION: Opthalmic
COMMON DOSAGE: 1 drop into affected eye once or twice daily (1 gtt qd or bid)
AUXILIARY LABEL:
- For the eye

GENERIC NAME: dipivefrin
TRADE NAME: Propine
ROUTE OF ADMINISTRATION: Opthalmic
COMMON DOSAGE: 1 drop into affected eye every 12 hours (1 gtt q12h)
AUXILIARY LABEL:
- For the eye

Prostaglandin Agonist. There is only one agent indicated to treat glaucoma in this classification. The medication latanoprost is kept in the refrigerator, unlike other ophthalmics. It is used to treat open-angle glaucoma and can be used to decrease intraocular pressure in patients who have not responded to the other agents available. The side effects of this medication include a possible change in iris color (becomes darker).

Drug Action. This medication reduces the intraocular pressure by increasing the outflow of the aqueous humor. Because this medication has not been used as long as the others discussed in this chapter, there are no long-term findings available. The action of the drug is not clear. There are, however, many unknown effects of this agent yet to be discovered.

> **GENERIC NAME:** latanoprost
> **TRADE NAME:** Xalantan
> **ROUTE OF ADMINISTRATION:** Opthalmic
> **COMMON DOSAGE:** 1 drop into affected eye once daily in the evening (1 gtt q pm)
> **AUXILIARY LABEL:**
> ■ For the eye
> **SPECIAL NOTE:** Unopened ophthalmic must be kept refrigerated. Once opened, it may be kept at room temperature for up to 6 weeks.

General Information. There are many combinations of ophthalmic medications available by prescription. These combinations lessen the number of application times and agents that patients need. It is imperative that eye solutions be kept sterile because foreign objects instilled into the eyes can cause damage or infection. Patients are counseled by the pharmacist to avoid touching the medication and contaminating it. In addition, most medications should not be instilled into the eyes while wearing contact lenses.

Antiinfection and Antiinflammatory Agents

The next classification of agents treats infections of the eye and other conditions that cause inflammation. There are a wide variety of conditions that affect the eyes such as bacterial, viral, and fungal infections and allergies. The course of treatment depends on identifying the microbe that has caused the infection. The two types of drugs used to treat these conditions are listed in Box 19.3.

Antiinflammatory Agents. Most of the agents used to decrease inflammation are solutions or suspensions. Suspensions need to be shaken well before use. Side effects include mild burning and or stinging on instillation.

Nonsteroidal Antiinflammatory Drugs (NSAIDs)

Drug Action. NSAIDs inhibit the enzyme cyclooxygenase, which is responsible for the synthesis (creation) of prostaglandins. Prostaglandins are directly related to the mechanisms that are responsible for inflammation and pain associated with it. These agents are available as an ophthalmic in solution only. Both flurbiprofen and suprofen are indicated for intraoperative miosis. Diclofenac and ketorolac may be used for the treatment of postoperative inflammation after cataract surgery. Ketorolac also relieves itching resulting from allergies.

BOX 19.3 MAIN TREATMENTS FOR INFLAMMATION AND INFECTION*

Antiinflammatory agents
NSAIDs
Corticosteroids
Decongestants and antihistamines (listed in Table 19.2)

Antiinfective agents
Sulfonamides
Aminoglycosides
Erythromycins
Antifungals
Antivirals

NSAIDs, Nonsteroidal antiinflammatory drugs.
*Antiinflammatories and antiinfectives use different classes of drugs to treat the condition depending on its cause.

CLASSIFICATION: ANTIINFLAMMATORY, NSAIDS
GENERIC NAME: flurbiprofen
TRADE NAME: Ocufen
ROUTE OF ADMINISTRATION: Opthalmic
COMMON DOSAGE: 1 drop into affected eye every 30 minutes beginning 2 hours before surgery
AUXILIARY LABELS:

■ For the eye
■ Use as directed

GENERIC NAME: suprofen
TRADE NAME: Profenal
ROUTE OF ADMINISTRATION: Opthalmic
COMMON DOSAGE: 2 drops into affected eye at 3, 2, and 1 hour before surgery
AUXILIARY LABELS:

■ For the eye
■ Use as directed

GENERIC NAME: diclofenac
TRADE NAME: Voltaren
ROUTE OF ADMINISTRATION: Opthalmic
COMMON DOSAGE: 1 or 2 drops into affected eye within 1 hour before surgery; after surgery: 1 drop into affected eye four times daily for 2 weeks (1 gtt qid × 2 weeks)
AUXILIARY LABELS:

■ For the eye
■ Use as directed

GENERIC NAME: ketorolac
TRADE NAME: Acular
ROUTE OF ADMINISTRATION: Opthalmic
COMMON DOSAGE: ocular itching: 1 drop four times daily (1 gtt qid); after cataract surgery: 1 drop into the eye(s) four times daily for 2 weeks (1 gtt qid × 2 weeks)
AUXILIARY LABELS:

■ For the eye
■ Use as directed

Corticosteroids. The corticosteroids are extremely potent agents used to relieve inflammation resulting from infection or injury. They are commonly used postoperatively to decrease swelling. These agents should not be used too long because they can influence the length of time it takes to heal. The dosage forms include solutions, suspensions, and ointments. Side effects may include burning, blurred vision, eye pain, or headaches.

Drug Action. There are many actions that steroids have on the body system including decreasing macrophage movement, kinin release, and other functions associated with swelling and pain. If they are used over a long period of time they can decrease antibody production.

CLASSIFICATION: ANTIINFLAMMATORY, CORTICOSTEROIDS
GENERIC NAME: prednisolone
TRADE NAME: AK-Pred (solution), Pred Forte* (suspension)
ROUTE OF ADMINISTRATION: Opthalmic
COMMON DOSAGE: 1 to 2 drops into affected eye two to four times daily (1 to 2 gtts bid to qid)
AUXILIARY LABELS:

■ For the eye

*Shake well before using

GENERIC NAME: dexamethasone
TRADE NAME: Decadron Phosphate(solution and ointment), *Maxidex(suspension)
ROUTE OF ADMINISTRATION: Opthalmic
COMMON DOSAGE: 1 to 2 drops into affected eye(s) hourly during the daytime and every 2 hours at night until inflammation decreases, then decrease as directed
AUXILIARY LABELS:

- For the eye
- Use as directed

SPECIAL NOTE: For ointment the patient should apply a thin ribbon to the inside of the eyelid on the same time schedule as the solution or suspension.

*Shake well before using

Decongestants and Antihistamines. Both decongestants and antihistamines are used to combat allergies. Antihistamines inhibit the release of histamine that results in common symptoms of itching and inflammation. Decongestants are used to dry out mucus caused by allergies and hay fever. In Table 19.2 lists decongestants and combination drugs that contain both decongestants and antihistamines. These are indicated for allergies resulting from pollen or other allergens.

Drug Action. Decongestants act on the specific receptors that cause constriction of the mucous membrane, thus lessening congestion. The drug action for antihistamines involves blocking the histamine receptors. Mast cells are responsible for histamine release when an allergen or antigen invades the body. By inhibition of the histamine receptors, the effects of seasonal allergies and other allergens can be lessened.

Antiinfective Agents

Conjunctivitis. The severe inflammation and discomfort of conjunctivitis can be treated with many different antibiotics. It is up to the physician to determine the medication depending on the cause of the infection. If the infection is viral, an agent such as vidarabine may be used. If the infection is fungal, natamycin may be prescribed. If the infection is bacterial, there are a wide variety of antibiotics that can be used depending on the specific microbe. For many bacterial infections a wide-spectrum antibiotic, such as gentamicin or ciprofloxacin, may be used. Other popular ophthalmics used to treat conjunctivitis and other infections of the eye are discussed in the following sections.

Sulfonamides. Sulfacetamide and sulfisoxazole are the two primary agents used to treat bacterial infections. Dosage forms include solutions, suspensions, and ointments. Side effects may include stinging of the eye on application. Sulfa-type preparations are also available in different strengths of combinations with antiinflammatories or decongestants such as the following:

TABLE 19.2 Ophthalmic Decongestants and Combinations*

Generic Name	Trade Name	Availability
Naphazoline	VasoClear, Cleareyes Soln	OTC
Naphazoline (decongestant) and	Naphcon-A Soln	OTC
pheniramine (antihistamine)	Naphoptic-A Solution	RX
oxymetazoline	Visine L.R.	OTC
Phenylephrine	Relief	OTC
Tetrahydrozoline	Visine	OTC
Olopatadine	Patanol Soln	RX

OTC, Over-the-counter; *RX,* prescription.
*Patients must read the package insert and follow manufacturer's recommended dosage. Dangerous side effects may occur if ophthalmic over-the-counter agents are used by patients with glaucoma.

- Sulfacetamide sodium and fluorometholone (antiinflammatory)
- Sulfacetamide sodium and phenylephrine (decongestant)
- Sulfacetamide sodium and prednisolone (antiinflammatory)

The actions of sulfonamides are bacteriostatic. Their range of microbes includes both gram-negative and gram-positive. They block the formation of folic acid required by microbes.

CLASSIFICATION: OPTHALMIC SULFONAMIDES

GENERIC NAME: sulfacetamide sodium

TRADE NAME: Bleph-10 (solution, ointment)

ROUTE OF ADMINISTRATION: Opthalmic

COMMON DOSAGE: 1 to 2 drops into lower eyelid every 1 to 4 hours initially (1 to 2 gtts q 1 to 4 hours); for ointment: apply a thin ribbon to lower eyelid for the same dosing as the solution

AUXILIARY LABELS:
- For the eye
- Use as directed

WARNING: This medication should not be used if solution becomes dark in color. Avoid contamination.

Aminoglycosides. Aminoglycosides are a very potent group of medications. Because of their wide spectrum of activity, they can also be used for some microbial resistant strains. Side effects and adverse effects include burning, stinging, and photosensitivity.

The drug action is the inhibition of bacterial protein synthesis. They are bactericidal in action and are used to treat both gram-negative and gram-positive microbes. Because these agents are extremely strong, the physician must determine the correct dosage based on the weight of the patient and the severity of the infection.

CLASSIFICATION: OPTHALMIC AMINOGYCOSIDES

GENERIC NAME: gentamicin

TRADE NAME: Genoptic (solution), Garamycin (ophthalmic ointment)

ROUTE OF ADMINISTRATION: Opthalmic

COMMON DOSAGE: solution: Instill 1 to 2 drops every 2 to 4 hrs;
ointment: Apply ½″ every 3 to 4 hours; 2 to 3 times daily

AUXILIARY LABELS:
- For the eye
- Use as directed

GENERIC NAME: tobramycin

TRADE NAME: Tobrex (solution and ointment)

ROUTE OF ADMINISTRATION: Opthalmic

COMMON DOSAGE: Solution: Instill 1 to 2 drops every 4 hours
Ointment: Apply 2 to 3 times daily

AUXILIARY LABELS:
- For the eye
- Use as directed

Erythromycin. The antiinfective erythromycin comes only in ointment form. Side effects may include stinging, burning, itching, and inflammation.

This agent is a bacteriostatic but can be bactericidal if used in high doses. It is used to treat mostly gram-positive and some gram-negative microbes. It is most often used to treat conjunctivitis. The ophthalmic ointment is also used as a prophylaxis in the eyes of newborns to prevent infection.

> **CLASSIFICATION: OPTHALMIC MACROCIDE**
> **GENERIC NAME:** erythromycin
> **TRADE NAME:** Ilotycin
> **ROUTE OF ADMINISTRATION:** Opthalmic
> **COMMON DOSAGE:** Instill ½″ 2 to 8 times daily, depending upon the type and severity of the eye infection
> **AUXILIARY LABEL:**
> - For the eye

Antifungals. Specific fungal infections must be treated with agents that can attack the specific metabolism of the invading fungus. The primary agent, Natamycin, is an aminoglycoside and a fungicidal agent. The only noted adverse effects are a possible sensitivity to the formulation. Safety has not been established in children and pregnant or lactating women.

Drug Action. The specific method of action involves the antifungal binding to cell membrane of the fungus. When this occurs, the stability of the membrane is jeopardized and the cell membrane breaks down, killing the fungus.

> **GENERIC NAME:** natamycin
> **TRADE NAME:** Natacyn (suspension)
> **ROUTE OF ADMINISTRATION:** Opthalmic
> **COMMON DOSAGE:** To treat fungal conjunctivitis, four to six applications are all that may be necessary
> **AUXILIARY LABELS:**
> - For the eye
> - Shake well before using

Antivirals. The three most common viral infections of the eye include herpes simplex, keratitis, and conjunctivitis. The aim of antivirals is to interrupt or alter synthesis (the making) of new virions at a specific step, thus rendering the virion inactive. Many of the viruses that affect the eyes are more common in persons with immunodeficiency such as those diagnosed with acquired immunodeficiency syndrome (AIDS). Side effects may be sensitivity to light, stinging, or mild burning sensation.

Drug Action. The general method of action for these antiviral agents is at the point where the attacking virus is using the host's deoxyribonucleic acid (DNA) to replicate. This results in a malformation of various components necessary for properly working virions. Therefore all agents are viricidal because they kill the virus.

> **CLASSIFICATION: OPTHALMIC ANTIVIRUS**
> **GENERIC NAME:** idoxuridine (IDU)
> **TRADE NAME:** Herplex
> **ROUTE OF ADMINISTRATION:** Opthalmic
> **COMMON DOSAGE:** initally, 1 drop into eye(s) every hour during the day and every 2 hours at night; may decrease over time as determined by physician
> **AUXILIARY LABELS:**
> - For the eye
> - Take as directed

> **GENERIC NAME:** vidarabine
> **TRADE NAME:** Vira-A (ointment)
> **ROUTE OF ADMINISTRATION:** Opthalmic
> **COMMON DOSAGE:** Apply thin ribbon of ointment to lower eyelid 5 times daily at 3-hour intervals
> **AUXILIARY LABELS:**
> - For the eye
> - Use as directed

GENERIC NAME: trifluridine
TRADE NAME: Viroptic (solution)
ROUTE OF ADMINISTRATION: Opthalmic
COMMON DOSAGE: 1 drop into affected eye every 2 hours while awake for a maximum of 9 drops, then treatment may decrease to 1 drop every 4 hours while awake (for 7 days) for a maximum of 7 drops per day
AUXILIARY LABELS:
- For the eye
- Use as directed
- Must be refrigerated

Miscellaneous Ophthalmic Agents. Agents such as artificial tears are commonly bought over-the-counter. They are used for the relief of dry eyes and irritation that may occur. Their ingredients include sodium chloride (NaCl), buffers to adjust for pH, and other additives to prolong their effects. The only dosage form is a solution, but they are available in various strengths and in combination with various ingredients. Although each tear product has somewhat different ingredients, they all contain NaCl and all are used for the same reasons.

Artificial tear inserts are also available by prescription for dry eye syndrome or severe keratoconjunctivitis by physician recommendation. Table 19.3 lists some of the most common types of artificial tears.

The Ears

The human ear is not only responsible for hearing but also for balance, equilibrium, and many communication skills. The ear is composed of three major sections—the external, middle, and inner ear (Figure 19.3).

EXTERNAL EAR

Working from the outside in, we begin with the most exterior area of the ear, called the auricle. This area is composed of cartilage and skin and serves as an entrance for sound waves. The next section is the auditory canal. This canal, measuring approximately 1 inch long, leads to the tympanic membrane (eardrum) inside the ear. This membrane has two major functions:

- Protection of the middle ear from foreign objects
- Transmission of sounds to the middle ear

The transmission is possible because of the vibration caused when sound hits the membrane, much the same way a drum skin vibrates, carrying the sound when struck with a drumstick. Cerumen (a waxy substance) is produced by glands at the tympanic membrane.

TABLE 19.3 Artificial Tears Products

Trade Name	Manufacturer	Ingredients
Tear Drop	Parmed	Polyvinyl alcohol, NaCl, EDTA, benzalkonium Cl
Artifical Tears	Various mfg	Polyvinyl alcohol, povidone, NaCl, chlorbutanol
Cellufresh	Allergan	Carboxymethylcellulose, NaCl, KCl, Na lactate
Refresh	Allergan	Polyvinyl alcohol, Povidone, NaCl
Just Tears	Blairex	Benzalkonium Cl, EDTA, polyvinyl alcohol, NaCl
Murine	Ross	Polyvinyl alcohol, povidone, benzalkonium Cl, dextrose, EDTA, NaCl, sodium bicarbonate, sodium phosphate

EDTA, Ethylenediamine tetraacetic acid.

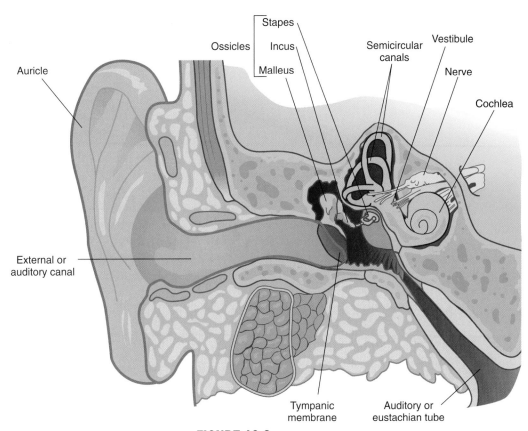

FIGURE 19.3 Anatomy of the ear.

MIDDLE EAR

Vibrations from the tympanic membrane are carried into the middle ear. This cavity (space) contains three small bony structures called ossicles. These are as follows:

- Malleus (hammer)
- Incus (anvil)
- Stapes (stirrup)

These three small bones are connected to each other and pass on the sound waves that enter the cavity. Another area in the middle ear is the eustachian tube. This tube leads to the nasopharynx. When swallowing, yawning, or movement of the jaw occurs, the eustachian tube opens and relieves the change in pressure between the outside and inside atmosphere.

TECH NOTE! When climbing altitudes in a car or plane, the eustachian tube relieves the decreased pressure from the outside by causing a pop of the ear. This brings equalization between the two pressure levels.

INNER EAR

After the transmission of sounds through the ossicles, the stapes (last bone) then continues the transfer of sound into the third section of the ear called the inner ear. This fluid-filled area is called the labyrinth and is composed of many components that process and transmit the audible sounds via nerve impulses to the brain where the sound is then interpreted. There are two important areas or divisions of the labyrinth:

Perilymph (bony labyrinth)	Composed of three main structures: cochlea, vestibule, and semicircular canal
Membrane division	Lines the bony division. Areas include sacs and tubes that run throughout the inner ear and aid in sound wave transference

The three main structures within the bony division are in very close proximity to each other and have very separate but important functions as described in Box 19.4. See Figure 19.4.

CONDITIONS AFFECTING THE EAR

There are various conditions that can affect the quality of hearing, including infections, ear wax accumulation, damage to the eardrum, and genetic defects. The following conditions are more common. The preparations that may be used to treat them follow.

Deafness

Deafness caused by factors other than genetic abnormalities include age and inflicted damage. There is a normal loss of hearing as one ages resulting from the effects of loud noises over the years. The small hairlike structures in the middle ear can break with loud noise. Unfortunately, they do not regenerate and over time a loss of hearing can occur. In the normal aging process, the hairs become less able to bend and transmission can be decreased. Although there is no medication that can increase hearing, there are hearing aids that can amplify sounds.

Otitis Media

This is an infection that occurs in the middle ear and is often associated with inflammation of the eustachian tube, which courses from the middle ear to the

---

BOX 19.4 THREE MAIN AREAS OF THE INNER EAR AND THEIR FUNCTIONS

Cochlea
This area is coiled and composes three fluid-filled canals. It is here that small hairlike structures are connected to the nerve that runs to the brain. As the sound waves enter, the hairs bend and create impulses that are transmitted to the nerve.

Vestibule
The vestibule is located between the cochlea and membrane division and is responsible for equilibrium and balance. It does this by hair-type cells that are affected by gravity when moved. Nerves carry this information to the brain, specifically to the cerebellum and midbrain areas. Thus equilibrium is maintained. This gives humans a sense of direction and orientation.

Semicircular Canal
There are three semicircular canals filled with a fluid that helps with the transfer of messages to a cranial nerve. Small hairlike fibers behave as sensors, moving back and forth as one moves forward, backward, or stops. The signals sent from two of these canals provide information to the brain about the orientation of the body when at rest, whereas the third canal sends information pertaining to the body when in motion.

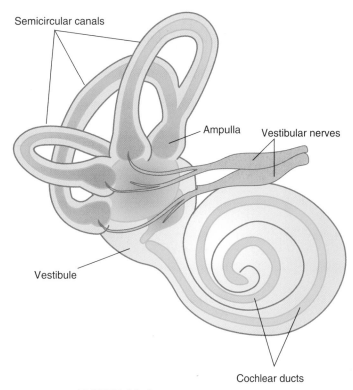

Semicircular canals

Ampulla

Vestibular nerves

Vestibule

Cochlear ducts

FIGURE 19.4 Anatomy of the inner ear.

nasopharynx. The lining of the middle ear and nasopharynx is a single continuous membranous structure. This is why a sore throat can lead to a middle ear infection, as is often seen in children. There are antiinfectives that can treat the infection. However, many times because of reoccurring infections in children, pediatricians insert small tubes that allow drainage from the middle ear and eustachian tube, which lessens infections.

Cerumen Buildup
As mentioned previously, the glands at the tympanic membrane naturally build up a waxy substance referred to as cerumen. See Figure 19.3. If excessive wax builds up or dries, it can impede hearing quality. It may be necessary for a doctor to remove this buildup to perform an examination or to improve hearing quality.

Ototoxicity
Some medications can cause toxic levels within the ears' lymph tissue that in turn may cause ear damage. A ringing or buzzing within the ears (tinnitus) can progress to permanent ear damage if left untreated. Balance may also be affected. Drugs listed in Table 19.4 have been noted to have ototoxic side effects when used in high doses or for long periods of time.

TABLE 19.4 Medications that Cause Ototoxicity

Aminoglycosides	Gentamicin, tobramycin
Erythromycins	Clarithromycin, erythromycin (macrolides)
Analgesics	Aspirin and NSAIDs
Loop diuretics	Furosemide, bumetanide, ethacrynic acid
Antineoplastics	Cisplatin
Quinine	Quinamm

NSAIDs, Nonsteroidal antiinflammatory drugs.

OTIC PREPARATIONS

Some of the conditions that affect the ears are infections. Most of these are from bacterial infections. Depending on the type of infection affecting the ears, certain preparations are available that may be bactericidal or bacteriostatic. Agents that are bactericidal kill the bacteria (see Chapter 29), whereas bacteriostatics hold the bacteria in stasis or stop any continued growth. Statics are used to assist the body in the battle against bacteria. Table 19.5 lists agents used on the ears and their indication. Almost all ear agents are combined ingredients containing several major ingredients. These include antibiotics, steroids, and other agents that help remove wax buildup. The names of the additives and their active ingredient in some of the otic preparations are given in Table 19.6.

All prescription agents used for the ear must be labeled with auxiliary labels "for the ear" and "external use only." Agents such as cerumenolytics should not be used by persons suffering from a perforated eardrum, swimmer's ear, or itching of the ear canal. As with all ear products, it is advisable to lie down on one side to allow the solution to enter into the ear canal.

TECH NOTE! It is common to see an ophthalmic prescribed for ear treatment. This is acceptable because all ophthalmics are sterile and can be used in the ear. However, otics cannot be used in the eye because they are not sterile.

TABLE 19.5 Ear Preparations*

Generic Name	Trade Name	Availability	Indication
Acetic acid	Domeboro	OTC	Used for external ear infections and prophylaxis of swimmer's ear
Benzocaine, benzethonium chloride, glycerin, PEG 300	Americaine	OTC	Used for pain within the ear caused by swimmer's ear and infections
Carbamide peroxide, glycerin, propylene glycol, sodium stannate	Debrox	OTC	Used to remove ear wax
Chloramphenicol	Chloromycetin Otic	RX	Used to treat ear infections caused by both gram-negative and gram-positive microbes
Desonide, acetic acid	Tridesilon	RX	Used to treat ear infections of the external canal
Triethanolamine, polypeptide, oleate-condensate	Cerumenex	OTC	Used to remove ear wax
Hydrocortisone, neomycin, polymyxin	Cortisporin Otic	RX	Used to treat superficial bacterial infections of the external auditory canal
Isopropyl alcohol, anhydrous glycerin	Swim-Ear	OTC	Used for swimmer's ear

OTC, Over-the-counter; *RX*, prescription.
*Many of the otics are combination drugs.

TABLE 19.6 Major Ingredients in Otic Preparations

Agents	Classification	Indication
Acetic acid	Antibacterial, antifungal	Infection
Boric acid		
Benzethonium chloride		
Desonide	Steroid	Antiinflammatory
Hydrocortisone	Steroid	Antiinflammatory
Phenylephrine	Vasoconstrictor	Decongestant

DO YOU REMEMBER THESE KEY POINTS?

- Main structures of the eye
- The function of rods and cones
- Conditions that can affect the eye
- What glaucoma is and the medications used to treat it
- Agents used to treat infections of the eye
- Main structures of the ear
- The three bony structures that make up the labyrinth of the inner ear
- Conditions that affect the ear
- Why children suffering from colds and flu often get ear infections
- Ear preparations
- Which medications for both eye and ear are available over-the-counter or by prescription
- What auxiliary labels are necessary for both eye and ear medications
- Why ear drops cannot be used in the eye

REVIEW QUESTIONS:

Multiple Choice

1. The cornea is responsible for
   A. The color of the eye
   B. Lubrication of the eye
   C. Protection of the eyeball
   D. Visual acuity

2. The substance that bathes the eye with nutrition is the
   A. Conjunctiva
   B. Aqueous humor
   C. Sphincter
   D. Blood vessels

3. Glaucoma is a condition of the eye that results from
   A. Narrowing of eye blood vessels
   B. A lack of aqueous humor
   C. Intraocular pressure
   D. Age

4. Glaucoma can be divided into three types; these are
   A. Acute congestive, chronic simple, and congenital
   B. Primary, secondary, and congenital
   C. Angle closure, open-angle, and chronic
   D. None of the above

5. Which of the medications that follow is not a beta-adrenergic blocker?
   A. Blocadren
   B. Betoptic
   C. Betagan
   D. Trusopt

6. Miotics act by
   A. Contraction of ciliary muscles increasing outflow of aqueous humor
   B. Inhibition of beta sites that then relax vessels allowing proper drainage of aqueous humor
   C. Inhibition of anhydrase thus lessening the formation of aqueous humor
   D. The drug action is not clear

7. Of the various antiinfectives used to treat eye conditions, which works as a bacteriostatic at low doses and as a bactericidal at high doses?
   A. Aminoglycosides
   B. Sulfacetamide sodium
   C. Erythromycin
   D. Natacyn

8. The cavity of the middle ear contains all the following structures except
   A. Cochlea
   B. Malleus
   C. Incus
   D. Stapes

9. The structure within the inner ear responsible for balance is the
   A. Semicircular canal
   B. Vestibule
   C. Cochlea
   D. A and B

10. The following ingredients are used to treat inflammation of the ear except
    A. Desonide
    B. Benzethonium chloride
    C. Phenylephrine
    D. Boric acid

True/False

*If the statement is false, then change it to make it true.

1. The eye is located in an area called the socket.
2. The back of the eye is oxygen-rich through blood vessels.
3. The occipital lobe in the brain is responsible for interpretation of images.
4. Conjunctivitis is inflammation of the cornea.
5. Otics may be prescribed to be used in the eye or ear.
6. The ossicles of the ear are located in the middle ear and are composed of four bones.
7. The eustachian tube connects the middle ear to the throat.
8. Debrox is an agent available over-the-counter for ear wax removal.
9. Otitis media is an infection or inflammation of the inner ear.
10. The tympanic membrane is a covering of the entrance of the middle ear.

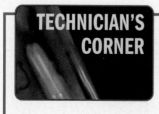
TECHNICIAN'S CORNER

Look up the following agents in *Mosby's Drug Consult* and list the following information on each one: normal dosage, strength, indication, and auxiliary labels that each one would require.

Neptazine	Burrows
Prefrin	Aurodin
Timolol	Ear Sol
Garamycin	Americaine otic

BIBLIOGRAPHY

Edmunds M: *Introduction to Clinical Pharmacology,* ed 3, St Louis, 2000, Mosby.
Drug Facts and Comparisons 1999, St Louis, 1999, Facts and Comparisons.
Hitner, Nagle: *Basic Pharmacology,* ed 4, New York, 1999, Glencoe.
McCuistion, Gutierrez: *Real World Nursing Survival Guide: Pharmacology,* Philadelphia, 2002, WB Saunders.
Mosby's Drug Consult, St Louis, 2004, Elsevier.
Salerno E: *Pharmacology for Health Professionals,* St Louis, 1999, Mosby.
Thiboudeau, Patton: *Structure and Function of the Body,* ed 11, St Louis, 2000, Mosby.

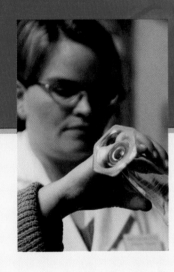

CHAPTER

20
Gastrointestinal System

Objectives

- Identify the anatomy of the digestive system that is covered in this chapter.

- List the most common conditions affecting the digestive system.

- List the trade and generic names of drugs covered in this chapter.

- Explain the differences between stool softeners, laxatives, and bulk-forming laxatives.

- Describe the drug action of the medications covered in this chapter.

- Explain the types of treatments used for ulcers, including non-medication treatments.

- Describe nonmedication treatments for ulcers.

- List common drug interactions between antacids and other medications.

- Distinguish between common ulcers and those caused by *Helicobacter pylori* and explain why the treatments are different.

- Explain causes of diarrhea, constipation, flatulence, and emesis.

- List the different types of treatments for each of the conditions discussed.

355

Absorption *The taking in of nutrients from food and liquids*

Amino acids *Molecules that makeup proteins*

Appendicitis *Inflammation of the appendix*

Carbohydrates *Chemical substances that include sugars, glycogen, starches, and cellulose with only carbon, hydrogen and oxygen makeup*

Chyme *The soupy consistency of food after mixing with stomach acids as it passes into the small intestines*

Constipation *The presence of dry, hard stools that may be decreased in frequency*

Diarrhea *Frequent, watery, loose stools*

Digestion *The mechanical, chemical, and enzymatic action of breaking food into molecules that can be used in metabolism*

Emesis *Vomiting*

Excretion *Elimination of waste products through stools and urine*

Gastritis *Inflammation of the stomach lining*

Ingestion *The act of taking in food or liquid*

Lipids *Fats and fatty acids*

Peptic ulcer *An ulcerative condition of the lower esophagus, stomach, or duodenum, usually resulting from the bacterium Helicobacter pylori (H. pylori)*

Peristalsis *The contraction and relaxation of the tubular muscles of the esophagus, stomach, and intestines that move food substances from the mouth to the anus*

Ulcer *A lesion on a mucous surface of the gastrointestinal (GI) tract*

Villus *A projection from the surface of a mucous membrane; in the gastric tract, these projections increase the surface area for the absorption of nutrients and liquids in the small inestines*

GASTROINTESTINAL DRUGS

Trade	Generic	Pronunciation	Trade	Generic	Pronunciation
H₂ Antagonists			**Antidiarrheal**		
Tagamet	cimetidine	sy-**met**-ta-deen	Lomotil	diphenoxylate/atropine	die-fen-**ox**-i-late
Zantac	ranitidine	ran-**nit**-ta-deen	Pepto Bismol	bismuth subsalicylate	**biz**-muth
Pepcid	famotidine	fa-**mo**-ta-deen	Kapectolin	kaolin/pectin	**kay**-oh-lin
Axid	nizatidine	nye-**zah**-tih-deen	Imodium	loperamide	low-**pear**-ah-myde
			Fibercon	polycarbophil	poly-**kar**-bow-phyl
Proton Pump Inhibitors			**Antinausea Antiemetics**		
Prilosec	omeprazole	oh-**mep**-rah-zole	Atarax	hydroxyzine	hi-**drox**-ah-zeen
Protonix	pantoprazole	pan-**tow**-prah-zole	Bonine, Antivert	meclizine	**meck**-la-zeen
Prevacid	lansoprazole	lan-**sew**-prah-zole	Dramamine	dimenhydrinate	die-men-**hi**-dra-nate
			Reglan	metoclopramide	mea-toe-**clow**-prah-myde
Anticonstipation			Compazine	prochlorperazine	pro-klor-**pear**-ah-zeen
Colace	docusate sodium	**dock**-you-sate	Transderm Scop	scopolamine	sko-**pole**-la-meen
Pericolace	casanthranol/docusate	kah-**san**-thrah-nole	**Antiflatulance**		
Dulcolax	bisacodyl	by-saw-**co**-dill	Mylicon	simethicone	sye-**meth**-i-cone
Senokot	senna	**sen**-ah	**Antiulcer**		
Metamucil	psyllium	fy-**sill**-ee-um	Carafate	sucralfate	soo-**kral**-fate
Citrucel	methycellulose	meth-ill-**cell**-you-lows			

Introduction

The digestive tract runs from the mouth to the end of the intestines and works to break down and absorb food and fluids. Foods are broken down from large items into small molecules that can be readily absorbed into the bloodstream and sent to areas of the body where they will be used for energy, synthesis of proteins, and enzymes for essential reactions. As food is broken down, nutrients are absorbed, and all nonessential food elements are excreted through the feces or urine. The common analogy used to describe the entire gastrointestinal (GI) system is as one long tube that runs though the body. This description is adequate for most of the functions that are covered in this chapter. There are various important functions that pharmacy technician students should be aware of. These areas are covered more thoroughly as they pertain to medications. Many conditions that affect the GI system (including digestion) are immediately recognized by the suffering patient, such as diarrhea. There are many medications that are available over-the-counter (OTC) to treat the symptoms of the digestive tract and the intestines. Because of the ease of self-treatment by purchasing OTC medications, many patients do not think it is necessary to ask their doctor or pharmacist about the possible interactions of these drugs and their legend (prescription) drugs. There are many interactions that need to be considered when filling new prescriptions for patients.

Form and Function of the GI System

The three main functions of the GI system are digestion, absorption, and metabolism. Within the GI tract, the various organs perform these functions 24 hours a day. The GI system is controlled by the parasympathetic nervous system. The parasympathetic nervous system is the part of the nervous system that balances with the sympathetic system in controlling many of the functions of the body (see Chapter 17). When we are at rest, the parasympathetic nervous system is at work in body systems such as the GI system. Each organ within the GI tract completes a specific task. This chapter examines the GI system from the time food is ingested until it is expelled. It also discusses additional organs, including the liver, pancreas, and gallbladder, that help the GI tract complete its task.

ANATOMY OF THE GI SYSTEM

The main organ one might think of when learning about the GI system is the stomach, yet by the time food has arrived to this organ it has already begun its transformation from a solid food. Let's begin by looking at the overall system of the GI tract (Figure 20.1). The organs discussed in this chapter, in sequence, are the mouth, salivary glands, pharynx, and esophagus (ingestion); followed by the stomach, small intestine, and large intestine (absorption); and finally the rectal area (excretion).

Ingestion

The mouth is the first apparatus of the human body where food is mixed manually. In addition to the action of the teeth chewing food into smaller pieces, salivary glands begin to secrete an enzyme called amylase that initiates the chemical breakdown of food. There are three pairs of salivary glands in the mouth that are responsible for the beginning of food breakdown—sublingual, submandibular, and parotid. The sublingual and submandibular glands are located below the tongue and jaw, respectively. The parotid glands are just in front of the ear (Figure 20.2).

Another function of the saliva besides enzymatic breakdown of food is to moisten the esophagus so that food can be easily swallowed. With the help from the tongue, the food is swallowed and makes its way into the pharynx. The pharynx connects

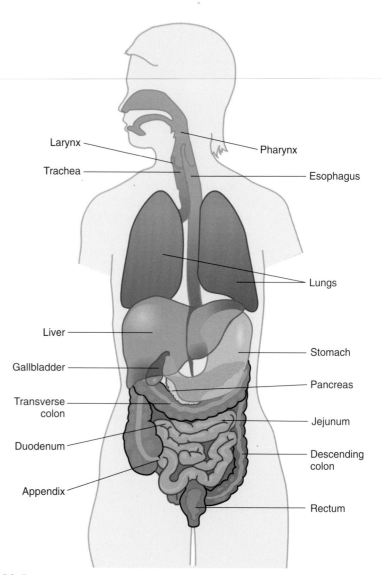

Larynx

Pharynx

Trachea

Esophagus

Lungs

Liver

Stomach

Gallbladder

Pancreas

Transverse colon

Jejunum

Duodenum

Descending colon

Appendix

Rectum

FIGURE 20.1 Anatomy of the GI system (including mouth, pharynx, esophagus, stomach, and intestines).

the mouth to the esophagus and contains the epiglottis. The function of the epiglottis is to close off the trachea so that food will not enter into the wrong tube. Food then makes its way to the stomach via peristalsis of the esophagus, pushing and moving the food downward into the stomach. As the food arrives in the stomach it enters into an acidic environment that will perform some of the chemical breakdown (Figure 20.3).

When activated by food, gastric juices are secreted in the stomach. The gastric juices are composed of intrinsic factor (IF) enzymes and hydrochloric acid (HCl) enzymes, which has a pH of 2 in the stomach lumen. Thus the stomach contents are extremely acidic and would irritate your skin if you were to come into contact with them. To help balance this extremely acidic pH, the inner mucosal lining of the stomach is alkaline for protection. An additional protective mucosal lining prevents the acid from eating through the stomach wall. (Another function of the stomach muscles is to help with digestion by a churning action that mixes the food.) The extremely acidic environment kills bacteria that have been ingested and helps activate the enzymes that break down food. An important chemical produced, pepsinogen, becomes an active enzyme in the stomach called pepsin. When

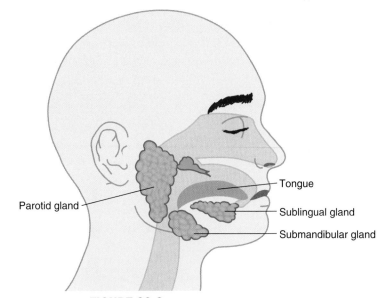

FIGURE 20.2 Major glands of the mouth.

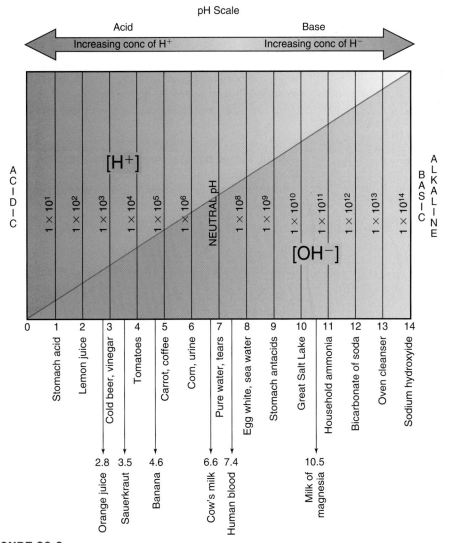

FIGURE 20.3 pH scale ranges from one (the most acidic) to 14 (the most basic). Normal human blood pH is about halfway between at 7.4 pH.

the churning and chemicals have broken down the solid substances into small bits, the acidic mixture left is referred to as chyme. The chyme then leaves the stomach and passes through the pyloric sphincter, the muscle that forms the division and opening into the small intestine. The pyloric sphincter must relax in order for the chyme to pass. This is a reflex action.

TECH NOTE! Intrinsic factor is a chemical needed to absorb vitamin B_{12}. A person born without the ability to secrete intrinsic factor must take a supplement for his or her entire life.

Absorption

Absorption of nutrients takes place from the food we eat. The vitamins and minerals move through the lining of the gut. Molecules of glucose, amino acids, and fatty acids begin to circulate into the body fluids. The blood becomes another avenue that nutrients must travel to reach their ultimate destination, the cells. Without the process of absorption, our cells would not be able to be nourished and would die. The overall process is called metabolism. Nutrients are used for energy and as building blocks for larger complex chemicals. The act of building molecules is known as anabolism, whereas breaking down molecules to release energy is known as catabolism. Together they are known as metabolism (see Chapter 30).

The small intestine is about 6 meters in length and is responsible for the final steps in the digestion of food. It also begins to absorb nutrients and then sends the remains into the large intestine. The structure of the intestines works perfectly for what it must do—absorb nutrients from the foods we eat. To do this it must be able to make contact with as much of the broken down food as possible and for as long as possible. It accomplishes this by being extremely long. Because there is limited space in a human body, it winds around, taking up much less space. In addition, the inside of the lining of the intestine is formed in such a way that it folds back and forth, again increasing the overall amount of surface area so that it has maximum exposure to the food (Figure 20.4).

The small intestine can be further divided into three sections—the duodenum, jejunum, and ileum. Each has its specific function and contribution to the breakdown and absorption of food. The duodenum is at the beginning of the small intestine and is about 25 cm long. It also is connected to the liver and pancreas from which it receives secretions that mix with the chyme from the stomach. The next section of intestine is the jejunum, which is much longer (about 2.5 m). The ileum is the last section, which measures about 3.5 m.

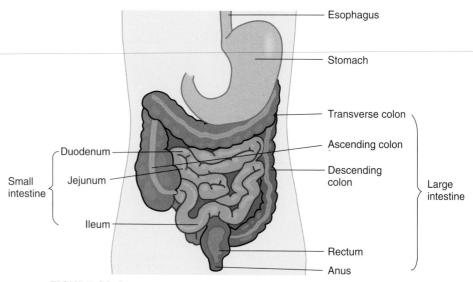

Esophagus

Stomach

Transverse colon

Ascending colon

Descending colon

Large intestine

Duodenum

Jejunum

Small intestine

Ileum

Rectum

Anus

FIGURE 20.4 Intestinal tract (including duodenum, jejunum, and ileum).

TABLE 20.1 Foods and Enzymes That Digest Them

Food	Enzyme*
Proteins	Peptidase
Sugars	Maltase, sucrase, lactase
Fats	Lipase

*Words ending in *-ase* indicate that the substance is an enzyme.

It is within these three areas that most of the food absorption takes place. Intestinal secretions have a more alkaline pH, allowing for better absorption of nutrients. Various enzymes continue to break down specific foods such as sugar, protein, and fat (Table 20.1). This enzymatic function of the stomach is very important because it allows the intestines to absorb the nutrients and chemicals from the foods we eat into the body for metabolic processes. However, this acidic environment also destroys many medications that enter into the stomach, which is why several medications either need special coating for protection or must be used in a different form such as parenteral so that they may bypass the stomach altogether.

The amount of secretions produced depends on how much food or chyme is present. In addition to the liver and pancreas, the gallbladder also helps in the digestion of food. The gallbladder releases bile that is stored by the liver and helps in the dispersion and absorption of fats.

Excretion

The large intestine follows the small intestine. Although it is much larger in circumference, it is not as long as the small intestine (only 1.5 m). The main sections of the large intestine include the cecum, colon, rectum, and anus. The colon takes up most of the length of the large intestine. Although absorption continues in the large intestine, it is limited to water and electrolytes. The substances moving through this portion of the intestine are not chyme but are transformed into solid fecal matter as water and electrolytes are absorbed into the bloodstream.

The rectum is the shortest section of the intestinal tract and connects to the anal canal. It is usually empty except during defecation. The amount of time for normal passage of fecal material can range from 3 to 5 days. Within the anal canal, the sphincter is under involuntary control and is responsible for the urge to defecate. The external anal sphincter is voluntary, giving the person control of the bowels.

Auxiliary Organ Functions

The chemical contribution from the auxiliary organs (pancreas, liver, and gallbladder) is only one function of many that these organs have. All three organs have ducts that lead to the duodenum. Here the enzymes from the pancreas meet the contents from the stomach and actively break down various foods. Foods such as proteins, carbohydrates, and fats must be broken down from complex molecules into simple molecules. Proteins are large molecules that are broken down into peptides first by pepsin in the stomach then by trypsin and chymotrypsin from the pancreas. Carbohydrates arrive in the stomach as large sugar molecules and are broken down into disaccharides, then in the duodenum into monosaccharides, where they can be absorbed and used for energy. Fats are not broken down very much until they reach the duodenum where they come into contact with bile produced by the liver and stored in the gallbladder. These long carbon chains of fat are more difficult to break down. They are first made water soluble by a process called emulsification then are further broken down by enzymes called lipases.

The appendix, attached to the cecum of the large intestine, is a small worm-shaped lymphatic structure that has no apparent function within the digestive system. If the lining of the appendix becomes inflamed, appendicitis results, which requires removal of the appendix (appendectomy).

Conditions Affecting the GI System

There are numerous conditions that can affect the GI system. These include commonly occurring and reoccurring conditions, such as heartburn, upset stomach, gastroesophageal reflux disease (GERD), constipation, and occasionally diarrhea. More severe illnesses, such as Crohn's disease, ulcers, and others, can be caused by consistent stress, which can worsen these conditions of the GI. Other GI conditions can be caused by bacterial infections, food allergies, and tumors, or may be caused by genetic defects, such as the lack of specific chemicals that are necessary for the proper function of this system. This section begins with a discussion of conditions of the mouth and then proceeds through the GI tract. The drugs used to treat each specific condition follow the condition and the symptoms description.

MOUTH AND THROAT

The mouth is subject to many kinds of bacteria on a daily basis. The lack of good oral hygiene is the most common reason for conditions affecting the mouth. Ulcers or inflammation of the gums can occur within the mouth cavity, causing pain and discomfort. In addition, the condition of the teeth plays an important role in the initial breakdown of food. The throat may become inflamed because of colds or the flu or through straining the vocal cords. Symptoms of inflammation include sore throat and fever. Treatments for the mouth and throat include mouthwashes, sprays, lozenges, or troches. Many agents contain alcohol or phenol bases. These agents are antiseptics and are good at killing bacteria. Benzocaines, phenols, and menthol have anesthetic effects. Other types of agents are listed in the following. Oral antibiotics may be swished and spit out or swallowed per doctor's orders.

TECH NOTE! The abbreviated term *s/s* means swish and swallow or can mean swish and spit. This is a common order for a nystatin oral suspension used for ulcers of the mouth or throat.

STOMACH

The high acid content of stomach fluids causes a number of stomach conditions. These conditions are more commonly known as upset stomach, indigestion, or heartburn. There are three main conditions that affect the stomach—hyperacidity, GERD, and peptic ulcers resulting from the bacterium *H. pylori*.

Hyperacidity is the occurrence of excessive acid secretion within the stomach. Conditions caused by hyperacidity include peptic and duodenal ulcers. Hyperacidity can result from the overproduction of acidic secretions or the decrease of chemicals that help deactivate excessive acidic secretions between meals. Small areas within the stomach lining are eroded away causing a sore that causes pain. GERD can occur when the cardiac sphincter (opening) at the top of the stomach relaxes. This allows acidic contents from the stomach to backup into the esophagus. This causes the burning sensation that most persons feel in their chest or throat. Antacids are the types of drugs normally used for both of these conditions

(Table 20.2). These agents decrease the acid content of the stomach. Most remedies can be purchased OTC.

Many OTC medications contain simethicone along with antacids, because of the common occurrence of flatulence (gas) that accompanies gastric upsets (Table 20.3). Gas can also be a side effect of the carbonates that are major ingredients in antacids. The following drugs are a small sample of the many agents that can be purchased.

In addition to antacids, histamine-2 (H_2) antagonists are used to treat GERD and ulcers. Agents such as cimetidine and ranitidine block H_2 receptors located within the lining of the stomach. A third type of agent used for GERD is proton pump inhibitors. These agents inhibit gastric acid secretion within the stomach lining by blocking the last enzymatic reaction before acid secretion takes place. This makes proton pump inhibitors very effective; thus they are usually prescribed for more severe cases of GERD. Currently, all medications for the treatment of GERDS are available by prescription only, although it may be just a matter of time before they too will get Food and Drug Administration (FDA) approval as an OTC drug.

TECH NOTE! H_2 antagonists' prescription counterparts are usually twice the strength of their OTC counterparts. For instance, Zantac OTC is 75 mg. If you wanted the same drug in a 150-mg strength, it would require a prescription. Likewise Tagamet 100 mg is OTC; the 300 mg strength is a legend drug. OTC remedies are not meant to treat ulcers or GERD but are for common heartburn.

TABLE 20.2 OTC Antacid Agents

Trade	Generic	Normal Dose
Milk of Magnesia	Magnesium hydroxide	5 to 15 mL qid
Alu-Cap	Aluminum hydroxide gel	1 cap tid prn
Tums	Calcium carbonate	1 to 2 tabs prn
Uro-Mag	Magnesium oxide	1 tid to qid
Riopan	Magaldrate	5 to 10 mL tid and hs
Combination Agents		
Gaviscon Chew tabs	Aluminum hydroxide, sodium bicarbonate	prn
Rolaids	Magnesium hydroxide, calcium carbonate	prn
Maalox Suspension	Aluminum hydroxide, sodium bicarbonate	prn
Titralac Ex-strength tabs	Calcium carbonate, saccharin	prn
Mylanta Gelcaps	Calcium carbonate, magnesium carbonate	prn

OTC, Over-the-counter.

TABLE 20.3 OTC Antiflatulance Agents

Trade	Generic	Common Dosage
Maalox Ex-strength tabs	Aluminum hydroxide, magnesium hydroxide, simethicone	Usually taken after meals or prn
Tempo tabs	Aluminum hydroxide, magnesium hydroxide, calcium carbonate, simethicone	Usually taken after meals or prn
Mylanta liq	Aluminum hydroxide, magnesium hydroxide, simethicone	Usually taken after meals or prn

Antacids Used to Treat Hyperacidity and GERD

Antacids include a variety of ion additives such as aluminum carbonate, sodium bicarbonate, calcium carbonate, magnesium hydroxide, and aluminum hydroxide. These ions each act in their own way to change the pH level in the stomach. Although both aluminum and magnesium are metallic cations, they differ in their side effects. Aluminum tends to cause constipation, whereas magnesium causes diarrhea. Compounds containing cations act as buffers, decreasing acidity within the stomach. Side effects vary depending on the various concentrations of these compounds. Most antacids contain a combination of the previously mentioned ions, thus reducing the probability of side effects such as diarrhea or constipation. Table 20.4 gives an example of key anions (−) used to alter pH. Three commonly used antacids are listed that are available OTC in both tablet and liquid forms.

TECH NOTE! Patients taking certain antibiotics such as tetracycline and ciprofloxacin should not take antacids containing magnesium or aluminum at the same time because they can decrease the absorption of the antibiotic.

Medications Used to Treat GERD

CLASSIFICATION: ANTACID
GENERIC NAME: magnesium hydroxide
TRADE NAME: Phillips, Milk of Magnesium (all)
ROUTE OF ADMINISTRATION: Oral
INDICATION: For the relief of hyperacidity and GERD
DRUG ACTION: Decreases acid secretions by binding to hydrogen ions
COMMON DOSAGE: Three to four times per day and at bedtime. Also given as needed
SIDE EFFECTS: Diarrhea. Also magnesium may bind to drugs causing a decrease in absorption

GENERIC NAME: aluminum hydroxide
TRADE NAME: Amphogel, Alu-Tab (all OTC)
ROUTE OF ADMINISTRATION: Oral
INDICATION: For the relief of hyperacidity and GERD
DRUG ACTION: Decreases acid secretions by binding to hydrogen ions
COMMON DOSAGE: Three times daily up to six times per day and as needed
SIDE EFFECTS: Constipation. Aluminum may slow the emptying of drugs from the stomach organ thus decreasing absorption in the intestines

TABLE 20.4 Example of Anions and Cation Combination Drugs Used for the Relief of GERD or Indigestion

Anions*	Combination Agents	Trade Name
Bicarbonate	Sodium bicarbonate	Alka Seltzer
Carbonate	Calcium carbonate	Tums
Citrate	Sodium citrate	Citra pH
Hydroxide	Aluminum magnesium hydroxide	Riopan

Cations	Combination Agents	Trade Name
Aluminum	Aluminum hydroxide	Alu-Cap
Magnesium	Magnesium hydroxide	Milk of Magnesia

GERD, Gastroesophageal reflux disease.
*The anions listed are normally combined with one of the two listed cations (+).

> **GENERIC NAME:** calcium carbonate
> **TRADE NAME:** Tums, Maalox, Mylanta (all OTC)
> **ROUTE OF ADMINISTRATION:** Oral
> **INDICATION:** For the relief of hyperacidity and GERD
> **DRUG ACTION:** Decreases acid secretions by binding to hydrogen ions
> **COMMON DOSAGE:** As needed
> **SIDE EFFECTS:** Minimal to none

Histamine-2 Antagonists. The prescription (RX) strength is the higher strength agent indicated next to the trade name and must be filled in the pharmacy. Although most of the prescription agents have normal dosages suggested by their manufacturer, many physicians allow patients to take cimetidine and ranitidine on an as-needed basis for indigestion.

Drug Action. H_2 antagonists bind to H_2 receptor sites, lowering acid secretions. Common side effects of histamine antagonists include possible GI upset and drowsiness.

> **TECH NOTE:** Histamine-1 receptors are located in the lungs, and agents used to treat the effects caused by histamine resulting from allergies are called antihistamines, whereas H_2 receptors are located in the stomach, and agents used to treat the effects of histamine are called H_2 antagonists.

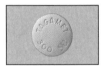

SmithKline
Beecham

> **CLASSIFICATION: H_2 RECEPTOR ANTAGONISTS**
> **GENERIC NAME:** cimetidine
> **TRADE NAME:** Tagamet (Rx: 300 mg, 400 mg, 800 mg), Tagamet HB (100 mg OTC)
> **INDICATION:** GERD, ulcer, duodenal ulcer prophylaxis (preventative therapy)
> **ROUTE OF ADMINISTRATION:** oral, intravenous (IV)
> **COMMON DOSAGE:** oral dosage Rx: 300 mg four times daily
> **AUXILIARY LABELS:**
> ■ Take with food
> ■ May cause drowsiness

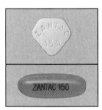

Glaxo Wellcome

> **GENERIC NAME:** ranitidine
> **TRADE NAME:** Zantac (Rx: 150 mg) Zantac 75 (OTC: 75 mg)
> **INDICATION:** GERD, ulcers, duodenal ulcer prophylaxis
> **ROUTE OF ADMINISTRATION:** oral, IV
> **COMMON DOSAGE:** 150 mg two times daily
> **AUXILIARY LABELS:**
> ■ Take with food
> ■ May cause drowsiness

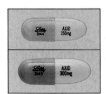

Lilly

> **GENERIC NAME:** nizatidine
> **TRADE NAME:** Axid Pulvules (RX: 150 mg, 300 mg), Axid AR (OTC: 75 mg)
> **INDICATION:** GERD, duodenal ulcer
> **ROUTE OF ADMINISTRATION:** oral
> **COMMON DOSAGE:** 150 to 300 mg once daily at bedtime
> **AUXILIARY LABEL:**
> ■ May cause dizziness and drowsiness

> **GENERIC NAME:** famotidine
> **TRADE NAME:** Pepcid (RX 20 mg, 40 mg) Pepcid AC (OTC: 10 mg)
> **INDICATION:** GERD, duodenal ulcer (OTC for heartburn, indigestion)
> **ROUTE OF ADMINISTRATION:** oral, IV
> **COMMON DOSAGE:** GERD: 20 mg twice daily up to 6 weeks
> **AUXILIARY LABELS:**
> ■ May cause dizziness and drowsiness
> ■ Special note: Suspension needs a "shake well" auxiliary label

Proton Pump Inhibitors. Proton pump inhibitors have similar indications for use in the treatment of GERD, although at this time they are available only by prescription. All of these agents are available as a delayed release form so that the patient is able to take them just once daily rather than having to take them at each meal. Drug action for all proton pump inhibitors is to block gastric acid secretions in the stomach.

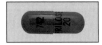

Merck

CLASSIFICATIONS: PROTON PUMP INHIBITORS
GENERIC NAME: omeprazole
TRADE NAME: Prilosec
INDICATION: peptic ulcer, *H. pylori*, duodenal ulcer; short-term use for esophagitis and GERD
ROUTE OF ADMINISTRATION: oral
COMMON DOSAGE: for GERD: 20 mg once a day for 4 to 8 weeks
SIDE EFFECTS: diarrhea
AUXILIARY LABELS:

- Take before meals
- Do not crush or chew capsule

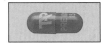

Tap Pharm

GENERIC NAME: lansoprazole
TRADE NAME: Prevacid
INDICATION: GERD, duodenal ulcer, gastric ulcer disease, erosive esophagitis
ROUTE OF ADMINISTRATION: oral
COMMON DOSAGE: for GERD: 15 mg once daily for up to 8 weeks
AUXILIARY LABELS:

- Take before meals
- Do not crush or chew capsules
- If capsule is opened and sprinkled onto food: do not chew or crush granules

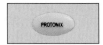

Wyeth-Ayerst

GENERIC NAME: pantoprazole
TRADE NAME: Protonix
INDICATION: GERD
ROUTE OF ADMINISTRATION: oral
COMMON DOSAGE: for GERD: 40 mg once daily for up to 8 weeks
AUXILIARY LABEL:

- Do not chew or crush tablet

GENERIC NAME: esomeprazole magnesium
TRADE NAME: Nexium
INDICATION: GERD
ROUTE OF ADMINISTRATION: oral
COMMON DOSAGE: 20 to 40 mg daily
AUXILIARY LABEL:

- Do not crush or chew

Peptic Ulcer Disease

H. pylori is a gram-negative bacillus. The bacterium can embed itself into the mucosal lining of the stomach, duodenum, and rectum. It is the cause of inflammation and peptic ulcers and is linked to cancer of the stomach. There are six laboratory tests that can be given to confirm the presence of *H. pylori*. They are listed in Table 20.5.

Medications to treat *H. pylori*, listed in Table 20.6, are the current treatments that have been approved by the FDA for eradication of *H. pylori*. Treatments consist of two, three, or four agents to be given simultaneously. The most effective

TABLE 20.5 Diagnostic Tests to Confirm *H. pylori*

Diagnostic Tests	Uses
Blood test	Confirms bacteria by elevated levels of antibody to *H. pylori*
Breath test	Carbon-labeled urea is given to patient. On exhaling, a change in the urea to ammonia detects the presence of bacteria
Tissue biopsy	After obtaining biopsy: four different laboratory tests can be run to confirm *H. pylori*

TABLE 20.6 *H. pylori* Agents

Regimens	Length of Tx
Amoxicillin (500 mg qid), clarithromycin, omeprazole	1 to 2 weeks
Tetracycline (500 mg qid), metronidazole, bismuth, omeprazole	1 week
Metronidazole (250 mg qid), amoxicillin, bismuth	1 to 2 weeks
Clarithromycin (500 mg tid/qid), omeprazole, metronidazole	1 week
Bismuth (525 mg qid), tetracycline, metronidazole	1 week
Omeprazole (20 mg bid), clarithromycin, amoxicillin, or tetracycline	2 weeks

combination is the four agents (bismuth, metronidazole, tetracycline, and omeprazole).

INTESTINAL CONDITIONS

Two of the most common symptoms affecting the intestinal tract are diarrhea and constipation. These can be caused by various infections of the GI system. Infections by bacteria, viruses, and parasites typically result in symptoms of diarrhea. Tumors and other obstructions can cause constipation; although most cases of diarrhea or constipation are isolated symptoms that can be treated with OTC medications. In addition, medications are among one of the most common causes of either diarrhea or constipation, and many physicians will prescribe stool softeners along with routine medications to alleviate potential problems.

Table 20.7 outlines major illnesses of the upper and lower intestines. Patients who require a bowel resection, such as for the removal of a tumor, may be required to wear a colostomy bag. These bags are attached to the abdominal wall with adhesive strips and allow for the emptying of the intestinal contents. The site of the colostomy varies depending on where the resection has taken place. The location of the colostomy determines the necessary replacement medications that a patient needs to take on a routine basis, such as laxatives or antidiarrheals. Because the intestinal tract is responsible for most of the nutrient absorption, if the colostomy site is close to the stomach, fewer nutrients can be absorbed through the intestine and must be provided to the patient. Other than having to empty the colostomy bag a few times during the day and changing the tubing twice weekly, a person can live a normal life with a colostomy.

Diarrhea

Treatment for diarrhea consists of agents that have an adsorbent and/or protectant quality. Activated attapulgite is most commonly used for its adsorbent and protectant ability, whereas bismuth has an adsorbent along with an antacid effect. These medications can be bought as OTC drugs and are considered safe by the FDA. As with any condition, if the symptoms do not disappear within a few days, it is advisable to visit the doctor to see if there is another underlying reason for the diarrhea. Diarrhea is also a very common side effect caused by medications. Bacteria can be another cause for diarrhea and can be deadly. Symptoms include watery stools, abdominal cramping, and general discomfort. As diarrhea continues, vital fluids as well as electrolytes are lost through the intestines. If these fluids are not replaced and the diarrhea brought under control, death can occur within days. Persons who are very susceptible to this danger are older adults and children. There are several agents, OTC and prescription, that can treat this condition (Table 20.8). OTC drugs include Kaopectate, FiberCon, and Pepto-Bismol. More potent drugs or controlled substances require a prescription. Agents such as Lomotil or Paregoric are meant for short-term use because they can become less effective with continued use. In some cases, the lack of normal intestinal

TABLE 20.7 Common Conditions Affecting the Gastrointestinal System

Condition	Definition	Symptoms	Treatment
Diverticular disease	Protrusions of the colon wall resulting from a weakened intestinal wall	Rectal bleeding, inflammation, and bowel obstruction	Surgery
Hemorrhoids	Lesions caused by enlargement and inflammation of veins in the rectum	Rectal bleeding, pain	Suppositories, creams, ointments
Crohn's disease	Congenital or acquired; chronic inflammation of the GI tract. Commonly occurs within the colon and terminal ileum	Abdominal pain, weight loss, diarrhea	Surgery or medications
Colitis	Congenital or acquired; inflammation of the intestines that commonly occurs in the large intestine	Rectal bleeding, pain	Surgery or medications

TABLE 20.8 Common OTC Antidiarrheal Agents

Trade Name	Ingredients	Common Dosage
Kaopectate	90 g kaolin, 2 g pectin	1 dose following each loose stool
Parepectolin	600 mg attapulgite, sucrose	1 dose following each loose stool up to 7 doses/day
Donnagel	600 mg attapulgite, saccharin, sorbitol	1 dose following each loose stool up to 7 doses/day
Diasorb	750 mg attapulgite, sorbitol	1 dose following each loose stool up to 3 doses/day
Imodium AD	2 mg loperamide	2 doses stat, then 1 dose following each loose stool up to 4 doses/day

OTC, Over-the-counter.

bacteria causes diarrhea. In this instance, a bacterial replacement therapy called *Lactobacillus* is used.

Medications Used to Treat Diarrhea

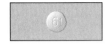

Searle

CLASSIFICATIONS: ANTIDIARRHEAL

GENERIC NAME: diphenoxylate w/atropine cv medication

TRADE NAME: Lomotil

ROUTE OF ADMINISTRATION: oral

INDICATION: acute or chronic diarrhea

DRUG ACTION: slows intestinal motility

COMMON DOSAGE: 2.5 to 5 mg qid, then prn

SIDE EFFECTS: dry mouth, dizzy, drowsy

AUXILIARY LABELS:

- May cause dizziness and drowsiness
- Do not drink alcohol
- Drink plenty of water

GENERIC NAME: loperamide

TRADE NAME: Imodium (Rx), Imodium AD (OTC)

ROUTE OF ADMINISTRATION: oral

INDICATION: acute or chronic diarrhea

DRUG ACTION: slows GI motility and increases viscosity of fecal matter

COMMON DOSAGE: 2 mg following each loose stool (Maximum 8 mg/day × 2 days)

SIDE EFFECTS: dizzy, drowsy, dry mouth

AUXILIARY LABELS:

- May cause dizziness and drowsiness
- Do not drink alcohol
- Drink plenty of water

GENERIC NAME: bismuth subsalicylate

TRADE NAME: Pepto-Bismol (OTC)

ROUTE OF ADMINISTRATION: oral

INDICATION: diarrhea and abdominal cramps

DRUG ACTION: antisecretory and antibacterial effects in GI

COMMON DOSAGE: 2 tablets or 30 mL (liquid) prn

SIDE EFFECTS: stools may appear grayish black

AUXILIARY LABELS:

- Drink plenty of water
- May cause dark stools
- Chew tablet before swallowing

Constipation

The lack of defecation or stools that are dry and very hard are the symptoms of constipation. This may be caused by a lack of fiber in the diet, a common problem in older adults. There are various classes of drugs used to treat this condition. Laxatives include bulk-forming types, stool softeners, hyperosmotic agents, and powerful stimulants. Bulk-forming agents work by absorbing water from the body to increase the moisture and overall bulk of the stools allowing for easier elimination. Stool softeners pull water and fatty compounds into the intestine to aid in elimination.

Hyperosmotic agents work by osmosis, increasing pressure within the bowels by drawing in water, similar to bulk-forming agents. For more stubborn bouts of constipation a stimulant may be used. These agents increase the peristalsis within the intestines (specifically the colon), which forces the contents out. Agents listed in Table 20.9 are examples of the many types of laxatives available. Bowel evacuants are used to empty the intestines before a procedure or surgery. Solutions that contain polyethylene glycol-electrolytes are loaded with replacement electrolytes because the intestines are not able to absorb the necessary ions from the expelled fecal material. Typically, the patient must drink approximately 4 L or 4000 mL of solution within a relatively short period of time. Other evacuants consist of a variety of laxatives to attain the same results.

Many gentle laxatives are available OTC, such as psyllium powder; however, there are some available OTC, such as Ex-Lax, that are very powerful. It is recommended to stay at home while taking these agents. Abdominal cramping is also a common occurrence if using more powerful laxatives. Persons who constantly take laxatives may eventually become dependent on them; therefore it is recommended to take them only as a short-term treatment. Nondrug treatments suggested to avoid constipation include the ingestion of adequate dietary fibers, found in fruits and vegetables, in the daily diet. Roughage also aids in good digestion and elimination. In addition to a well-balanced meal plan, drinking plenty of water also helps prevent constipation.

TABLE 20.9 Laxatives

Anticonstipation Agents	Ingredients	Normal Dosage	ROA
Over the Counter **Laxative**			
Milk of Magnesia	Magnesium hydroxide	30–60 mL prn	po
Sodium phosphates	Sodium phosphate, sodium biphosphate	20–30 mL prn	po
Stimulants			
Ex-Lax	Phenolphthalein	1 dose qhs	po
Bulk-Producing Laxatives			
FiberCon	500 mg calcium	qd-qid (max 6 g/day)	po
Enemas			
Fleet Bisacodyl	Bisacodyl	1 dose qd	pr
Fleet mineral oil	Mineral oil	1 dose qd	pr
Bowel Evacuants			
Fleet Prep Kit 1	45 mL Phospho-Soda	1 dose	po
	4 bisacodyl tablets		po
	1 bisacodyl suppository		pr
Prescription			
Laxative			
Cephulac	Lactulose	15–30 mL qd	po
Bowel Evacuants			
Golytely	PEGES, sodium sulfate, sodium bicarb, sodium chloride, potassium chloride	1 dose (4L)	po

ROA, Route of administration; *PEG*, poly ethylene glycol; *po*, by mouth; *pr*, per rectum.

Bulk-Forming Medications

CLASSIFICATION: BULK-FORMING LAXATIVES
GENERIC NAME: psyllium (OTC)
TRADE NAME: Metamucil
INDICATION: constipation
ROUTE OF ADMINISTRATION: oral
DRUG ACTION: holds water within the intestine allowing stools to pass
COMMON DOSAGE: prn
SIDE EFFECTS: n/a
SPECIAL NOTES: also used to reduce cholesterol levels in persons with hyperlipidemia

All laxatives should be used only as short-term treatments for constipation.

CLASSIFICATION: SURFACTANT
GENERIC NAME: docusate sodium (OTC) AKA: DSS
TRADE NAME: Colace
INDICATION: constipation
ROUTE OF ADMINISTRATION: oral, rectal (enema)
DRUG ACTION: retains fat and water in bowels allowing stools to pass
COMMON DOSAGE: orally 50 to 500 mg once daily
SIDE EFFECTS: n/a

GENERIC NAME: bisacodyl (OTC)
TRADE NAME: Ducolax
INDICATION: constipation
ROUTE OF ADMINISTRATION: oral, rectal (suppository or enema)
DRUG ACTION: acts on increasing intestine mucosal lining and water softening stools
COMMON DOSAGE: one rectally once daily as needed
SIDE EFFECTS: n/a

GENERIC NAME: senna (OTC)
TRADE NAME: Senokot
INDICATION: constipation (Also used for constipation from opioid agents)
ROUTE OF ADMINISTRATION: oral
DRUG ACTION: irritates intestinal wall and causes osmotic gradient, softening stools
COMMON DOSAGE: 30 mg one to two times per day
SIDE EFFECTS: n/a

GENERIC NAME: glycerin (OTC)
TRADE NAME: Glycerin
INDICATION: constipation
ROUTE OF ADMINISTRATION: rectal
DRUG ACTION: irritates intestinal wall and causes osmotic gradient, softening stools; rectal lubricant
COMMON DOSAGE: one suppository rectally once daily as needed
SIDE EFFECTS: n/a

OTHER CONDITIONS

Emesis

Although most people have experienced nausea and vomiting at one time or another, it is usually an isolated event. Persons who are subjected to chemotherapeutic agents as a part of cancer treatment must deal with extreme nausea and vomiting. The chemotherapy agents damage the lining of the stomach and other areas of the body, causing emesis as a common side effect. This violent reaction of the body is controlled from the medulla oblongata located within the brain. Known as the chemoreceptor trigger zone or nausea zone, this small area can be activated by smell, pain, medication, motion sickness (caused by relay from the inner ear), and even emotions. When the chemoreceptor trigger zone is activated, chemical signals are sent via the nervous system to the vomit center (Figure 20.5), which then relays the message down to the stomach where muscles of the diaphragm, stomach, esophagus, and the salivary glands working together cause the vomiting reflex. Drugs used to treat this condition are referred to as antiemetics.

Most antiemetics require a prescription because of their effects on the chemoreceptor trigger zone, which is located near the respiratory center of the brain. When this area is inhibited it can cause a decrease in respiration. Agents that do not affect the chemoreceptor trigger zone can be bought OTC and are usually used for motion sickness. All of the following agents are available by prescription or OTC. For the following agents only the normal oral dosages are given.

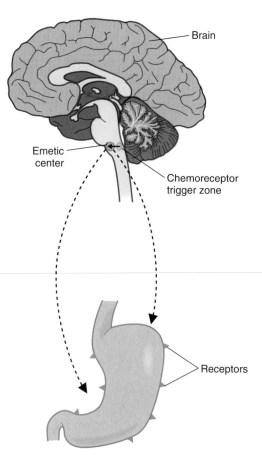

FIGURE 20.5 Chemoreceptor trigger zone. Located in the brain, the chemoreceptor trigger zone is responsible for signaling the emetic center, which causes the vomiting reflex.

Antiemetic Medications
Legend Drugs

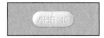

A.H. Robins

CLASSIFICATION: ANTIEMETIC
GENERIC NAME: metoclopramide
TRADE NAME: Reglan
INDICATION: for the relief of nausea and vomiting
ROUTE OF ADMINISTRATION: oral, IV
DRUG ACTION: blocks dopamine receptors in chemoreceptor trigger zone and increases GI motility
COMMON DOSAGE: nonchemotherapy dosing: 10 mg before meals and at bedtime as needed
SIDE EFFECTS: diarrhea, drowsy, restlessness
AUXILIARY LABELS:

- May cause dizziness and drowsiness
- Alcohol may intensify this effect

GENERIC NAME: thiethylperazine maleate
TRADE NAME: Torecan
INDICATION: for the relief of nausea and vomiting
ROUTE OF ADMINISTRATION: oral, IV
DRUG ACTION: inhibits chemoreceptor trigger zone and vomit center
COMMON DOSAGE: 10 mg once to three times daily as needed
SIDE EFFECTS: dizzy, drowsy, dry mouth, rash, fever, headache
AUXILIARY LABELS:

- May cause dizziness and drowsiness
- Alcohol may intensify this effect
- Drink plenty of water

GENERIC NAME: trimethobenzamide
TRADE NAME: Tigan
INDICATION: for the relief of nausea and vomiting
ROUTE OF ADMINISTRATION: oral, rectal, IV
DRUG ACTION: depresses the chemoreceptor trigger zone
COMMON DOSAGE: 250 mg tid to qid
SIDE EFFECTS: dizzy, drowsy, diarrhea, headache, blurred vision
AUXILIARY LABELS:

- May cause dizziness and drowsiness
- Alcohol may intensify this effect
- Drink plenty of water

CLASSIFICATION: ANTICHOLINERGIC
GENERIC NAME: scopolamine
TRADE NAME: Trasnderm-scop
INDICATION: for the relief of nausea and vomiting
ROUTE OF ADMINISTRATION: IM, IV, SC, topical
DRUG ACTION: affects chemoreceptor trigger zone directly by blocking serotonin in brainstem and GI tract
COMMON DOSAGE: apply 1 patch behind ear 4 hours before stimulation every 3 days
SIDE EFFECTS: dizzy, drowsy, headache
AUXILIARY LABELS:

- May cause dizziness and drowsiness
- Alcohol may intensify this effect

CLASSIFICATION: SEROTONIN RECEPTOR ANTAGONIST

GENERIC NAME: ondansetron Hydrochloride

TRADE NAME: Zofran

INDICATION: for the relief of nausea and vomiting, used with chemotherapy

ROUTE OF ADMINISTRATION: oral, injectable

DRUG ACTION: affects chemoreceptor trigger zone directly by blocking serotonin in brainstem and GI tract

COMMON DOSAGE: 8 mg 30 minutes before chemotherapy treatment then 8 mg 8 hours after dose followed by 8 mg every 12 hours for several days

SIDE EFFECTS: fever, headache, constipation, diarrhea

AUXILIARY LABELS:

- Take as directed
- Do not drink alcohol

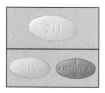

Roerig

CLASSIFICATION: ANTICHOLINERGICS

GENERIC NAME: meclizine

TRADE NAME: Antivert, Bonine Antiver/50 RX only

INDICATION: to relieve nausea and vomiting resulting from motion sickness

ROUTE OF ADMINISTRATION: oral

DRUG ACTION: affects the labyrinth within the inner ear decreasing stimulation

COMMON DOSAGE: 12.5 to 25 mg 1 hour before exposure to stimulus

SIDE EFFECTS: dizzy, drowsy, dry mouth

SPECIAL NOTES: meclizine is also available in 25-mg and 50-mg tablets but requires a prescription

GENERIC NAME: dimenhydrinate

TRADE NAME: Dramamine

INDICATION: to relieve nausea and vomiting resulting from motion sickness

ROUTE OF ADMINISTRATION: oral, IM, IV

DRUG ACTION: affects the labyrinth within the inner ear decreasing stimulation

COMMON DOSAGE: 50 to 100 mg every 4 to 6 hours

SIDE EFFECTS: dizzy, drowsy, dry mouth

*OTC strength

Flatulence

More commonly called gas, flatulence can be caused by the byproduct of microbial breakdown of food (see Chapter 29). Also, certain foods are known to produce gas such as broccoli, onions, and garlic. Symptoms are discomfort and pain within the abdominal cavity. The only OTC medication used for the treatment of gas is simethicone. This medication comes in tablets, chew tablets, and liquid for children.

Antiflatulence Medications

CLASSIFICATION: ANTIFLATULENT

GENERIC NAME: simethicone

TRADE NAME: Gas-X; Mylecon

INDICATION: for the relief of gas and abdominal distension caused by gas

ROUTE OF ADMINISTRATION: oral

COMMON DOSAGE: 40 to 80 mg up to four times daily as needed

SIDE EFFECTS: none

General Information

Because the GI system can be affected by outside forces, such as bacteria, viruses, parasites, medications, and emotions, this system is a complicated one. There are numerous OTC remedies available to consumers to treat a variety of symptoms. As the median age increases across America and around the world, there is an increase in the amount of routine medication that is taken to help deter illness. Imbalances that affect the GI system can alter the amount of nutrients the body can absorb and the chain reaction that allows for the chemical breakdown of food. If this chain reaction breaks down, side effects may occur. By reducing stress, eating a well-balanced diet, and exercising, the GI tract is better able to remain in good working condition. However, those who are diagnosed with a more severe condition have many medications and sometimes surgery available to treat their illness. If at all possible, it is important to take care of the GI system before problems occur.

DO YOU REMEMBER THESE KEY POINTS?

- The major parts that make up the digestive system
- The pH of the stomach and its importance
- The function of the stomach and intestines
- The major conditions covered in this chapter that affect the GI system
- The agents used to treat common conditions such as indigestion
- The ingredients used in antacids
- The generic names of the medications covered in this chapter
- The difference between GERD and *H. pylori* infection
- The treatment for *H. pylori* infection
- The difference between laxatives such as cathartics and stool softeners

REVIEW QUESTIONS:

Multiple Choice

1. The three main functions of the GI system include all of the following except
   A. Digestion
   B. Absorption
   C. Secretion
   D. Metabolism
   E. All of the above are functions

2. Auxiliary organs to the GI system include all those listed except
   A. Pancreas
   B. Liver
   C. Gallbladder
   D. Appendix
   E. All of the above are auxiliary organs

3. The function of the epiglottis is to
   A. Break down food particles
   B. Digest food
   C. Block off the tracheal tube
   D. Aid in peristalsis

4. The pH of the stomach is acidic and its function is to
   A. Help in digestion by breaking down food into chyme
   B. Help move food through the intestines
   C. Help the absorption of food in the stomach
   D. Help in metabolism

5. The pyloric sphincter is located _____ and allows chyme to pass when _____.
   A. At the top of the stomach; relaxed
   B. At the base of the stomach; tense
   C. At the opening of the small intestine; tense
   D. At the opening of the small intestine; relaxed

6. The duodenum, jejunum, and the ileum make up the
   A. Stomach
   B. Small intestine
   C. Large intestine
   D. Adjacent organs to the GI system

7. Bile is made by the _____ and stored by the _____.
   A. Gallbladder; liver
   B. Liver; gallbladder
   C. Pancreas; gallbladder
   D. Liver; pancreas

8. Excretion takes place mainly in the _____.
   A. Stomach
   B. Small intestine
   C. Large intestine
   D. Rectum

9. A person diagnosed with GERD may be placed on which of the following medications?
   A. Antacids
   B. H$_2$ antagonists
   C. Proton pump inhibitors
   D. All of the above

10. Ulcers that can be attributed to hyperacidity include all those listed except
   A. Peptic
   B. Duodenal
   C. GERD
   D. *H. pylori*

True/false

*If the statement is false, then change it to make it true.

1. Chyme is an acidic mixture of small food particles.

2. Anabolism is the breaking down of molecules, whereas catabolism is the building of molecules; each representing a part of metabolism.

3. Proteins are broken into simple sugars by enzymatic actions.

4. Most antacids should be given twice daily, once in the morning and at bedtime.

5. Simethicone is an antacid that is added to many stomach medications.

6. H$_2$ receptors are located in the lungs.

7. Carbonates are used to balance pH concentrations.

8. The drug action for proton pump inhibitors is that they inhibit gastric secretions and block enzymes.

9. Aluminum and magnesium both can cause diarrhea as a side effect.

10. *H. pylori* is a gram-positive microbe that infects the esophagus.

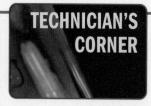
TECHNICIAN'S CORNER

A. A patient comes in to fill a prescription in your pharmacy. The prescription calls for codeine 30 mg. Take 1-2 tablets every 4 to 6 hours as needed for pain. The quantity indicates #100.

   What OTC medication was probably prescribed by the physician or will be suggested by the pharmacist at the time of consultation and why?

B. A patient who tested positive for *H. pylori* comes into the pharmacy and gives you a prescription for the following agents:
   Clarithromycin
   Omeprazole
   Metronidazole

Question: What would be the recommended strengths and the dosing of these medications? Also give the length of time the medications should be taken and how it is determined whether they should be stopped?

BIBLIOGRAPHY

Drug Facts and Comparisons 1999, St Louis, 1999, Facts and Comparisons.

McKenry L, Salerno E: *Pharmacology in Nursing,* ed 21, St Louis, 2001, Mosby.

Goodman G, Gillman L: *The Pharmacological Basis of Therapeutics,* ed 8, Elmsford, NY, 1990, McGraw Hill.

Koda-Kimble M, Young L: *Applied Therapeutics: The Clinical Use of Drugs,* ed 7, Philadelphia, 2001, Lippincott.

Mosby's Drug Consult, St Louis, 2004, Elsevier.

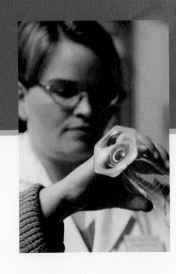

21

Urinary System

Objectives

- Describe the location and function of the kidneys.

- Explain the functions of the nephrons.

- Describe the location and function of the bladder.

- Differentiate between secretion and reabsorption.

- List the most common conditions that affect the urinary system.

- Describe the drug action of various diuretics discussed in this chapter.

- List the most commonly used diuretics.

- Describe dialysis treatments and the medications that are given with them.

- List the auxiliary labels necessary when filling diuretic prescriptions.

- List the major medications for dialysis.

Terms And Definitions

Acidification *The conversion to an acid environment*

Acidosis *The increase of acid content in the blood resulting from the accumulation of acid or loss of bicarbonate; the pH of blood is lowered*

Alkalosis *The increase of alkalinity in the blood resulting from the accumulation of alkali or reduction of acid content; the pH of blood is raised*

Blood urea nitrogen (BUN) *A test that measures the nitrogen in the blood in the form of urea*

Congestive heart failure (CHF) *Accumulation of blood in the circulatory due to inefficient pumping of the heart*

Dialysis *The passage of a solute through a semipermeable membrane to remove toxic materials and to maintain fluid, electrolyte, and pH levels of the body system when the kidneys no longer work*

Diuresis *The secretion and passage of large amounts of urine from the body*

Diuretics *An agent that increases urine output and diuresis*

Edema *A local or generalized condition in which body tissues retain excessive amounts of tissue fluid*

Excretion *The elimination of waste products from the body*

Hyperkalemia *An excessive amount of potassium in the blood*

Hypokalemia *An abnormally low concentration of potassium in the blood*

Incontinence *Loss of control over excretion of urine or feces*

Micturition *Urination*

Nocturia *Having to urinate excessively at night*

Pyelonephritis *Inflammation of the kidney and renal pelvis*

Urinary retention *The inability to empty the bladder completely*

Urea *The main nitrogenous constituent of urine and final product of protein metabolism; formed in the liver*

Uremia *The buildup of urea and other nitrogenous products within the body that would normally be excreted by healthy kidneys*

Urolithiasis *Kidney stones*

COMMONLY USED DRUGS FOR THE URINARY SYSTEM

Trade	Generic	Pronunciation	Trade	Generic	Pronunciation
Thiazide and Similar Drugs			**Potassium-Sparing Diuretics**		
Diuril	chlorothiazide	klor-oh-**thigh**-ah-zide	Aldactone	spironolactone	spear-own-oh-**lak**-tone
Hygroton	chlorthalidone	klor-**thal**-ah-doan	Aldactazide	spironolactone w/HCTZ	
Lozol	indapamide	in-**dap**-ah-myde	Dyrenium	triamterene	try-**am**-tur-een
Esidrix	hydrochlorothiazide	high-drow-klor-oh-**thigh**-ah-zide	Dyazide, Maxzide	triamterene w/HCTZ	
Zaroxolyn	metolazone	me-**toe**-lah-zone	Midamor	amiloride	ah-**mill**-or-ide
			Moduretic	amiloride w/HCTZ	
Loop Diuretics			**Potassium Replacement Supplements**		
Bumex	bumetanide	byew-**met**-ah-nide	K-Dur, Slow-K, K-Lor	potassium chloride	
Demadex	torsemide	**tore**-sea-myde	K-Lyte	potassium bicarbonate/ citrate	
Lasix	furosemide	feur-**oh**-sah-myde			
Osmotic Diuretics			**Dialysis Agents**		
Diamox	acetazolamide	ah-see-ta-**zoe**-la-myde	Epogen, Procrit	epoetin	eh-**poh**-ee-tin
Mannitol	mannitol	**man**-ah-tol			

HCTZ, Hydrochlorothiazide.

Introduction

The kidneys are located inside the upper abdominal cavity on either side of the vertebra as shown in Figure 21.1. The right kidney is located a little lower than the left because the liver is located directly above. A fibrous connective tissue called the renal fascia holds the kidneys stationary. The shape of the kidneys is similar to the shape of a kidney bean with a small indentation called the hilus. Blood enters the kidneys at the hilus via the renal artery and is filtered in the kidney. Important ions such as sodium (Na) and chloride (Cl) are reabsorbed into the body and circulatory system. The renal vein and ureter leave the kidney at the hilus. The renal vein returns the blood to the body after it has undergone the filtering process. The ureter carries wastes removed from the blood to the bladder where the waste is stored for excretion.

The bladder is similar to a holding tank that can expand. When the bladder becomes full we feel the urge to urinate. The urine is eliminated through the

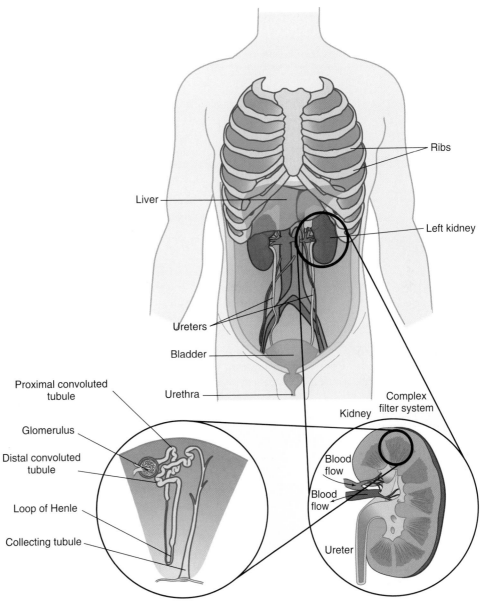

FIGURE 21.1 Anatomy of urinary tract and nephrons.

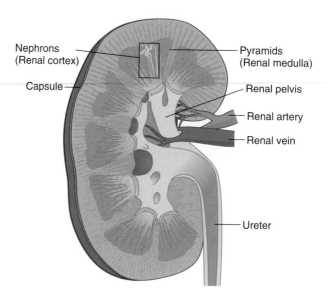

FIGURE 21.2 Anatomy of the kidney.

urethra, which is a shorter tube leading from the bladder to the outside of the body (Figure 21.2).

Function of the Kidneys

The kidneys play an important role in our daily lives. All the food and drink that is consumed is metabolized by the liver and ultimately carried to the kidneys where filtration is carried out and important nutrients and chemicals are allowed to reenter the body system for cellular use. The remaining waste is eliminated in a process called excretion. Excretion is one of the four major important functions of the body:

1. Absorption. The intake of liquids, solids, and gases into the body fluids and tissues
2. Distribution. The way in which chemicals or drug agents are separated throughout the body
3. Metabolism. How chemical changes and all transformations occur within the body system. It includes anabolism (building up processes) and catabolism (breaking down processes)
4. Excretion. The elimination of chemicals and substances from the body system

The bladder has walls that can expand to hold up to 1000 ml (1 L) of urine if necessary. The body excretes about 960 ml of urine per day. Urine contains urea, which is produced by the liver. It is a form of nitrogen which, on standing for a period of time, changes to ammonia. This gives urine its ammonia odor. The kidneys also have an important function: balancing the fluid content of the body. Most of the body is composed of fluids such as water, blood, and plasma and various ions such as chloride (Cl), potassium (K), and sodium (Na). The kidneys balance ions within the blood and eliminate excess ions in the blood. When excess ions are present in the bloodstream, certain conditions such as acidosis or alkalosis can occur. Acidosis is when too many free hydrogen ions are present, and alkalosis occurs when too many hydroxide ions are present. The blood urea nitrogen (BUN) test is used to determine the levels of acid in the patient's system. Patients who have kidney conditions or those who are taking medications that may weaken the effectiveness of the kidneys may have this test done. Although the kidneys are only about the size of a fist, they manage to filter about 50 gallons (6400 ml) of blood products everyday. Plasma travels through an amazing 140 miles of tubules contained inside the kidneys.

NEPHRON FUNCTION

The portion of the kidneys that does the work of separation is the nephrons. Each kidney contains millions of microscopic nephrons (Figure 21.3). Each nephron is shaped like an inverted pyramid with many twists and turns of its tubules; the nephrons work 24 hours a day. The following is a step-by-step look into the filtering process by following the blood as it enters the kidney:

1. The renal artery containing blood enters the kidneys where it divides into smaller and smaller vessels until it becomes an afferent arteriole, which in turn enters Bowman's capsule and becomes capillaries. The capillaries are called a glomerulus. Bowman's capsule (which resembles a baseball glove) covers the glomerulus.

2. Blood cells, platelets, and large proteins are not allowed to pass through the capillaries of the glomerulus into Bowman's capsule. Only plasma can pass through the glomerulus. Plasma is composed of all the contents of blood other than the cells and platelets. However, some of the components of plasma are still to large to leave the capillaries, such as albumins and globulins. Other components of plasma include toxins that may build up in the blood. These are so small that they can easily leave the capillaries and enter the Bowman's capsule.

3. The filtrate from Bowman's capsule travels down the descending tubule called the proximal convoluted tubule and back up the ascending tubule called the distal convoluted tubule. The u-turn part of the nephron is called the loop of Henle.

4. As the filtrate passes through the nephron tubules, various nutrients and important chemical ions such as chloride, potassium, and water are pulled out of the filtrate and returned to the plasma to be used for cellular nourishment. At the same time other ions in the tubules (such as those in excess) are excreted.

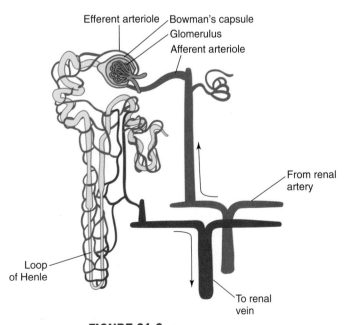

FIGURE 21.3 Nephron anatomy.

5. The filtrate, now called urine, travels to the collecting ducts where it leaves the nephron.
6. The ducts empty directly into the ureter.
7. The ureter goes directly to the bladder.
8. The bladder empties the urine into the urethra and the urine travels out of the body.

Tubular Reabsorption

The first function of the nephrons is tubular reabsorption. This is a process in which important molecules are separated from the filtrate into their individual components. Some of these molecules are eventually excreted in urine, whereas others such as glucose (sugar), water, sodium, chloride, and amino acids (proteins) reenter the plasma. This takes place at various points in the proximal convoluted tubule, distal convoluted tubule, and in the loop of Henle (Figure 21.4).

The kidneys balance the acid-base content of the body. There are two mechanisms that affect the balance of ions. The first is ion exchange. Sodium ions are pulled out of the tubules and are exchanged for hydrogen ions. As sodium builds up on the outside of the proximal convoluted tubules, it creates an osmotic gradient and water molecules are drawn toward the higher concentration of sodium. This is called osmosis (Figure 21.5). The overall effect is a decrease in excreted water. Ion exchange can also take place in the distal convoluted tubule. As sodium ions exit the nephron tubule, they are exchanged for potassium ions. In the loop of Henle, there is a different mechanism. This mechanism is called active trans-

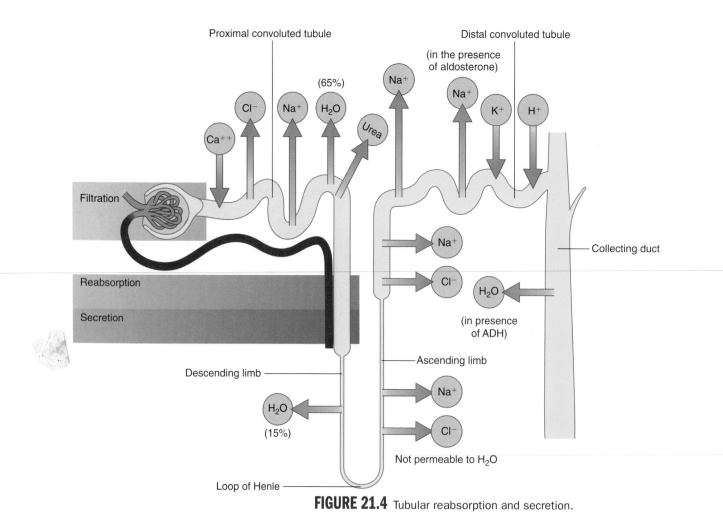

FIGURE 21.4 Tubular reabsorption and secretion.

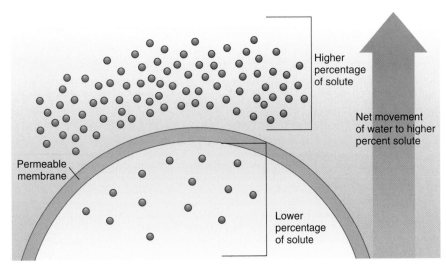

FIGURE 21.5 Also known as an osmotic gradient, the smaller water molecules gravitate toward the highly concentrated sodium ions.

port. Instead of an exchange of ions, there is a one-way uptake of sodium and chloride from the loop of Henle. These ions return to the circulatory system. Most of the sodium that enters the renal system is returned to the circulatory system.

TECH NOTE! Sodium helps conduct nerve impulses and balance fluid through reabsorption in the kidneys.

Tubular Secretion

Tubular secretion is another major function of the nephrons. This function takes place throughout the nephron. Various ions, toxins, and water are secreted into to the collecting duct. First, molecules such as toxins, water-soluble molecules, and excess or unnecessary chemicals are excreted. Weak acids, such as aspirin and penicillin, weak bases, such as narcotic analgesics, and antihistamines are the types of chemicals that are secreted and eliminated. The second function of secretion is to allow the kidneys to regulate the pH of the body through urine acidification. Acidification is the process of eliminating extra hydrogen ions through the urine. This is why urine has an acid content between a pH of 4 and 5, whereas the blood's pH is maintained at approximately 7.4.

As hydrogen ions are taken into the nephron tubules, they combine with other molecules to produce bicarbonate. This is then released into the bloodstream where it regulates the overall pH of the body, helping to maintain homeostasis. Bicarbonate is a buffer. A buffer has the ability to bind hydrogen (which creates a basic environment) or release hydrogen (which creates an acidic environment by liberating a base) balancing the blood pH. To put it another way, an acid can release hydrogen ions, whereas a base can remove hydrogen by binding the hydrogen to itself. The extra hydrogen ions are taken into the tubules and eventually excreted.

Conditions Affecting the Urinary System

It seems as though it would be impossible for people to survive very long without the constant functioning of both kidneys; however, many people live with just one kidney. The kidneys are so efficient that as little as 20% of them need to be working

TABLE 21.1 Conditions Affecting the Urinary System

Anuria	Lack of urine: less than 100 ml over 24 hours
Cystitis	Inflammation of the bladder
Edema	Increase in fluid in cells, tissues, and/or cavities
Hyperkalemia	Excessive increase in potassium in the blood
Hypokalemia	Excessive decrease in potassium in the blood
Incontinence	Lack of control of urination or feces
Oliguria	Little urine output: Between 100 ml and 400 ml over 24 hours
Polyuria	Excessive or large volume of urine within a certain time
Pyelonephritis	Inflammation of the kidney
Renal failure	Kidney no longer functions
Uremia	Excess urea in the blood
Urethritis	Inflammation of the urethra
Urolithiasis	Kidney stones made of calcium or salts
Urinary tract infection (UTI)	Infection of the urinary tract caused by microorganisms

for survival. This does not mean that a person does not have to watch diet, medications, and activities, but many people can live normal lives with only one kidney or a partial kidney functioning. In some cases, however, dialysis or even kidney transplants may be necessary. The bladder can also create problems if there is residual urine that does not leave the body. This can lead to infection of the kidneys.

Other conditions that can affect the kidneys and urinary system in general include blockages or infections of the kidney, ureter, bladder, and urethra. Drinking plenty of water is one of the most effective ways of taking care of the urinary system because it helps to cleanse the body of toxins and other unwanted chemicals. Other common conditions affecting the urinary system are listed in Table 21.1.

RENAL FAILURE

There are many possible causes that can lead to renal failure such as accidents, toxic agents, genetic diseases, or certain illnesses. For example, persons who are at high risk of renal failure include those with human immunodeficiency virus (HIV), diabetes mellitus, leukemia, Hodgkin's disease, and those with genetic predispositions. A common genetic disease that can cause renal failure is polycystic renal disease. This disease can affect a person in childhood or in adulthood. The kidney becomes enlarged and filled with cysts, and, if progression is fast, the kidney eventually fails. In many cases, the deterioration of the kidneys can at least be decreased through the use of medications.

Older people suffer from acute renal failure more often than younger adults. As a kidney ages, it is less able to compensate for fluid imbalances of the body. Cardiovascular disease, diabetes mellitus, and other diseases are the most common causes of renal failure in older people. As renal failure progresses, every part of the body is affected because of the buildup of waste products and an imbalance of fluids. Some of the symptoms of end-stage renal disease are listed in Table 21.2.

EDEMA

Millions of people suffer from edema caused by congestive heart failure (CHF) or hypertension. In CHF, the heart muscle is weakened by disease. This decreases

TABLE 21.2 End Stage Renal Disease Symptoms*

System	Effect
Cardiovascular	Hypertension, CHF
Respiratory	Pulmonary edema, dyspnea
GI	Nausea, vomiting, GI bleed
Endocrine	Hyperthyroidism
Eye	Hypertensive retinopathy
Nervous	Fatigue, confusion, seizures

CHF, Congestive heart failure; *GI*, gastrointestinal.
*Other symptoms include problems with the skin, nerves, blood, and metabolism and psychological problems.

its efficiency, and as the blood is pumped less and less through the body, the following signs and symptoms may occur:

- Edema in the extremities, such as the legs, ankles, feet, and hands, and edema in the liver, abdominal cavity, lungs, and other areas of the body
- Chest pain resulting from the decreased oxygen to and increased workload of the diseased heart
- Fatigue, dyspnea, and orthopnea from the lack of oxygen in the body

In CHF, when the kidneys get signals that there is a lack of blood content in the body, they try to solve the problem by retaining fluid. This in turn puts more work on the heart, creating the vicious cycle of CHF. Only with the use of medications can a person suffering from CHF extend his or her life. There is no cure. Persons suffering from hypertension must be especially careful because the condition may eventually damage the veins within the heart muscle, which can lead to CHF.

Depending on the disorder of the urinary system, different treatments or medications are prescribed by a physician. In the next section, we discuss the types of treatments and medications used for urinary conditions.

URINARY TRACT INFECTIONS

Noscomial Infection

One of the most common conditions that can affect the urinary system is a urinary tract infection (UTI). Many of the infections are nosocomial in origin. This means the infection was picked up while the patient was in the hospital for a different reason. Most of these types of nosocomial infections are due to catheterization or cystoscopic examinations. Regardless of the cause it is important to determine the specific organism in order to prescribe the proper medication. Infections of the kidney are called pyelonephritis, whereas a bladder infection is called cystitis.

KIDNEY STONES

Kidney stones are experienced by hundreds of thousands of Americans every year. Although stones are most commonly found in persons between the ages of 20 and 55, they can affect anyone. They occur at a somewhat higher percentage in Caucasians than African Americans, and they tend to run in families. There are different types of stones and each one has a specific treatment; therefore it is imperative that a urologist determines which one is the cause. The different types of stones are listed in Table 21.3 along with their characteristics and treatments.

TABLE 21.3 Types of Kidney Stones

Type	Possible Cause	Characteristic	Treatment
Cystine	Genetic	Decreased absorption of cystine in GI tract causes buildup	Penicillamine, potassium citrate
Uric acid	Gout, genetic	Seen more in men, especially Jewish men	Potassium citrate, change diet
Struvite	UTI	Seen more in women	Antimicrobials, surgery
Calcium phosphate	Hyperparathyroidism	Appearance of both struvite or oxalate stones	Treat hyperparathyroidism, alkaline urine
Calcium oxalate	Genetic, idiopathic hypercalcuria	Small stones, seen more in men	Increase water intake, decrease oxalate in diet

GI, gastrointestinal; UTI, urinary tract infection.

Treatments for Urinary System Conditions

DIALYSIS

When a person has lost too much of their kidney function, has end stage renal disease, and a transplant is not an option, dialysis is the only alternative. Although transplants are relatively common and have a high rate of success, unfortunately there are not enough donors to supply kidneys. There are many patients whose names are on transplant waiting lists for years. While they wait, dialysis is the patients' option. Sometimes a transplant may not be an option because the donor's kidneys are not compatible with the recipient's. Also, many times people do not want to have surgery to replace their kidneys.

Dialysis is the cleansing of the blood for patients with end stage renal disease. This treatment replaces the normal kidney function of removing wastes and balancing fluids. There are two major methods in use today, hemodialysis and peritoneal dialysis. A newer third type, nocturnal dialysis, may be yet another choice. Although each of these types of dialysis has drawbacks, they keep people alive. Drawbacks include the additional medications that patients must take to further balance pH and fluids, the inconvenience of having to be stationary for a length of time, and the fact that even sophisticated machinery cannot perform as efficiently as one's own kidneys.

Hemodialysis requires the patient to visit a clinic or hospital for treatment. The patient is hooked up by a vein shunt (needle puncture with a reinforced opening) to a machine that takes a small but steady stream of blood from the body and cleans it of impurities using a mechanical filtration system. Patients undergoing this treatment feel very good afterwards; however, over time the body builds up toxins again and they begin to feel ill. Although the length of treatment varies, it normally takes around 5 hours two to three times weekly.

Peritoneal dialysis is an alternative to hemodialysis. The patient is hooked up to a bag of osmotic solution. A catheter plug is implanted into the abdominal cavity for administration and removal of the solution. The osmotic solution flows into the peritoneal cavity. The peritoneal membrane is a thin lining that encases the organs of the abdomen, including the stomach, liver, spleen, and kidneys. The osmotic solution works in the same fashion as the sodium gradient works in the kidneys. As the solution is allowed to fill the cavity, wastes are pulled into the solution where they can be drained from the cavity into an empty bag attached to the abdominal wall on the outside. This treatment usually is done on a daily basis to keep toxins to a minimum. Treatments can be done at home; however, it

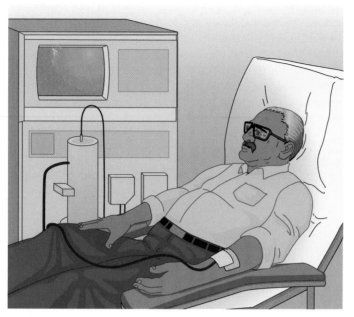

Hemodialysis

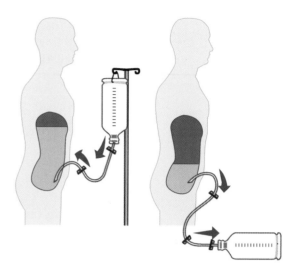

Continuous ambulatory peritoneal dialysis

FIGURE 21.6 Types of dialysis.

can be done in clinics if the patient cannot afford a home health nurse to assist him or her (Figure 21.6).

Nocturnal dialysis is a newer treatment that is being tested here in the United States. It allows the patient to receive treatment while sleeping. Because it can be done very slowly over the course of the night, the patient keeps the system at a steadier state of wellness. Patients do not have to wait between treatments, which is when they begin to feel the effects of toxic buildup nor do they have to visit clinics or be immobilized for hours at a time. Although this treatment may sound like the best option, the patient must have a full hemodialysis system in the bedroom, which is both costly and unwieldy. Also, he or she must be able to troubleshoot problems with the machinery if there is a malfunction. Finally, the patient must have a home health nurse to help with the treatment.

People on dialysis have to be careful of their fluid and salt intake. With any of these treatments there is a loss of ions and nutrients that must be replaced with supplements each time dialysis is performed. One of the most common side effects of dialysis is anemia. For this condition iron and erythropoietin are given to the patient. Iron increases the oxygen-carrying capacity of the hemoglobin. Hemoglobin is a protein within the red blood cells that carries oxygen with the help of iron. Both iron and erythropoietin agents are listed in the following.

Replacement Therapy for Dialysis

CLASSIFICATION: MINERAL

GENERIC NAME: ferrous sulfate

TRADE NAME: Feosol

ROUTE OF ADMINISTRATION: oral

INDICATION: dialysis, also for iron deficiency

COMMON DOSAGE: hemodialysis (900 mg); peritoneal dialysis (500 to 900 mg)

SIDE EFFECTS: constipation, black stools

AUXILIARY LABEL:

■ May cause black stools

SPECIAL NOTE: Iron supplements are normally taken with a stool softener to counteract the side effect of constipation

CLASSIFICATION: BLOOD FORMER
GENERIC NAME: epoetinaefa (erythropoietin)
TRADE NAME: Epogen, Procrit
ROUTE OF ADMINISTRATION: subcutaneous or intravenous (IV)
INDICATION: dialysis
COMMON DOSAGE: for dialysis patients: 75 units/kg three times weekly
SIDE EFFECTS: HTN, headache, nausea and vomiting
SPECIAL NOTE: erythropoietin must be kept refrigerated

TREATMENT OF EDEMA

The main drugs used for the treatment of edema include diuretic thiazides, thiazide-like agents, loop diuretics, potassium-sparing agents, carbonic anhydrase inhibitors, and osmotics. Each classification is discussed along with its drug action and a listing of each medication.

Thiazides and Thiazide-like Agents

The drug action of these agents is the equal increase of urinary excretion of the ions sodium and chloride. They do this by inhibiting the normal process of reabsorption within the ascending tubule following the loop of Henle and in the early distal tubules. They also increase the loss of potassium and bicarbonate. Their onset of action is rapid. Because of the loss of potassium, a potassium supplement must be taken concurrently with this type of medication. Common side effects for all thiazides include frequent urination. For this reason they are normally to be taken early in the day to avoid nocturia.

The normal dosage given is for an adult maintenance dose for edema.

CLASSIFICATION: THIAZIDE OR THIAZIDE-LIKE DIURETICS
GENERIC NAME: indapamide
TRADE NAME: Lozol
ROUTE OF ADMINISTRATION: oral
COMMON DOSAGE: 2.5 mg once daily
SIDE EFFECTS: headache, dizziness, upset stomach
AUXILIARY LABELS:
- Take with food or milk
- Do not crush tablet

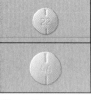

Novartis

GENERIC NAME: hydrochlorothiazide
TRADE NAME: Esidrix
ROUTE OF ADMINISTRATION: oral
COMMON DOSAGE: 25 to 100 mg daily or intermittently
SIDE EFFECTS: may cause gastrointestinal (GI) upset and photosensitivity
AUXILIARY LABELS:
- Take with food or milk
- May cause photosensitivity

GENERIC NAME: chlorothiazide
TRADE NAME: Diuril
ROUTE OF ADMINISTRATION: oral, IV
COMMON DOSAGE: 0.5 to 1 g once or twice daily
SIDE EFFECTS: may cause photosensitivity
AUXILIARY LABELS:
- Take with food or milk
- May cause photosensitivity

GENERIC NAME: metolazone
TRADE NAME: Zaroxylyn
ROUTE OF ADMINISTRATION: oral
COMMON DOSAGE: 5 to 20 mg once daily
SIDE EFFECTS: may cause photosensitivity
AUXILIARY LABELS:

■ Take with food or milk
■ May cause photosensitivity

Loop Diuretics

Loop diuretics inhibit reabsorption of sodium and chloride in the proximal convoluted tubule and distal convoluted tubule and within the loop of Henle. Because of the strong action of these agents, a great deal of potassium is lost with urination. They are normally prescribed to be taken early in the day to avoid nocturia.

CLASSIFICATION: LOOP DIURETICS
GENERIC NAME: bumetidine
TRADE NAME: Bumex
ROUTE OF ADMINISTRATION: oral
COMMON DOSAGE: 0.5 to 2 mg one to two times daily
SIDE EFFECTS: may cause GI upset, dizziness, lightheadedness
AUXILIARY LABELS:

■ Take with food or milk
■ May cause dizziness

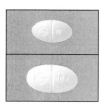

Boehringer
Mannhein

GENERIC NAME: torsemide
TRADE NAME: Demadex
ROUTE OF ADMINISTRATION: oral, IV
COMMON DOSAGE: 10 to 20 mg once daily
SIDE EFFECTS: may cause dizziness, lightheadedness
AUXILIARY LABELS:

■ May cause dizziness
■ May cause photosensitivity
SPECIAL NOTE: Torsemide does not need to be taken with food or milk

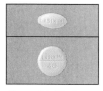

Hoescht Marion
Roussel

GENERIC NAME: furosemide
TRADE NAME: Lasix
ROUTE OF ADMINISTRATION: oral, IV
COMMON DOSAGE: 20 to 80 mg daily
SIDE EFFECTS: may cause GI upset
AUXILIARY LABEL:

■ Take with food or milk

Potassium-Sparing Agents

Because potassium-sparing agents work primarily in the distal convoluted tubule and inhibit sodium reabsorption, which decreases potassium loss, they do not cause large amounts of potassium to be lost in the urine. With these types of agents it is recommended that patients avoid large quantities of potassium-rich foods.

Combination drugs composed of the listed potassium-sparing and thiazide or loop diuretics are given in Table 21.4 along with their indication, dosage form, and auxiliary labels.

TABLE 21.4 Combination Diuretics

Generic	Trade	DF	Strength	Normal Dosage	Auxiliary Label
Amiloride/HCTZ	Moduretic	Tab	5 mg/50 mg	1-2 tabs daily	Take with food Photosensitivity
Spironolactone/HCTZ	Aldactazide	Tab	25 mg/25 mg	1-8 tabs daily	Take with food Photosensitivity
	Aldactazide	Tab	50 mg/50 mg	1-4 tabs daily	Take with food Photosensitivity
Triamterene/HCTZ	Dyazide	Cap	37.5 mg/25 mg	1-2 caps daily	Take with food Photosensitivity
	N	Cap	50 mg/25 mg	1-2 twice daily	Take with food Photosensitivity
	Maxzide-25	Tab	37.5 mg/25 mg	1-2 tabs daily	Take with food Photosensitivity
	Maxzide	Tab	75 mg/50 mg	1 tab daily	Take with food Photosensitivity

DF, Dosage form; *HCTZ*, hydrochlorothiazide.

CLASSIFICATION: POTASSIUM-SPARING DIURETICS
GENERIC NAME: amiloride
TRADE NAME: Midamore
ROUTE OF ADMINISTRATION: oral
COMMON DOSAGE: 5 mg per day
SIDE EFFECTS: may cause GI upset, dizziness, headache, visual disturbances
AUXILIARY LABELS:
- Take with food
- May cause dizziness

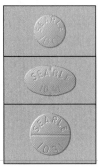

Searle

GENERIC NAME: spironolactone
TRADE NAME: Aldactone
ROUTE OF ADMINISTRATION: oral
COMMON DOSAGE: for edema: 25 to 200 mg per day
SIDE EFFECTS: may cause drowsiness, mental confusion
AUXILIARY LABEL:
- May cause dizziness and drowsiness

GENERIC NAME: triamterene
TRADE NAME: Dyrenium
ROUTE OF ADMINISTRATION: oral
COMMON DOSAGE: 100 mg twice daily after meals
SIDE EFFECTS: may cause GI upset, headache
AUXILIARY LABEL:
- Take after meals

Carbonic Anhydrase Inhibitors

Carbonic anhydrase inhibitors inhibit the enzyme carbonic anhydrase. Carbonic anhydrase inhibitors include acetazolamide, dichlorphenamide, and methazolamide. They inhibit hydrogen ion secretion by the renal tubule causing an increase in urination of sodium, potassium bicarbonate, and water. Most of these agents are more commonly used to treat glaucoma (see Chapter 19), although acetazolamide can also be used for the treatment of edema resulting from CHF. Side effects include possible GI upset, photosensitivity, and drowsiness.

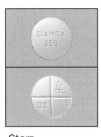

Starz

CLASSIFICATION: CARBONIC ANHYDRASE INHIBITOR
  GENERIC NAME: acetazolamide
  TRADE NAME: Diamox
  ROA: oral, IV, IM
  COMMON DOSAGE: 250 to 375 mg once daily
  AUXILIARY LABELS:
  ■ Take with meals
  ■ May cause dizziness

Osmotics

Osmotics inhibit tubular reabsorption of water by increasing the osmolarity of the glomerular filtrate. They are used for prophylaxis of acute renal failure when the glomerular filtration is reduced. Agents such as urea, glycerin, and isosorbide are also used for glaucoma. Table 21.5 lists osmotics and their normal dosages.

TREATMENT OF UTIs

The most common bacterial infections are those that cause UTIs. Because the urethra is much shorter in women than in men, women are more susceptible to contract infections from bacteria entering the urethra. Another cause of UTIs is catheterization. Infection of the kidney is called glomerulonephritis or pyelonephritis, whereas those in the bladder are referred to as cystitis. The symptoms of an upper (kidney) UTI include lower back pain, stomach pain, nausea, vomiting, and headache. Symptoms of lower (bladder) UTIs include frequent but small amounts of urine, dysuria, and sometimes incontinence. As discussed earlier, if the infection is acquired within the hospital, it is referred to as a nosocomial infection. Most of these are caused by gram-negative microbes. The most common agents used to treat UTIs are listed in Table 21.6. Often a physician will give the patient instructions to take an initial large dose called a loading dose (LD) before the normal dosage regimen. This is done to quickly bring the antibiotic within the system up to therapeutic levels so that it can begin to assist the body in fighting off the infection. The drug action for these antibiotics is given in Chapter 24.

TREATMENT OF INCONTINENCE

A common urinary condition that affects millions of Americans is incontinence. Older adults are more prone to this condition, as well as women in general. Women who have multiple pregnancies tend to develop this condition later in life.

TABLE 21.5 Osmotics

Generic	Trade	DF	Strength	Normal Dosage
Mannitol	Osmitrol	Injection	5%, 10%, 15%, 20%, 25%	20-200 g over 24 hours
Urea	Ureaphil	Injection	40 g/150 ml	30% soln by slow IV infusion not to exceed 4 ml/min
Glycerin	Osmoglyn	Oral solution	50%	1 to 2 g/kg, 1 to 1.5 hr before surgery
Isosorbide	Ismotic	Oral solution	45%	1 to 3 g/kg two to four times a day as needed

DF, Dosage form; *IV,* Intravenous.

TABLE 21.6 Treatments for Urinary Tract Infections

Generic	Trade	Normal Dosage
Sulfonamides		
Sulfamethoxazole	Gantanol	2 g LD, then 1 g every 8 to 12 hours
Sulfisoxazole	Gantrisin	2-4 g LD, then 750 mg-1.5 g every 6 hours
Sulfadiazine	Generic only	2-4 g LD, then 1 g every 4 to 6 hours
Fluoroquinolones		
Ciprofloxacin	Cipro	250-500 mg every 12 hours
Norfloxacin	Noroxin	400 mg every 12 hours
Ofloxacin	Floxin	200 mg every 12 hours from 3 to 10 days
Enoxacin	Penetrex	200 mg every 12 hours for 7 to 14 days
Miscellaneous Antiinfectives		
Nitrofurantion	Macrodantin	50-100 mg every 6 hours
Methenamine	Mandelamine	1 g four times daily

LD, Loading dose.

TABLE 21.7 Types of Incontinence

Type	Possible Causes	Possible Treatment
Stress	Relaxed pelvic muscles because of lower estrogen levels, multiple pregnancies	Kegel exercises, weight loss, vaginal estrogen creams or rings
Urge	CNS disorders such as Alzheimer's disease, Parkinson's disease, tumors, and bladder disorders	Anticholinergic agents; treat underlying cause or condition; vaginal estrogen creams
Reflex	CNS disorder	Treat underlying cause or condition; surgery; Alpha-adrenergic blockers
Functional	Age: Older adults lose mobility and balance	Change in environment, timed voiding, or implement a care plan for person
Overflow	Hyperplasia, bladder neck obstruction following surgery	Catheterization, bethanechol to increase bladder contractions; Surgery

CNS, Central nervous system.

Table 21.7 lists the types of incontinence along with possible treatments. The most common treatment for most types of incontinence is the Kegel exercise. This is an exercise that involves the pelvic floor muscles. It requires that the patient tighten the muscles around the pelvis in the same fashion as he or she would to hold urine and can be done either standing or sitting. The exercise is usually done in sets of ten, ten times daily over several weeks. Often incontinence can be overcome if the patient seeks help from his or her physician. If it cannot be corrected by exercise or medication, surgery (in some cases) can alleviate the problem.

DO YOU REMEMBER THESE KEY POINTS?

- The location of the kidneys
- The function of the kidneys
- The major components of the kidney and urinary system
- The functions of the glomerulus
- What conditions require dialysis and the types available
- The various types of medications that dialysis patients must receive
- The drug action of diuretics
- The major conditions affecting the urinary system and their treatments

REVIEW QUESTIONS:

Multiple Choice

1. Blood enters the kidneys through the
   A. Renal fascia
   B. Renal artery
   C. Renal vein
   D. Hilus

2. All of the following are components of the nephron except
   A. Glomerulus
   B. Urethra
   C. Bowman's capsule
   D. Loop of Henle

3. When taking loop diuretics, it should not be necessary to take which of the following supplements?
   A. Potassium
   B. Calcium
   C. Multivitamins
   D. A, B, and C

4. The _____ is where sodium is actively transported along with chloride.
   A. Proximal convoluted tubule
   B. Distal convoluted tubule
   C. Loop of Henle
   D. Glomerulus

5. Edema is commonly associated with all of the following conditions except
   A. Hypertension
   B. CHF
   C. Glaucoma
   D. Nephritis

6. Buffers have the ability to prevent
   A. Large changes in pH
   B. Edema
   C. Renal failure
   D. Blood loss

7. Plasma is a component of
   A. Buffers
   B. Water
   C. Blood
   D. Dialysis

8. Which of the following classifications of medications include diuretics?
   A. Blood formers
   B. Thiazides
   C. Carbonic anhydrase inhibitors
   D. B and C

9. Active transport is when
   A. Sodium is exchanged for hydrogen
   B. Potassium is exchanged for sodium
   C. Sodium and chloride leave the nephron
   D. Bicarbonate leaves the nephron

10. Loop diuretics and thiazides both
    A. Have a slow mechanism of action
    B. Cause a loss of potassium
    C. Cause a loss of sodium
    D. Must be taken with a potassium-sparing agent

True/False

*If the statement is false, then change it to make it true.

1. The connective tissue that holds the kidneys in place is called the peritoneal membrane.

2. All food is metabolized and excreted by the kidneys.

3. When giving thiazide diuretics, a potassium replacement is not necessary.

4. A BUN test measures the uric nitrogen content within the liver.

5. Urine is collected in the glomerulus and transported to the bladder.

6. Weak acids and bases are reabsorbed via the nephron.

7. Waste products from the kidneys are called urine.

8. Urine pH is between 4 and 6, which is acidic.

9. The two mechanisms of reabsorption involve ion exchange and active transport.

10. Epoetin is given to dialysis patients to counteract iron deficiency.

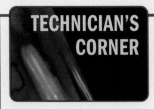

TECHNICIAN'S CORNER

Ms. Lewis went to the doctor because of swelling in her legs and shortness of breath. After blood tests and a physical examination she was diagnosed with CHF. The doctor prescribed the following medications to be filled in the pharmacy:

> Spironolactone 25 mg 1 q am
> Furosemide 20 mg 1 tablet q am

Question:

What are the classifications of these medications, and what auxiliary labels will you place on the vial? Also, what medication did the doctor omit that you would bring to the attention of the pharmacist?

BIBLIOGRAPHY

Drug Facts and Comparisons 1999, St Louis, 1999, Facts and Comparisons.

Lacy C, et al., *Drug Information Handbook,* Hudson, Ohio, 2000–2001, Lexi-Comp.

Lewis S, et al., *Medical Surgical Nursing Assessment,* ed 5, St Louis, 2000, Mosby.

Mosby's Drug Consult, St Louis, 2004, Elsevier.

Salerno E, *Pharmacology for Health Professionals,* St Louis, 1999, Mosby.

Stedman's Concise Medical Dictionary for Health Professionals, ed 3, Baltimore, 1997, Williams & Wilkins.

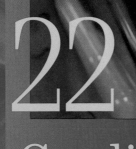

22

Cardiovascular System

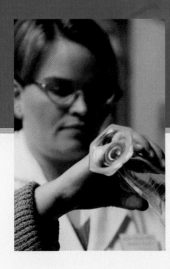

Objectives

- Describe the location and function of the heart.

- Name the four chambers of the heart.

- Explain how the heart receives nourishment.

- List the major disease states of the heart.

- Explain the possible causes of coronary artery disease (CAD), congestive heart failure (CHF), and hypertension.

- List the three types of angina.

- Describe how hypertension and hyperlipidemia can contribute to heart conditions.

- List the drugs used for heart conditions.

- List the drugs used for hypertension.

- Describe the indications for and mechanisms of the following classifications of drugs:
  Angiotensin-converting enzyme (ACE) inhibitors
  Anticoagulants
  Beta-blockers
  Calcium channel blockers
  Nitrates
  Thrombolytics

TERMS AND DEFINITIONS

Arrhythmia *Irregular rhythm of the heart*

Artery *A vessel that carries oxygenated blood from the heart to the tissues of the body*

Capillary *Extremely small vessel that connects the ends of the smallest arteries (arterioles) to the smallest veins (venules), where exchanges of nutrients and wastes, O_2 and CO_2 occur; blood vessels at cellular level*

Coagulate *To solidify or change from a fluid state to a solid state*

Diuretic *An agent that increases urine excretion*

Edema *A condition in which the body tissues contain an excessive amount of tissue fluid*

Enzymes *Proteins that act as a catalyst causing metabolic reactions to take place at a faster rate within the body*

Thrombin *An enzyme that is formed in coagulating blood from prothrombin; this reacts with fibrinogen converting it into fibrin, which is essential in the formation of blood clots; tested by performing a prothrombin time (PT) or partial thromboplastin time (PTT) blood test*

Thrombolytic *Medication used to break up a thrombus or blood clot*

Vein *A vessel that carries deoxygenated blood to or toward the heart*

CARDIOVASCULAR DRUGS

Brand	Generic	Pronunciation	Brand	Generic	Pronunciation
Antihypertensives			Brevibloc	esmolol	**es**-moe-lol
Aldomet	methyldopa	meth-ill-**doe**-pah	Trandate	labetalol	lah-**bet**-ah-lol
Cardura	doxazosin	docks-**ah**-zoe-sin	Kerlone	betaxolol	be-**tax**-oh-lol
Catapres	clonidine	**klon**-ih-deen			
Hytrin	terazosin	tear-**aye**-zoe-sin	**Calcium Channel Blockers**		
Minipress	prazosin	**pray**-zoe-sin	Cardizem	diltiazem	dill-**tea**-ah-zem
Only generic	reserpine	re-**sir**-peen	Calan,	verapamil	ver-**ap**-ah-mill
Apresoline	hydralazine	high-**dral**-ah-zeen	Isoptin		
			Procardia	nifedipine	nye-**fed**-ih-peen
Antiarrhythmic			Cardene	nicardipine	nye-**kar**-de-peen
Pronestyl	procainamide	pro-**cane**-ah-myd	Plendil	felodipine	fe-**low**-de-peen
Lanoxin	digoxin	di-**jox**-in	Nimotop	nimodipine	nye-**moe**-di-peen
ACE inhibitors			**Anticoagulant Agents**		
Vasotec	enalapril	eh-**nal**-ah-prill	Coumadin	warfarin	**war**-fair-in
Prinivil, Zestril	lisinopril	lih-**sin**-oh-prill	Liquaemin	heparin	**hep**-ah-rin
Lotensin	benazepril	ben-**ayz**-ah-prill			
Monopril	fosinopril	foe-**sin**-oh-pril	**Antianginals**		
Accupril	quinapril	**kwin**-a-pril	Imdur	isosorbide mononitrate	eye-soe-**sor**-bide mono-**ny**-trate
Capoten	captopril	**cap**-tow-pril	Isordil	isosorbide dinitrate	eye-soe-**sor**-bide dye-**ny**-trate
Angiotensin II Antagonist			Tridil,	nitroglycerin	nye-troe-**glis**-sir-rin
Cozaar	losartan	low-**sar**-tan	Nitrostat		
Diovan	valsartan	val-**sar**-tan			
Beta-blockers			**Antihyperlidimic Agents**		
Tenormin	atenolol	ay-**ten**-oh-lol	Questran	cholestyramine	koe-lee-**sty**-rah-meen
Inderal	propranolol	pro-**pran**-oh-lol	Lopid	gemfibrozil	gem-**fib**-row-zil
Lopressor	metoprolol	meh-toe-**pro**-lol			

CARDIOVASCULAR DRUGS—cont'd

Brand	Generic	Pronunciation	Brand	Generic	Pronunciation
Mevacor	lovastatin	**low**-vah-stat-in	**Coagulants**		
Zocor	simvastatin	sym-vah-**stat**-in	Mephyton	phytonadione	fy-toe-na-**dye**-own
Pravachol	pravastatin	**prav**-ah-stat-in	Protamine	protamine	**pro**-toe-mean
Lipitor	atorvastatin	a-tore-va-**stat**-in			
			Thrombolytics		
Vasodilators			Activase tPA	alteplase	**al**-tee-plase
Nitrostat	nitroglycerin	nye-troe-**glis**-sir-rin	Abbokinase	urokinase	your-oh-**kin**-ase
Isordil	isosorbide	eye-soe-**sore**-bide	Streptase	streptokinase	strep-toe-**kye**-nase
Transderm Nitro	nitroglycerin patches	nye-troe-**glis**-sir-rin			

Introduction

The cardiovascular system is a network of many complex interactions. It involves the blood, lungs, arteries, and veins of the body and the heart muscle itself. Millions of people die each year from heart disease; however, millions are living normal lives because of the advancements made in medicine. In addition, there is an awareness of heart health in the public because of health organizations. People are living longer because of their lifestyle changes and medications and the advancements of new surgical techniques. We begin with an overview of the anatomy of the heart, followed by the most common conditions that affect the heart. The last section is on the treatments available—the focus is on the medications. Technicians fill many prescriptions for heart medications over their careers and it is important to learn basic information about the classifications to assist the pharmacist.

Location and Anatomy of the Heart

The heart is located in the chest cavity between the lungs. It is a large muscle that initiates systemic arterial pulse waves, causing blood to circulate throughout the body and supply it with nutrition and oxygen. Extending from the heart are large transport tubes called arteries. These arteries flow into smaller tubes called arterioles and then ultimately into very small tubes called capillaries. It is from capillaries that oxygen and nutrients are exchanged throughout the tissues (Figure 22.1).

A normal heart beats anywhere from 60 to 100 times per minute and is about the size of a person's fist. It is surrounded by connective tissue called the pericardium, which in turn is anchored by ligaments to the chest wall and diaphragm. The heart is composed of three main layers:

1. **Endocardium** (inside): The endocardium has a smooth accordion-pleat-like surface, which allows the heart wall to collapse when it contracts.
2. **Myocardium** (muscle): The myocardium is the heart muscle that contracts.
3. **Epicardium** (outside): The epicardium is the outer layer of the heart. It is also the inner layer of the pericardium. The coronary arteries that supply the heart with oxygenated blood and the coronary veins that return deoxygenated blood to the heart are located in the epicardium.

OXYGENATION

The heart has two pumps, each of which is composed of two chambers (Figure 22.2). The first two chambers are the right atrium and the right ventricle. Blood circulates through the body exchanging oxygen, nutrients, and other substances to tissues and organs. The blood returns to the heart via two large veins called the superior

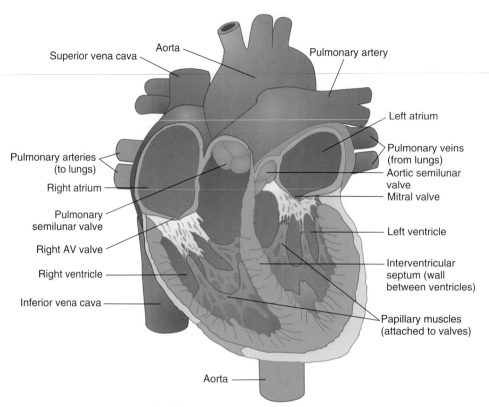

FIGURE 22.1 Anatomy of the heart.

and inferior vena cava. The superior vena cava brings blood from the upper portion of the body, and the inferior vena cava brings blood into the heart from the lower portion of the body. The blood travels through the right atrium into the right ventricle. The right ventricle contracts, expelling blood into the pulmonary arteries that go to the lungs where blood is fully oxygenated by the air that we breathe (see Chapter 18). The left atrium of the heart then receives the fully oxygenated blood from the lungs via the pulmonary veins. Blood is then passed into the left ventricle through the mitral valve. The left ventricle then contracts, expelling the blood into the aorta. In the aorta the blood initiates a pulse wave that carries it to all parts of the body (Figure 22.3). Although the heart is a very efficient organ, it still must be oxygenated just like other organs. The main arteries that supply blood to the heart are called the coronary arteries.

CARDIAC CONDUCTION SYSTEM

The cardiac conduction system provides the electrical charge that makes the heart pump. It is a lifetime battery that keeps our heartbeats in rhythm. This cardiac conduction system is run by to two nodes: the sinoatrial (SA) and atrioventricular (AV). The SA node is located in the upper right atrium wall (this is where the impulse begins). The signal is then sent down to the AV node, located in the septum between the right atrium and the right ventricle. As the cardiac impulse is sent from the SA to the AV node, it also is sent out to the muscle fibers that run throughout the atria. From the AV node the impulse goes to the ventricles to initiate a ventricular beat by stimulation of the bundle branches and Perkinje Fibers (Figure 22.4).

The Cardiac Cycle

The series of events that occur for one complete heartbeat is called the cardiac cycle. This cycle is composed of two sequences:

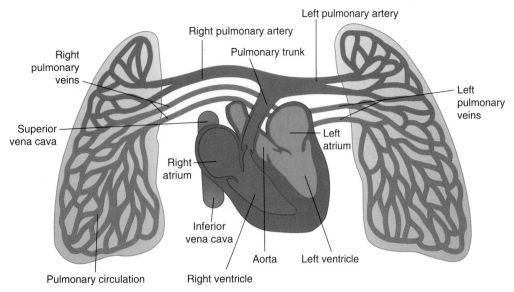

FIGURE 22.2 Blood oxygenation.

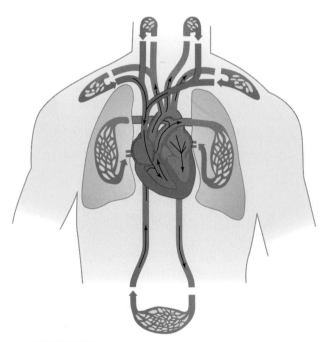

FIGURE 22.3 Circulation of blood through the body.

1. Systole—The myocardium squeezes blood from the heart chamber into the pulmonary artery or aorta.
2. Diastole—Blood is allowed to refill the chambers (relaxation). During diastole, the atria contract to pack 20% more blood into the ventricles. Most of your blood supply is cycled every minute through the heart.

Conditions Affecting the Heart

There are many heart conditions that affect millions of people each year. Because of the advancements made in the area of health, including the importance of lifestyle choices on our health, new medications, and new surgical techniques available, people are living longer lives. Box 22.1 lists some of the most common cardiovascular conditions along with a brief description.

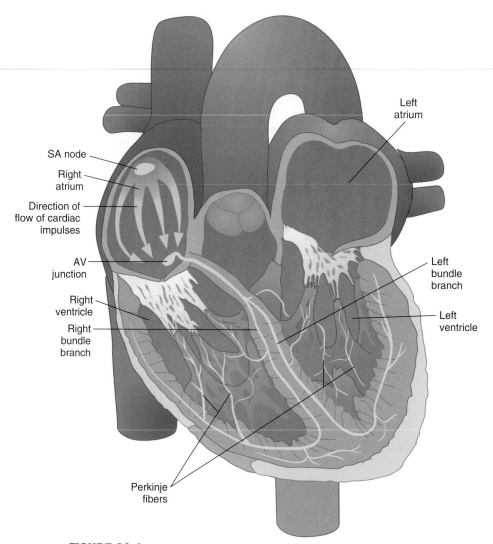

FIGURE 22.4 Conduction system. *SA*, Sinoatrial; *AV*, atrioventricular.

BOX 22.1 CONDITIONS AND DEFINITIONS

Angina pectoris	Pain and pressure in the chest caused by a lack of proper blood flow and oxygenation to the heart muscle
Arrhythmia	Irregular heartbeats resulting from a malfunction in the conduction system
Arteriosclerosis	A disease of the arterial vessels resulting from thickening, hardening, and loss of elasticity in the arterial walls
Atherosclerosis	A form of arteriosclerosis resulting from cholesterol-lipid calcium deposits in the walls of the arteries
Congestive heart failure	A condition in which the heart is unable to pump the amounts of blood needed to meet the requirements of the body; normally abbreviated CHF
Coronary artery disease	A term used to describe blood vessels disorders that affect the coronary arteries; normally abbreviated CAD
Hyperlipidemia	High or excessive amounts of lipid (fat) in the blood that leads to arteriosclerosis and atherosclerosis
Hypertension	High blood pressure, which is considered a systolic reading of >140 mm Hg or >90 mm Hg diastolic over several readings
Myocardial infarction	An event in which part of the heart muscle dies because of interruption or cessation of blood flow
Prehypertensive state	Blood pressure 120/80 to 140/90
Thrombosis	The formation of a blood clot within the vascular system

It is important to see how all of these conditions are related to one another, so we briefly discuss the differences and similarities between the conditions listed.

CORONARY ARTERY DISEASE

Coronary artery disease (CAD) is associated with atherosclerosis. This condition can be the result of a lifelong buildup of small plaques mainly composed of lipids (fats) especially cholesterol. Although these lipids can build up anywhere in the large arteries of the body they also tend to accumulate in the arteries throughout the heart. Atherosclerosis has been linked to high blood pressure. For example, small injuries can occur in the vessel wall. As lipids pass by they attach and begin to build up along the wall of the artery, eventually blocking the site altogether. Although much of the damage to the heart may be done in adulthood, lipid deposits have been observed in young children as well. Over time if these fatty deposits build up, a thrombus can be generated that can block the artery. This causes myocardial infarction (MI). There are many risk factors that can be linked to the development of atherosclerosis and eventual CAD. These include hypertension, age, gender, race, and genetics. Although these traits cannot be altered there are several factors that can be altered, such as a fatty diet, no exercise, smoking, and stress.

TECH NOTE! Arteriosclerosis is characterized by hardening and loss of elasticity of the arterial vessels. There are three forms of this condition: atherosclerosis, sclerosis of the arterioles, and calcific sclerosis of the medial layer of the arteries. Of these three types, atherosclerosis is the most common type, which causes angina, transient ischemic attacks (TIAs), stroke, or even a myocardial infarction resulting from the formation of a thrombus (clot).

Hyperlipidemia

Hypderlipidemia is the increase of lipids in the bloodstream and is the precursor to atherosclerosis. When discussing fats (lipids) in the body, the purpose of cholesterol, one type of lipid, is an important aspect. Cholesterol is produced by the body and is vital for making steroid hormones and cell membranes. When people eat foods that are high in fat they also are ingesting too much cholesterol and other fatty acids, which our bodies cannot eliminate. Instead these fatty substances float throughout the bloodstream where they can latch onto large arteries and middle-sized arteries of the heart and brain. Therefore it is important that regular checkups include a blood test to reveal the amount of cholesterol in the bloodstream. A generic type of test indicating the overall cholesterol levels is normally done; a cholesterol level below 200 mg/dL indicates an overall low cholesterol, 200 to 239 mg/dL indicates a borderline high reading, and a level at or above 240 mg/dL is a high value. In the case of a borderline or above normal level, a more in-depth look at the low-density lipoprotein (LDL) and high-density lipoprotein (HDL) would probably be indicated. The guidelines for specific cholesterol readings are listed in the following chart. (Values are derived from blood tests or serum of the blood in adults.)

LDL		HDL
<130	Good	>75
130–159	Borderline	36–44
>160	High	26–35

Another type of cholesterol not normally mentioned in laboratory values is very low density lipoproteins (VLDL). The level of VLDL is an indicator of the amount of LDL because it is a precursor to LDL. Other factors that will determine the treatment approach include family history, lifestyle habits, and the patient's personal medical history. The good cholesterol HDL are transporters of fat from tissues. Bad cholesterol LDL carry around lipids (fat) that can attach to artery walls causing atherosclerosis.

Hypertension

Hypertension is defined as persistent high blood pressure. High blood pressure is a prevalent problem in the United States affecting millions of Americans. This disease is also known as the "silent killer" because there are no obvious signs of its presence.

Why and How Hypertension Occurs. Hypertension is a result of various factors. Either the heart is diseased and the blood flow is decreased or another organ, such as the kidney, is not working properly, causing edema (a buildup of watery fluids). When the kidneys are not working properly, the concentration of ions such as sodium (Na) can increase throughout the body system. (Remember that water follows salt because of the higher concentration; therefore when an increase in salt occurs, the patient retains water, resulting in edema.) Whatever the cause of hypertension, the result is that the heart must work much harder to pump blood through the chambers and out into the body. Hypertension can also result from various conditions and risk factors such as those listed in Box 22.2.

The continuous overload on the coronary system also adds to the development of atherosclerosis (hardening of the arteries) and can cause small ruptures of vessels within the heart. Common signs of high blood pressure can be confused with other causes not associated with hypertension such as edema, blurred vision, headache, and shortness of breath. Another important factor that patients should be made aware of by their physician and pharmacist is that many over-the-counter (OTC) agents can affect their blood pressure. This includes antihistamines, decongestants, and ingredients in many different cold and allergy remedies.

Blood Pressure Readings. Everyone should have their blood pressure taken many times throughout their lifetime to evaluate blood pressure for elevations or to seek medical attention if necessary. A person with a systolic blood pressure reading of more than 140 mm Hg is considered to have hypertension. A prehypertensive state is considered when blood pressure reaches 120/80. There are three categories of hypertension based on diastolic readings and two categories based on systolic readings, as explained in Box 22.3. Blood pressure units are read by mm Hg, which is millimeters of mercury. Even a mild case of hypertension can lead to problems in later life because of the extra work placed on the heart. Blood pressure readings should be taken a few times during each visit to the doctor to obtain an average for each specific person's blood pressure because it does vary depending on different factors such as emotions and physical activity.

BOX 22.2 COMMON CONDITIONS THAT CAN LEAD TO HYPERTENSION (HTN)

Common conditions for hypertension
Heart condition
Hyperthyroidism
Kidney conditions

Increased risk factors which can lead to hypertension
1. Genetic
   Age
   Gender
   Race
2. Lifestyle
   Diet
   Anxiety
   Alcohol consumption
   Sodium intake

BOX 22.3 CLASSIFICATION OF BLOOD PRESSURE MEASUREMENTS

First or Top Measurement (Systolic Blood Pressure)
Normal: less than or equal to 115 mm Hg
Prehypertensive state: between 120 and 140 mm Hg
High: greater than 160 mm Hg

Second or Bottom Measurement (Diastolic Pressure)
Prehypertensive state: between 80 and 90 mm Hg
Mild Hypertension: 90 to 100 mm Hg
Moderate Hypertension: 105 to 115 mm Hg
Severe Hypertension: greater than 115 mm Hg

Angina Pectoris

Angina pectoris results from a decrease in blood flow to the heart, which results in pain in the chest. These pains can vary from minor to severe. Decreased blood flow can be caused by factors such as hardening of the arteries (atherosclerosis), hypertension, cigarette smoking, and diabetes. Environmental and genetic influences can also play a role in acquiring angina (chest pain). There are three types of angina:

1. Classic angina
2. Variant angina
3. Unstable angina

In classic angina the patient can experience short ischemic episodes of pain, in which a mild deficiency of oxygen has occurred. Patients may feel as though there is a weight on the chest accompanied with a sharp pain. This pain can occur in the chest, neck, arms, teeth, and jaw. Many times this type of an anginal attack occurs after exercise or excessive activity.

Another type of angina is variant angina. This type may not be related to atherosclerosis; instead the patient experiences spasms of the coronary artery. This is very painful and may occur even at rest.

The third type is unstable angina, which may worsen in a person with a known history of anginal attacks. Unstable angina is mainly caused by obstruction of the arteries, which increases over many years.

All three types of anginal pain are treated with medications such as nitrates. In addition to medications, the patient may be required to make certain lifestyle changes that may decrease these attacks. In addition, surgery may be performed to bypass the blockage.

Myocardial Infarction

If coronary blood flow to an area of the heart becomes entirely blocked because of a thrombus or embolism, that area of heart muscle cannot receive the necessary oxygen. This results in the death of that part of the muscle. Depending on the severity of the blockage, the patient may have an MI from which he or she can recover from over time or a massive MI that weakens the heart permanently or may even result in death.

Arrhythmias

A person with CAD can develop arrhythmias (irregular heartbeats), also known as dysrhythmias. As previously discussed in the section on the conduction system, the heart beats in a rhythm. This is done via special fibers, which run throughout the heart. The pacemaker is located in the SA node. There are many factors that influence the efficient working of the pacemaker, including chemical balance. If there is an imbalance resulting from chemicals or oxygen, then irregular heartbeats can occur. Most patients will receive short-term treatment in the emergency room. Once stabilized they may be sent home. If so, there are long-term medications that can be given to help keep the heart beating regularly.

Congestive Heart Failure

Congestive heart failure (CHF) is usually a progressive disease. There are very effective treatments to help patients with CHF, but there is no cure. A common heart disease of older people, CHF occurs when the heart cannot pump as vigorously thus delivering less blood throughout the body. Edema complicates CHF because the kidneys compensate for the lack of blood flow by retaining more fluid in the body. This fluid adds more work for the heart, further weakening it.

Thrombosis

When bleeding occurs, the body prevents bleeding to death by forming blood clots. It is a normal body function aimed at stopping hemorrhage and starting the healing process. Unfortunately our bodies can also form unwanted blood clots that can appear in areas such as the heart or brain. This can occur because of an overactive clotting mechanism or narrowing of the arteries, such as those in persons with atherosclerosis. An obstructed blood vessel to the brain can cause a stroke (also known as a brain attack). When it strikes the heart muscle, it can cause an MI or heart attack.

An embolus is a blood clot that has broken away from the thrombus (main clot) and has traveled through the body to another area where it can become lodged and create a blockage. The body produces chemicals that prevent clotting. Sometimes, however, the body needs additional help in preventing blood clots. This is when prophylactic treatment would be given. A prophylactic is an agent or treatment that is aimed at prevention, in this case preventing a clot.

Hypotension

A person suffering from hypotension has low blood pressure as opposed to high blood pressure. A common problem that people can experience is orthostatic hypotension. This is caused by standing up quickly from a sitting or lying position. This occurs because a large amount of blood remains in the lower extremities. When one stands quickly, the blood returning to the heart is decreased considerably, and the body responds by raising the heartbeat, compensating for the lack of blood flow. This results in a feeling of lightheadedness. Side effects of hypotension include syncope (fainting) and/or vertigo (dizziness). For persons who suffer often from this condition, physicians may recommend midodrine, which causes vasoconstriction, raising blood pressure.

Treatments and Medications for the Cardiovascular System

TREATMENT OF HYPERLIPIDEMIA

Because hyperlipidemia is known to lead to atherosclerosis, it is important to obtain an accurate cholesterol level. Factors such as family history and lifestyle are important parts of the assessment as well. These may indicate the likelihood of experiencing further problems. Through diet and exercise many people can lower their lipid content. On occasion a physician may suggest niacin, which is available OTC to lower the cholesterol. For persons at high risk because of family history or those who have high levels that do not decrease through diet and exercise, there are agents available (referred to as antihyperlipidemics). In severe cases, bypass surgery may be indicated for those persons who might not be responding to medications and lifestyle changes or those who have had an MI.

Antihyperlipidemics

The classes of drugs that make up the antihyperlipidemics include the bile acid sequestrants and HMG-CoA reductase inhibitors. Bile acid sequestrants, such as cholestyramine, increase the loss of cholesterol specifically LDL through **increased** defecation. There are many agents that effectively help reduce cholesterol in this manner. HMG-CoA reductase agents such as lovastatin, simvastatin, and pravastatin are referred to as the **statins**. They specifically inhibit an enzyme responsible for one of the first steps in the overall conversion of fats into cholesterol. They raise the HDL levels and decrease the LDL and VLDL cholesterol levels. There are other agents such as gemfibrozil that work specifically to lower VLDL cholesterol levels by the inhibiting the extraction of free fatty acids, which reduces the ability of the liver to produce triglycerides. This agent also increases HDL; however, the specific mechanism of action is not well known. Nicotinic acid (OTC agent) reduces cholesterol, triglyceride, and VLDL levels, which leads to an overall decrease in LDL levels; the exact mechanism is not well known. The recommended maintenance dose for an adult is listed in the following.

CLASSIFICATION: BILE ACID SEQUESTRANTS

    GENERIC NAME: cholestyramine

    TRADE NAME: Questran

    ROUTE OF ADMINISTRATION: oral (powder)

    COMMON DOSAGE: 4 g once or twice daily

    SIDE EFFECTS: constipation, flatulence

    AUXILIARY LABELS:

- Do not chew or crush tablets
- Take before meals

    *SPECIAL NOTE: powder form should be mixed into 60 to 180 mL of liquid. Other medications should be taken 4 to 6 hours apart from cholestyramine to avoid interference of absorption.

    GENERIC NAME: colestipol

    TRADE NAME: Colestid

    ROUTE OF ADMINISTRATION: oral

    COMMON DOSAGE: 5 to 30 g per day (may be given in divided doses)

    SIDE EFFECTS: constipation, flatulence

    AUXILIARY LABELS:

- Do not chew or crush tablets
- Take before meals

    *SPECIAL NOTE: powder form should be mixed into at least 90 mL of liquid. Other medications should be taken 4 to 6 hours apart from cholestyramine to avoid interference of absorption.

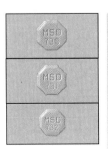

Merck

CLASSIFICATION: HMG-COA REDUCTASE INHIBITORS

    GENERIC NAME: lovastatin

    TRADE NAME: Mevacor

    ROUTE OF ADMINISTRATION: oral

    COMMON DOSAGE: 10 to 80 mg daily in single or divided doses

    SIDE EFFECTS: may cause photosensitivity, gastrointestinal (GI) upset

    AUXILIARY LABELS:

- May cause photosensitivity
- Take with meals

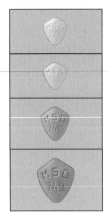

Merck

GENERIC NAME: simvastatin
TRADE NAME: Zocor
ROUTE OF ADMINISTRATION: oral
COMMON DOSAGE: 5 to 40 mg once daily
SIDE EFFECTS: may cause photosensitivity
AUXILIARY LABELS:
■ May cause photosensitivity

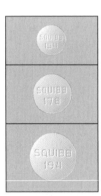

Bristol-Myers
Squib

GENERIC NAME: pravastatin
TRADE NAME: Pravachol
ROUTE OF ADMINISTRATION: oral
COMMON DOSAGE: 10 to 40 mg once daily at bedtime
SIDE EFFECTS: may cause photosensitivity
AUXILIARY LABEL:
■ May cause photosensitivity

GENERIC NAME: atrovastatin
TRADE NAME: Lipitor
ROUTE OF ADMINISTRATION: oral
COMMON DOSAGE: 10 to 80 mg once daily
SIDE EFFECTS: may cause photosensitivity
AUXILIARY LABEL:
■ May cause photosensitivity

Parke-Davis

CLASSIFICATION: FIBRIC ACID ANTIHYPERLIPIDEMIC
GENERIC NAME: gemfibrozil
TRADE NAME: Lopid
ROUTE OF ADMINISTRATION: oral
COMMON DOSAGE: 600 mg twice daily before morning and evening meals
SIDE EFFECTS: may cause dizziness, blurred vision
AUXILIARY LABEL:
■ May cause dizziness

CLASSIFICATION: MISCELLANEOUS ANTIHYPERLIPIDEMIC
GENERIC NAME: nicotinic acid
TRADE NAME: Niaspan RX (Niacin OTC [read package insert for dosage])
ROUTE OF ADMINISTRATION: oral
COMMON DOSAGE: 1 to 2 g three times daily with or following meals
SIDE EFFECTS: may cause photosensitivity
AUXILIARY LABEL:
■ May cause photosensitivity

TREATMENT OF ARRHYTHMIAS

The medications used in treating arrhythmias are called antiarrhythmic agents. Quinidine sulfate, procainamide, disopyramide, and verapamil are common agents that may be prescribed. See the following for a complete list of medications and their indications. In severe cases in which medications cannot correct the continuing problem of arrhythmias, a pacemaker implant may be the only alternative.

Drug Action

All of these agents work on the conduction system and induce regular heartbeats. Lidocaine is used in an emergency situation to treat arrhythmias resulting from MIs and other conditions. Both quinidine sulfate and procainamide slow down the speed of the conduction system and are used for tachycardias (rapid heartbeat) and other arrhythmias. The injectable form of procainamide is normally used in life-threatening tachycardia episodes in an emergency. Disopyramide slows the heart rate. Again, the injectable form is used in life-threatening tachycardias similar to procainamide. Verapamil slows the conduction system at the AV node and stabilizes cardiac rhythm.

CLASSIFICATION: ANTIARRHYTHMICS
  GENERIC NAME: quinidine sulfate, quinidine gluconate
  TRADE NAME: Quinidex (oral), Quinalan (IV)
  ROUTE OF ADMINISTRATION: sulfate, gluconate (injectable[IM, IV]), and polygalacturonate (oral tabs)
  COMMON DOSAGE: 200 to 300 mg three to four times daily
  SIDE EFFECTS: GI upset; do not crush or chew sustained-release tablets
  AUXILIARY LABELS:
  - Take with food
  - Take as directed

TECH NOTE! Serious medication errors can occur because of the similar names of quinidine and quinine. Quinine is an antimalarial agent; quinidine is a cardiac agent. These two medications often sit close to one another on a pharmacy shelf and have been mistaken for one another. This can result in a dangerous error.

GENERIC NAME: procainamide
TRADE NAME: Pronestyl
ROUTE OF ADMINISTRATION: oral, injectable (IM, IV)
COMMON DOSAGE: to be determined by physician based on weight and age of patient
SIDE EFFECTS: no major effects unless patient does not adhere to dosing schedule
AUXILIARY LABEL:
- Take as directed

Searle

GENERIC NAME: disopyramide
TRADE NAME: Norpace
ROUTE OF ADMINISTRATION: oral
COMMON DOSAGE: 100 to 200 mg q6h or 300-SR-q12h
SIDE EFFECTS: dry mouth, dizziness, difficulty urinating, constipation, blurred vision
AUXILIARY LABELS:
- Do not break or chew tablet
- May cause dizziness
- Take as directed

GENERIC NAME: Lidocaine
TRADE NAME: Xylocaine
INDICATION: acute management of ventricular arrhythmias
ROUTE OF ADMINISTRATION: injection or intravenous (IV) drip
COMMON DOSAGE: for IV infusion 50 to 100 mg at a rate of 25 to 50 mg per minute
***SPECIAL NOTE:** this medication is kept in emergency rooms and other areas where crash carts are located. They are used in code blue situations. In the emergency department and intensive care units a code blue occurs when a patient is having a heart attack or stops breathing.

TREATMENT OF CONGESTIVE HEART FAILURE

The most common treatment for CHF is cardioglycosides. The only one available in the United States is digoxin. Diuretics are also commonly used in addition to glycosides to treat the edema that normally accompanies CHF.

Drug Action

Cardioglycosides increase the forcefulness of the pumping of the heart but not the oxygen requirements. Specifically, it inhibits the sodium potassium pump, which works within the heart to increase contractility. In arrhythmias, there is a suppression of the AV node that increases regularity of the heartbeat and decreases conduction speed and force (velocity); thus (in both cases) the heart works smarter, not harder. It is very important that patients take their medications exactly as directed. Diuretics are often prescribed concurrently. They increase urine output, thus decreasing the overall fluid retention (See Chapter 21) and allowing the heart to work more easily.

CLASSIFICATION: CARDIAC GLYCOSIDE
GENERIC NAME: digoxin
TRADE NAME: Lanoxin
INDICATION: treatment of CHF and certain arrhythmias
ROUTE OF ADMINISTRATION: oral, injectable (intravenous, intramuscular)
COMMON DOSAGE: 0.125 to 0.25 mg (This dosage must be based on body weight and normal renal function for age of patient)
SIDE EFFECTS: nausea and vomiting, diarrhea, dizziness
AUXILIARY LABELS:
- Take as prescribed
- Do not stop taking medication without consulting physician
***SPECIAL NOTE:** the antidote for an overdose of digoxin is Digibind. This agent binds to the digoxin molecule and it is then excreted from the body. This treatment must be done in the emergency department and is available in injectable form only.

TECH NOTE! The pharmacy tech should reinforce the fact that the pulse should be taken each day prior to taking digitalis. If the pulse is below 60, the patient should call a physician prior to taking the medicine.

Diuretics Used for CHF-Related Edema. There are different diuretic agents used to help reduce edema. With thiazides and loop diuretics an important consideration is the large amount of potassium lost in the urine. For this reason both classes of drugs may be supplemented with potassium. Diuretics are also given along with one or more of the listed agents to decrease the effects of sodium retention. Frequent urination leading to a decrease in edema is the main outcome with the use of diuretics. A major side effect of certain diuretics is the

BOX 22.4 CLASSIFICATION OF DIURETIC AGENTS

Thiazides
Loop diuretics
Potassium-sparing diuretics
Carbonic anhydrase inhibitors
Osmotic diuretics

loss of potassium along with the urine. An example is the agent hydrochlorothiazide. There are, however, agents that are known as *potassium sparing*. These include agents such as triamterene and hydrochlorothiazide and others listed in Box 22.4. A maximum of two examples of each type of diuretic are given because a more extensive list is provided in Chapter 21.

Thiazides. Thiazide agents are used to increase urinary excretion. They are indicated for use in patients with edema resulting from CHF, hypertension, and other conditions. Their side effects are similar and include frequent urination, GI upset, and possible photosensitivity. Each medication's auxiliary label is noted along with the normal dosage for an adult at maintenance.

CLASSIFICATION: THAZIDE AND THAZIDE-LIKE DIURETICS
   GENERIC NAME: chlorothiazide
   TRADE NAME: Diuril
   ROUTE OF ADMINISTRATION: oral, injectable (IV, IM)
   COMMON DOSAGE: 0.5 to 1 g once or twice daily (qd or bid)
   AUXILIARY LABELS:
- Take with food or milk
- May cause photosensitivity

   GENERIC NAME: Metolazone
   TRADE NAME: Zaroxolyn
   ROUTE OF ADMINISTRATION: oral
   COMMON DOSAGE: 2.5 to 5 mg once daily (qd)
   AUXILIARY LABELS:
- Take with food or milk
- May cause photosensitivity

Loop Diuretics. Loop diuretics work specifically in the loop of Henle within the renal tubules (see Chapter 21). They work rapidly and cause large amounts of urine to be excreted. They are often prescribed for patients who have edema caused by CHF and hypertension. Their side effects include increase in urination, possible GI upset, orthostatic hypotension, and photosensitivity. Because these agents work rapidly, it is advised that the patient take them in the morning or early in the day.

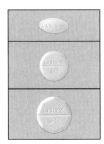

Hoescht Marion
Roussel

CLASSIFICATION: LOOP DIURETICS
   GENERIC NAME: furosemide
   TRADE NAME: Lasix
   ROUTE OF ADMINISTRATION: oral, injectable (IV, IM)
   COMMON DOSAGE: 20 to 80 mg daily (qd)
   AUXILIARY LABELS:
- Take with food or milk
- May cause photosensitivity

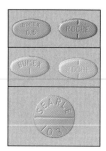

Roche

GENERIC NAME: bumetanide

TRADE NAME: Bumex

ROUTE OF ADMINISTRATION: oral, injection (IM, IV)

COMMON DOSAGE: 0.5 to 2 mg daily (qd)

AUXILIARY LABELS:

- Take with food or milk
- May cause photosensitivity

Potassium-Sparing Diuretics (K + sparing). Potassium-sparing agents work to eliminate urine by way of interrupting the sodium reabsorption within the distal tubules of the kidney. Because of their place of action they do not cause a large amount of potassium to be excreted along with the urine. Their side effects are similar to other diuretics with possible GI upset, but they may also cause dizziness, drowsiness, headache, and diarrhea. Following are a few of commonly used agents.

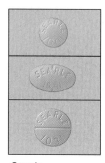

Searle

CLASSIFICATION: POTASSIUM-SPARING DIURETICS

GENERIC NAME: spironolactone

TRADE NAME: Aldactone

ROUTE OF ADMINISTRATION: oral

COMMON DOSAGE: 50 to 100 mg daily (qd)

AUXILIARY LABELS:

- Take with food or milk
- May cause dizziness and drowsiness

GENERIC NAME: triamterene

TRADE NAME: Dyrenium

ROUTE OF ADMINISTRATION: oral

COMMON DOSAGE: 100 mg twice daily (bid)

AUXILIARY LABEL:

- Take after meals

Carbonic Anhydrase Inhibitors. Carbonic anhydrase inhibitors specifically inhibit the enzyme carbonic anhydrase. These agents work to reduce edema by inhibiting the hydrogen ion secretion by the renal tubule, which causes the loss of ions such as sodium and potassium. Acetazolamide also is used to reduce intraocular pressure, which is the cause of glaucoma (see Chapter 19).

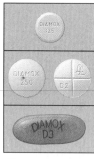

Starz

CLASSFICATION: CARBONIC ANHYDRASE INHIBITORS

GENERIC NAME: acetazolamide

TRADE NAME: Diamox

ROUTE OF ADMINISTRATION: oral, injectable (IM, IV), topical (otic)

COMMON DOSAGE: 250 to 375 mg once daily (qd)

AUXILIARY LABELS:

- Take with food or milk
- May cause photosensitivity
- May cause dizziness and drowsiness

Osmotic Diuretics. Osmotic diuretic agents eliminate excess water weight by increasing the osmolarity of the glomerular filtrate, which has the effect of decreasing tubular reabsorption of water. Certain agents such as mannitol are available in injection only and can be used for IOP as well as for edema caused by acute renal failure and when the glomerular filtration is dangerously reduced.

CLASSIFICATION: OSMOTIC DIURETICS

GENERIC NAME: mannitol

TRADE NAME: Osmitrol

ROUTE OF ADMINISTRATION: injection (IV)

COMMON DOSAGE: usual adult dose ranges from 20 to 200 g over a 24-hour period

AUXILIARY LABEL:

- None: Given in the hospital

GENERIC NAME: glycerin
TRADE NAME: Osmoglyn
ROUTE OF ADMINISTRATION: oral
COMMON DOSAGE: 1 to 2 g/ kg 1 to 1.5 hours before surgery
AUXILIARY LABEL:
■ None: Given in the hospital

TREATMENT OF HYPERTENSION

Treatment of hypertension is given by a "step-care" approach. There are four steps that are based on the severity of the condition. As shown in an example in Table 22.1, diet is usually indicated with or without medication because foods high in fat, sodium, or tyramine are a leading contributor to hypertension. The main agents used for high blood pressure are antihypertensive medications such as methyldopa, doxazosin, clonidine, terazosin, and prazosin. Other agents used to treat high blood pressure include diuretics and vasodilators. People who have high blood pressure are not always aware of their condition because of the lack of signs or symptoms. Therefore compliance in taking medication as directed can be a problem. Because they do not physically feel bad, patients do not take their medications.

Reducing salt intake and alcohol consumption, as well as exercising and abstaining from smoking, has been proven to reduce hypertension, therefore reducing the workload on the heart. However, even with these types of interventions, hypertension still may not be controlled. If medication is required to control hypertension, the initial drug therapy may include diuretics. Along with a diuretic there are many medications available that are very effective in controlling hypertension, including angiotensin-converting enzyme (ACE) inhibitors, beta-blockers, and calcium channel blockers. These medications are covered separately including their drug action, side effects, and commonly used auxiliary labels on prescription vials.

THE ABCs OF HEART MEDICATIONS

Because there are many different agents used to treat heart conditions, such as CAD and hypertension, it is important to learn about the medications and

TABLE 22.1 Example of Four-Step Approach to Controlling High Blood Pressure

Therapy	Medication
Step 1	
Separate or in combination	
Weight reduction*	None
ACE inhibitors	Captopril
Beta-blockers	Propranolol
Calcium channel blockers	Verapamil
Diuretics	Furosemide
Step 2: Additional Medication	
Adrenergic blockers	Clonidine
Step 3: Additional Medication	
Vasodilators	Hydralazine

ACE, Angiotensin-converting enzyme.
*A change in diet is indicated regardless of which medications are used. Fat consumption, salty foods, and foods containing tyramine should be decreased. Often fluid restriction may also be recommended.

remember the information. An easy way of remembering the types of medications used to treat the heart conditions discussed in this chapter is to remember "ABCs." This stands for the common classifications of agents used to treat heart conditions. Although there are more classifications of agents available, this is a simplified way to begin to remember them.

Angiotensin Converting Enzyme Agents (ACE Inhibitors)

ACE inhibitors are a set of agents that help reduce blood pressure by causing a decrease of pressure in the arteries. Certain enzymes produced by the kidneys ultimately help produce ACE, which increases sodium content. This allows for further increases of fluid retention. ACE inhibitors stop these enzymes from causing vasoconstriction that would normally result in high blood pressure caused by the sodium imbalance. Side effects for ACE inhibitors may include headache, hypotension, nausea, or vomiting.

CLASSIFICATION: ANGIOTENSIN CONVERTING ENZYME AGENTS

GENERIC NAME: enalapril

TRADE NAME: Vasotec

INDICATION: mild to severe hypertension

ROUTE OF ADMINISTRATION: oral, injectable (IV)

COMMON DOSAGE: oral: 10 to 40 mg daily in once or twice divided doses (qd or bid) for hypertension

AUXILIARY LABEL:
- Take as directed

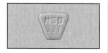

Merck

GENERIC NAME: lisinopril

TRADE NAME: Prinivil, Zestril

INDICATION: hypertension

ROUTE OF ADMINISTRATION: oral

COMMON DOSAGE: oral: 40 mg once daily (qd)

AUXILIARY LABEL:
- Take as directed

GENERIC NAME: benazepril

TRADE NAME: Lotensin

INDICATION: hypertension

ROUTE OF ADMINISTRATION: oral

COMMON DOSAGE: 20 to 40 mg once or twice daily (qd or bid)

AUXILIARY LABEL:
- May cause dizziness or drowsiness

GENERIC NAME: captopril

TRADE NAME: Capoten

INDICATION: hypertension

ROUTE OF ADMINISTRATION: oral

COMMON DOSAGE: 25 mg twice or three times daily (bid or tid)

AUXILIARY LABELS:
- Take before meals
- May cause dizziness or drowsiness

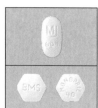

Bristol-Myers Squibb

GENERIC NAME: fosinopril

TRADE NAME: Monopril

INDICATION: hypertension

ROUTE OF ADMINISTRATION: oral

COMMON DOSAGE: 20 to 40 mg once daily (qd)

AUXILIARY LABELS:
- Take before meals
- May cause dizziness

Angiotensin II Receptor Antagonist

These agents work by inhibiting the effects of angiotensin II receptors located vascular muscles. This in turn lowers blood pressure via antagonistic effects on vasoconstriction. There are no major side effects.

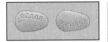

Merck

CLASSIFICATION: ANGIOTENSIN II RECEPTOR ANTAGONIST

> **GENERIC NAME:** losartan
> **TRADE NAME:** Cozaar
> **ROUTE OF ADMINISTRATION:** oral
> **COMMON DOSAGE:** 50 mg once daily
> **AUXILIARY LABEL:**
> - Take as directed

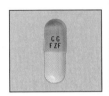

Ciba-Geigy

> **GENERIC NAME:** valsartan
> **TRADE NAME:** Diovan
> **ROUTE OF ADMINISTRATION:** oral
> **COMMON DOSAGE:** 80 to 320 mg once daily
> **AUXILIARY LABEL:**
> - Take as directed

Beta-Blocking Agents

Beta-Blockers are a set of agents that are effective because they block various enzymes, such as epinephrine, that can cause high blood pressure. There are two sites where beta-blockers work, beta-1 and beta-2 receptor sites. Beta-1 receptors are located in the heart, whereas beta-2 receptors are located in the lungs and deep arteries. The actions of medications can be specific or nonspecific. Nonspecific agents affect both beta-1 and beta-2 sites.

A nonspecific agent would not be recommended if a person were suffering from asthma or another type of respiratory problem. When beta-2 sites are inhibited, breathing airways can be restricted; therefore it is up to the physician to determine the appropriate agent for the patient. Side effects include dizziness, hypotension, and diarrhea.

CLASSFICATION: BETA-BLOCKING AGENTS

> **GENERIC NAME:** atenolol
> **TRADE NAME:** Tenormin
> **INDICATION:** hypertension, angina pectoris, after MI
> **ROUTE OF ADMINISTRATION:** oral, injection (IV)
> **COMMON DOSAGE:** 50 mg once daily (qd)
> **AUXILIARY LABELS:**
> - Take as directed
> - May cause dizziness

> **GENERIC NAME:** propranolol
> **TRADE NAME:** Inderal
> **INDICATION:** hypertension, angina, arrhythmias, and migraines
> **ROUTE OF ADMINISTRATION:** oral, injection (IV)
> **COMMON DOSAGE:** For hypertension 40 mg twice daily (bid)
> **AUXILIARY LABELS:**
> - Take as directed
> - May cause dizziness

> **GENERIC NAME:** metoprolol
> **TRADE NAME:** Lopressor
> **INDICATION:** hypertension, angina pectoris, arrhythmias
> **ROUTE OF ADMINISTRATION:** oral, injectable (IV)
> **COMMON DOSAGE:** Oral: 100 to 450 mg per day either twice or three times (bid or tid)
> **AUXILIARY LABELS:**
> - Take as directed
> - May cause dizziness

GENERIC NAME: pindolol
TRADE NAME: Visken
INDICATION: hypertension
ROUTE OF ADMINISTRATION: oral
COMMON DOSAGE: maximum of 60 mg daily
AUXILIARY LABELS:

- Take as directed
- May cause dizziness

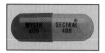

Wyeth-Ayerst

GENERIC NAME: acebutolol
TRADE NAME: Sectral
INDICATION: hypertension, ventricular arrhythmias
ROUTE OF ADMINISTRATION: oral
COMMON DOSAGE: 400 to 800 mg daily (qd)
AUXILIARY LABEL:

- Take as directed

Calcium Channel Blockers

Calcium channel blockers work by decreasing calcium intake by the heart and blood vessels. Calcium is used by the heart to stimulate the conduction system (the electrical pump). When the calcium channel is blocked by these agents, the heart rate slows, which decreases stress on the heart muscle. Common side effects include dizziness, drowsiness, and blurred vision in varying degrees depending on the specific agent.

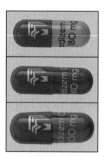

Hoechst Marion Roussel

CLASSIFICATION: CALCIUM CHANNEL BLOCKERS
GENERIC NAME: diltiazem
TRADE NAME: Cardizem CD
INDICATION: angina pectoris, chronic stable angina, essential hypertension
ROUTE OF ADMINISTRATION: oral, injectable (IV)
COMMON DOSAGE: oral: for hypertension, 180 to 360 mg daily in divided doses; either three or four times a day (tid or qid)
AUXILIARY LABELS:

- Take as directed
- Do not crush or chew tablet (For sustained-released tablets)

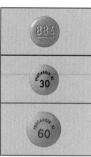

Pfizer; Miles

GENERIC NAME: nifedipine
TRADE NAME: Procardia, Adalat
INDICATION: chronic stable angina, hypertension
ROUTE OF ADMINISTRATION: oral
COMMON DOSAGE: for hypertension, 30 or 60 mg once daily
AUXILIARY LABELS:

- Take as directed
- Do not chew or break tablet (For sustained-released tablets)

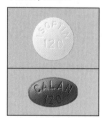

Searle; Knoll

GENERIC NAME: verapamil
TRADE NAME: Calan, Isoptin
INDICATION: angina, chronic atrial flutter or fibrillation, essential hypertension
ROUTE OF ADMINISTRATION: oral, injectable (IV)
COMMON DOSAGE: oral: for hypertension, 80 mg three times daily (tid); for sustained released 120 mg or 240 mg once daily
AUXILIARY LABELS:

- Take with food
- Take as directed

GENERIC NAME: amlodipine
TRADE NAME: Norvasc
INDICATION: hypertension, chronic stable angina, variant angina
ROUTE OF ADMINISTRATION: oral
COMMON DOSAGE: for hypertension 5 to 10 mg once daily (qd)
AUXILIARY LABEL:

■ Take as directed

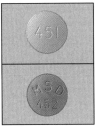
Merck

GENERIC NAME: felodipine
TRADE NAME: Plendil
INDICATION: hypertension
ROUTE OF ADMINISTRATION: oral
COMMON DOSAGE: 2.5 to 10 mg once daily
AUXILIARY LABELS:

■ Take as directed
■ Do not crush or chew tablet

TREATMENT OF ANGINAL ATTACKS

Nitrates, calcium channel blockers, and beta-blockers are commonly used to treat anginal attacks. Probably one of the most prescribed antianginal agents is nitroglycerin. Millions of people carry nitroglycerin sublingual tablets in their pockets or purses in the event of an anginal attack. There are many dosage forms for nitroglycerin, including capsules, topical patches, paste, and sublingual spray. The sublingual tablets and injectable forms are used for emergencies.

Drug Action

Nitrates are vasodilators that dilate the arteries to permit an increase of blood flow through the heart muscle. They also reduce the workload of the heart. Because more oxygenated blood is allowed to enter the arteries, less blood is returned to the heart, thereby decreasing the workload. Isosorbide and nitroglycerin are the two types of agents used for the treatment of angina. Both agents are available as sublingual tablets, which are very effective because of their rapid absorption; the medication bypasses the GI system and enters directly into the bloodstream for a more rapid onset of action. The sublingual route has several benefits. First, the drug is not inactivated by stomach acid (many medications are rendered less active because of the low pH of the stomach). Second, the sublingual route provides faster onset of action (oral medications usually take at least 20 to 30 minutes to work, which is too long for a patient experiencing severe chest pain). A common prescription order can be seen in Figure 22.5.

Nitroglycerin is good for only 6 months after opening the container. In addition, it must be kept in a dry area and in a light-protected glass container to prevent the active agent from breaking down. A list of the nitrate agents and their dosage forms are provided in Table 22.2. Sublingual dosages are kept at the patient's bedside for emergency relief of angina attacks. The nitroglycerin transdermal patches are normally applied once daily in the morning and taken off at bedtime to decrease the possibility of tolerance to the medication. Ointment tubes are available in 60 g, 30 g, and 1 g unit dose sizes tubes. The ointment also comes with papers premarked in half-inch increments for delivering the proper amount of ointment. The ointment is squeezed onto the paper in increments of one half inch to 2 inches, similar to toothpaste placed on a toothbrush. The translingual spray is used if an anginal attack occurs. The patient sprays one or two metered doses under the tongue with a maximum of three sprays in a 15-minute period.

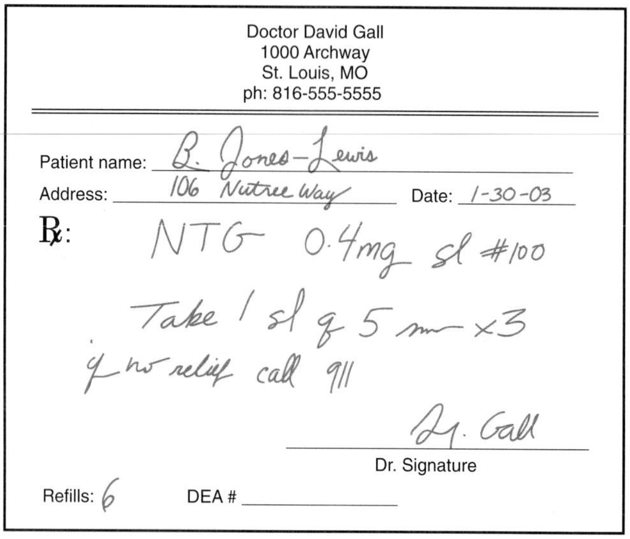

Doctor David Gall
1000 Archway
St. Louis, MO
ph: 816-555-5555

Patient name: B. Jones-Lewis

Address: 106 Nutree Way   Date: 1-30-03

Rx:

NTG 0.4mg sl #100

Take 1 sl q 5 min x3

if no relief call 911

D. Gall
Dr. Signature

Refills: 6   DEA # _____

FIGURE 22.5 Nitroglycerin sublingual tablet prescription.

TABLE 22.2 Common Nitrate Agents

Trade	Generic	Dosage Form	Normal Usage
Tridil	Nitroglycerin	Injectable	Emergency
Ntg in D5W	Nitroglycerin	Injection solution	Emergency
Nitrostat	Nitroglycerin	Sublingual tablets	Emergency
Nitrogard	Nitroglycerin	Buccal tablets	Routine med
Nitrong	Nitroglycerin	SR tabs	Routine med
Nitrobid	Nitroglycerin	SR capsules	Routine med
Nitro-Dur, Transderm	Nitroglycerin	Nitro patches	Routine med
Nitro-Bid	Nitroglycerin	Ointment 2% with papers	Routine med
Monoket, ISMO	Isosorbide mononitrate	Tablets, extended release tablets	Routine med
Isordil	Isosorbide dinitrate	Sublingual tablets, chewable tablets	Emergency
Sorbitrate, Isordil	Isosorbide dinitrate	Tablets, capsules, tablets SR	Routine med

Med, Medication; *SR,* sustained release; *tab,* tablet.

TECH NOTE! When filling nitroglycerin, never take the tablets out of the glass container they come in. Instead the glass container must be placed within a larger plastic vial on which the label is attached. Other containers include the box type, which holds four small glass vials each containing 25 tablets and which has a space on the box for the drug label.

TREATMENT OF BLOOD CLOTS

Drug Action of Anticoagulants

Clots are formed by fibrin, a type of binding string that holds blood cells together. Heparin converts blood-clotting fibrin into another substance similar to warfarin. Each drug works at a different site within the body and blocks the formation of blood clots. However, once a clot is formed, heparin, warfarin (Coumadin), or aspirin cannot be used for treatment. A thrombolytic must be administered as soon as possible.

The medications used for a thrombosis are emergency agents that include streptokinase, urokinase, and tissue plasminogen activator (tPA). These agents' dosage forms are injectable only and are kept in areas within a hospital such as emergency, surgery, and intensive care units. A patient does not normally need more than one dose, and the sooner the drug is administered to the patient, the better the outcome.

To prevent blood from coagulating (binding together), anticoagulants may be prescribed. There are two kinds of anticoagulants, heparin and warfarin. Heparin is available in injectable form only. It inhibits thrombosis by inactivating a factor (called Xa) as well as by preventing the conversion of prothrombin to thrombin. This stops the coagulation mechanism. Heparin is prepackaged by manufactures in 20,000 unit bags of 500 mL or can be made in various units from a wide variety of vial strengths. Heparin cannot be given orally because stomach acids destroy it. For example, patients who are admitted into the hospital with an MI or stroke may be placed on a heparin IV drip to prevent any blood clotting. Heparin is very effective and is intended for short-term use in a hospital setting. Some patients are sent home on a low molecular weight heparin, such as enoxaparin, which is an IM injection. The patient may be counseled by a nurse on how to administer this injectable IM dose. This low dose heparin is normally given for up to 14 days for prophylactic treatment against embolisms.

Another type of anticoagulant is warfarin. This agent is available in both injectable and oral dosage forms. Unlike heparin, oral warfarin is also indicated for long-term use and is always taken once a day. Warfarin interferes with the liver's synthesis of vitamin K-dependent coagulation factors (II, VII, IX, and X). Prothrombin time (PT) tests must be done to monitor how long it takes the blood to form clots while the patient is on this medication. It is vital that a patient not be overdosed on warfarin or the patient can bleed to death internally. Warfarin has many interactions with other drugs and with certain foods. Any drug that may increase the potency of warfarin must be avoided as well as those that counteract the effectiveness of this medication.

TECH NOTE! Foods such as broccoli cause coagulation. Therefore persons who normally do not eat broccoli and who begin to take warfarin should avoid large amounts of broccoli because it will counteract the effectiveness of warfarin. Persons who normally eat broccoli may continue to do so because lab results will be based on the blood coagulation time of a person who eats broccoli.

There are also many OTC agents that are used to prevent thrombosis. One of the best known and popular is aspirin. The advantage of taking aspirin over warfarin is the lower amount of interactions between drugs and food. However, only a doctor can determine which is best for a patient. In addition, the anticoagulant effect of aspirin lasts for 7 days.

TECH NOTE! Aspirin should not be taken with warfarin because it increases the effectiveness of this anticoagulant, which may result in internal bleeding.

CLASSIFICATION: ANTICOAGULANTS
GENERIC NAME: heparin
TRADE NAME: Liquaemin
ROUTE OF ADMINISTRATION: injectable forms only (IV, SC)
SIDE EFFECTS: possible hemorrhage (PT must be monitored closely)
ANTIDOTE: Phytonadione injection (vitamin K)

GENERIC NAME: warfarin
TRADE NAME: Coumadin
ROUTE OF ADMINISTRATION: oral, injectable (IV)
SIDE EFFECTS: because of possible hemorrhage (PT must be monitored closely)
ANTIDOTE: Phytonadione injection (vitamin K)

TABLE 22.3 Antiplatelet Agents

Generic	Trade	Common Prophylaxis Dosage
Aspirin	Aspirin	81 to 325 mg once daily
Dipyridamole	Persantine	75 to 100 mg 4 times daily
Ticlopidine	Ticlid	250 mg twice daily, with food
Clopidogrel	Plavix	75 mg qd

Antiplatelet Agents. Antiplatelet drugs work mainly on arterial thrombi, which are made of platelet aggregates (particles). The drugs most commonly used to treat these types of clots are listed in Table 22.3.

Drug Action of Thrombolytics

Streptokinase (Streptase) is an enzyme extracted from bacteria that destroys clots after they are formed. Urokinase (Abbokinase) is another type of lytic agent that is retrieved from a human protein that also reduces thrombosis. The newest agent is alteplase (Activase, or tPA), a natural enzyme that is normally produced by the body to dissolve blood clots. It binds to fibrin within a thrombus and converts the entrapped plasminogen to plasmin, dissolving the clot. This enzyme is isolated and prepared for parenteral use. Of the three agents, alteplase is the most expensive at well over $1000 per dose. These medications have specific uses and are intended for use as soon as possible after an MI to break up the clot.

NONPHARMACOLOGICAL TREATMENT FOR MYOCARDIAL INFARCTION

The many available medications for patients after MI have been discussed previously in this chapter. With the continued use of a variety of agents and a change in lifestyle, many patients live a normal life-span. However, if the patient's MI was severe, surgery, such as bypass surgery, may be necessary. Bypass surgery creates new routes for blood flow to the heart muscle. Veins are transplanted from the legs and rerouted around the damaged vessel within the heart. Newer techniques allow surgeons to conduct bypass surgery without opening the chest wall. This less invasive technique enables the patient to recover more quickly. For more information on new innovative treatments in cardiac surgery visit the American Heart Association online (www.heartassociation.org).

DO YOU REMEMBER THESE KEY POINTS?

- The location of the heart
- How blood flows through the heart
- The layers of the heart muscle
- Conditions that affect the heart
- Causes for heart problems such as CHF, CAD, and hypertension
- Treatments for conditions affecting the heart
- Common side effects for medications mentioned in this chapter
- Types of diuretics and their mechanism of action
- The effects of OTC medications for persons suffering from hypertension
- The types of angina and the medications used to treat them
- The difference between the use of anticoagulants and thrombolytics

REVIEW QUESTIONS:

Multiple Choice

1. The average adult heart beats _____ times per minute.
   A. 50
   B. 70
   C. 90
   D. 100

2. The artery responsible for supplying the heart muscle with oxygen is called the
   A. Pulmonary artery
   B. Aorta
   C. Coronary artery
   D. Myocardial passageway

3. The cardiac conduction system is responsible for
   A. Providing the electrical charge to the heart muscle
   B. Oxygenating the blood
   C. Receiving blood from the body
   D. None of the above

4. A condition in which fluid builds up within tissues is known as
   A. Myocardial infarction
   B. Angina pectoris
   C. Congestive heart failure
   D. Hypertension

5. Factor(s) that may effect the condition of atherosclerosis is/are
   A. Lifestyle
   B. Family history
   C. Smoking
   D. All of the above

6. If Mr. Low has a blood pressure of 165/95, he would have
   A. Low blood pressure
   B. Normal blood pressure
   C. Slightly high blood pressure
   D. High blood pressure

7. ACE inhibitors is an abbreviation for
   A. Activating coronary electrical site inhibitors
   B. Altering and converting enzyme inhibitors
   C. Angiotensin-converting enzyme inhibitors
   D. Anginal converting enzyme inhibitors

8. Beta-blockers are effective because they work by
   A. Blocking receptor sites in the heart
   B. Blocking receptor sites in the heart and kidneys
   C. Activating receptor sites in the heart and lungs
   D. Activating receptor sites in the heart and kidneys

9. Calcium channel blockers are effective because they work by
   A. Blocking both channel one and two receptors
   B. Reducing cardiac conduction
   C. Speeding up the heart to pump more blood
   D. None of the above

10. Which instruction is NOT patient information necessary about taking oral nitroglycerin medications?
    A. Take with food
    B. Keep medication within the original container
    C. Take as needed for chest pain; max 3 times in 15 minutes, if no relief, then call 911
    D. Keep medication out of direct sunlight

11. Streptase, Abbokinase, and tPA are all classified as
    A. Vasoconstrictors
    B. Vasodilators
    C. Prophylaxis thrombolytics
    D. Thrombolytics

12. The common lifespan of nitroglycerin (once opened) is
    A. 3 months
    B. 6 months
    C. 12 months
    D. None of the above

13. The four chambers of the heart are
    A. Right and left: upper and lower atrium
    B. Right and left: atrium and superior and inferior vena cava
    C. Right and left: atrium and ventricle
    D. None of the above

14. The medication that dissolves blood clots is called
    A. Heparin   C. tPA
    B. Aspirin   D. Warfarin

15. Heparin cannot be given orally because
    A. It takes too long to work
    B. It is used only for emergencies
    C. It is degraded by gastric juices
    D. It binds directly to blood products

True/False

*If the statement is false, then change it to make it true.

1. The heart pumps only oxygenated blood.

2. Oxygenated blood returns from the lungs via the pulmonary artery.

3. The epicardium is the outer layer of the heart muscle, and it protects the heart.

4. The vena cava is the large artery that carries blood to the body system.

5. Two major types of lipoproteins that should be monitored are HDL and LDL.

6. HDL stands for high-density lipoproteins and is considered bad cholesterol.

7. Cholesterol has no benefit to the human body.

8. The fibers that control the conduction system are called the pacemaker.

9. Congestive heart failure can be cured by surgery.

10. Hypertension is also known as the silent killer.

11. Nitrates are agents that cause vasoconstriction.

12. Aspirin is a thrombolytic agent.

13. Calcium channel blockers are often the first line of treatment for angina.

14. An embolism is a thrombosis or clot which has moved from its origin.

15. Aspirin has more side effects than either heparin or warfarin.

16. Beta-blockers increase blood pressure thus helping the heart beat stronger.

17. ACE inhibitors increase blood pressure thus helping the heart beat faster.

18. Nitroglycerin must be kept in a glass container.

19. All diuretics cause a loss of potassium through frequent urination.

20. Edema is a condition of inflammation of the tissues resulting from hyperlipidemia.

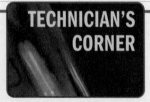

TECHNICIAN'S CORNER

Mrs. Lewis comes into the pharmacy with several prescriptions. Using a comprehensive drug reference, such as *Facts and Comparisons or Mosby's Drug Consult*, look up the medications listed and determine what Mrs. Lewis may be suffering from. In addition, for each of the medications, classify each one and transcribe into laymen's terms as though you were preparing a prescription label.

    Zocor 5 mg qd #30
    Digoxin 125 mcg qd #30
    Furosemide 40 mg bid #60
    K-Dur 20 mEq bid #60
    Albuterol INH 1 to 2 puffs prn SOB #17 g
    NTG 0.4 mg sl prn cp, 1 q 5 min, mr × 3 over 15 min, then call 911 4/#25s
    Atenolol 25 mg qd #30

BIBLIOGRAPHY

Drug Facts and Comparisons 1999, St. Louis, 1999, Facts and Comparisons.

Lacy C, et al., *Drug Information Handbook,* Hudson, Ohio, 2000-2001, Lexi-Comp.

Lewis S, et al., *Medical Surgical Nursing Assessment,* ed 5, St. Louis, 2000, Mosby.

Mosby's Drug Consult, St Louis, 2004, Elsevier.

Stedman's Concise Medical Dictionary for Health Professionals, ed 3, Baltimore, 1997, Williams & Wilkins.

CHAPTER 23

Reproductive System

Robert M. Fulcher and Eugenia M. Fulcher

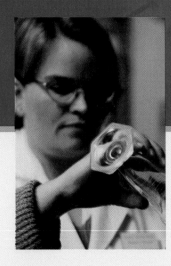

Objectives

- Describe the organs of the male and female reproductive tract and their locations.

- Describe the male and female hormones and their roles in the body.

- List the common conditions affecting the male reproductive system and the medications used to treat these conditions.

- List the common conditions of the female reproductive system and the medications used to treat these conditions.

- Describe hormone replacement therapy in the female and list the medications used for hormone replacement.

- List the different types of oral contraceptives.

- List other types of contraception and the advantages and disadvantages of each.

- Describe the medications that are used as abortifacients.

Abortifacients *Any treatment that causes abortion of a fetus*

Amenorrhea *Absence or suppression of menses*

Androgens *Male hormones*

Benign prostatic hypertrophy *Nonmalignant enlargement of prostate gland*

Chloasma *Hyperpigmentation of skin, limited or confined to a certain area, usually found on the face during pregnancy*

Depot *An area of the body where a substance can accumulate or be stored for later distribution; in pharmacy, medications are provided in depot form to allow slow absorption in the body*

Dysmenorrhea *Painful menstruation*

Endometriosis *Condition in which tissue resembling endometrium is found outside the uterine cavity, usually in the pelvic area*

Endometrium *Mucous lining of the uterus*

Fallopian tube *Narrow passage between the ovary and the uterus*

Fertilization *The process by which a sperm unites with an ovum to create a new life*

Gametes *Sex cells or ova and sperm*

Inert ingredient *An ingredient that has little or no effect on body functions*

Menopause *Cessation of menstruation; a natural phenomenon in which a woman passes from a reproductive state to a nonreproductive state*

Negative feedback *A self-regulating mechanism in which the output of a system has input or control on the process; a factor within a system that causes a corrective action to return the system to normal range*

Oocytes or ova *The female reproductive germ cells*

Palliative *Brings relief but does not cure*

Therapeutic *Curative treatment that is effective*

REPRODUCTIVE SYSTEM DRUGS

Trade Name	Generic Name	Pronunciation	Trade Name	Generic Name	Pronunciation
Androgens			**Estrogens**		
Histerone, Testex, Transderm, Androderm	testosterone	tes-**toss**-te-rone	Estrace, Estraderm, Climara	estradiol	ess-tra-**dye**-ol
Halotestin	fluoxymesterone	floo-**ox**-ee-mes-ter-one	Delestrogen	estradiol valerate	ess-tra-**dye**-ol val-er-ate
Oreton, Testred	methyltestosterone	meth-ill-tes-**toss**-te-rone	Estratab, Menest	esterified estrogen	ess-ter-i-**fide** es-tro-gin
			Estratest	esterified estrogens/ methyltestosterone	ess-ter-i-**fide** es-tro-gins/meth-ill-tes-**toss**-te-rone
Adrenergic Antagonists for Benign Prostatic Hypertrophy					
Hytrin	terazosin	ter-**ay**-zoe-sin	Premarin	conjugated estrogens	**con**-ju-gate-ed **es**-tro-gins
Cardura	doxazosin	dox-**ay**-zoe-sin			
Flomax	tamsulosin	tam-sue-**lo**-sin	Prempro, Premphase	esterified estrogens/ medroxyprogesterone	ess-ter-i-**fide** es-tro-gins/me-drox-ee-proe-**jess**-ter-one
Other Medications for Benign Prostatic Hypertrophy					
Proscar	finasteride	fin-**ass**-te-ride			

REPRODUCTIVE SYSTEM DRUGS—cont'd

Trade Name	Generic Name	Pronunciation	Trade Name	Generic Name	Pronunciation
Ogen, Ortho-Est	estropipate	ess-troe-**pye**-pate	***Triphasic Combinations***		
			Tri/Norinyl, Ortho-Novum 7/7/7	ethinyl estradiol/ norethindrone	eth-i **nill** ess-tra-**dye**-ol/nor-eth-**in**-drone
Progestins					
Crinone, Gesterol	progesterone	pro-**jess**-ter-one	Triphasil, Tri-Levlen	ethinyl estradiol/ levonorgestrel	eth-i-**nill** ess-tra-**dye**-ol/lev-o-nor-**jess**-trel
Provera, Amen, Cycrin, Depo-Provera	medroxyprogesterone	me-drox-ee-proe-**jess**-te-rone			
Hylutin	hydroxyprogesterone	hye-drox-ee-proe-**jess**-te-rone	Ortho Tricyclin	ethinyl estradiol/ norgestimate	eth-i-**nill** ess-tra-**dye**-ol/nor-**jess**-ti-mate
Micronor, Norlutin	norethindrone	nor-eth-**in**-drone			
Ovrette	norgestrel	nor-**jess**-trel	***Estrophasic Combinations***		
			Estrastep	ethinyl estradiol/ norethindrone	eth-i-**nill** ess-tra-**dye**-ol/nor-eth-**in**-drone
Oral Contraceptives					
Monophasic Combinations					
Loestrin, Ovcon, Genora, Ortho-Novum, Norinyl	ethinyl estradiol/ norethindrone	eth-i-**nill** ess-tra-**dye**-ol/nor-eth-**in**-drone	**Long-Acting Contraceptives**		
			DepoProvera	medroxyprogesterone	me-drox-e-pro-**jess**-te-rone
Ortho-Evra	ethinyl estradiol/ norelgestramin	eth-i-**nill** ess-tra-**dye**-ol/nor-**jess**-ti-min	Lunelle	medroxyprogesterone/ estradiol	me-drox-e-pro-**jess**-te-rone/ess-tra-**dye**-ol
Alesse, Levlen	estinyl estradiol/ levonorgestrel	ess-**tin**-ill ess-tra-**dye**-ol/lev-o-nor-**jess**-trel			
			Spermicidals		
Lo-Ovral, Ovral	estinyl estradiol/ norgestrel	ess-**tin**-ill ess-tra-**dye**-ol/nor-**jess**-trel	Delfen, Koromex, Emko	nonoxynol-9	non-**ox**-i-nol
Desogen, Ortho-Cept, Mircette	estinyl estradiol/ desogestrel	ess-**tin**-ill-ess-tra-**dye**-ol/des-o-**ges**-trol	**Medications for infertility**		
			Clomid	clomiphene	**kloe**-mi-feen
Levora, Ortho-Cyclin	estinyl estradiol/ norgestimate	ess-**tin**-ill ess-tra-**dye**-ol/nor-**jess**-ti-mate	Pergonal, Humegon	menotropin	men-o-**trop**-in
			Parlodel	bromocriptine	bro-mo-**crip**-tin
Demulin	estinyl estradiol/ ethynodiol	**ess**-**tin**-ill ess-tra-**dye**-ol/eh-the-no-**dye**-ol	**Miscellaneous Medications for the Reproductive System**		
			Emergency Contraceptives		
Ortho-Novum 1/50, Norinyl, Genora 1/50	mestranol/ norethindrone	**mess**-tra-nol/nor-eth-**in**-drone	Plan B, Ovrette	progestin	pro-**jess**-tin
			Preven	estrogen/progestin	**ess**-tro-gin/pro-**jess**-tin
Alesse-28, Necon 1/35, Ortho-Novum 1/35	estrogen/progestin	**ess**-tro-gen/pro-**jess**-tin			
			Drugs for endometriosis		
Biphasic Combinations			Zoladex	goserelin	goe-**ser**-a-lin
Ortho-Novum 10/11, Nelova 10/11	ethinyl estradiol/ norethindrone	eth-i-**nill** ess-tra-**dye**-ol/nor-eth-**in**-drone	Lupron	leuprolide	loo-**pro**-lide
			Synarel	nafarelin	naf-a-**rell**-in
			Drugs for erectile dysfunction		
			Viagra	sildenafil	sil-**den**-a-fil

Introduction

The major function of the reproductive system is the production of offspring or the survival of the species. This organ system operates interdependently with other systems such as the endocrine system (for the hormones necessary to function properly) and the urinary system (especially in the male). In both men and women, the functions of reproduction are divided between the primary and secondary, or accessory, organs. The primary reproductive organs are the gonads (ovaries or testes), which are necessary to produce the gametes or sex cells (ova or sperm). The gonads are also responsible for the secretion of the hormones that provide gender characteristics of the male or female. The secondary reproductive organs include the structures necessary for transport and sustenance of the gametes and also those organs necessary for the sustenance of the developing fetus in the female.

MALE REPRODUCTIVE SYSTEM

In the male, the reproductive system is very closely tied to the urinary system. The urethra passes through the penis and is surrounded by the prostate gland. The testicles are responsible for the production of sperm after puberty and for the immediate storage of these cells. Once sperm production begins, it continues throughout the lifetime of the male. After formation, the sperm pass through the epididymis, where they mature, and into the vas deferens where peristaltic movements move them into the proximal portion. The sperm then enter the ejaculatory duct. The prostate and bulbourethral glands secrete fluids to nourish the sperm, to enhance their motility and viability, and to provide a slightly alkaline environment that will neutralize the acidic environment of the vagina. Finally the sperm and fluids pass through the urethra in the penis for ejaculation during sexual intercourse (Figure 23.1).

Male sex hormones are stimulated by the gonadotropin releasing hormone (GnRH) of the anterior pituitary gland that then stimulates the formation of luteinizing hormone (LH), also called interstitial cell stimulating hormone (ICSH) in the male, and follicle stimulating hormone (FSH). ICSH then promotes the growth of interstitial cells in the testes and stimulates the cells to secrete testosterone. Testosterone and FSH stimulate spermatogenesis in the testicles (Figure 23.2).

Male sex hormones are collectively called androgens, with testosterone being the most abundant androgen. At puberty, the androgens stimulate the formation

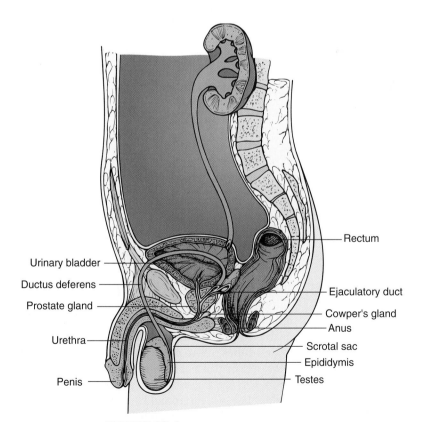

FIGURE 23.1 Male reproductive system.

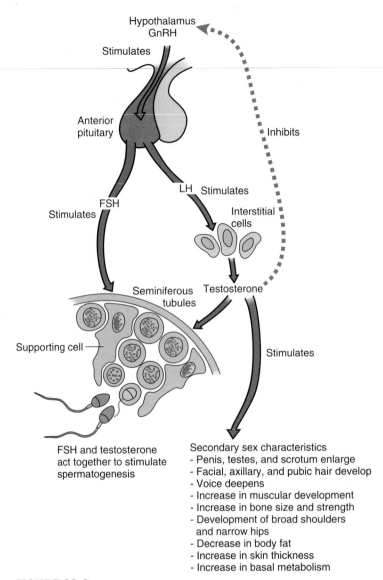

Hypothalamus
GnRH

Stimulates

Anterior
pituitary

Inhibits

LH Stimulates

FSH

Stimulates

Interstitial
cells

Seminiferous
tubules

Testosterone

Supporting cell

Stimulates

FSH and testosterone
act together to stimulate
spermatogenesis

Secondary sex characteristics
- Penis, testes, and scrotum enlarge
- Facial, axillary, and pubic hair develop
- Voice deepens
- Increase in muscular development
- Increase in bone size and strength
- Development of broad shoulders
  and narrow hips
- Decrease in body fat
- Increase in skin thickness
- Increase in basal metabolism

FIGURE 23.2 Function of testes in response to hormone stimulation.

of secondary male characteristics, such as increased muscle mass, deepening of the voice, and growth of facial hair.

FEMALE REPRODUCTIVE SYSTEM

The female reproductive system produces and transports ova from the ovary through the fallopian tube into the uterus, which will house a fertilized ovum. After puberty, the female ovary matures an egg each month although recent science indicates that more than one egg may mature. At birth, the female ovary contains all the eggs that the female will ever have. Thus, females do not produce ova throughout life but only mature those that are available. When an egg is mature, it is gathered by the fimbriated end of the infundibulum of the fallopian tube. The fallopian tubes are in constant motion, but at ovulation their activity increases, and currents in the peritoneal fluid are created to propel the egg into the fallopian tube. During the next 7 days, the ovum is moved down the fallopian tube where it may become fertilized by a sperm. Because an ovum is only viable for 24 to 38 hours, most fertilization occurs in the fallopian tube. At the end of the tube is the uterus that will house the fertilized ovum or slough the ovum and endometrium

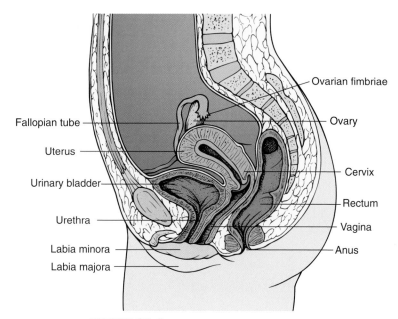

FIGURE 23.3 Female reproductive system.

as menses if fertilization has not occurred. This cycle begins at puberty and continues until menopause, or for a period of about 40 years (Figure 23.3).

As in the male, the GnRH from the anterior pituitary begins the secretion of the hormones necessary for ovulation. FSH and LH stimulate the ovaries to secrete estrogen and progesterone. These female hormones found in the endocrine system are controlled by negative feedback and are secreted in cycles, unlike the continuous secretion of sex hormones in males (Figure 23.4). The level of female hormones peaks when a woman is in her 20s and then gradually decreases throughout life.

The accessory organs of the female reproductive tract are the mammary glands or breasts. This tissue is also regulated by hormonal secretions. At puberty the increase in estrogen stimulates the development of glandular tissue, causing an accumulation of adipose tissue, and progesterone stimulates the development of the duct system that will be used during milk production.

The chief drugs that affect the reproductive system are hormones. Some agents stimulate secretions, whereas others inhibit the action of certain hormones. Medication therapy for conditions of the reproductive tract can be very complicated because hormone levels must be considered and must remain fairly constant. However, many of the drug names are familiar. Female hormones are used to treat some conditions of the male reproductive tract, such as prostate and testicular cancer, and male hormones are used to treat endometrial or breast cancer, endometriosis, and fibrocystic disease in the female. The inhibition of the natural hormones in either gender is brought about by the use of the hormones of the other gender, much like negative feedback in which the stimulating hormone is inhibited. Remember that the hypothalamus cannot distinguish between hormones naturally produced by the body and those that are administered as medications; therefore, the body will react to the medication in the same manner as it reacts to synthetic and naturally occurring hormones.

Medications Related to Male Hormones

Testosterone provides a sense of well-being, mental stability, and energy. It also provides the body with a resistance to fatigue. Natural testosterone that is used for medicinal purposes is obtained from the testes of bulls. Androgens that are

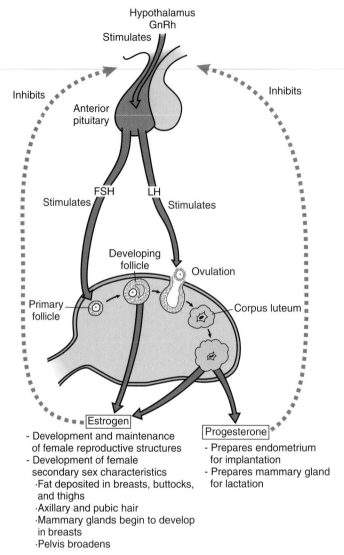

Hypothalamus
GnRh
Stimulates

Inhibits

Inhibits

Anterior
pituitary

FSH   LH
Stimulates   Stimulates

Developing
follicle

Ovulation

Primary
follicle

Corpus luteum

Estrogen

- Development and maintenance
  of female reproductive structures
- Development of female
  secondary sex characteristics
  ·Fat deposited in breasts, buttocks,
  and thighs
  ·Axillary and pubic hair
  ·Mammary glands begin to develop
  in breasts
  ·Pelvis broadens

Progesterone

- Prepares endometrium
  for implantation
- Prepares mammary gland
  for lactation

FIGURE 23.4 Function of ovaries in response to hormone stimulation.

produced synthetically are called anabolic steroids—medications that are used to build muscle mass. Because of the misuse and abuse of anabolic steroids, the Drug Enforcement Agency (DEA) has placed anabolic steroids on the Schedule III list of controlled medications.

Androgens are used to produce male secondary sex characteristics and to maintain the male reproductive structures. Therefore, androgens are used to treat hypogonadism or infertility resulting from a low sperm count. The increase in sperm count is achieved through the suppression of negative feedback, causing an increased secretion of testosterone, FSH, and ICSH.

Male hormones are also used as palliative agents in treating male reproductive tumors. In addition to an increased feeling of well-being, the androgens increase bone density and lean body mass. Because of the ability of androgens to reverse tissue wasting, these hormones are often used to reverse the debilitating affects of diseases and the wasting that comes from long-term use of corticosteroids. These medications tend to decrease pain levels, make the male more alert, and increase appetite. These actions lead to an overall feeling of increased well-being.

Male hormones can be used for treating some female breast tumors that grow faster in the presence of estrogen. Androgens suppress the effects of estrogen, thus preventing rapid growth of these tumors. Sometimes the medications may even cause the tumor to atrophy. Other uses of androgens in females are to suppress postpartum breast engorgement and fibrocystic disease by causing atrophy of the breasts. For the woman with endometriosis, androgens cause suppression of the endometrium and thus prevent the excessive uterine bleeding that is found with the disease.

Adverse reactions to testosterone medications include nausea, vomiting, and diarrhea. Blood levels of calcium, sodium, phosphorus, potassium, and cholesterol may become elevated. Hypoglycemia, pruritus, jaundice, and alterations in libido may also occur with continued use of testosterone. With men, breast engorgement, impotence, male pattern baldness, and acne are expected. Women receiving androgen therapy for prolonged periods of time may have amenorrhea or menstrual irregularities. Hot flashes, headaches, sleep disorders, increased libido, vaginitis, and masculinization are also found. Changes in the voice (lowering of the voice) are often permanent, whereas other symptoms such as loss of breast mass, increased facial and body hair, and increased muscle mass may reverse when the testosterone therapy is discontinued. Masculinization does not seem to occur with short-term use of androgens by women with such conditions as postpartum engorgement of the breasts.

Patients taking androgens should be informed that weight gain and headaches are common but a weight gain of more than 2 pounds may require medications to rid the body of edema. Taking the medications with food will help decrease undesired gastrointestinal symptoms. Patients taking anticoagulants and hypoglycemics may require smaller doses of these medications when taking androgens. Androgens are divided into two groups: those from natural sources and those from synthetic sources.

CLASSIFICATION OF ANDROGENS

Natural Androgens

GENERIC NAME: testosterone (short and long acting)
TRADE NAME: Testoderm, AndroGel, Androderm, Depo-Testosterone, Depotest
INDICATION: androgen replacement therapy, palliation of female mammary cancer, male hypogonadism
ROUTE OF ADMINISTRATION: implantable pellet, gel, transdermal patch
COMMON DOSAGE: short acting: 25 to 30 mg 2 to 3 times/week
long acting: 50 to 400 mg q2 to 4 weeks

GENERIC NAME: testosterone propionate
TRADE NAME: Testex
INDICATION: androgen replacement therapy, male hypogonadism, palliation of female breast cancer
ROUTE OF ADMINISTRATION: injectable
COMMON DOSAGE: 50 to 400 mg q2 to 4 weeks

Synthetic Androgens

GENERIC NAME: fluoxymesterone
TRADE NAME: Halotestin
INDICATION: male hypogonadism, female breast cancer
ROUTE OF ADMINISTRATION: oral tablet
COMMON DOSAGE: 5 to 20 mg/day

GENERIC NAME: danazol
TRADE NAME: Danocrine
INDICATION: endometriosis and fibrocystic disease in women
ROUTE OF ADMINISTRATION: oral tablet
COMMON DOSAGE: 400 mg bid

GENERIC NAME: methyltestosterone
TRADE NAME: Oreton, Adroid-25, Testred
INDICATIONS: hypogonadism, breast cancer in women
ROUTE OF ADMINISTRATION: oral and buccal tablets
COMMON DOSAGE: 10 to 50 mg qd

GENERIC NAME: stanozolol
TRADE NAME: Winstrol
INDICATION: aplastic anemia, weight gain
ROUTE OF ADMINISTRATION: oral tablet
COMMON DOSAGE: 2 mg tid

GENERIC NAME: nandrolone
TRADE NAME: Durabolin
INDICATION: breast cancer, anemias resulting from aplastic anemia
ROUTE OF ADMINISTRATION: injectable
COMMON DOSAGE: 50 to 100 mg/week

Medications for benign prostatic hypertrophy are used to decrease the mass of an enlarged prostate gland. Benign prostatic hypertrophy occurs in about 73% of men by the age of 70. The goal of treatment for benign prostatic hypertrophy is to relieve the bothersome symptoms such as urinary tract infections, hesitancy on urination, a decrease in the stream of urine, postvoiding dribbling, frequency, and nocturia. Some of the medications, such as finasteride, promote shrinkage of the prostate, whereas the alpha-adrenergic blockers relax the smooth muscle of the prostatic tissue to reduce obstruction.

Antiandrogen

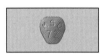

Merck

GENERIC NAME: finasteride, dutasteride
TRADE NAME: Proscar, Avodart
INDICATION: benign prostatic hypertrophy
ROUTE OF ADMINISTRATION: oral capsule
COMMON DOSAGE: 5 mg qd
NOTE: This drug is teratogenic so a form of contraception should be used, if applicable.

Alpha-Adrenergic Blockers

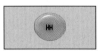

Abbott

GENERIC NAME: terazosin
TRADE NAME: Hytrin
INDICATION: benign prostatic hypertrophy
ROUTE OF ADMINISTRATION: oral tablet
COMMON DOSAGE: 1 to 10 mg qd

GENERIC NAME: tamsulosin
TRADE NAME: Flomax
INDICATION: benign prostatic hypertrophy
ROUTE OF ADMINISTRATION: oral capsule
COMMON DOSAGE: 0.4 mg daily

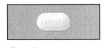

Roerig

GENERIC NAME: doxazosin
TRADE NAME: Cardura
INDICATIONS: benign prostatic hypertrophy, mild hypertension
ROUTE OF ADMINISTRATION: oral capsule
COMMON DOSAGE: 1 mg qid

Medications Related to Female Hormones

Like testosterone secretion in the male, estrogen and progesterone secretion responds to the secretions of the anterior pituitary gland. Gonadotropin-releasing hormone (GnRH) stimulates follicle stimulating hormone (FSH) and luteinizing hormone (LH) to cause the ovaries to secrete estrogen and progesterone. Unlike testosterone in the male, these hormones follow cyclic patterns each month beginning at puberty and continuing until menopause when hormone secretion decreases. During premenopause, the ovaries gradually decrease estrogen production, and in the childbearing years gradually cease.

Estrogens are the dominant form of medical therapy that is used to treat conditions such as abnormal uterine bleeding resulting from hormone imbalance, abnormal ovulation, and infertility. Estrogens are also used for hormone replacement therapy. One of the main uses of estrogen preparations is for oral contraception. Estrogens also have effects on bone and cardiovascular function and cause reduced levels of low-density lipoproteins and thus raise levels of high-density lipoproteins to lower the risk of cardiac disease. Estrogens support the development and maintenance of the reproductive organs and the secondary sex characteristics and have profound influences on the menstrual cycle. In the male, estrogens are used to treat prostate and breast cancer.

Estradiol is the major natural estrogen that is produced by the ovaries. Used for hormone replacement therapy in the naturally postmenopausal woman or in the woman who is experiencing a surgical menopause, estradiol is usually combined with progestins because of the increased risk of endometrial and breast cancer when combination medications are not used. Estrogen replacement therapy seems to protect the female against coronary and vascular disease; thus, the values of the medications must be weighed against the known risks, such as thromboembolytic diseases and increased risk for neoplasms. Most replacement therapy is in conjugated doses from natural sources such as from the urine of pregnant mares or from placentas, but estrogens may also be synthetically formulated. The naturally occurring estrogens, such as estrone, estradiol, and estriol, are steroids that are converted to estriol by the body. Some of the synthetically formulated products are steroidal in nature, whereas others are nonsteroidal.

Estrogens are available in several forms; and some forms are unique such as implants, vaginal inserts, and nasal sprays. The most common forms are oral and injectable preparations in either water or oil base. The oil-based medications, called *depot* medications, are prepared to prolong the action by allowing absorption in the fatty tissue for slow distribution. Transdermal preparations are applied to the skin to provide continuous daily release of the medication. Drug-laden vaginal rings are pressed into the vaginal canal for the continuous release of medications into the local tissues. Other local administrated estrogens include vaginal inserts and creams that provide absorption of hormones at the local site. The choice of preparation to be used is dependent on the reason for use, cost, reliability of the patient to use it correctly, and the convenience of use. Most estrogens are prescribed at the lowest dose needed to provide the desired effect over the shortest period of time.

The primary actions of estrogens are to maintain reproductive structures such as ova production and to provide secondary sex characteristics. Estrogens also assist with the retention of calcium and phosphorus for bone production in the postmenopausal state. In women, estrogens are used to treat hypogonadism; for postpartal breast engorgement or lactation; to relieve symptoms of menopause (natural or surgical); and to relieve symptoms of dysmenorrhea, endometriosis, and dysfunctional uterine bleeding. In men, estrogens are used for inoperable prostate and testicular cancer. The increased estrogen in males causes feminization to occur, including voice changes, breast enlargement, loss of body hair, testicular and penile atrophy, and impotence. The feminization and impotence of males are usually reversed on termination of medication.

In the female, adverse effects may include chloasma, photosensitivity, nausea, vomiting, bloating, and risk of gallbladder disease. Infertility, dysmenorrhea, breast tenderness and enlargement, and increased susceptibility to thrombolytic disease are also commonly seen effects. Although estrogens induce a feeling of well-being, high levels tend to cause depression that may progress to psychosis. In addition, estrogens may aggravate asthma, epilepsy, migraines, heart disease, urinary tract diseases, and increase the symptoms of diabetes mellitus.

ESTROGEN PREPARATIONS

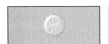

Bristol-Myers
Squibb

GENERIC NAME: estradiol
TRADE NAME: oral: Estrace; transdermal: Estraderm, Vivelle, Climara; vaginal ring: Estring
INDICATIONS: menopausal symptoms, female hypogonadism
COMMON DOSAGE: oral: 0.5 to 2 mg daily in cycles, transdermal: 0.05- to 1-mg patch applied once or twice a week; vaginal ring: change ring every 3 months

GENERIC NAME: estradiol valerate
TRADE NAME: Delestrogen, Gynogen-LA
INDICATIONS: menopausal symptoms, female hypogonadism, prostate cancer
ROUTE OF ADMINISTRATION: injectable
COMMON DOSAGE: 5 to 20 mg q2 to 4 weeks

GENERIC NAME: estradiol cypionate
TRADE NAME: Depo-Estradiol, Depogen, Dura-Estrin
INDICATIONS: menopausal symptoms, female hypogonadism, postmenopausal osteoporosis, prostate cancer, metastatic breast cancer
ROUTE OF ADMINISTRATION: injectable
COMMON DOSAGE: 5 to 20 mg q2 to 4 weeks

GENERIC NAME: esterified estrogen
TRADE NAME: Estratab, Menest
INDICATIONS: menopausal symptoms, female hypogonadism, breast cancer
ROUTE OF ADMINISTRATION: oral tablet
COMMON DOSAGE: 0.3 to 1.25 mg qd

GENERIC NAME: esterified estrogen with methyltestosterone
TRADE NAME: Estratest
INDICATIONS: menopausal symptoms, female hypogonadism, breast cancer
ROUTE OF ADMINISTRATION: oral tablet
COMMON DOSAGE: 1.25 to 2.5 mg qd

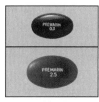

Wyeth-Ayerst

GENERIC NAME: conjugated estrogens
TRADE NAME: Premarin
INDICATIONS: menopausal symptoms, osteoporosis prevention, prostate cancer, breast cancer, hypogonadism, atrophic vaginitis
ROUTE OF ADMINISTRATION: oral tablets, injectable, vaginal cream
COMMON DOSAGE: oral: 0.3 to 2.5 mg qd in cycles; injectable: 25 mg IM; vaginal cream: 2 to 4 g vaginally as directed in cycles

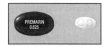

Wyeth-Ayerst

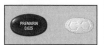

Wyeth-Ayerst

GENERIC NAME: esterified estrogen with medroxyprogesterone
TRADE NAME: Prempro, Premphase
INDICATIONS: menopausal symptoms, osteoporosis prevention, prostate cancer, breast cancer, hypogonadism, atrophic vaginitis
ROUTE OF ADMINISTRATION: oral tablet
COMMON DOSAGE: 0.625 mg/2.5 mg to 0.625 mg/5 mg

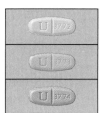

Pharmacia &
Upjohn

GENERIC NAME: estropipate
TRADE NAME: Ogen, Ortho-Est
ROUTE OF ADMINISTRATION: oral tablet
INDICATIONS: menopausal symptoms, prostate cancer, osteoporosis, hypogonadism
COMMON DOSAGE: 0.75 mg to 3 mg qd in cycles

GENERIC NAME: chlorotrianisene
TRADE NAME: TACE
INDICATIONS: menopausal symptoms, vaginitis, female hypogonadism, prostate cancer
ROUTE OF ADMINISTRATION: oral capsule
COMMON DOSAGE: 12 to 24 mg daily in cycles

GENERIC NAME: diethylstilbestrol (DES)
TRADE NAME: none
INDICATIONS: prostate cancer, breast cancer, postcoital contraception
ROUTE OF ADMINISTRATION: oral tablet
COMMON DOSAGE: 1 to 3 mg daily for prostate cancer; 15 mg daily for breast cancer; 25 mg bid ×5 days for postcoital contraception

PROGESTIN

Progesterone, naturally occurring as progestin, is the female hormone secreted from day 14 through day 28 of the menstrual cycle. This hormone has many functions including changing the secretions of the cervix, reducing uterine contractility, and maintaining the corpus luteum. Other actions include stimulating the development of ducts and glands of the breasts in preparation of lactation; however, progestin does not cause lactation.

Progestins may also be made synthetically; natural and synthetic forms have similar pharmacological effects on the body. Placentas are one of the natural sources for obtaining progestins. Because the liver rapidly metabolizes progestin preparations, oral administration of natural preparations is not indicated. Injected forms are usually placed in an oil base to delay the absorption and thus prolong effects. Synthetically produced preparations are different from natural progesterone and are called either progestins or progestogens. The synthetic form is most often used rather than the natural forms because synthetics are more effective. Given both by injection and orally, the action of synthetic progestin is prolonged over progesterone, and the oral administration is effective because the synthetically made progestin is not rapidly metabolized by the liver.

Progestins are used for treating amenorrhea and abnormal uterine bleeding from hormone imbalances, for contraception, in combination with estrogen for hormone replacement therapy in menopause, and as therapy for renal and endometrial cancer. When used with estrogen for contraception, the dosage of progestin is measured in milligrams, whereas the estrogen component is measured in micrograms. Used to treat infertility, progesterone and progesterone-like products cause negative feedback and with the gonadotropic hormones stimulate the development of ova and subsequent ovulation.

The side effects of progestins include weight gain, stomach pain and cramping, swelling of the face and legs, headaches, mood swings, anxiety, weakness, rashes, acne, and insomnia. Menstrual changes and breast tenderness may occur, and liver dysfunction and phlebitis are more severe adverse reactions. Glucose intolerance is seen in women who are prone to diabetes mellitus, and fetal teratogenic effects have occurred.

GENERIC NAME: progesterone
TRADE NAME: Crinone, Gesterol
INDICATIONS: amenorrhea, abnormal uterine bleeding
ROUTE OF ADMINISTRATION: injectable, vaginal gel
COMMON DOSAGE: 5 to 10 mg qd × 6 to 8 days for abnormal uterine bleeding

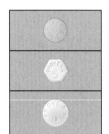

Pharmacia &
Upjohn

GENERIC NAME: medroxyprogesterone
TRADE NAME: oral: Provera, Amen, Cycrin; injectable: Depo-Provera
INDICATIONS: endometrial hyperplasia, secondary amenorrhea, abnormal uterine bleeding; Depo-Provera: contraception
COMMON DOSAGE: 2 to 10 mg qd × 5 to 10 days for amenorrhea, abnormal bleeding; Depo-Provera: 150 mg q 3 months as contraceptive

GENERIC NAME: hydroxyprogesterone
TRADE NAME: Hylutin
INDICATIONS: amenorrhea, abnormal uterine bleeding
ROUTE OF ADMINISTRATION: injectable
COMMON DOSAGE: 375 mg q 4 weeks for amenorrhea, uterine bleeding

GENERIC NAME: norethindrone
TRADE NAME: Micronor, Norlutin
INDICATIONS: amenorrhea, abnormal uterine bleeding, endometriosis, contraception, prevention of endometrial hyperplasia with estrogen therapy
ROUTE OF ADMINISTRATION: oral tablet
COMMON DOSAGE: 2.5 to 10 mg in cycles for amenorrhea, 0.35 mg qd for contraception, 5 mg for prevention of endometrial hyperplasia

CONTRACEPTIVES

Oral contraceptives are used as a means of birth control by preventing fertilization of an ovum and the subsequent pregnancy. Contraception may be accomplished through pharmacological methods such as oral contraceptives (Figure 23.5) or medication-laden devices, such as vaginal rings, patches, or intrauterine devices (Figure 23.6). Nonpharmacological methods such as surgery, the rhythm method, and mechanical devices may also be used. Of the different methods of birth control, the oral contraceptives have the highest incidence of side effects—from nausea and vomiting to menstrual abnormalities to thrombolytic diseases. Barrier methods have the least side effects but are not as effective as hormone-based medications (Figure 23.7).

Oral contraceptives are relatively safe when used by nonsmokers who have normal cardiovascular function. Combination oral contraceptives consist of both

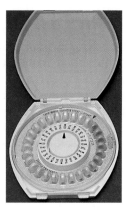

FIGURE 23.5 Typical packaging of oral contraceptives.

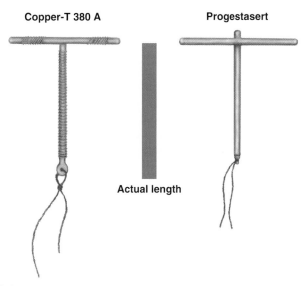

Copper-T 380 A   **Progestasert**

Actual length

FIGURE 23.6 Intrauterine device (IUD) that has progestin (Progestasert) implanted.

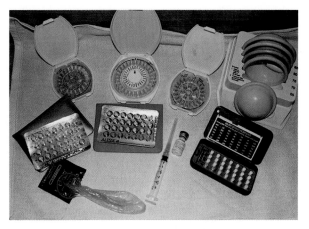

FIGURE 23.7 Common contraceptives, including barrier and medicinal methods: condoms, diaphragm, oral contraceptives, and parenteral contraceptives.

estrogen and progestin to inhibit ovulation. The progestin only contraceptives are called "minipills." The combination medications are the most often prescribed contraceptives and are almost 100% effective. The combination medications are available in monophasic, biphasic, triphasic, and estrophasic formulas. In the monophasic regimen, the daily doses of estrogen and progestin remain constant throughout the menstrual cycle. In the biphasic regimen, the estrogen remains constant but the progestin dose is increased in the second half of the cycle. The triphasic regimen divides the menstrual cycle into three phases, and the amount of progestin changes in each phase. The estrophasic cycle has a constant amount of progestin and the estrogen component is gradually increased throughout the cycle.

The side effects of oral contraceptives include thromboembolism, increased susceptibility to myocardial infarction, and stroke. These medications can increase blood sugar levels, and gallbladder disease, acne, and hirsutism may develop.

The effectiveness of oral contraceptive use is dependent on taking the medication as prescribed. The medication is started on the fifth day of the menstrual cycle and should be taken at the same time of the day for 21 days. If a single dose of the contraceptive is missed, the chance of ovulation is small. However, the risk of pregnancy increases with each dose missed. If one dose is missed, it should be taken on the next day. If two doses are missed, two tablets should be taken on each of the next two days. If three doses are missed, a new cycle of medications should be started 7 days after the last pill was taken, and additional forms of birth control are needed during the first 2 weeks of the new cycle.

Most oral contraceptives are in tablet form, whereas some are available as transdermal patches. Some contraceptives are given by injection for safety and each injection is effective for 3 months. These injections, used in persons who may be noncompliant with oral dosage forms, prevent pregnancy in three ways: by suppressing ovulation, by thickening the cervical mucus, and by altering the endometrium to discourage implantation. The adverse reactions are typical of progestins. Oral contraceptives provide no protection against sexually transmitted diseases, and this is an important factor in patient education.

TECH NOTE! Oral contraceptives should be taken at the same time each day. Oral contraceptives may increase blood glucose levels; thus, a person with diabetes mellitus should be monitored closely. Additional methods of contraception should be used during the initial cycle of oral contraceptives. Some oral contraceptives are packaged in 21-tablet packs, whereas others have 21 tablets of the medication and 7 tablets that are either an iron preparation or an inert tablet.

Contraceptive medications are listed in the following sections. For drugs separated with a slash, the first drug listed is the estrogen component and second drug is the progestin component.

Monophasic Medications

GENERIC NAME: ethinyl estradiol/norethindrone
TRADE NAME: Loestrin, Ovcon, Brevicon, Ortho-Novum, Norinyl, Genora
ROUTE OF ADMINISTRATION: oral tablets in cycle pack
COMMON DOSAGE: these medications are supplied in various strengths of estrogen/progestin; the estrogen is in mcg, the progestin in mg

GENERIC NAME: ethinyl estradiol/drospirenone
TRADE NAME: Yasmin
ROUTE OF ADMINISTRATION: oral tablets in cycle pack

GENERIC NAME: ethinyl estradiol/norelgestromin
TRADE NAME: Ortho-Evra
ROUTE OF ADMINISTRATION: transdermal patch

TECH NOTE! Transdermal patches for contraception should be applied to the upper arms, back, abdomen, or buttocks. The patch should be applied and worn for 1 week; a new patch should be applied on the same day of the week that the first patch was applied. The fourth week should be patch free.

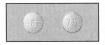

Wyeth-Ayerst

GENERIC NAME: estinyl estradiol/levonorgestrel
TRADE NAME: Levlen, Nordette
ROUTE OF ADMINISTRATION: 28-day cycle pack

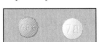

Wyeth-Ayerst

GENERIC NAME: estinyl estradiol/norgestrel
TRADE NAME: Lo-Ovral, Ovral
ROUTE OF ADMINISTRATION: oral tablets in 28-day cycle pack

GENERIC NAME: estinyl estradiol/desogestrel
TRADE NAME: Desogen, Ortho-Cept, Mircette
ROUTE OF ADMINISTRATION: oral tablets in 28-day cycle pack

GENERIC NAME: estinyl estradiol/norgestimate
TRADE NAME: Levora, Ortho-cyclin
ROUTE OF ADMINISTRATION: oral tablets in 28-day cycle pack

GENERIC NAME: estinyl estradiol/ethynodiol diacetate
TRADE NAME: Demulen
ROUTE OF ADMINISTRATION: oral tablets in 28-day cycle pack

GENERIC NAME: mestranol/norethindrone
TRADE NAME: Genora 1/50, Norinyl, Ortho-Novum
ROUTE OF ADMINISTRATION: oral tablets in 28-day cycle pack

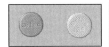

Ortho-McNeil

GENERIC NAME: estrogen/progestin
TRADE NAME: Necon 1/35, Ortho-Novum 1/35, Alesse-28
ROUTE OF ADMINISTRATION: oral tablets in 28-day cycle pack

Biphasic Medications

GENERIC NAME: ethinyl estradiol/norethindrone
TRADE NAME: Ortho-Novum 10/11, Necon 10/11
ROUTE OF ADMINISTRATION: oral tablets in 28-day cycle pack

Triphasic Medications

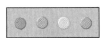

Ortho-McNeil

GENERIC NAME: ethinyl estradiol/norethindrone
TRADE NAME: Tri-Norinyl, Ortho-Novum 7/7/7
ROUTE OF ADMINISTRATION: oral tablets in 28-day cycle pack

Berlex

GENERIC NAME: ethinyl estradiol/levonorgestrel
TRADE NAME: Triphasil, Tri-Levlen
ROUTE OF ADMINISTRATION: oral tablets in 28-day cycle pack

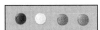

Wyeth-Ayerst

GENERIC NAME: ethinyl estradiol/norgestimate
TRADE NAME: Ortho-TriCyclen
ROUTE OF ADMINISTRATION: oral tablets in 28-day cycle pack

Estrophasic Medications

GENERIC NAME: ethinyl estradiol/norethindrone
TRADE NAME: Estrostep
ROUTE OF ADMINISTRATION: oral tablets in 28-day cycle pack

Progestin-Only Medications

GENERIC NAME: norethindrone
TRADE NAME: Micronor, Nor-QD
ROUTE OF ADMINISTRATION: oral tablets in 28-day cycle pack

GENERIC NAME: norgestrel
TRADE NAME: Ovrette
ROUTE OF ADMINISTRATION: oral tablets in 28-day cycle pack

Long-Acting Contraceptives

GENERIC NAME: medroxyprogesterone
TRADE NAME: Depo-Provera
ROUTE OF ADMINISTRATION: injectable
COMMON DOSAGE: injection every 3 months

Intrauterine Progesterone Contraception

GENERIC NAME: progesterone
TRADE NAME: Progestasert
ROUTE OF ADMINISTRATION: intrauterine device (IUD)

Other Contraceptives

Other contraceptives include spermicides that have the active ingredient nonoxynol-9. These contraceptives are available as foam, jelly, gel, cream, suppository, and vaginal film. The correct use of a spermicide is essential for contraceptive efficacy. The spermicide must be applied before coitus but no more than 1 hour in advance of sexual intercourse. Spermicides may be purchased without a prescription and must be applied each time intercourse is anticipated.

TECH NOTE! Douching should be postponed for at least 6 hours after intercourse when using spermicides.

Barrier devices are nonpharmacological methods of birth control, although a prescription may be written for cervical caps and diaphragms to ensure proper fitting. These devices include male and female condoms (Figure 23.8), cervical caps, and diaphragms (Figure 23.9). The most commonly used is the male condom. Three materials are used in the manufacture of male condoms: latex, polyurethane, and lamb intestine. Lubricants containing mineral oil can decrease the barrier strength of condoms.

TECH NOTE! Lamb intestine condoms do not provide effective protection against the transmission of viruses and bacteria.

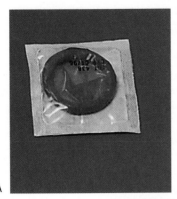
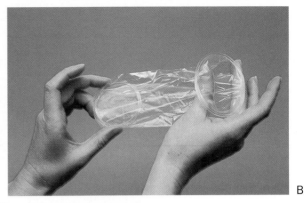

FIGURE 23.8 **A**, Male condom. **B**, Female condom.

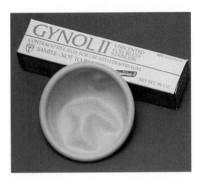

FIGURE 23.9 Contraceptive diaphragm.

Barrier types of contraception for women include the condom, which is a loose-fitting tubular polyurethane pouch with flexible rings at both ends, and the diaphragm, which is a soft rubber cap with a metal spring that fits over the cervix. Before a diaphragm is inserted, it should be filled with spermicide to completely block the cervix from sperm access. The cervical cap, another contraceptive device, is a small cup-shaped barrier that fits directly over the cervical rim and is held in place by suction.

Table 23.1 provides information on the types of contraception and their efficacy.

TECH NOTE! Patches and vaccines for men and women are currently under development. In testing, the male vaccine has been shown to be 99% effective against sperm production. The vaccine for men requires weekly injections of testosterone.

Postcoital, or emergency, forms of contraceptives (ECP) may be either "morning-after pills" or the "abortion" pill to prevent pregnancy after intercourse. To be effective, the first dose of morning-after medication must be taken within 72 hours of unprotected sexual intercourse. A second dose is then taken 12 hours after the first dose. These medications should not be used as a routine type of contraception because of the potential side effects, but they should be used for sexual attacks, contraception failure, or the like.

The morning-after pill is a high-dose contraceptive formulated of either progestin only, estrogen only, or both of these. The combined form of ECPs is about 75% effective but one side effect is nausea and vomiting as if the woman was pregnant. The progestin ECP requires only one tablet and is packaged under the name of Plan B. Plan B is more effective than combined estrogen and progestin forms.

TABLE 23.1 Contraceptive Methods: Risks, Complications, and Failure

Type	Risk/Potential Complications	Failure Rate (%)
Periodic abstinence	Sexual frustration, STDs	20
Calendar abstinence	Sexual frustration, unexpected ovulation, STDs	9-23
Withdrawal (coitus interruptus)	Anxiety, frustration, inability to relax, pregnancy, STDs	19
Vasectomy	Bruising, edema, pain, infection, psychological problems, STDs	0.15
Tubal ligation	Typical abdominal surgical risks, STDs	0.40
Injectible progestogen	Menstrual changes, weight gain, headaches, STDs	0.30-1
Intrauterine devices	Spotting, increased bleeding, uterine cramping, PID, STDs	1-5
Oral contraceptive (estrogen/progesterone tablets)	Nausea, headaches, dizziness, spotting, weight gain, breast disease, ovarian cysts, fluid retention, mood changes, cardiovascular problems, STDs	1-5
Male condom	Allergic reactions, decreased sensitivity, loss of spontaneity, STDs	3-15
Female condom	Visibility, loss of spontaneity	21
Diaphragm	Allergy, toxic shock, vaginal irritation, cervical erosion	4-25
Cervical cap	Allergy, toxic shock, vaginal irritation, cervical erosion	4-25
Sponge	Allergy, toxic shock, vaginal dryness, vaginal irritation	15-30
Spermicides (alone)	Allergy, unpleasant smell or taste	10-25
Douche	Infection, local irritation, STDs	40
None	Pregnancy, STDs	85

ECPs may lead to infertility, breast tenderness, chest pain, shortness of breath, blurred vision, and jaundice. If pregnancy is not terminated by the use of this medication, the woman who took the ECPs should consider an abortion because ECPs are teratogenic to a fetus.

RU-486, mifepristone, is known as the abortion pill. It acts as an antiprogestin. Because progesterone is necessary for establishment and maintenance of pregnancy, RU-486 as an antagonist to progesterone prevents the maintenance of the pregnancy. For safety, this medication must be used within the first 9 weeks of pregnancy. Because of the abortifacient effects of the medication, the administration of RU-486 must be performed by a qualified health care professional, and a prescription will not be written for dispensing by a pharmacist.

Miscellaneous Medications Used in the Reproductive System

Infertility is the decreased ability to reproduce. Anovulation is a cause of infertility that can be corrected by pharmaceutical means. Agents are given to promote maturation of the Graafian follicle and the production of ovulation to release an ovum.

CLASSIFICATION

Antiestrogen

> **GENERIC NAME:** clomiphene
> **TRADE NAME:** Clomid
> **INDICATION:** female infertility
> **ROUTE OF ADMINISTRATION:** oral tablet
> **COMMON DOSAGE:** 50 mg qd × 5 days

LH and FSH Stimulants

> **GENERIC NAME:** menotropin
> **TRADE NAME:** Pergonal, Humegon
> **INDICATION:** stimulate follicles to mature in infertility
> **ROUTE OF ADMINISTRATION:** injectable
> **COMMON DOSAGE:** 75 to 150 U of FSH/LH

> **GENERIC NAME:** urofollitropin
> **TRADE NAME:** Metrodin
> **INDICATION:** stimulate follicle maturity in males and females
> **ROUTE OF ADMINISTRATION:** oral tablet
> **COMMON DOSAGE:** 75 mg qd × 1 week

Ergot Alkaloid

> **GENERIC NAME:** bromocriptine
> **TRADE NAME:** Parlodel
> **INDICATION:** stimulate follicle maturity
> **ROUTE OF ADMINISTRATION:** oral tablet
> **COMMON DOSAGE:** 2.5 to 7.5 mg/day with food

Sildenafil (Viagra) was introduced in 1998 for the treatment of impotence. This medication was initially released for use as a cardiovascular agent to lower blood pressure. Today this medication is used for erectile dysfunction by increasing blood flow to the penis and causing penile rigidity. Sildenafil should be taken as a single dose of 50 mg 1 hour before sexual activity and not more than once a day. The side effects include headaches, flushing of the skin, gastrointestinal symptoms, nasal congestion, and diarrhea. Patients taking nitrates should not take sildenafil because of the dangerous decrease in blood pressure.

DO YOU REMEMBER THESE KEY POINTS?

- Hormones mimicked by the medications used in reproductive tract therapy
- Conditions that androgens are used to treat
- The danger of synthetically produced androgens
- Uses of testosterone therapy in the male; uses of estrogen therapy in the female
- Action of medications used to treat benign prostatic hypertrophy
- Forms of oral contraceptive preparations
- Packaging of oral contraceptive for ease of compliance
- Uses of progestin therapy
- Method of wearing transdermal contraceptive patches
- Method of taking oral contraceptives; method for taking oral contraceptives after missed doses
- Hormones found in combination oral contraceptives
- Forms of contraception other than oral tablets
- Dangers of sildenafil

REVIEW QUESTIONS:

Multiple Choice

1. The primary reproductive organs in the female are
   A. Uterus
   B. Ovaries
   C. Testes
   D. A and B

2. What are the male sex hormones collectively called?
   A. Estrogens
   B. Androgens
   C. Progestins
   D. Testosterones

3. What is the major natural hormone produced by women?
   A. Estradiol
   B. Androgen
   C. Progestin
   D. All of the above

4. Which one of the following is used to obtain progestin naturally?
   A. Urine of mares
   B. Testes of bulls
   C. Placentas
   D. None of the above

5. Which of the following are classified on the controlled substances list as Schedule III drugs?
   A. Estrogens
   B. Androgens
   C. Anabolic steroids
   D. All of the above

6. Testosterone is used to treat which of the following?
   A. Hypogonadism in females
   B. Hypogonadism in males
   C. Breast and endometrial cancer in females
   D. B and C

7. Estrogens are used to treat which of the following?
   A. Menopausal symptoms
   B. Hypogonadism in males
   C. Hypogonadism in females
   D. A and C

8. Medications used to treat benign prostatic hypertrophy include
   A. Antiandrogens
   B. Estrogens
   C. Androgens
   D. Alpha-adrenergic blockers
   E. A and D

9. There are four combination forms of oral contraceptives containing estrogen and progestins. In which of the combinations does estrogen gradually increase throughout the cycle?
   A. Monophasic
   B. Biphasic
   C. Triphasic
   D. Estrophasic
   E. None of the above

10. If two tablets of oral contraceptives are missed and not taken at the correct time, what is the correct procedure?
   A. Don't worry about the missed medication, just discard the medication not taken
   B. Take the two extra tablets with the next dose of medication
   C. Take two tablets with the next two doses at the regular time
   D. Take the two extra tablets at the end of the cycle

True/False

*If a statement is false, then change it to make it true.

1. The female produces ova just as males produce sperm.

2. Fertilization of the ovum occurs in the uterus.

3. Patients on androgens should be told that a weight gain may occur because of the accumulation of fluids.

4. Progestins used with estrogen for contraception are measured in milligrams, and the estrogens are measured in micrograms.

5. In biphasic oral contraceptives, the progestin is increased in the first half of the cycle.

6. Transdermal estrogen patches should be worn on a hairless area of the body such as the upper arms, back, abdomen, or buttocks.

7. Oral contraceptives are effective against sexually transmitted disease.

8. A prescription for RU-486 will be brought to the pharmacy for dispensing.

9. Sildenafil is safe for use by all men and may be used as often as necessary.

10. All types of contraception have approximately the same effectiveness.

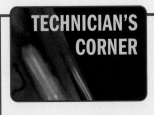

TECHNICIAN'S CORNER

A 55-year-old male patient with diabetes mellitus, hypertension, and coronary artery disease presents a prescription to the pharmacy for sildenafil (Viagra). When you, the pharmacy technician, review his medication history you find that the following medications are taken on a regular basis:

Glucotrol-XL 5 mg daily
metformin 500 mg tid
Tenormin 50 mg daily
Lipitor 20 mg qam
Isordil 10 mg bid

Is the Viagra safe for dispensing with the previously listed medication history? Which of the medications are in a correct dosage? Which medications could be given with sildenafil? Which are contraindicated with sildenafil, if any? What should you as a pharmacy technician do if this prescription is presented for dispensing?

BIBLIOGRAPHY

Applegate EJ: *The anatomy and physiology learning system,* 2nd ed, Philadelphia, 2000, WB Saunders.

Clayton BD, Stock YN: *Basic pharmacology for nurses,* 12th ed, St. Louis, 2001, Mosby.

Fulcher EM, Soto C, Fulcher RM: *Pharmacology: principles and applications,* Philadelphia, 2003, WB Saunders.

Leifer G: *Introduction to maternity and pediatric nursing,* 4th ed, Philadelphia, 2003, WB Saunders.

Mosby's medical, nursing, and allied health dictionary, 6th ed, St. Louis, 2002, Mosby.

Classifications
of Drugs

24 *Antiinfectives*

25 *Antiinflammatories and Antihistamines*

26 *Vitamins and Minerals*

27 *Vaccines*

28 *Oncology Agents*

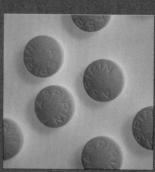

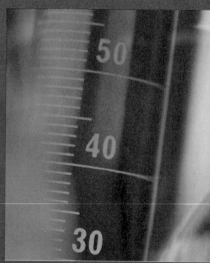

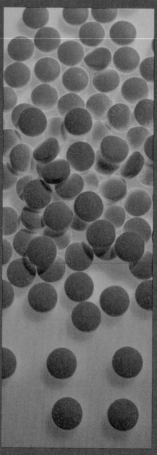

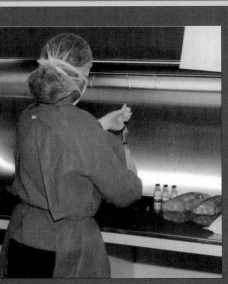

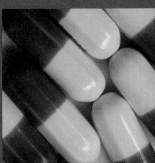

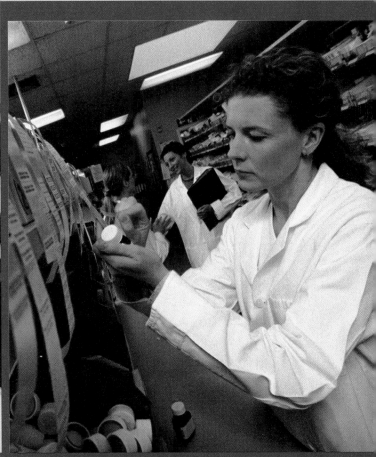

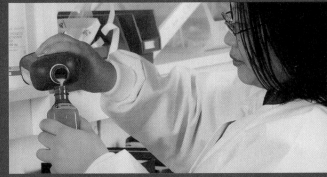

24

Antiinfectives

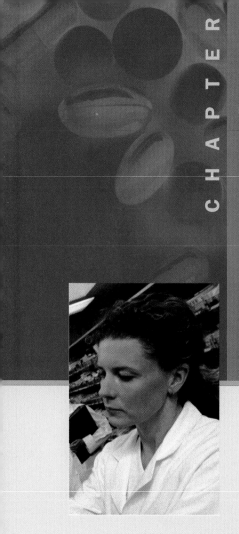

Objectives

- Discuss the history of antibiotics/antibacterials.

- Understand the main causes of infections.

- List the various methods of transmission.

- Explain the reasons for antibiotic resistance.

- List the various generations of penicillins and cephalosporins.

- Describe the differences in the generations of antibiotics.

- Be able to describe the drug action for the various antibiotics discussed.

- List the common side effects of the antibiotics described in this chapter.

- Describe the types of infections caused by bacterial, fungal, and protozoan microbes.

- Describe the types of conditions caused by viruses.

- Distinguish between different antibiotics used for bacterial, fungal, and protozoan infections and antiviral agents used for viral infections.

- Differentiate between helminthic-type infestations and typical bacterial, fungal, and other parasitic infections.

- List the products used to treat infestations by helminths.

- Distinguish between gram-negative and gram-positive microbes and agents used to treat them.

- Distinguish between bacteriostatic and bactericidal effects of various agents discussed.

Antibiotic *Chemical agents produced by organisms used to treat infections*

Antibiotic spectrum *The variety of microbes that a particular antibiotic can treat. Broad-spectrum agents can treat many different types of organisms, whereas narrow-spectrum agents treat only a selected few*

Antimicrobial *Chemicals agents produced by scientists to prevent growth of or kill microorganisms*

Bacteria *Unicellular organisms*

Bactericidal *Agents that kill bacteria*

Bacteriostatic *Agents that prevent the growth of bacteria but do not kill the microbe*

Fungicide *Agents that kill fungus*

Gram-negative bacteria *Bacteria that are unable to keep crystal violet stain when washed in acid alcohol*

Gram-positive bacteria *Bacteria that are able to keep crystal violet stain when washed in acid alcohol*

Helminth *Multicellular worm*

Inhibit *To stop or hold back; to keep a reaction from taking place*

Morphology *Appearance including shape, size, structure, and Gram stain characteristics of organisms; study of organisms without regard to their functions*

Mycosis *Fungal disease*

Normal flora *Microorganisms that reside harmlessly in the body and do not cause disease, but rather may aid the host organism*

Nosocomial infection *An infection acquired while hospitalized*

Parasites *Organisms that require a host for nourishment and reproduction*

Protozoa *Kingdom Protista; unicellular organism; Kehara parasites*

Symbiotic *A close relationship between two species*

Synthesis *The formation of chemical components within the body system*

Vector *The living entity by which infections are transferred but which does not itself have the disease, as a mosquito bite transfers malaria; in this case the mosquito is the vector*

Viruses *Organisms that cannot replicate without the necessary components from a host; live inside other living cells to attain necessary nutrients*

ANTIINFECTIVES

Trade	Generic	Pronunciation	Trade	Generic	Pronunciation
Penicillins			Unipen	nafcillin	naf-**sil**-lin
1st Generation			Staphcillin	methicillin	meth-ah-**sil**-lin
Penicillin G	penicillin G	pen-ah-**sil**-lin	Prostaphlin	oxacillin	ox-ah-**sil**-lin
Penicillin V	penicillin V	pen-ah-**sil**-lin	**2nd Generation**		
			Omnipen, Unipen	ampicillin	amp-ah-**sil**-lin
Penicillinase Resistant			Unasyn	ampicillin/sulbactam	amp-ah-**sil**-lin
Tegopen	cloxacillin	klox-ah-**sil**-lin	Amoxil	amoxicillin	a-mox-ah-**sil**-lin
Dynapen	dicloxacillin	die-klox-ah-**sil**-lin	Augmentin	amoxicillin/clavulanate	a-mox-ah-**sil**-lin

ANTIINFECTIVES—cont'd

Trade	Generic	Pronunciation	Trade	Generic	Pronunciation
3rd Generation			**Aminoglycosides**		
Geocillin	carbenicillin	car-ben-ah-**sil**-lin	Amikin	amikacin	am-ah-**kay**-sin
Ticar	ticarcillin	tie-car-**sil**-lin	Garamycin	gentamicin	jent-ah-**my**-sin
Timentin	ticarcillin/clavulanate	tie-car-**sil**-lin	Kantrex	kanamycin	cane-ah-**my**-sin
			Nebcin	tobramycin	tow-bra-**my**-sin
4th Generation			Streptomycin	streptomycin	strep-tow-**my**-sin
Mezlin	mezlocillin	mez-low-**sil**-lin	**Antifungal**		
Pipracil	piperacillin	pie-**per**-ah-sil-lin	Diflucan	fluconazole	flew-**kone**-ah-zole
Zosyn, Tazocin	piperacillin/tazobactam	pie-**per**-ah-sil-lin	Sporanox	itraconazole	it-trah-**kone**-ah-zole
			Nizoral	ketoconazole	kee-toe-**kone**-ah-zole
Cephalosporin Agents			Monistat	miconazole	my-**kone**-a-zole
1st Generation			Flagyl	metronidazole	met-roh-**neye**-die-zole
Ancef	cefazolin	seh-**faz**-oh-lyn	Lotrimin	clotrimazole	kloe-**trim**-ah-zole
Keflex	cephalexin	sef-ah-**lex**-in	**Antiprotozoan Agents**		
Velosef	cephradine	**sef**-rah-deen	Vermox	mebendazole	me-**ben**-dah-zole
			Biltricide	praziquantel	pra-ze-**quan**-tell
2nd Generation			Aralen	chloroquine	**klor**-o-kwin
Ceclor	cefaclor	**sef**-ah-klor	Lariam	mefloquine	**mef**-low-kwin
Monocid	cefonicid	seh-**fon**-eye-sid	Daraprim	pyrimethamine	pie-rye-**meth**-ah-mean
Cefotan	cefotetan	sef-o-**tea**-tan	Primaquine	primaquine	**prim**-ah-queen
Mefoxin	cefoxitin	**cef**-ox-eye-tin	Yodoxin	iodoquinol	eye-oh-do-**kwin**-ole
Cefzil	cefprozil	cef-**pro**-zil	**Antituberculin**		
Zinacef	cefuroxime	cef-your-**ox**-zeem	Myambutol	ethambutol	eh-**tham**-byoo-toll
			INH	isoniazid	eye-so-**nye**-ah-zid
3rd Generation			Rifadin	rifampin	**riff**-am-pin
Suprax	cefixime	ceh-**fich**-zeem	**Antiviral**		
Cefobid	cefoperazone	cef-o-**pear**-ah-zone	Pentam	pentamidine	pen-**tam**-eye-deen
Vantin	cefpodoxime	cef-poe-**dox**-zeem	Zovirax	acyclovir	aye-**sye**-kloe-vee
Fortaz	ceftazidime	**cef**-taz-eye-deem	AZT	zidovudine	zye-**doe**-vue-deen
Cefizox	ceftizoxime	cef-tah-**zox**-zeem	Epivir	lamivudine	la-**miv**-you-deen
Rocephin	ceftriaxone	cef-try-**ax**-zone	Foscavir	foscarnet	fos-**car**-net
			Viracept	nelfinavir	nell-**fin**-ah-veer
4th Generation			Videx	didanosine	dye-**dan**-oh-seen
Maxipime	cefepime	**cef**-eye-peem	Crixivan	indinavir	in-**dih**-nah-veer

Introduction

The body has a built-in defense mechanism called the immune system that identifies and kills foreign bodies that have invaded the body. However, if a microorganism cannot be destroyed by our immune systems, then help from antibiotics may be necessary. Infections can occur when the invading microorganisms grow rapidly and the body cannot fight off the invader. This may be due to factors such as a weakened immune system. If the invading organism gets out of hand, antibiotics can help. The word antibiotic literally means "against life." They are made from either natural or synthetic substances that can inhibit or destroy microorganisms. The term antimicrobial refers specifically to substances produced by scientists that are used against human infections. However, both terms are used interchangeably in the medical field.

Although it may seem reasonable that bacteria are an unnecessary component for a healthy life, in reality, this is not true. Within the intestines of a normal human body, billions of microbes reside. We refer to these microbes as the normal flora, and their function is a symbiotic one; that is to say, both entities benefit from each other. The human gut provides a warm, nutrient-rich environment for the bacteria to survive, and the bacteria aid in the digestion and absorption of food, from which humans benefit. Other areas of the human body in which bacteria can be found are in the mouth and throat. However, if the microbial growth does not stay in balance, then even our own normal flora can cause us to become ill. This can occur if our immune system is weakened and cannot keep the bacteria in balance.

Antibiotics have a bacteriostatic or bactericidal effect on microbes. Those agents that arrest the development or stop growth of microbes are considered bacteriostatic. When antibiotics are "static" they do not kill mature cells. Instead, they inhibit (stop) any new growth, allowing the body's immune system to kill off the remaining microbes. With a bactericidal agent the microorganisms are killed.

This chapter discusses a brief history of antibiotics, followed by a description of each body system along with the types of infections that are most commonly seen. Finally, the drugs used to treat various conditions are listed along with their drug action, side effects, auxiliary labels, and any special notes that pharmacy technicians should be acquainted with. More information on microorganisms can be found in Chapter 29.

History of Antibiotics

IMPORTANT "FIRSTS" IN ANTIBIOTIC THERAPY

In the 1930s, the first antibiotic, sulfa (sulfanilamide), was discovered. This agent was found to cure staphylococcus infections via bacteriostatic action. With the mass production of sulfa drugs, thousands of military personnel were saved from death from infections during World War II. Sulfas were the first antibiotics produced and were considered a miracle drug; thus they were used often and without regard to the possibility of resistance. Resistance allows a microorganism to decrease the action of antibiotics. As patients took their sulfa drug and began to feel better, they would stop taking their medication. This allowed the remaining microbes to build up a type of immunity to the sulfa drug. The next time the infection appeared, the bacteria were more resistant to the antibiotic. As this trend repeated, more bacteria became resistant, eventually making it impossible to kill them with normal antibiotic therapy. It was not until decades later that researchers found out that microbes have the ability to alter their genetic makeup. Therefore, because of the overuse and misuse of antibiotics, new strains of bacteria made the antibiotic ineffective. By the 1960s, sulfa drugs were obsolete; however, they have found a limited yet useful place in antibiotic treatment and are used for urinary tract and certain respiratory infections. It is important, however, to always take antibiotics for the full course of treatment, as prescribed.

THE DISCOVERY OF PENICILLIN

Most people associate penicillin with the mold that forms on bread. Alexander Fleming was an English physician who discovered penicillin by accident. As he worked on his laboratory experiments, he inadvertently contaminated an agar plate with mold called Penicillium *notatum*. As the mold grew within the agar plate, he observed a ring of clearance being formed around the *Penicillium* species. The ring was produced by chemicals emitted from the mold into the agar plate. The chemicals had killed off the surrounding microorganisms (Figure 24.1). This is called the zone of clearance. This substance was eventually isolated and became what we now know as penicillin. Penicillin agents have been around since the

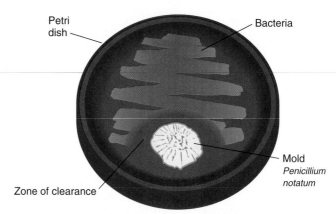

FIGURE 24.1 A petri dish is prepared with nutrient-rich agar. This nutrient feeds the bacteria that are placed on the plate. The penicillium colony can be seen with an area of clearance where the bacteria cannot grow. This occurs because the penicillium inhibits the bacterial growth.

1940s and are very effective, having a bactericidal effect toward gram-positive bacteria more than toward gram-negative bacteria.

Advancements in the science world concerning antiinfectives have increased the current treatments to include more than one dozen classifications of antiinfectives and more than 100 individual drugs that are available to combat a range of infections.

GRAM STAIN

A man by the name of Hans Christian Gram developed the Gram stain procedure in 1883. It is still in use today to determine the morphology of bacteria. The morphology refers to the shape and appearance of microorganisms. Gram-positive bacteria have a thick outer membrane made of peptidoglycan links. Penicillin molecules enter into these links and break them, which kills the microorganism. Gram-negative organisms have a different type of cell wall and are therefore harder to kill (see Chapter 29). There are several antibiotics, especially newer antibiotics, that can kill gram-negative microorganisms.

MODERN ANTIBIOTICS

Because microorganisms have the ability to alter their genetic makeup enough to deter the effects of many antibiotics, stronger antiinfectives have needed to be developed. A different class or generation of antibiotic is used to overcome these organisms. Antibiotics were altered chemically to be more effective against different microbial infections. Some microbes were able to make penicillin ineffective. These specialized bacteria are referred to as penicillinase-producing microbes. However, there have been advances made in strengthening penicillins by additives such as clavulanate (used with amoxicillin) to make Augmentin and sulbactam (used with ampicillin) to make Unasyn. These agents inhibit the penicillinase enzymes from breaking down the antibiotic. This renders the penicillinase-producing microbes susceptible to the antibiotic. There are many antibiotics available to treat a wide variety of infections; these are covered in the next section.

Types of Infections and Their Treatments

COMMON INFECTIONS

Infections can appear anywhere on or within the body. Some are more common because of exposure to the environment, foods we eat, and contact with others. The most common types of organisms that attack the major body organs are outlined in Box 24.1.

The internal body is normally a sterile environment; however, this does not include areas that are open to the outside (air) or those that contain outside substances. Many areas within the body are subject to bacterial, viral, and parasitic infections. Those areas open to the outside are susceptible to infections. The common areas most likely to become infected include the following:

Male and female genital systems (sexually transmitted diseases [STDs])
Gastrointestinal (GI) tract
Respiratory system, upper and lower
Skin
Nose and mouth
Eyes and ears

SEXUALLY TRANSMITTED DISEASES

STDs can be caused by various bacteria, protozoal organisms, and viruses. They can do permanent damage to internal organs and must be treated with the correct antibiotic or antiviral medication. Examples of the most common types of STDs and their treatments are listed in Table 24.1.

GASTROINTESTINAL INFECTIONS

The stomach is subjected to food that normally carries many different bacteria. The highly acidic environment within the stomach usually destroys any bacteria, but if the stomach lining is injured or if the stomach juices are not strong enough to kill microbes, they may settle in the gut, causing infections. One of the major infections of the stomach is from the bacterium *Helicobacter pylori*, also known as *H. pylori*. This bacterium can be eradicated by a triple drug therapy. The primary antibiotics that are used include tetracycline, sulfamethoxazole/trimethoprim (Septra), or metronidazole. These antibiotics have a bactericidal effect on the bacilli. Other areas susceptible to infections include the mouth, throat, and trachea.

Microbes can also infiltrate areas of the body that do not come into contact with air; these microbes are referred to as anaerobic microbes. Microbes that can live in air are aerobic, those that do not live in air are anaerobic, and the types of microbes that can tolerate oxygen to a degree are called facultative anaerobes.

BOX 24.1 TYPES OF MICROORGANISMS

Bacteria
Fungi
Protozoa
Viruses*
Multicellular microscopic parasites

*Not technically an organism.

TABLE 24.1 Common Sexually Transmitted Diseases and Treatments

Sexually Transmitted Disease	Species	Morphology	Symptoms	Drug Treatment
Chlamydia	*Chlamydia trachomatis*	Gram-negative obligate intracellular microbe	Sterility of both sexes	Tetracycline, doxycycline, erythromycin, zithromax
Genital herpes	*Herpes labialis*	Enveloped virion or naked viral capsomere	Fever, headaches, genital blisters, mortality in newborns if active	Acyclovir
Gonorrhea	*Neisseria gonorrhoeae*	Gram-negative diplococci	White discharge from penis in men, painful urination, sterility in both sexes	Ceftriaxone, doxycycline, ciprofloxacin, erythromycin
Syphilis	*Treponema pallidum*	Gram stain is variable, spirochete	Damages the nervous and circulatory systems	Penicillin G, procaine PCN, tetracycline doxycycline
Trichomoniasis	*Trichomonas vaginalis*	Flagellate	Causes a thin, malodorous discharge, often asymptomatic	Metronidazole

PCN, Penicillin.

The type of antibiotic that is prescribed depends on the type of microbe that is causing the infection.

RESPIRATORY INFECTIONS

Infections of the respiratory system can occur in any part of the respiratory system. When we breathe, small particles and microorganisms can be inhaled on dust. These include bacteria, fungi, and viruses. These can settle within the airways and cause infection. Common symptoms of a respiratory infection include wheezing, coughing, and shortness of breath (see Chapter 18).

One of the most serious respiratory infections is pneumonia, which affects more than 4 million Americans annually. Pneumonia is an infection of the lungs. Infectious pneumonia can be caused by bacteria, viruses, fungi, parasites, and chemicals. Pneumonia acquired within the hospital or nursing home is referred to as a nosocomial infection. Many elderly persons who are bedridden for long periods of time are at high risk of acquiring pneumonia, as well as people with chronic conditions such as emphysema, bronchitis, asthma, and immunosuppressive disorders.

Unlike pneumonia, tuberculosis (TB) is a highly contagious respiratory infection that is caused by the bacterium *Mycobacterium tuberculosis*. TB causes inflammation, abscesses, necrosis, and fibrosis of the respiratory system and can spread to other parts of the body as well. Because of the increase in immunodeficiency from human immunodeficiency virus (HIV) and acquired immunodeficiency syndrome (AIDS), TB has been increasing. There are an estimated 10 to 15 million Americans with TB, and there are more than 1.7 billion infected worldwide. Symptoms include chronic coughing, fever, sweating, and weight loss. It is diagnosed in the United States by a tuberculin skin test but must be confirmed by a sputum test that isolates the bacteria.

Fungal infections are more prone to infect patients with other major illness such as cystic fibrosis and those whose immune systems are compromised, such as persons with AIDS, cancer patients on chemotherapy, or patients on multiple antibiotics. These are normally acquired while in the hospital or nursing home. The two most common fungal infections of this type are *Candida albicans* and *Aspergillus fumigatus*.

Bacterial infections secondary to chemical exposure include those toxins that are inhaled in fumes. For example, if inhaled, asbestosis causes scarring of the lungs, decreasing the capacity of the lungs to take in oxygen. It can eventually cause emphysema, pulmonary edema, and even cancer. These in turn can lead to infections within the respiratory system.

NOSOCOMIAL INFECTIONS

Most hospitalizations are a result of illness, trauma, or surgery, or to conduct tests to determine the cause of a problem. Nursing homes are necessary for long-term care of older adults and severely ill persons. Infections that are acquired within hospitals or nursing homes are known as nosocomial infections, and they can be deadly. Hand sanitization and hand washing are the major steps for the prevention of nosocomial infections. See Appendix F. Patients having conditions that weaken their immune system and who are bedridden are more susceptible to infection. Nosocomial infections can be bacterial, fungal, or viral; they are hard to fight.

INFECTIONS OF THE SKIN

Skin abrasions, cuts, and scrapes are a common occurrence with growing children and should be cleaned and kept free of bacteria that can infect the area and cause disease. Diabetics are at high risk for infections of the skin. Because of the lack of blood flow to the extremities in some diabetics, minor injuries to the feet can get infected and cause septic infections that can cause gangrene. For these types of infections, hospitalization and treatment with strong antibiotics may be necessary.

Fungal infections are common on the skin surface because fungi need a high concentration of oxygen to live. A common fungal infection is *Tinea pedis*, or athlete's foot. For this condition there are several over-the-counter (OTC) medications available.

INFECTIONS OF THE NOSE AND MOUTH

The nose and mouth come in constant contact with air-borne microbes. Colds and the yearly flu (influenza) are common conditions experienced by most people at one time or another. For minor colds and flulike symptoms, OTC products can bring some relief of the symptoms experienced. Unfortunately, because viruses cause colds and flu, antibiotics are useless against them. If the normal (bacterial) flora within the mouth, nose, or throat should grow out of control, antibiotics may be prescribed. In addition to bacteria, there are some antivirals and antifungals to treat a variety of infections.

INFECTIONS OF THE EYES AND EARS

The eyes and the ears are susceptible to infections because they are exposed to the environment. The eyes are most often infected by bacteria or viruses. The most common eye infection is conjunctivitis. Conjunctivitis is an inflammation of the lining of the eyelids and cornea called the conjunctiva. Within the eyelids, styes may appear, as well as a discharge of pus. The eye may swell and close. Seasonal allergies can also cause conjunctivitis. If an infection of the underlying cornea develops, it is called keratitis.

Otitis media is a very common ear infection that many babies and young children experience. There are two types of otitis media or middle ear infection—acute and chronic. The acute form is normally caused by a bacterial infection that begins as an upper respiratory tract infection that proceeds to infect the ear. The chronic form is due to repeated infections. Both cause inflammation of the tympanic membrane and are very painful. Chronic otitis media may also result from rupture of the tympanic membrane. See Table 24.2 for a list of ophthalmic and otic antiinfectives.

TABLE 24.2 Otic and Ophthalmic Antiinfectives

Generic	Trade	Classification	Indication	Dosage Forms	Auxiliary Label
Otic Agent					
Chloramphenicol	Chloromycetin	Antiinfective	External ear infections	Solution, ointment	For the ear
Ciprofloxacin	Cipro-NC	Flouroquinolones	External ear infections	Solution	For the ear
Ophthalmic Agents					
Chloramphenicol	Chloroptic	Chloramphenicol	Superficial ocular infections	Solution, ointment	For the eye
Ciprofloxacin	Ciloxan	Fluoroquinolones	A broad spectrum of gram +/− microorganisms	Solution, ointment	For the eye
Erythromycin	Ilotycin	Macrolide	Neonatal prophylaxis of *Neissera gonorrhoeae* or *Chlamydia trachomatis*/ ocular infections	Ointment	For the eye
Gentamicin	Garamycin	Aminoglycoside	A broad spectrum of gram +/− microorganisms	Solution, ointment	For the eye
Idoxuridine	Herplex	Antiviral	Herpes simplex virus keratitis	Solution, ointment	For the eye
Natamycin	Natacyn	Antifungal	Conjunctivitis, keratitis, blepharitis from fungal infection	Solution	For the eye
Neomycin, polymyxin B sulfate, bacitracin	Neosporin	Triple antibiotic	Superficial ocular infections	Solution, ointment	For the eye
Norfloxacin	Chibroxin	Fluoroquinolones	A broad spectrum of gram +/− microorganisms	Solution	For the eye
Oflaxacin	Ocuflox	Fluoroquinolones	Conjunctivitis, corneal ulcers that are caused by susceptible organisms	Solution	For the eye
Polymyxin B sulfate	Aerosporin	Antibiotic	Susceptible gram negative organisms	Solution	For the eye
Sulfacetamide	Bleph-10, Sulamyd	Sulfonamide	Susceptible gram +/− organisms	Solution, ointment	For the eye
Sulfisoxazole	Gantrisin	Sulfonamide	Acute otitis media and susceptible gram +/− organisms	Solution	For the eye
Tifluridine	Viroptic	Antiviral	Herpes simplex virus keratoconjunctivitis	Solution	For the eye
Tobramycin	Tobrex	Aminoglycoside	A broad spectrum of gram +/− microorganisms	Solution, ointment	For the eye
Vidarabine	Vira-A	Antiviral	Herpes simplex virus keratoconjunctivitis	Ointment	For the eye

Antibiotic Treatments

There are many types of microorganisms that can cause infections. Antibiotics are often referred to as wide-spectrum or narrow-spectrum agents. This refers to the variety of microorganisms that they can stop or kill. A narrow-spectrum agent typically covers mostly gram-positive microbes, whereas wide-spectrum agents cover many gram-positive and gram-negative microorganisms. Another important morphological characteristic is whether the organism shape is a rod, coccus, spirillum, or other type. Once the microorganism is identified, a physician can determine the best antibiotic to use for the infection. There are several classifications of antibiotics. In addition to those agents listed at the beginning of the

TABLE 24.3 Antibiotic Reference Table 1

Type of Infection	Treatment	Conditions
Gram-positive cocci (spherical-shaped microbe) aerobic and anaerobic		
Staphylococcus	Penicillin G	Throat infections, cuts, sepsis
Streptococcus	PCN G, PCN VK	Strep throat, pneumonia, sepsis
UTIs	PCN G, ampicillin	Sepsis
Gram-negative cocci (spherical-shaped microbe) aerobic and anaerobic		
Gonorrhea (STD)	Ceftriaxone	Pneumonia, pelvic inflammatory disease
Meningitis	PCN G	Inflammation of the covering of the brain and spinal cord
Pneumonia	Unasyn, Augmentin	Lungs, alveoli
Gram-positive bacilli (rod-shaped microbe) aerobic and anaerobic		
Pneumonia	PCN G	Lungs, alveoli
Bacteremia	Vancomycin	Sepsis of the blood
Gangrene	PCN G	Necrosis
Gram-negative bacilli (rod-shaped microbe) aerobic and anaerobic		
UTI	Cephalosporins, sulfa, ampicillin, gentamicin	Ureters, urethra, bladder
Bacteremia	Ampicillin, glycosides, cephalosporins	Sepsis, stomach infections
Pneumonia	4th generation PCN, aminoglycoside	Lungs, alveoli

PCN, Penicillin; *UTI*, urinary tract infection; *STD*, sexually transmitted disease.

chapter, there are several more that cover specific gram-negative and/or gram-positive microorganisms.

Table 24.3 lists some of the most common types of infections based on their bacterial morphology and their treatments. This includes the outcome of a Gram stain, the microbe's shape, and where the microbe is located.

PENICILLIN

Penicillin antibiotics are taken from two different molds, *Penicillium notatum* and *Penicillium chrysogenum*. They are grown in laboratories and are synthetically altered to fight off many microorganisms. The drug action of penicillin is bactericidal toward microbes that are currently reproducing. They disrupt the formation of the cell wall so that the bacteria cannot keep a constant osmotic gradient and lyses (breaks open). Penicillin-type agents cover mostly gram-positive organisms. Because penicillins are susceptible to degradation from stomach acids, it is important that they be taken 1 to 2 hours before or after meals.

For some infections, such as those that can affect the GI system, more potent antibiotics are required. In this case, broader spectrum "cillins" such as ampicillin and carbenicillin can kill both gram-positive and some gram-negative organisms.

TECH NOTE! Gram-positive microbes have a different cell wall than gram-negative microbes. Antibiotics can kill microbes by breaking down their cell walls. The reason they do not kill human cells is because human cells do not have a cell wall.

Mild side effects make these agents a good choice. However, if someone has a penicillin allergy, other agents must be used. If penicillin is given to a person suspected of having an allergy, a skin test can be performed to see if there is any sensitivity. Nausea, vomiting, and diarrhea; headache; sore mouth or rashes; pain; and fever may be signs of allergic reaction. One of each generation of penicillins is listed along with their individual information. Each drug's normal dosage is the recommended oral adult dosage.

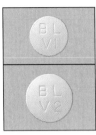

Bristol-Myers Squibb

CLASSIFICATION: ANTIBACTERIAL, PENICILLIN
GENERIC NAME: penicillin V potassium
TRADE NAME: Veetids
GENERATION: 1st generation penicillin
ROUTE OF ADMINISTRATION: oral
INDICATION: pneumonococcal pneumonia, streptococcal pharyngitis, syphilis, gonorrhea
DOSAGE FORMS: tablet, oral solution
COMMON DOSAGE: 125 to 500 mg orally every 6 to 8 hours
AUXILIARY LABELS:
- Take on an empty stomach
- Take until gone

SPECIAL NOTE: liquid should have a "shake well and refrigerate" auxiliary label
14 day expiration date after reconstitution if stored in refrigerator

GENERIC NAME: ampicillin
TRADE NAME: Omnipen, Polycillin
GENERATION: 2nd generation penicillin
ROUTE OF ADMINISTRATION: oral
INDICATION: skin/soft tissue infections, otitis media, sinusitis, respiratory, GI, meningitis, septicemia, and endocarditis prophylaxis
DOSAGE FORMS: capsules, suspension, injectable
COMMON DOSAGE: 250 to 500 mg orally every 6 hours
AUXILIARY LABELS:
- Take on an empty stomach
- Take until gone

SPECIAL NOTE: suspension should have a "shake well and refrigerate" auxiliary label
14 day expiration after reconstitution if stored in refrigerator

GENERIC NAME: ticarcillin
TRADE NAME: Ticar
GENERATION: 3rd generation penicillin
ROUTE OF ADMINISTRATION: injectable (IM, IV)
INDICATION: drug-resistant or severe skin infections, bone/joint infections, septicemia, respiratory infections, urinary tract infections (UTIs)
DOSAGE FORMS: injectable only
COMMON DOSAGE: 3 g intravenous (IV) every 4 to 6 hours; 200 mg/kg daily or 15 to 40 g daily q4h
SPECIAL NOTE: after reconstitution, drug is good for 72 hours if kept in the refrigerator

CEPHALOSPORINS

Cephalosporins are less affected by stomach acids; therefore, they can be taken with meals. Although cephalosporins are not exactly like penicillins, there is a 10% chance of an allergic reaction for those who have penicillin allergies.

TECH NOTE! It is normal for a physician to write for a loading dose of an antibiotic followed by a lower routine dose. The reason for a loading dose is to bring the antibiotic up to its therapeutic level as quickly as possible.

An example of one cephalosporin from each generation is listed in the following. In addition, the common dosage forms and dosages are listed, as well as any special notes of which technicians should be aware.

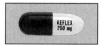

Dista

CLASSIFICATION: CEPHALOSPORINS
 GENERIC NAME: cephalexin
 TRADE NAME: Keflex
 GENERATION: 1st generation cephalosporin
 ROUTE OF ADMINISTRATION: oral
 INDICATIONS: most infections, cystitis, skin/soft tissue infections, streptococcal pharyngitis
 DOSAGE FORMS: tablet, capsules, suspension
 COMMON DOSAGE: 250 mg to 1 g orally every 6 hours
 AUXILIARY LABEL:

- Take until gone

 SPECIAL NOTE: suspension should have a "shake well and refrigerate" auxiliary label
  14 day expiration date after reconstitution if stored in a refrigerator

Glaxo Wellcome

 GENERIC NAME: cefuroxime
 TRADE NAME: Ceftin (Tab), Axetil (Susp), Zinacef (INJ)
 GENERATION: 2nd generation cephalosporin
 ROUTE OF ADMINISTRATION: oral, IM
 INDICATIONS: most infections, UTI, gonorrhea
 DOSAGE FORMS: tablet, suspension, injectable
 COMMON DOSAGE: 250 to 500 mg orally twice daily
 AUXILIARY LABEL:

- Take until gone

 SPECIAL NOTE: suspension should have a "shake well and refrigerate" auxiliary label

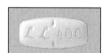

Lederle

 GENERIC NAME: cefixime
 TRADE NAME: Suprax
 GENERATION: 3rd generation cephalosporin
 ROUTE OF ADMINISTRATION: oral
 INDICATION: most infections, gonorrhea
 DOSAGE FORMS: tablet, suspension
 COMMON DOSAGE: 400 mg orally once daily or divided every 12 hours
 AUXILIARY LABEL:

- Take as directed

 SPECIAL NOTE: suspension should have "shake well" auxiliary label. Storage and Stability: May be kept at room temperature for up to 14 days

 GENERIC NAME: cefepime
 TRADE NAME: Maxipime
 GENERATION: 4th generation cephalosporin
 ROUTE OF ADMINISTRATION: IV
 INDICATION: skin infections, UTI, moderate to severe pneumonia; wide range of gram-negative bacilli and other microorganisms
 DOSAGE FORMS: injectable
 COMMON DOSAGE: most infections: 1 to 2 g IV every 12 hours for 5 to 10 days
 SPECIAL NOTE: drug is stable 7 days if refrigerated

Penicillin and cephalosporins are popular agents used to fight off bacterial infections caused by both gram-negative and gram-positive microbes. However, there are other classes of antibiotics available, such as those listed in Table 24.4. These medications are used depending on the specific microbe that has been isolated. A culture is taken of the area infected, and, by using various laboratory methods, the specific microbe in most cases can be identified (see Chapter 29). In addition, the organism is tested for its sensitivity to various antibiotics; thus the

TABLE 24.4 Antibiotic Reference Table 2

Antibiotic	Trade	Generic	Effects	Normal Adult Dosage
Aminoglycosides	Garamycin	Gentamicin	Mostly gram-negative microbes: bactericidal	Normally based on peak/ tough levels: See F&C
	Kantrex	Kanamycin	Mostly gram-negative microbes: bactericidal	1g q6h, max 3-4 days
	Amikin	Amikacin	Mostly gram-negative microbes: bactericidal	15g/kg/day IV/IM q6-8h
	Nebcin	Tobramycin	Mostly gram-negative microbes: bactericidal	3g/kg/day IV/IMq8h
Carbapenem	Merrem	Meropenem	Broad spectrum: bactericidal	1g IV q8h
	Primaxin	Imipenem-Cilastatin	Broad spectrum: bactericidal	250mg IV q6-8h 500mg IV q6-8h
Monobactams	Azactam	Aztreonam	Broad spectrum: bactericidal	500mg-1g IV q8-12h: 2g IV q6-8h
Fluoroquinolones	Cipro	Ciprofloxacin	Broad spectrum: bactericidal	250-750g po q12h; 200-400g IV q12h
	Noroxin	Norfloxacin	Broad spectrum: bactericidal	200-400g po/IV q12h
	Trovan	Trovafloxacin mesylate/ alatrofloxacin mesylate	Broad spectrum: bactericidal	100-200g po q24h; 200-300g IV q24h
	Levaquin	Levofloxacin	Broad spectrum: bactericidal	500g IV/po q24h
Lincosamides	Cleocin	Clindamycin	Gram-positive microbes; anaerobes: bacteriostatic	150-300g po q6h; 300-600g IV q6-12h
	Lincocin	Lincomycin	Gram-positive microbes; anaerobes: bacteriostatic	500g po q6-8h; 600g IV q12h-qd
Macrolides	Biaxin	Clarithromycin	Broad spectrum: bactericidal/ bacteriostatic	250-500g po q12h
	E-Mycin	Erythromycin	Broad spectrum: bactericidal/ bacteriostatic	Dosage varies depending on what type of erythromycin is given: see F&C
	Zithromax	Azithromycin	Broad spectrum: bactericidal/ bacteriostatic	250-500mg po qd
Spectinomycin	Trobicin	Spectinomycin	Specific for gonorrhea* bactericidal	2g IM/IV × 1 dose
Tetracyclines	Achromycin	Tetracycline	Broad spectrum: bacteriostatic	250-500g po q6-12h
	Vibramycin	Doxycycline	Broad spectrum: bacteriostatic	100g po qd to bid
Vancomycin	Vancocin	Vancomycin	Active against gram-positive: bactericidal/ bacteriostatic	125-500g po q6-8h; 500mg IV q12h

F&C, Drug Facts and Comparisons; IM, intramuscular; IV, intravenous; po, by mouth.

right drug can be used. If the microbe cannot be isolated or the infection is severe, doctors may give a broad-spectrum antibiotic in hopes that it will cover the microbe in question. In addition to this alternative type of treatment, a combination of agents can be used to cover many different species of bacterial infections.

MYCOBACTERIUM AND MYCOBACTERIAL TREATMENT

Two main infections in humans caused by a mycobacterium are TB and leprosy. (*Mycobacterium* is closely related to bacteria but is considered a different species than those that fit into the general class of bacteria.) Both of these conditions are chronic. Leprosy (Hansen's disease) is an infectious disease that is caused by *Mycobacterium leprae*. In the past, it affected millions of people across the world, with most cases in Asia and Africa. Recently, the disease has progressively decreased. Noticeable skin lesions appear. Ulceration of the feet and loss of hand function may occur, and corneal abrasions may cause blindness. This condition can be treated with dapsone (bacteriostatic) and clofazimine (bactericidal).

TB is a disease that was known as the wasting disease because it robs a person of breath and strength. Eventually, death occurred. It was responsible for thousands of deaths throughout history, but in the 1960s TB was disappearing as new drugs were invented to eradicate the disease. Unfortunately many people quit taking their medication once they felt better; thus the microbe was able to withstand low doses of antibiotics until it became resistant. Now, entering the new millennium, TB is once again occurring in staggering numbers. It is estimated that two thirds of prisoners have TB. Millions of people are dying each year, and, for those persons who acquire the resistant strain, there is no medication available to combat this deadly disease. It is prevalent here in the United States as well as around the world.

TECH NOTE! Visit CDC.gov/mmwr (Mortality and Morbidity Weekly Report) to see what type of outbreaks occur in the United States and the world.

There are a few antituberculin-type medications that are used to treat TB, but they must be taken for the full course of treatment. This can last from 6 months to years depending on test results and must not be stopped regardless of how well the person feels. As the microbes are decreased, the person begins to feel better, but if the medication is stopped the microbe reoccurs and it is stronger and much harder to kill (Table 24.5).

AMINOGLYCOSIDES

Aminoglycosides are among the strongest antibiotic agents in use today. They are bactericidal to many varieties of gram-negative microorganisms. The drug action for parenteral aminoglycosides is their ability to bind to ribosomes of the microor-

TABLE 24.5 Antituberculin Agents

Generic	Trade	Dosing Regimen	Length of Time
Isoniazid	Abbreviation: INH	300 mg qd	6-24 months
Rifampin	Rifadin	600 mg qd	Months to years
Ethambutol	Myambutol	800 mg to 1.6 g qd	Months to years
Pyrazinamide	Pyrazinamide	1-2 g qd	Months to years
Cycloserine	Seromycin	750 mg to 1 g qd	Bacteriostatic: used for retreatment
Kanamycin	Kantrex	500 mg to 1 g qd	Bactericidal: used for retreatment

ganism stopping the protein synthesis, which ultimately causes the death of the organism. Many of these medications come in parenteral (IV) form only and are used mainly in hospitals for severe infections. Often, they are given with other antibiotics to further their microbial coverage. Because aminoglycosides have a narrow range between therapeutic and toxic serum levels, careful calculations must be made to determine the appropriate dosage. This is done by evaluation of the patient's blood levels of antibiotic, drawn at specific times (called peak and trough levels). In this way the patient's clearance of the aminoglycoside drug can be seen and changes can be made in the dosage or dosing time if necessary. Patients with renal disease and older adults are more susceptible to toxic levels of these agents because of decreased excretion. A sample of the types of agents most commonly seen by technicians is listed in the following along with their specifics.

CLASSIFICATION: AMINOGLYCOSIDE
GENERIC NAME: amikacin
TRADE NAME: Amikin
INDICATION: serious infections such as *Pseudomonas*, *Proteus*, *Serratia*, and various gram-positive bacilli that cause bone and respiratory infections, endocarditis, and septicemia
DOSAGE FORMS: injection 50 mg/mL in 2-mL and 4-mL vials; 250 mg/mL in 2-mL and 4-mL vials
COMMON DOSAGE: based on weight of patient: normally 5 to 7.5 mg/kg/dose every 8 hours
SPECIAL NOTE: stable for 2 days if refrigerated after mixing into appropriate solution

GENERIC NAME: gentamicin
TRADE NAME: Garamycin (IV), Genoptic (Ophthalmic), G-myticin (Topical)
INDICATION: for gram-negative organisms such as *Pseudomonas*, *Proteus*, *Serratia*, gram-positive staphylococcus; bone and respiratory tract infections, skin and soft tissue infections, UTI and abdominal infections, and eye infections caused by susceptible bacteria
DOSAGE FORMS: infusion, ophthalmic ointment, solution, topical cream
COMMON DOSAGE: based on weight of patient: for UTI: 1.5 mg/kg/dose IV; ophthalmic: instill $\frac{1}{2}$-in. ointment 2 to 3 times daily every 3 to 4 hours or gttsii in infected eye tid to qid; topical: apply 3 to 4 times per day to affected area(s)
AUXILIARY LABELS:
■ For ophthalmic: For the eye
■ For topical cream: Topical use only
SPECIAL NOTE: IV solution does not need to be refrigerated before or after mixing into solution. Stability is 24 hours only after mixing

GENERIC NAME: tobramycin
TRADE NAME: Nebcin (IV), Tobrex (ophthalmic), TOBI (Inhalation)
INDICATION: for susceptible gram-negative bacilli including *Pseudomonas aeruginosa*. Ophthalmic use for superficial infections to the eye from susceptible bacteria
DOSAGE FORMS: infusion, ophthalmic ointment, solution, inhalation solution
COMMON DOSAGE: based on weight of patient; for UTI: 1.5 mg/kg/dose IV; ophthalmic: instill ointment 2 to 3 times daily every 3 to 4 hours; for inhalation 60 to 80 mg 3 times daily
AUXILIARY LABEL:
■ For ophthalmics: For the eye
SPECIAL NOTE: after reconstitution of powder, IV is stable for 96 hours if refrigerated

ADDITIONAL ANTIBIOTICS

The following agents are commonly used antibiotics for a variety of infections. Their classification, drug action, and indications, as well as generic and trade names are listed in Table 24.6.

TABLE 24.6 Antibiotic Reference Table 3

Class	Generic	Trade	Indication	Drug Action
Tetracyclines*				
	doxycycline	Vibramycin	Severe infections	IPS*
	tetracycline	Achromycin	such as	
	minocycline	Minocin	respiratory,	
			GI, and skin	
Fluoroquinolones†				
	ciprofloxacin	Cipro	TB, respiratory,	IBDNAS*
	levofloxacin	Levaquin	and UTIs	
	ofloxacin	Floxin		
	norfloxacin	Noroxin		
Macrolides				
	azithromycin	Zithromax	Respiratory, genital,	IPS*
	clarithromycin	Biaxin	GI, and skin	
	erythromycin	Emycin, Ery-Tab	infections	
	erythro ethylsuccinate	EES		
	erythromycin state	Erythrocin		
Carbapenems				
	imipenem/cilastin	Primaxin	Serious infections	IBCWS*
Monobactam				
	aztreonam	Azactam	Wide-spectrum gram-negative aerobic organisms	IBCWS*
Vancomycin				
	vancomycin	Vancocin	Serious/severe infections	IBCWS*

GI, Gastrointestinal; *IBCWS*, inhibits bacterial cell wall synthesis; *IBDNAS*, interferes with bacterial DNA synthesis; *IPS*, inhibits protein synthesis; *TB*, tuberculosis; *UTI*, urinary tract infection.
*Auxiliary labels: Take on an empty stomach. Take with plenty of water. Avoid dairy products. Avoid antacids. Avoid direct sunlight.
†Auxiliary labels: Do not take antacids. Avoid iron/zinc supplements 4 hours before or 2 hours after taking domestication.

ANTIFUNGALS

Fungi are plantlike organisms that can grow on cloth, food, showers, people, or in any warm moist environment. They absorb nutrients from either the environment or hosts such as animals and humans. Most conditions caused by fungi tend to affect the outside of the body and are not life threatening but do cause great annoyance. A systemic infection is much more serious. This is when the fungus invades inside the body. For these types of infections, more potent agents are used (Table 24.7).

Candida *Infections*

A common fungi species that resides inside the human body is *Candida albicans*. Although this fungal species is found within a human's normal flora, if it gets out

TABLE 24.7 Antifungals

Generic	Trade	Type of Infection	Drug action	Indications
Amphotericin B	Fungizone	Candidiasis, fungal septicemia, cryptococcal meningitis	Affects fungus cell membrane causing lysing to occur; both bactericidal and bacteriostatic	Systemic mycosis
Clortrimazole	Lotrimin, Gyne-Lotrimin	Candidiasis, *Tinea*	Alters cell membrane permiability	Vaginal, oral, and topical fungal infections
Fluconazole	Diflucan	Cryptococcal meningitis	Affects biosynthesis-inhibiting growth; both bactericidal and bacteriostatic	Esophageal, UTI, and vaginal mycosis
Flucytosine	Ancobon	*Candida* spp., fungal pneumonia, septicemia	Inhibits DNA synthesis and metabolism of pyrimidine; bactericidal	Serious mycosis
Griseofulvin	Fulvicin U/F, Grisovin F/P	*Tinea* infections	Inhibits cell mitosis; bactericidal	Ringworm, toes/ fingernail mycosis
Itraconazole	Sporanox	Histoplasmosis, blastomycosis	Affects biosynthesis inhibiting growth; bactericidal	Lung infections
Ketoconazole	Nizoral	*Tinea* infections	Affects biosynthesis inhibiting growth; bactericidal	Systemic mycosis
Miconazole	Monistat, Monistat IV, Monistat-Derm	Candidiasis	Affects biosynthesis inhibiting growth; bactericidal	Skin, vaginal mycosis
Nystatin	Mycostatin	*Candida albicans*	Affects fungus cell membrane causing lysing to occur; bactericidal	Vaginal, intestinal mycosis
Terbinafine	Lamisil	Onychomycosis, *Tinea* infections	Inhibits cell wall synthesis; bactericidal	Skin, toes, fingernail mycosis

UTI, Urinary tract infection.

of control because of a weakened immune system or because of use of potent antibiotics, it can cause serious effects.

There are different species of *Candida*. Depending on the specific species, they are responsible for infections of the mouth, vagina, or under the fingernails and toenails. When fungal infections occur on the skin surface, they are referred to as dermatophytic infections. The agents used are applied directly to the skin unless the infection has advanced into the bloodstream, then parenteral antifungals must be used. Topical agents are available in different dosage forms—lotions, creams, ointment, powders, and sprays. A person can use what works best for him or her. Many antifungal agents are available OTC. There are many OTC medications available to treat mild cases of mycosis (fungus infections). Some of the agents listed are either fungicidal (kills fungi) or fungistatic (inhibits further growth) depending on the organism they are used for.

Tinea Infections

One of the most common conditions caused by a fungus is dermatophytosis, caused by fungi from the genera *Trichophyton*, *microsporum* or *Epidermophyton*. Tinea pedis (foot) is also known as athlete's foot. If it appears on the scalp, it is known as tinea capitis or ringworm. If it appears on babies in the groin area, it is called tinea cruris or diaper rash.

BOX 24.2 PARASITIC ORGANISMS AND THEIR DESCRIPTION

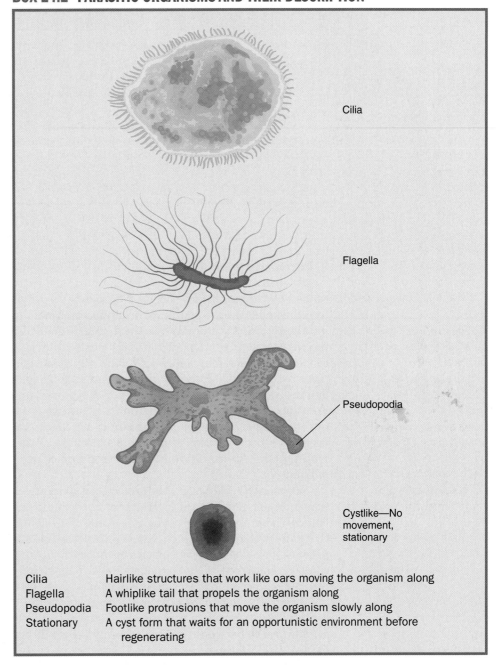

Cilia	Hairlike structures that work like oars moving the organism along
Flagella	A whiplike tail that propels the organism along
Pseudopodia	Footlike protrusions that move the organism slowly along
Stationary	A cyst form that waits for an opportunistic environment before regenerating

Parasites

Parasites are organisms that benefit at the expense of another. The host is the organism that is being used by the parasite. Under the Kingdom Protista, the Phylum Sporozoa consists of parasitic organisms. The morphology (characteristics) of an organism depends on whether they are multicellular or unicellular and how they are transmitted. How these organisms are distinguished from each other depends on several factors such as morphology and locomotion (movement) as listed in Box 24.2. The life cycles of many of the organisms that affect humans are explained in Chapter 29. Some major conditions that can occur from protozoa are listed in Table 24.8.

TABLE 24.8 Protozoal Infections and Their Treatments

Species	Disease name	Transmission	Treatment
Toxoplasma gondii	Toxoplasmosis	Contaminated food, water, feces of a bug or cat; sand flies, tsetse flies also carry the disease	Pyrimethamine sulfdiazine Trimethoprim/ sulfamethoxazole Pentamidine (IV) Azithromycin
Plasmodium vivax	Malaria	Female mosquitoes	Chloroquine Quinine Mefloquine Primaquine

Parasitic Conditions

Protozoa. Many protozoa are human parasites. Amebiasis is an infection caused by the protozoan species *Entamoeba histolytica*. The cyst form is transferred via fecal-oral routes. Symptoms can include abdominal pain, nausea, flatulence, and fatigue. Treatments include iodoquinol, which rids the body of the infestation. Another protozoan disease that is more dangerous to humans is toxoplasmosis. The species *Toxoplasma gondii* is transferred via uncooked meat or cysts that may be present in cat feces. Although the symptoms may be mild in most adults, it can be deadly to both infants and the unborn fetus. Treatment includes pyrimethamine and sulfadiazine. Trichomoniasis is caused by the species *Trichomonas vaginalis*. It affects the vaginal area; the cervical area becomes red and inflamed. These protozoa can also infect both the female and male urethra. Metronidazole is the drug of choice and must be used by both sexual partners.

Helminths (Worms). Helminths are parasitic worms. They are not microscopic organisms, but the procedures used to diagnose infections are done in a clinical laboratory. These parasites are multicellular. The two major worms that affect Americans are roundworms (nematodes) and flatworms (platyhelminthes). There are 50 species of roundworms that can infect humans. Many can be transferred in undercooked meat. There are species that can lodge in the intestine or lymph nodes, causing harm to the host. Hookworms are another type of roundworm and are transferred via feces infected with the worm through skin contact. For example, if someone walks on soil that has been contaminated with human feces that contains hookworms, they will enter through the skin of the foot.

Flatworms are further divided into tapeworms and flukes. Many flatworms live by feeding off of dead matter or small organisms and are not harmful to humans. Tapeworms reside in the intestines of most vertebrates where they absorb digested food from the host. Eating undercooked meat can transfer them to humans. Flukes have an interesting life cycle that involves freshwater snails and humans. People who drink water from feces-contaminated water can acquire flukes. Many helminth diseases are caused by undercooked meat or contaminated water and soil. Most helminth infections occur in people who live in areas where sanitation is nonexistent or in people who are not aware of the problem with eating raw meat. The species, symptoms, and treatments are listed in Table 24.9.

Parasitic Treatments. There are only a few ways to deal with parasites—kill them and wash them away, rid them from the body alive or dead, or surgically

TABLE 24.9 Antihelminthes and Their Treatments

	Species or Disease Name	Symptoms	Treatment
Phylum Nematoda			
Roundworms	Trichinosis	Inflammation	Diethylcarbamazine, ivermectin
Hookworms	Ankylostoma duodenale, *Necator americanus*	Anemia, weakness, fatigue	Mebendazole, albendazole, pyrantel
Pinworms	*Enterobius vermicularis*	Anal itching	Mebendazole, albendazole, pyrantel
Bladder worm	Cysticercus	Forms a cyst that can be as large as an orange; symptoms vary depending on area infected	Praziquantel
Phylum Platyhelminthes			
Tapeworms	*Taenia saginata, Taenia solium*	Diarrhea, weight loss, perforation of intestine	Praziquantel, niclosamide
Flukes	Schistosomiasis	Loss of blood in feces	Praziquantel

remove them. Whichever mechanism is used, the main goal is to remove them from the body. All agents used to rid the parasites from the body are oral dosage forms; therefore hospitalization is rarely necessary. In addition, the dosage regimen is normally short term, and treatment can be done in just a few oral doses.

All parasites can cause damage to the tissues or organs that they invade. Although parasites may weaken the host, most parasites do not kill their host, because this would cut off their food and shelter. Listed in Table 24.10 are the main antihelminthic agents and their drug action.

Malaria

Malaria is a sporozoan infection with symptoms consisting of fever, chills, sweating, headache, and nausea. The cycle of chills, fever, and sweating varies depending on the particular pathogen. The genus *Plasmodium* has four different species that are responsible for malaria. Some cause severe side effects, such as the species *falciparum*, which can cause death. The human body, the site of sporozoan reproduction, is called the reservoir. Transmission is usually via an infected mosquito, but the sporozoa can also be transmitted by infected needles or syringes or by blood transfusion. The incubation period ranges from 1 week to 1 month depending on the species.

Malaria is a major health problem in more than 100 countries. Reported cases of malaria are responsible for more than 1 million deaths annually. Approximately 1200 cases are diagnosed in the United States annually. The prevention and control of malaria consists of controlling mosquitoes by using insect repellants, filling in water holes where mosquitoes breed, and using insecticides.

The diagnosis of malaria is made based on blood smears. Chloroquine phosphate is used as treatment when possible. However, if the strain is resistant to chloroquine, other agents such as mefloquine, doxycycline, or primaquine can be used.

TABLE 24.10 Antihelminthic Agents Action of Drug and Common Dosage

Generic	Trade	Drug Action	Common Dosage
Diethylcarbamazine	Hetrazan	Cidal: increases the loss of filariae, decreases ability to produce more	2-3 mg/kg po tid
Mebendazole	Vermox	Vermicidal: stops glucose uptake in worm	100 mg po bid × 3 days
Niclosamide	Niclocide	Cidal: affects mitochondria, decreases metabolism	8 g × 1 dose or 2 g po qd × 1 week (depends on type of worm infestation)
Oxamniquine	Vansil	Cidal: causes worms to move to liver where they are killed	12-15 mg/kg po × 1 (dose may vary depending on type of worm infestation)
Praziquantel	Biltricide	Paralysis: causes loss of calcium and eventual paralysis of worm, which is then flushed out	25 mg/kg pd tid × 1 day
Pyrantel	Antiminth	Paralysis: causes depolarization and eventual paralysis of worm, which is then flushed out	11 mg/kg po × 1 dose May be repeated in 2-3 weeks if necessary
Thiabendazole	Mintezol	Vermicidal: inhibits essential enzymes causing death	25 mg/kg po bid × 2 days

ANTIVIRALS

Viruses are organisms that cannot live outside their host. They are unlike bacteria or any other organisms because of their structure and design. Viruses are classified by the following criteria:

1. Nucleic acid makeup (single- or double-stranded DNA or RNA)
2. Size
3. Host it infects
4. Enveloped or naked

There is still debate within the biological community as to whether viruses should be classified as a living organism because they differ in most criteria that are used to classify living organisms. All living organisms replicate or reproduce themselves with their own set of blueprints or DNA; however, viruses do not. They require a host's DNA to replicate. Unlike parasites, viruses either kill the host's cell on leaving or bud off, allowing further reinfections. Another major difference between the Kingdom Protista and viruses is that they do not have the ability to reproduce themselves in the same way that other organisms do. Most organisms reproduce sexually or asexually; however, viruses cannot reproduce by themselves. They must use their host's components to replicate. The virus's makeup is closely related to a human's DNA. Therefore, when agents are used to destroy a virus, they can inadvertently destroy human cells along with the virions. There are many different types of viral diseases that both plants and animals can contract. For animals these include chickenpox, colds, influenza, polio, rabies, warts, HIV, AIDS, and some types of cancer.

The following analogy will help explain viral replication. Let's say you have been given the key to an automobile manufacturing plant, but instead of making one of the cars normally made in the plant, you want a truck specialized to fit your needs. You have all the necessary components within the auto shop, but the outcome will be different from what is normally manufactured in the plant. This is the same type of action that a virion (one virus particle) has on your body. It invades your cells and uses your components to assemble its own blueprints. There are five steps in the invasion and spread of virions. The steps are as follows:

1. Attachment: This is a lock-and-key mechanism that allows virions to attach to specific host cells
2. Injection of nucleic acids: Either the whole virion will enter the cell or it will inject its nucleic acids to begin the replication process
3. Synthesis: This is when the virion takes over the cell's controls and begins to use them to make its own necessary enzymes and proteins to replicate its RNA or DNA and component parts
4. Assembly: Once all the parts are made then the parts are assembled to create a new virion. Millions of new virions are assembled and readied for transport
5. Spread via lyse or budding: When the assembly is completed the virions leave the manufacturing plant (host cell) and continue to reinfect other cells

There are agents that can slow down and, in some cases, kill viruses. To interrupt the process outlined previously in the manufacturing plant analogy, an antiviral agent can affect the virus by the processes listed in Box 24.3.

TECH NOTE! Did you know there are even smaller virus type particles called viroids? They have only a single strand of RNA. Fortunately, they do not affect humans but have been found in plant species. They are responsible for the destruction of many plants and important food crops.

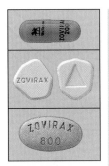

Glaxo Wellcome

CLASSIFICATION: ANTIVIRAL
  GENERIC NAME: acyclovir
  TRADE NAME: Zovirax (Glaxo Wellcome)
  DOSAGE FORMS: tablet, capsules, injectable, suspension, ointment
  DRUG ACTION: interferes with DNA synthesis of the virion by inhibiting viral replication
  SIDE EFFECTS: headache, dizziness, rash, nausea
  AUXILIARY LABELS:
  ■ Suspension: Shake well
  ■ Ointment: Topical use only
  SPECIAL NOTE: suspension is banana flavored

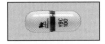

Glaxo Wellcome

CLASSIFICATION: ANTIRETROVIRAL
  GENERIC NAME: zidovudine
  TRADE NAME: Retrovir (AKA: AZT)
  DOSAGE FORMS: tablet, capsule, injection, syrup
  DRUG ACTION: zidovudine is an analog of thymidine that interferes with the HIV viral RNA-dependent DNA polymerase (enzymes), which results in the inhibition of viral replication
  SIDE EFFECTS: headache, weakness, abdominal pain, diarrhea, nausea, anemia
  AUXILIARY LABEL:
  ■ Take as directed
  SPECIAL NOTE: syrup is strawberry flavored

Colds/Flu

Everyone gets a cold now and then without much concern, and it is common knowledge that there is no cure for the common cold. The reason is that colds are caused by viruses. Viruses, as you may have learned, mutate very well; therefore they change each year. New products claim to decrease the chance or severity of colds, but the cold still rules. The good news is that although it is inconvenient, in a healthy person it is not deadly. Influenza is another type of virus that affects millions of people each year. This condition, unlike the common cold, causes death in many older adults and immunocompromised persons every

BOX 24.3 ANTIVIRAL MECHANISMS OF ACTION

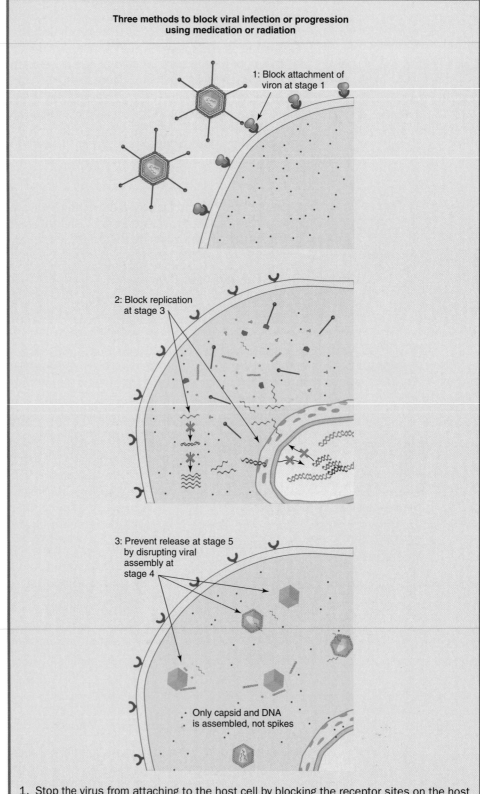

Three methods to block viral infection or progression using medication or radiation

1: Block attachment of viron at stage 1

2: Block replication at stage 3

3: Prevent release at stage 5 by disrupting viral assembly at stage 4

Only capsid and DNA is assembled, not spikes

1. Stop the virus from attaching to the host cell by blocking the receptor sites on the host cell or by blocking the sites on the virion
2. Stop the replication process within the host cell thus inhibiting the virion from making its necessary components
3. Disrupt the assembly of virion particles as they are being assembled within the host cell thus rendering an incomplete virion particle

year. For this reason, vaccines, which contain the viruses that are most likely to cause influenza that year, are given each year (in late fall or early winter) to persons who are at higher risk. These include older adults, health care workers, and immunocompromised persons such as those who are on chemotherapy or those with HIV or AIDS.

HIV/AIDS

Since the 1970s, HIV (the resulting disease is called AIDS) infections have been increasing. HIV is a bloodborne, sexually transmitted virus. Although there are many agents now available to treat AIDS, there is no cure for this disease. The virion does not cause death, but instead it renders the host too weak to fight off any infection; thus a person with AIDS will succumb to common illnesses. The HIV virus attacks the immune system of humans. It can be transmitted by bodily fluids containing the virus. Simple sexual safety steps, which include having both partners tested for HIV before sexual activities, or wearing condoms, reduce the chances of acquiring HIV. In medical settings, protective wear such as gloves and face shields are used to decrease the risk of contamination. HIV could be transmitted to a nurse or doctor via fluids such as blood or even vaginal secretions. New syringes are also now in use to decrease the possibility of needle sticks.

TECH NOTE! Remember that HIV is the virus. A positive test result for HIV is considered the precursor to AIDS.

In the beginning stages of HIV, the body will weaken because of the virus replication process within the immune system. Specifically the number of T4 lymphocytes decreases; the infected person is diagnosed as having AIDS when the T-cell count is less than 200.

It has been estimated that the onset of AIDS can occur up to 20 years after acquiring HIV. However, the virus is always contagious. All agents that are available to treat both HIV and AIDS are aimed at controlling the progression of the disease but cannot cure it. Therefore the only way to avoid this disease is to prevent contracting it.

Miscellaneous Viral Conditions

Papillomavirus. The papillomavirus is a virus that causes the common wart. Most warts disappear on their own within 6 months. There are many agents available OTC such as Wart-Off, to treat warts if they do not go away on their own (see Chapter 9 for additional information about OTC).

Herpes Viruses. There are three main types of herpes: herpes simplex type 1 and type 2 and herpes zoster. Their activities within the human body vary as outlined in Box 24.4.

Herpes type 1 causes blisters on the surface of the skin. It can also cause blindness if left untreated. Herpes type 2 causes infections in both adults and neonates.

BOX 24.4 TYPES OF HUMAN HERPES VIRUSES

Herpes simplex
  Type 1   Causes disease of the mouth, face, skin, esophagus, or brain
  Type 2   Causes disease of the rectum, genital, meninges

Herpes zoster
  Shingles   Lesions on the skin surface appearing on torso, arms, and legs
  Chicken pox Childhood disease: the body will normally produce immunity against reinfection

If a mother has an active case of herpes type 2 when the baby is being born, the neonate can acquire the virus. Herpes zoster affects the nerves endings, and results in severe pain. It also causes lesions on the skin surface, referred to as shingles. This form of the virus tends to have cyclical reinfections. Chicken pox is also caused by herpes zoster, although after infection, the body may build up an immunity (see Chapter 27) so that the virus cannot cause reinfection.

There are two types of immunity, either active or passive. Active immunity occurs if the immunity is from antibodies produced by the body. This can be either natural or artificial. An example of active natural immunity is when children are exposed to a child with the measles; those who then acquire the virus from the child who has the measles have contracted measles in a natural way. Artificial natural immunity is when the dead or attenuated (weakened) virus is given as an injection. The second type of immunity, passive, can be either natural or artificial. An example of passive natural immunity is when antibodies are passed in a passive fashion, for example, from mother to the newly born child providing immunity for up to 3 months. Passive artificial immunity is when an injection of either the antibodies or immune globulin is given. These antibodies and globulins are prepared in a laboratory.

DO YOU REMEMBER THESE KEY POINTS?

- The generations of penicillins and cephalosporins
- The drug actions of the drugs discussed in this chapter
- What types of bacteria are good and where they reside
- How the Gram stain is done and what it indicates
- What causes tuberculosis and the treatment
- What are some of the most common fungal infections
- How viruses proliferate
- The three mechanisms of destroying or stopping viruses

REVIEW QUESTIONS:

Multiple Choice

1. Penicillin agents are most effective against which type of microbes?
   A. Gram positive
   B. Gram negative
   C. Gram positive and fungus
   D. Gram positive and viruses

2. The difference in the "generations" of penicillin and cephalosporin agents is that
   A. Generations determine the spectrum of gram-negative and gram-positive microbes that they work against
   B. Generations determine the types of microbes that they work against
   C. Generations determine the length and course of treatment
   D. Generations are determined by when they were discovered

3. The following diseases are caused by STDs except
   A. Chlamydia
   B. Syphilis
   C. Trichomoniasis
   D. Trichinosis

4. The following conditions are *always* caused by viruses except
   A. Colds
   B. Warts
   C. HIV
   D. Pneumonia

5. A person with an allergy to penicillin that has a UTI would most likely be treated with which of the following agents?
   A. 2nd generation penicillin
   B. 3rd generation penicillin
   C. Cephalosporin
   D. Aminoglycoside

6. All of the following agents are 3rd generation cephalosporins except
   A. Cefepime
   B. Cefixime
   C. Ceftizoxime
   D. Cefprozil

7. The condition marked by corneal abrasions and skin lesions that are progressive are symptoms of
   A. STDs
   B. Tuberculosis
   C. HIV
   D. Hansen's disease

8. The most common treatment for TB is the combination regimen of
   A. Penicillin G and gentamicin
   B. INH, rifampin, and ethambutol
   C. Kanamycin, cycloserine, and isoniazid
   D. Amikacin, kanamycin, and rifampin

9. Fungus grows best in or on
   A. Shower floors
   B. In very dry environments
   C. On clothes
   D. On cooked food

10. Antiparasitic agents work by all of the methods listed except
    A. Killing the parasite
    B. Killing the host
    C. Ridding the body of the live parasite
    D. Paralyzing the parasites, then flushing them out of the body

11. One way to avoid a parasitic infestation is to
    A. Cook all meat thoroughly
    B. Do not drink from rivers or streams
    C. Wash your hands before eating food
    D. All of the above

12. The following antihelminthic agents are vermicidal except
    A. Thiabendazole
    B. Oxamniquine
    C. Praziquantel
    D. Mebendazole

13. Malaria is a disease that is caused by
    A. Mosquitoes
    B. Blood transfusions
    C. Tropical climates
    D. Sporozoan species

14. Antiviral agents' actions include all of the following except
    A. They can interrupt the attachment of the virion to the host cell
    B. They can affect the replication phase of the virion within the host cell
    C. They can affect the assembly of the viral parts within the host cell
    D. They can lyse open the viral particles before they reach the host cell

15. Influenza is most dangerous to all of the following groups of people except
    A. Babies
    B. Older adults
    C. Immunosuppressed
    D. Adults aged 18–25 years

16. The type of herpes that is closely related to chicken pox is
    A. Herpes type 1
    B. Herpes type 2
    C. Herpes simplex
    D. Shingles

True/False
*If the statement is false, then change it to make it true.

1. All microbes cause disease.
2. Bacteriostatic agents kills microbes, whereas bactericidal agents only stop the growth.
3. Anaerobic organisms need oxygen to survive, whereas aerobic organisms do not.
4. A nosocomial infection is an infection within the nose such as a cold.
5. Tinea pedis is a viral infection affecting the feet.
6. Terbinafine is normally used to treat fungal infections such as onychomycosis.
7. The most common form of fungus found as part of the normal flora is the species *Candida albicans*.

8. All parasites cause problems for the host because they benefit at the expense of another.

9. The STD *Trichomonas vaginalis* is a parasitic infection.

10. AIDS causes similar conditions such as HIV.

11. Not all herpes viruses are contagious.

12. Chicken pox is a childhood disease that will bring about passive immunity.

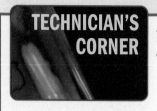

TECHNICIAN'S CORNER

Use a reference book to determine the following information about the listed antiinfective agents:

Use
Necessary auxiliary label
Dosage forms
Routes of administration

Agents:

Zidovudine
Ethambutol
Miconazole
Ticarcillin/clavulanate
Maxipime

BIBLIOGRAPHY

Center for Disease Control web site *http://www.cdc.gov/travel/malinfo.htm* accessed Jan. 30, 2003.

Drug Facts and Comparisons 1999, St Louis, 1999, Facts and Comparisons.

Goodman G, Gillman L: *The Pharmacological Basis of Therapeutics*, ed 8, Elmsford, NY, 1990, McGraw Hill.

McKenry L, Salerno E: *Pharmacology in Nursing*, ed 21, St Louis, 2001, Mosby.

Mosby's Drug Consult, St Louis, 2004, Elsevier.

Shannon M, et al.: *Health Professional's Drug Guide 2002*, Upper Saddle River, NJ, 2002, Prentice Hall.

Thibodeau, Patton: *Structure & Function of the Body*, ed 11, St Louis, 2000, Mosby.

CHAPTER 25

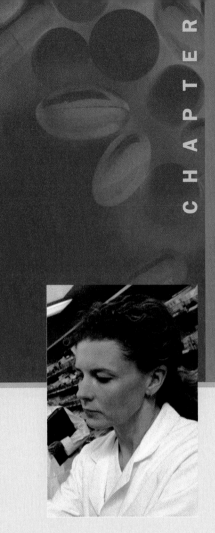

Antiinflammatories and Antihistamines

Objectives

- List both generic and trade names of the medications discussed in this chapter.

- Describe the symptoms of inflammation.

- Differentiate between steroidal and nonsteroidal antiinflammatories.

- List the major side effects of the agents discussed.

- List the major cells that are activated from the immune system to repair damaged cells.

- List the major inflammatory conditions.

- List the drug action of pain receptors.

- List the major medications used in the treatment of arthritis, rheumatoid arthritis, osteoarthritis, and other major conditions.

- Describe the symptoms of asthma and the classifications of drugs used to treat asthma.

- Explain the use of inhalers as opposed to nebulizers and when they are used.

TERMS AND DEFINITIONS

Anaphylactic shock *A severe allergic reaction that causes blood pressure to decrease rapidly, the heart to go into ventricular tachycardia, and the airways to close; a medical emergency that will cause death if not treated immediately*

Antigen *A substance that is capable of stimulating an immune response*

Bradykinins *Chemicals produced by the body, responsible for inflammation and pain*

Debride *To remove dead or damaged tissue*

Dermatitis *Inflammation of the skin associated with itching and burning*

Erythema *Redness of the skin resulting from capillary dilation*

Histamine *A substance that interacts with tissues, producing an allergic reaction*

NSAIDs *Nonsteroidal antiinflammatory drugs*

Over-the-counter (OTC) *Medications that can be bought without a prescription*

Rhinitis *Inflammation of the lining of the nose; runny nose*

Steroids *Messenger chemicals produced by the body that help fight inflammation and pain*

Systemic *Pertaining to the entire body rather than to individual body parts*

Urticaria *A skin eruption of itching wheals*

Vasodilation *Widening of the blood vessels that allows for increased blood flow*

ANTIINFLAMMATORY AGENTS

Trade	Generic	Pronunciation
Aspirin-Like Agents		
Indocin	indomethacin	in-doe-**meth**-ah-sin
Trilisate	choline magnesium trisalicylate	**coe**-leen mag-**knee**-see-um try-sall-**ih**-sa-late
Clinoril	sulindac	**suh**-lin-dack
Meclomen	meclofenamate	mea-kloe-**fen**-ah-mate
Nonsteroidal Antiinflammatory Drugs (NSAIDs)		
Bayer	aspirin*	**ass**-pur-rin
Motrin, Advil*	ibuprofen	eye-bu-**pro**-fen
Aleve*	naproxen	nah-**prox**-sin
Anaprox	naproxen sodium	nah-**prox**-sin **so**-di-um
Orudis*	ketoprofen	key-toe-**pro**-fin
Ansaid	flurbiprofen	flur-**bip**-row-fin
Toradol	ketorolac	key-toh-**row**-lack
Nalfon	fenoprofen	fen-oh-**pro**-fen
Daypro	oxaprozin	ox-ah-**pro**-sin
Relafen	nabumetone	na-**byoo**-me-tone
Lodine	etodolac	ee-toe-**doe**-lak
Cyclooxygenase Inhibitors (COX-2 Inhibitors)		
Celebrex	celecoxib	ce-lee-**cox**-ib
Vioxx	rofecoxib	row-fe-**cox**-ib

Trade	Generic	Pronunciation
Corticosteroids		
Deltasone	prednisone	**pred**-nis-own
Solu-Medrol, Medrol	methylprednisolone	meth-il-pred-**nis**-oh-lone
Bronchodilators (Asthma Agents)		
Aluvent	metaproterenol	met-a-proe-**tear**-e-nol
Azmacort	triamcinolone	trye-am-**sin**-oh-lone
AeroBid	flunisolide	floo-**nis**-oh-lide
Flovent	fluticasone	floo-**tik**-a-sone
Pulmicort	budesonide	byoo-**des**-oh-nide
First-Generation Antihistamine Drugs		
Benadryl*	diphenhydramine	die-fen-**hi**-dra-meen
Chlor-Trimeton*	chlorpheniramine	klor-fen-**ear**-ah-meen
Periactin	cyproheptadine	sye-pro-**hep**-tah-deen
Tavist*	clemastine	**klee**-mas-teen
Second-Generation Drugs		
Allegra	fexofenadine	fex-oh-**fen**-ah-deen
Zyrtec	cetirizine	sea-**tur**-eye-zeen
Claritin*	loratadine	lor-at-**tah**-deen
Atarax, Vistaril	hydroxyzine	high-**drox**-ie-zeen

*Over the counter

474

Introduction

Unlike many other conditions, there are several medications available over-the-counter (OTC) that are used to treat inflammation. Aside from the common cold, muscle pain resulting from inflammation is one of the leading causes for self-medication. Most pharmacies sell more OTC NSAIDs and analgesics than any other type of agent. This is partially due to the hectic lifestyle many people live and the accessibility of OTCs. Although many OTCs are considered safe and effective, they can cause adverse side effects if taken inappropriately, especially when the patient may be taking other medications concurrently or if he or she has a preexisting condition. In addition, there are many legend drugs that can make a person feel better; however, these too can have serious side effects if not taken correctly.

In this chapter we explore the conditions caused by inflammation and the use of both steroidal and nonsteroidal medications to treat inflammation. We also briefly cover the major conditions associated with allergies and other inflammatory conditions of the airways, as well as agents used to treat them. We begin by taking a look at the structures of antiinflammatory agents and their derivatives to understand the differences between them. We then explore the types of conditions that occur and the most common agents used to treat them.

Inflammation

Inflammation can be caused by infection, allergic reactions, or injury. Inflammation is a necessary response if the body is to heal itself.

Along with the obvious swelling effects of inflammation, there are other effects that are felt rather than seen. Thousands of years ago the Romans described the symptoms of inflammation as redness, swelling, heat, pain, and the eventual loss of function of the affected area. The body tries to repair the damages with the help of blood and cells and natural chemicals. Some chemicals send messages to the smooth muscles causing vasodilation, allowing more blood to reach the affected area. Because the blood rushes in, the area is warmer. Areas surrounding the damaged area may not be able to adapt to the increase in blood, resulting in edema (buildup of fluids) within the surrounding tissues. Specialized cells are sent to the area, and the repair process begins. Table 25.1 lists some of the major types of cells that make up our immune system and their effects on the body system.

There are many different chemicals contained in the body's cells that have a role in inflammation. Each has a specific job to perform. One such chemical found in many cells is an enzyme called cyclooxygenase. This enzyme produces various hormones called prostaglandins, which are responsible for other chemical reactions that cause inflammation, pain, and increased temperature. Aspirin is one agent that inhibits cyclooxygenase pathways and thereby stops the production of prostaglandin.

Inflammation can only occur in living tissue; therefore if an area undergoes necrosis (death of the tissue), such as necrosis of the hands or feet from frostbite, there will be no apparent swelling of the tissue. Instead, as blood flow diminishes, the skin will turn black, and because the tissue has no blood supply, the area will need debriding to prevent the infection from spreading further.

There are two different types of inflammation—acute and chronic. Acute inflammation only lasts a few days and the body usually can recover without any help from medication. Chronic inflammation can arise from an acute case of inflammation or from of an injury. It can occur locally, such as at a cut on the surface of the skin, or systemically within areas of the body. When inflammation becomes

TABLE 25.1 Immune Cell Responses in Injury

Name of Cell or Molecule	Type of Cell Involved	Effects
Antibodies	Produced by B lymphocytes in response to an antigen. Memory cells previously produced increase in population to fight off infection. Found in the blood.	Can neutralize or destroy antigens in different ways such as by coating or lysing the antigen. They can stimulate phagocytosis and prevent the antigen from adhering to host cells.
Fibrinogen	A globulin found in blood plasma.	Helps in coagulating blood.
Granulocytes	Mature leukocyte cells that contain granules, including neutrophils and other types of immune response cells.	Fights off infection.
Leukocytes	White blood cells formed in bone marrow, including granulocytes and nongranulocytes.	Fights off infection and tissue damage. They destroy foreign organisms and also clean up damaged cells by phagocytosis.
Lymphocytes	White blood cells formed in the spleen and bone marrow.	Adhere to endothelial cells: intensify inflammation by causing direct cell injury and promoting formation of antibodies that increase the inflammatory response.
Monocytes	Large type of leukocyte.	Eventually become macrophages. Macrophages are one of the first line of defenses in the inflammatory process.
Neutrophils	Mature white blood cells in the granulocytic series, comprise more than 50% of the leukocytes present in the body.	Adhere to damaged site to protect against infection by destroying infectious microbes; also destroy antigens.
Macrophages	Large cells called phagocytes that secrete cytokines.	Ingest dead tissue, bacterial cells, or dying cells.

TABLE 25.2 Types of Inflammation

Condition	Location of Inflammation	Notes
Pneumonia	Lungs	Alveolar spaces swell
Pericarditis	Heart	Lining of the heart swells
Strep throat	Throat lining	Caused by bacterial infection
Abscess	Organs or tissues	Pus- or liquid-filled spaces
Colitis	Colon (large intestine)	Bacterial or ulcerous
Ulcer	Epithelial lining such as in the stomach or duodenum	Peptic ulcers and duodenal ulcers

chronic, the site of injury may swell again and a low grade fever can result. Table 25.2 describes types of inflammation.

Chronic inflammation can cause damage to the affected sites or internal organs. As the body heals, it leaves behind scar tissue. This scar tissue can alter the normal workings of the body system. For instance, if the heart becomes scarred, it may not work as well in pumping or circulating the blood. If the fallopian tubes are scarred by pelvic inflammatory disease, the woman may become sterile. Inflammation can also damage the kidneys to the extent that the person needs dialysis. Along with inflammation there can be varying degrees of pain associated with the swelling.

Pain

Everyone experiences pain at some time as the result of injury. Each person's perception of pain is specific to him or her and cannot be measured by scientific methods. Most pain lasts only a short time. However, if the pain is persistent (lasts for 3 months or longer), it is called chronic pain. When consulting a health care provider, a patient may be asked to rate the severity of pain using a numerical scale from 1 to 10. The number 1 indicates very little pain and 10 indicates severe pain. If pain is severe, it may be called acute pain. Most muscle or tendon sprains result in acute pain and last only a few weeks. Cancer pain can be severe and chronic. With prolonged pain, either acute or chronic, the psychological health of the person in pain can be affected. Many cancer patients are given pain medications that are dosed on a schedule (such as every 6 or 8 hours) in order to minimize pain. Pain that resurfaces before the scheduled dose time is called breakthrough pain. Most pain medications used to treat cancer patients are controlled substances and are discussed in Chapter 28.

For pain caused by inflammation, a variety of medications can be used to relieve it, including NSAIDs. These medications can play an important part in the reduction of pain through their mechanism of action. The following sections include a brief overview of the types of medications used to treat inflammation including one of the first antiinflammatory agents—aspirin. Refer to the glucocorticoid section of this chapter for a more in-depth review of the chemicals that play a part in the inflammatory process.

THE HISTORY OF ASPIRIN

In England in the early 1800s, it was reported that the bark from the willow tree was effective as a pain, fever, and inflammation reducer. Many cultures had known this for centuries but it was not until the early 1800s that the medical community began to isolate the active ingredients. A French chemist by the name of Henri Leroux found that a bitter glycoside was responsible for the bark's medicinal properties. This chemical was referred to as salicin. When this chemical breaks apart, it creates glucose (sugar) and salicylic alcohol. The salicylic alcohol ultimately can be broken down into acetylsalicylic acid (ASA).

Scientists were aware of the effects of salicin and wanted to know exactly how it produced these effects. For the effects of decreasing pain, they discovered that it inhibits prostaglandins. Prostaglandins, produced naturally by the body, are a group of hormonal chemicals that are responsible for pain, inflammation, and the elevated temperature associated with injury. Although salicin helps decrease inflammation, pain, and the heat associated with injury, it will not lower body temperature caused from normal activities, such as exercising.

As this new information became available, salicin was considered a miracle drug and was used to treat illnesses such as gout, inflammation from injury, and pain and to reduce high fever, which could cause death. The first company to market this miracle agent was the Bayer Company in 1899. They called their new wonder drug aspirin. Since then there have been many new drugs introduced into the marketplace that work similarly, although aspirin is still a popular drug because of how well it works.

TECH NOTE! Aspirin contains a chemical called acetylsalicylic acid. This chemical inhibits prostaglandins. This inhibition decreases inflammation and helps decrease pain and fever.

WHAT IS ASPIRIN USED FOR?

One of the most common uses of aspirin is for the prevention of strokes or heart attacks. Aspirin decreases platelet aggregation (blood clotting). If a clot occurs in

TABLE 25.3 Various Strengths of Aspirin Available

Trade Name	Strength	Dosage Form
Maximum Bayer	500 mg	Tablet, caplet
Arthritis Foundation Pain Reliever	500 mg	Tablets
Ecotrin	325 mg	EC tablet, caplet
Extra Strength Bayer EC	500 mg	EC tablet, caplet
Aspergum	227.5 mg	Gum tablet
1/2 Halfprin	165 mg	EC tablet
Bayer Low Adult Strength	81 mg	Tablet
Ecotrin Adult Low Strength	81 mg	Tablet
Halfprin	81 mg	Tablet
Heartline	81 mg	Tablet
St. Joseph Adult Chewable Aspirin	81 mg	Chewable tablet

EC, Enteric coated; *OTC*, over-the-counter.
Enteric coated: a film coating protects the stomach from irritation.

the brain, it can cause a stroke. If the clot occurs in the blood vessels of the heart, it can cause a heart attack. If it occurs in the lungs, it can cause a pulmonary embolism. All of these conditions are life threatening. Many physicians prescribe 81 to 325 mg per day to decrease blood clotting (Table 25.3). Anticoagulation medication is often called a "blood thinner."

Aspirin comes in a dose of 975 mg (Easpirin), and is a prescription drug. Although aspirin is a very inexpensive and effective agent against fever, pain, and inflammation, it should not be given to children, especially those with flulike symptoms because of Reye's syndrome, which may occur following chickenpox or upper respiratory infection. Reye's syndrome is a childhood disease that causes vomiting, lethargy, and encephalopathy, which can lead to coma and death. For children suffering from the chicken pox or flulike symptoms, acetaminophen (Tylenol) can be given without fear of Reye's syndrome.

Aspirin has a maximum dosing range that should not exceed 4 g per day. A common side effect is upset stomach. Therefore an auxiliary label "take with food" should be affixed to any aspirin prescription. In addition, persons on anticoagulation agents normally should not take aspirin because it increases the anticoagulation effects of the prescribed agent, which may result in internal bleeding. Pharmacists should counsel patients any time an anticoagulant is prescribed.

SALICYLATES

There are various salicylate chemical combinations that can be prescribed for pain resulting from rheumatoid arthritis and other more serious conditions. Some of the more common agents are listed in Table 25.4.

NONSTEROIDAL ANTIINFLAMMATORY AGENTS

Aspirin is a salicylate drug and the prototype agent for the newer NSAIDs. Although NSAIDs have a different chemical structure than aspirin, they have the same basic benzene ring attached to a (acid) carboxyl group as seen in Figure 25.1. There is a close similarity between the structure of aspirin and aspirin-like drugs and NSAIDs. All of these agents have analgesic, antipyretic, and antiinflammatory properties that make them very popular in the retail marketplace. There are more than a dozen NSAIDs available in prescription form and about four differ-

TABLE 25.4   Conditions Treated and Common Dosing of Aspirin or Aspirin-like Agents

Availability	Type of Salicylate Agent	Condition/Symptoms	Dosing
OTC/RX	Aspirin	Antipyretic/analgesic	325 mg up to 650 mg q4h prn, 975 mg (RX)
RX	Disalcid	Antipyretic/analgesic	3 g/day in divided doses
OTC	Sodium salicylate	Antipyretic/analgesic	325 to 650 mg q4h
RX	Sodium thiosalicylate (Hyrex)	Gout	100 mg q3-4h × 2 days, then 100 mg qd until symptoms disappear
		Muscle pain	50 to 100 mg qd
		Rheumatic fever	100 to 150 mg q4-8h × 3 days, then 100 mg bid until symptoms disappear
OTC	Choline salicylate	Antipyretic/analgesic	870 mg q 3-4h
		Rheumatoid arthritis	870 mg to 1.74 g qid
RX	Diflunisal (Dolobid)	Mild to moderate pain	500 mg q8-12h
		Osteoarthritis/rheumatoid arthritis	250 to 500 mg bid

OTC, Over-the-counter; *RX,* prescription.

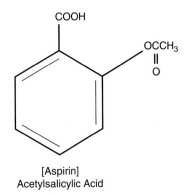

FIGURE 25.1 Chemical structure of aspirin.

ent types of medications available OTC. In contrast, most aspirin is sold OTC by dozens of different manufacturers in various strengths and dosage forms and in combinations with other drugs.

NSAIDs can be used for mild to moderate pain. They have several positive effects on the body, such as the following:

1. They are not addictive, unlike controlled substances
2. They decrease pain (analgesic)
3. They decrease fever (antipyretic)
4. They decrease inflammation (antiinflammatory)
5. Many can be purchased OTC

Their method of action includes inhibition of cyclooxygenase, which is the enzyme responsible for the formation of prostaglandins and bradykinins. These chemicals are responsible for pain and inflammation. NSAIDs also have an antipyretic effect by acting on the hypothalamus (the body thermostat). Wide variations have been documented among different NSAIDs, even if they are related and in the same chemical family. Because each type of NSAID tends to work differently, if one brand does not work, another one might.

TABLE 25.5 NSAIDs, COX-1, COX-2, and Similar Agents

Generic	Brand	Adult Dosage	Note
Aspirin	Bayer**	325 to 1000 mg q4-6 h	Max 4 g qd
Celecoxib	Celebrex††	100 to 200 mg q12-24 h	Max 400 mg qd*
Choline Magnesium trisalicylate	Arthropan**	1 to 1.5 g q12 h	Max 4 g qd
Etodolac	Lodine††	200 to 400 mg q6-12 h	Max 1.2 g qd
Fenoprofen	Nalfon††	200 mg q4-6 hr	Max 3.2 g qd
Flurbiprofen	Ansaid††	50 to 100 mg q6-12 h	Max 300 mg qd
Ibuprofen	Motrin*	300 to 800 mg q6-8 h	Max 3.2 g qd
Indomethacin	Indocin††	25 to 50 mg q8-12 h	Max 200 mg qd
Ketoprofen	Orudis†	12.5 to 75 mg q6-8 h	Max 300 mg qd
Ketorolac	Toradol††	15 to 60 mg q6 h	Max 120 mg (IM or IV)
		10 mg q4-6 h	Max 120 mg qd (PO)
Meclofenamate	Meclomen††	50 to 100 mg q4-6 h	Max 400 mg qd
Nabumetone	Relafen††	1 g q12-24 h	Max 2 g qd*
Naproxen	Naprosyn Aleve**	275 to 500 mg q12 h	Max 1.25 g qd
Naproxen sodium	Anaprox†	250 to 50 mg q12 h	Max 1.5 mg qd
Piroxicam	Feldene†	20 mg q24 h	Max 20 mg qd
Rofecoxib	Vioxx††	12.5 to 50 mg q24 h	Max 50 mg qd*
Sulindac	Clinoril††	150 to 200 mg q12 h	Max 400 mg qd
Tolmetin	Tolectin††	200 to 600 mg q6-8 h	Max 1.8 g qd

NSAIDS, Nonsteroidal antiinflammatory drugs; *COX*, cyclooxygenase; *IM*, intramuscular; *PO*, oral.
*May decrease stomach upset.
**OTC only.
†Have OTC and Rx strengths.
††Rx only.

NSAIDs are used to treat many different types of conditions and chronic illnesses such as the following:

1. Muscle pain
2. Rheumatoid arthritis
3. Bone pain such as in osteoarthritis
4. Premenstrual syndrome

Millions of people use OTC and legend NSAIDs to treat various inflammatory conditions. However, overuse of these agents can cause major problems. NSAIDs can worsen stomach problems such as gastroesophageal reflux disease. They can also cause ulcers if used for a long time. All NSAIDs should be taken with food to prevent stomach problems. In addition, they can increase bleeding and should not be used by those taking warfarin or other anticoagulants. Table 25.5 lists some of the common NSAIDs and aspirin-like agents. Lower dosages of some of these agents are available OTC (see Chapter 9).

TECH NOTE! Pregnant women should not take warfarin at any time during pregnancy because it can pass through the placenta. Heparin does not cross the placenta.

DRUG ACTION OF CYCLOOXYGENASE (COX-1 vs. COX-2)

Cyclooxygenase (COX) is an enzyme that works along a pathway that synthesizes prostaglandins and other compounds. It is a substance found in all tissues where it helps regulate many processes. COX has two forms, COX-1 and COX-2. COX-1 is present in most tissues and helps to take care of many normal functions including protecting gastric mucosa and promoting platelet aggregation. COX-2 is found mainly at sites of tissue injury where it helps sensitize receptors to pain and mediates inflammation. It is also located within the brain where it affects fever and pain perception. Therefore COX-1 can be thought of as taking care of the more normal processes, whereas COX-2 takes care of the processes when pain and discomfort are present.

First generation NSAIDs inhibit both COX-1 and COX-2 enzymes, which results in a decrease in inflammation, pain, and fever. The only benefit of inhibiting COX-1 enzymes is to protect against myocardial infarction (heart attacks) by reduction in platelet aggregation, which lowers the chances of blood clotting. Unfortunately, the negative side of inhibiting COX-1 enzymes is that they have serious side effects such as gastric erosion, ulceration, bleeding, and renal damage.

Second generation NSAIDs are COX-2 selective, thus reducing inflammation, pain, and fever without the side effects of COX-1 inhibitors or first generation NSAIDs.

Acetaminophen (Tylenol) is not included in antiinflammatories because, although it does affect COX enzymes in an inhibitory way by relieving pain and fever, it does not alleviate inflammation.

Other chemicals in the body are able to help with the reduction of inflammation, such as corticosteroids. Whereas NSAIDs suppress inflammation by inhibiting prostaglandin production, the glucocorticoids not only inhibit prostaglandin synthesis but also suppress inflammation.

GLUCOCORTICOIDS (STEROIDS)

There are different types of steroids produced by the body. They are secreted from the endocrine glands and are chemical messengers of the body. The main gland that produces steroids is the adrenal gland. The adrenal cortex makes both glucocorticoids and mineralocorticoids (both are referred to as corticosteroids). Another steroid, corticotropin, secreted by the anterior pituitary gland, is a regulator of the adrenal gland. Steroids have an important role in the maintenance of the body system. The imbalance of normal steroid levels can cause various diseases. Because of the common use of high-dose glucocorticoids, we focus on these agents in this chapter.

The glucocorticoids have two major effects on the body, both physiological and pharmacological. When low doses are given, a physiological effect is seen (for treatment of adrenocortical insufficiency). When high doses are given, pharmacological effects are seen. This involves the ability of these agents to decrease inflammatory conditions caused by various types of arthritis, such as rheumatoid arthritis and osteoarthritis. Other uses include treatment of asthma and certain types of cancer, and suppression of the immune response in organ transplant recipients.

Because of their strong effects on the immune system, corticosteroids can cause many serious side effects if they are taken over long periods of time, taken inappropriately, or stopped abruptly. To understand why this can happen we first must review the mechanism of action of high-dose steroids.

Glucocorticoid therapy has the same effects as naturally produced glucocorticoids. It affects protein, fat, and glucose metabolism within the body. It raises the blood glucose levels. One way in which this is accomplished is by decreasing the metabolism of proteins by converting them into glucose. The overall effect reduces muscle mass and bone density and causes thinning of the skin. Glucocorticoid therapy also causes fat redistribution by alteration of fat metabolism. This can lead to the appearance of a "moon face," a symptom of Cushing's disease.

Normally the release of glucocorticoids in the body is regulated by a negative feedback system. For example, when a physiologically stressful event occurs the brain sends signals to the adrenal glands. Glucocorticoids and other chemicals, such as prostaglandins and leukotrienes, are released into the body system and reduce inflammation.

Although glucocorticoids are very effective in reducing inflammation, they can have adverse effects if their secretion is prolonged. Stressful events, such as surgery,

Doctor Frank DeStefano
Suite 100
Pine Grove, CA 94222
ph: 916-555-4242

For: _Michael Sewollen_   Date: _9-19-02_

Address: _44 Round St._   PH: _____

℞:

Prednisone 10mg tab   Quantity

_QS_

_1 20mg qd × 10d, 15mg qd × 10d,_
_10mg qd × 10d, 5mg qd × 10d,_

QS=
Quantity sufficient:
i.e., pharmacy to
calculate amount
needed for course
of Rx.

M.D. Signature

DEA # _AD 1245997_   Refills _∅_

FIGURE 25.2 Prednisone taper prescription.

high doses, or prolonged use of glucocorticoid medications, may cause a suppression of lymphocytes, which may in turn lower resistance to infections. Other side effects may include increased appetite, increased bruising, insomnia, restlessness, anxiety, hypotension, and headache.

Adrenal Effects of Steroid Agents

Glucocorticoids are essential to the wellness of the body. One problem of long-term use of steroids is the body's ability to produce glucocorticoids on its own is decreased and eventually may stop altogether. Depending on the length of time that steroids are used, the body can take from days to a year to begin production of glucocorticoids. When it is determined that it is time to discontinue a steroid, it must be done slowly to allow the body to begin production of glucocorticoids by tapering the dose over a month or more. An example of a tapered order is given in Figure 25.2.

There are several routes of administration for steroids: oral, parenteral (intravenous [IV], intramuscular [IM], subcutaneous [SC]), topical, and inhalation. Prescriptions are normally written for the smallest effective amount of steroids as well as the least amount of time necessary to treat the condition. Side effects of oral dosages include gastrointestinal (GI) upset; therefore all steroids should have the auxiliary label "take with food." Because dosages are varied based on the severity of the condition and patient's health, we have not included them in the drug monographs in this chapter. An example of common agents used to treat inflammation and pain are listed in the following.

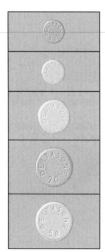

Pharmacia &
Upjohn

CLASSIFICATION: STEROIDAL AGENTS

GENERIC NAME: prednisone

TRADE NAME: Deltasone

INDICATION: for the treatment of a wide variety of diseases such as adrenocortical insufficiency and respiratory, GI, and neoplastic diseases. Also used for allergic, inflammatory, and autoimmune conditions

DOSAGE FORMS: tablets, solution, syrup

GENERIC NAME: hydrocortisone (Available in many different forms, such as hydrocortisone acetate, butyrate, cypionate, sodium phosphate, valerate, and sodium succinate)
TRADE NAME: Cortef (oral), Hytone (topical), Kenalog (aerosol), Anusol-HC (suppository), Cortenema (enema), Solu-Cortef (injectable)
INDICATION: oral: management of adrenocortical insufficiency, relief of inflammation of dermatosis, and adjunctive treatment of ulcerative colitis; suppositories for hemorrhoids
DOSAGE FORMS: injectable; aerosol; topical forms: ointment, cream, lotion; oral forms: tablet, solution, syrup, suspension

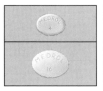

Pharmacia & Upjohn

GENERIC NAME: methylprednisolone sodium succinate
TRADE NAME: Medrol (oral), Depo-Medrol (injectable)
INDICATION: antiinflammatory or immunosuppressive agents used to treat a variety of diseases; also used after bone marrow transplants
DOSAGE FORMS: injection as acetate or sodium succinate; tablet, tablet dose pack (tapered dose)

GENERIC NAME: triamcinolone acetonide
TRADE NAME: Aristocort (topical), Azmacort (inhalent), Kenalog (aerosol), Nasacort (nasal)
INDICATION: systemic use: adrenocortical insufficiency, rheumatic disorders, allergic states, respiratory diseases, and other diseases requiring antiinflammatory or immunosuppressive effects; nasal spray: treatment of seasonal allergic rhinitis; inhalation: control of bronchial asthma and related bronchospastic conditions
DOSAGE FORMS: oral tablet, syrup; aerosol; spray; topical; injection as acetonide, diacetate, hexacetonide

Asthma

Millions of Americans suffer from asthma, a chronic inflammatory disorder of the airways that can occur in childhood or adulthood. Because of many environmental factors, the incidence of asthma is increasing. Smoking, sickness such as cold or flu, animal dander, environmental contaminants, and even stressful situations can cause the onset of an asthmatic attack. Because of the inflammation of the lining and constriction of the bronchioles that occurs during an attack, a person can die if not treated quickly.

After the airway is exposed to an irritant, different cells within the body (mast cells, T lymphocytes, neutrophils, and epithelial cells) are altered. Various chemicals that are released from these cells cause the smooth muscle in the airway to become inflamed. Epithelial layers become damaged and mucous membranes secrete large amounts of mucus. All of these events contribute to the overall decrease in normal breathing. An acute attack of asthma has been known to cause anaphylaxis if not treated quickly. Anaphylaxis is a severe allergic condition in which the smooth muscles of the body, including the airways, constrict and the capillaries dilate. Death may occur if untreated. Fortunately, there are many medications available to treat asthma. However, there is currently no cure for this common disease.

AGENTS USED TO TREAT ASTHMA

The most common medications used to treat acute asthma are beta-adrenergic agonists. These can be used along with bronchodilators such as corticosteroids. The effects of beta-adrenergics is to dilate the bronchial airways. There are short- and long-acting agents that work effectively. In addition to beta-adrenergic agents, corticosteroids are also commonly used. These agents are available in inhalant or parenteral (injectable) forms. Corticosteroids can be both short term and long term. Other agents that can be used to treat asthma are anticholinergics. Anticholinergics may be administered parenterally (by injection); however, the most

TABLE 25.6 Asthma Agents

Trade	Generic	Adult Dose of Inhalent	Route of Administration	Specific Targets
Short Acting beta-2-Agonists (Sympathomimetics)				Relaxes bronchial smooth muscle. Specifically affects beta-2 sites
Proventil, Ventolin	Albuterol	1-2 puffs q4-6h	PO, Inh	
Bronkosol	Isoetharine	1-2 puffs q4h	Inh	
Maxair	Pirbuterol	1-2 puffs q6h	Inh	
Adrenaline	Epinephrine	1-2 puffs qid	SC, Inh	
Alupent	Metaproterenol	1 puff q4h	PO, Inh	
Isuprel	Isoproterenol	2-3 puffs q3-4h	Inh, IV	
Brethine	Terbutaline	max 12/d	PO, Inh, IV	
Atrovent	Salmeterol	2 puffs qid		
Corticosteroid Agents				Inhibits certain enzymes that are responsible for inflammation. Stabilizes lysosomal membranes
Vanceril, Beclovent	Beclomethasone	2 puffs q6-8h	Inh	
Pulmicort	Budesonide	1-2 puffs bid	Inh	
Azmacort	Triamcinolone	2 puffs qid	Inh	
AeroBid	Flunisolide	2 sprays each nostril bid	Nasal	
Flovent	Fluticasone	1 puff bid	Inh	
Anticholinergics				
Atrovent	Ipratropium bromide	1-2 puffs qid	NEB	
Leukotriene Agonists				Blocks leukotriene receptors, stops anaphylaxis
Singulair	Montelukast	10 mg daily (4 mg and 5 mg Pediatric)	PO, chew tab	
Accolate	Zafirlukast	20 mg bid	PO	
Prophylactics				Used in the prevention of asthma attacks. It inhibits the release of histamine, leukotrienes, and other inflammatory producing cells
Intal	Cromolyn sodium	1 spray or cap qid	NEB, Inh, Nasal	

Inh, Inhalent; *IV*, intravenous; *NEB*, nebulizer; *PO*, orally; *SC*, subcutaneous; *Nasal*, nasal spray.

common route is inhalation. There are two methods of inhalation—a nebulizer or a metered-dose inhalant. Table 25.6 presents examples of inhalants used for asthma prophylaxis and attacks.

Sympathomimetics not only reduce inflammation of the bronchi but also relieve spasms within the smooth muscle of the airway. Because these agents mimic the sympathetic system, they affect both alpha-receptors and beta-receptors. Alpha-receptors are located in the smooth muscles of the lungs, whereas beta-receptors are located in the heart. These agents can be used to treat bronchitis and emphysema as well as asthma. Side effects of these agents can range from lightheadedness to increased heart rate.

Xanthine agents also work on the smooth muscle of the bronchioles. The main difference between sympathomimetics and xanthine agents is their route of administration. Xanthine agents such as aminophylline and theophylline are given in oral and parenteral form, not as inhalants like the sympathomimetics. Parenteral theophylline can worsen heart conditions, such as arrhythmias. Indications include symptomatic relief or prevention of bronchial asthma and other associated bronchial disorders. Auxiliary labels include "take with food," "do not chew or crush tablets," "take as directed."

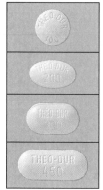

Schering

CLASSIFICATION: ANTIASTHMATICS
   GENERIC NAME: theophylline
   TRADE NAME: Theo-Dur, Slo-bid
   DOSAGE FORMS: oral: tablet, capsule, syrup, elixir, solution, sustained released tablets and capsules; injectable: theophylline in 5% dextrose

   GENERIC NAME: aminophylline
   TRADE NAME: Phyllocontin
   DOSAGE FORMS: oral: tablet, liquid; rectal: suppositories; injection

Leukotrienes are substances that cause the smooth muscle of the bronchi to contract, causing labored breathing. Zafirlukast, montelukast, and zileuton work to decrease bronchoconstriction of the airways. They can also be given to prevent asthma attacks caused by pollen, dander, cold air, or other antigens if taken before contact is made. The auxiliary label is "take as directed."

   GENERIC NAME: zileuton
   TRADE NAME: Zyflo
   DOSAGE FORMS: tablets

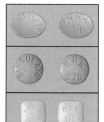

Merck

   GENERIC NAME: montelukast
   TRADE NAME: Singulair
   DOSAGE FORMS: tablets and chewable tablets (PED: 4 mg to 5 mg chewable)

Corticosteroids, unlike the agents mentioned previously, are not to be used over a long period of time, but are normally used short-term to treat asthma. They help the other agents stop the asthmatic response of bronchiole constriction. Because administered corticosteroids replace the body's steroid production, they have special dosing requirements. Commonly used inhalers along with normal dosages are listed for the treatment of asthma in adults. Always remember that all MDIs need a "shake well" auxiliary label.

   GENERIC NAME: beclomethasone
   TRADE NAME: Beclovent, Vanceril
   INDICATION: chronic asthma
   DOSAGE FORMS: aerosol
   COMMON DOSAGE: Beclovent: 2 inhalations 3 to 4 times daily; Vanceril: 2 puffs twice daily

   GENERIC NAME: flunisolide
   TRADE NAME: AeroBid
   INDICATION: chronic asthma
   DOSAGE FORMS: aerosol
   COMMON DOSAGE: 2 puffs twice daily

   GENERIC NAME: triamcinolone acetonide
   TRADE NAME: Azmacort
   INDICATION: chronic asthma
   DOSAGE FORMS: aerosol
   COMMON DOSAGE: 2 puffs 3 to 4 times daily or 4 puffs 2 times daily

Cromolyn sodium is the only agent considered an antiasthmatic and anti-allergic agent. It prevents mast cells from releasing histamine, which is one cause of asthmatic symptoms. Cromolyn is inhaled via a metered-dose inhaler (MDI), nebulizer, or a nasal inhaler. The use of cromolyn can prevent allergic reactions from occurring if taken before contact with the allergen. The nasal inhaler is available OTC.

> **GENERIC NAME:** cromolyn sodium
> **TRADE NAME:** Intal
> **INDICATION:** severe bronchial asthma, prevention of exercise-induced bronchospasm, allergic rhinitis
> **DOSAGE FORMS:** inhalation solution, aerosol spray, nasal solution, capsules for inhalation
> **AUXILIARY LABEL:** inhalers: "Shake well before using"

Most patients with asthma are given a prescription for an inhaler and they keep it close by for emergencies. The specific administration method takes practice and is usually explained by the doctor or pharmacist. The inhaler must be shaken before use.

Because it is difficult for many patients to dose themselves correctly, there are devices called an Aerochamber or spacers that fit over the end of the mouthpiece of the inhaler. As the dose of medicine is released from the inhaler, it fills the spacer and the patient can slowly and more accurately inhale more of the drug.

TECH NOTE! To find out if an inhaler is empty, simply place it into a bowl of water. The empty container will float; a partial container will have only one end floating; and a full container will drop to the bottom of the bowl.

Nebulizer treatments are given by a respiratory therapist in a hospital if ordered by the physician, or they can be used at home with proper training. Many of the agents, such as metaproterenol and albuterol, are available in unit dose containers that deliver only one dose. The exact number of drops can be placed into the nebulizer reservoir. The machine creates a steam that is filled with the medication. The drug is inhaled via a nose and mouth mask, allowing for deep, thorough inhalation treatments.

Antihistamines

Antihistamine agents are used to decrease inflammation and irritation from allergens. Allergens are also known as antigens. They are substances that are capable of stimulating an immune response. Millions of Americans suffer from seasonal allergies, as well as allergies from other common substances. Some commonly found substances are listed in Table 25.7.

TABLE 25.7 Types of Antigens

Manmade Chemicals	Natural Occurring Chemicals	Miscellaneous
Detergents, cleaners	Venom from snake bites or bee stings	Dust
Topical agents such as soaps, lotions, creams	Heavy molecular weight compounds such as blood or Dextran	Large lacerations
Drugs	Pollen	Animal dander

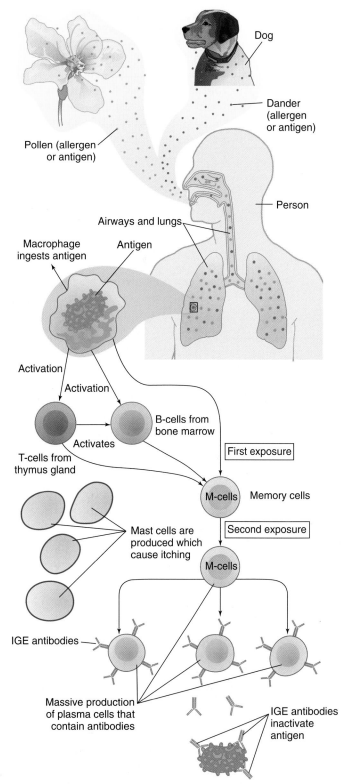

FIGURE 25.3 Events that take place in an allergic reaction, from the first exposure to an antigen to the allergic reaction.

ALLERGIC MECHANISM

When the body first comes into contact with any antigens, the body produces immunoglobulin E (IgE) antibodies that attach to mast cells. These sensitized mast cells are found in tissues of the GI tract, skin, and the respiratory tract. They attach to the mast cells throughout the body waiting for the next stimulation from antigens. Histamine-1 receptors are found in the lower respiratory tract and skin, whereas histamine-2 receptors are located in the GI tract. With the second exposure to an antigen, the antigen binds to the IgE antibodies on the mast cells (Figure 25.3). This binding causes a release of the contents of the mast cells. Histamine is released and binds to histamine receptor sites in tissues causing an allergic response that commonly includes coughing, sneezing, wheezing, and rash. More severe reactions can include decreased blood pressure, migraine headache, bronchiolar constriction, increased heart rhythm, and anaphylactic shock.

Histamine can produce a drop in blood pressure because it can dilate small blood vessels and capillaries. This dilation can then stimulate pain receptors in the head causing severe headaches or migraines. Histamine also causes bronchoconstriction making it difficult to breathe. In extremely severe reactions, the airways of a person can become swollen and closed—anaphylactic shock. This can result in death if not treated immediately.

ANTIHISTAMINE REACTIONS

When an allergic reaction takes place, antihistamines decrease the release of histamines by binding the antigen to the mast cells. There are two ways in which allergic reactions can be blocked:

1. Mast cells are prevented from releasing histamine
2. Histamine-1 receptors are blocked from interacting with histamine

Antihistamine drugs specifically block histamine-1 receptors. These agents are commonly found in cold and cough medications because of their ability to dry secretions (some antihistamines work against cholinergic responses of the nervous system). These agents are classified as anticholinergics (see Chapter 17).

Histamine-2 receptors are located in the GI tract—the stomach and intestines. Foods that cause an allergic reaction can result in vomiting, diarrhea, and cramps. A different class of drugs is used to treat this type of allergic reaction. The histamine-2 blockers, called H_2 antagonists, block the receptor sites within the GI tract. These medications are discussed in Chapter 20.

There are two generations of antihistamines. The first-generation drugs are considered nonspecific antihistamines. They were found to bind to both histamine-1 and histamine-2 receptors. Many can cause sedation because of their effect on the central nervous system (CNS) if used in higher concentrations. Some of the first-generation agents also decrease nausea, vomiting, and motion sickness by their actions on the CNS. Second-generation antihistamines became available more recently. These agents can affect histamine-1 receptors specifically, thus they do not cause the same amount of sedation. Examples of the two generations of antihistamines are given in Table 25.8 along with their common uses.

Medications that can be taken to prevent an allergic response by stabilization of the mast cell membranes include cromolyn, Zyrtec, and Allegra. These are legend (prescription) drugs. OTC medications, such as Benadryl and Claritin, are available as well. For the most severe reactions that cause swelling of the airways, epinephrine is given either by inhalation or, if necessary, by injection to open the airways. The main side effects experienced when taking antihis-

TABLE 25.8 Antihistamine Agents

Trade	Generic	Dosage Form	Uses
Benadryl*	Diphenhydramine	Cap, tab, soln(s), injection	Allergies, sedation
Chlor-Trimeton*	Chlorpheniramine	Tab, syrup, injection	Allergies
Tavist 1.25* 2.68[†]	Clemastine	Tab, syrup	Allergies
Phenergan[†]	Promethazine	Tab, syrup, suppositories, injection	Allergies, sedation, antiemetic, motion sickness
Atarax, Vistaril[†]	Hydroxyzine	Tab, cap, syrup, injection	Allergies, sedation (PO), antiemetic (IV)
Claritin*	Loratadine	Tab, syrup	Allergies
Second-Generation Drugs			
Zyrtec[†]	Cetirizine	Tab, syrup	Allergies

Cap, Capsule; *tab*, tablet.
*OTC
[†]Rx

tamines include drowsiness, dry mouth, constipation, urinary retention, sedation, and increase in intraocular pressure.

DRUG INTERACTIONS

The effects of drugs that suppress the CNS will increase if used with first-generation antihistamines. Alcohol should not be consumed if one is taking antihistamines because it can intensify drowsiness. Some antibiotics such as macrolides, ketoconazole, and itraconazole can intensify the effects of second-generation antihistamines. All first-generation antihistamines should be given an auxiliary label that states "may cause drowsiness." All OTC antihistamines have labeling that cautions consumers of their ability to cause drowsiness.

ASTHMA TREATMENT DOSAGE FORMS

Asthma is a serious condition. If left untreated, asthma can lead to anaphylactic shock, which often results in death. Most medications used for the treatment of severe asthma and other similar conditions of the respiratory system are legend drugs. There is a wide range of agents that can be used with multiple routes of administration. The more common route for adults is by inhalation. In young children, oral liquid is more commonly used. An MDI is convenient and can easily be kept in a purse or pocket for emergency use. For a more thorough treatment, nebulizers can be used at home or may be given in a clinic or hospital by respiratory therapy. Finally, in severe cases, there are parenteral medications, such as xanthines, that can be used.

DO YOU REMEMBER THESE KEY POINTS?
- The commonly used agents for each of the conditions discussed in this chapter
- What chemicals produced by the body cause inflammation
- What chemicals can be used to reduce inflammation
- What are the risks of taking steroids
- How should steroids be discontinued
- What are the symptoms associated with asthma
- Why asthma is considered an inflammatory condition
- What types of agents are used to treat asthma

- What causes the symptoms of seasonal allergies
- What over-the-counter remedies are available to treat allergies
- What are the side effects of most agents used to treat allergies

REVIEW QUESTIONS:

Multiple Choice

1. Inflammation is caused by all of the following except
   A. Infection
   B. Temperature
   C. Allergic reactions
   D. Injury

2. All of the following symptoms accompany inflammation except
   A. Swelling
   B. Pain
   C. Redness
   D. Dizziness

3. Nonspecific antihistamines are used for all of the following symptoms except
   A. Sleepiness
   B. Motion sickness
   C. Allergies
   D. All of the above

4. The enzyme that is responsible for pain, inflammation, and fever is
   A. Prostaglandin
   B. Acetylsalicylic acid
   C. Cyclooxygenase
   D. Inflammatory disease

5. Histamine-1 receptors are located in the
   A. GI system
   B. Skin
   C. Bronchioles
   D. Both B and C

6. Aspirin should not be given to children because
   A. It can cause Reye's syndrome in children with flulike symptoms
   B. It can cause vomiting
   C. It can cause lethargy
   D. All of the above

7. Aspirin is often given to patients who have had a heart or brain attack because
   A. It stops inflammation and infection
   B. It lowers body temperature
   C. It decreases chances of blood clotting
   D. It speeds up the flow of blood

8. Common side effects of steroidal use include
   A. Ability to bruise easier
   B. Easier to get an infection
   C. Increase in heart rate
   D. All of the above

9. Those cells that contain histamine are called
   A. IgE antibodies
   B. Antihistamines
   C. Mast cells
   D. Immune cells

10. Corticosteroids are available in all dosage forms except
    A. Injectable
    B. Inhalent
    C. Liquid
    D. Tablet
    E. All of the above

True/False

*If the statement is false, then change it to make it true.

1. All antiinflammatory agents are legend drugs.

2. Edema is a result of blood rushing to the damaged tissue or organ.

3. Promethazine suppositories are commonly used for allergies.

4. Acetylsalicylic acid increases inflammation.

5. All aspirin strengths are available over-the-counter.

6. All NSAIDs work the same; therefore if one does not work, none of them will.

7. Corticosteroids are used solely for asthma patients.

8. Alpha-adrenergic agents affect the bronchiole tubes by causing dilation.

9. Asthma is genetically inherited, or only affects persons who smoke.

10. Antihistamine agents bind to mast cells and stop all allergic reactions.

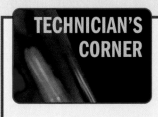

TECHNICIAN'S CORNER

Transcribe the following order into layperson terms and answer the following questions. Prednisone order as follows:

Give orally 30 mg bid × 2 days, 25 mg bid × 2 days, 20 mg bid × 2 days, 15 mg bid × 2 days, 10 mg qd × 2 days, 5 mg bid × 2 days, 5 mg qd × 2 days, stop. How many tablets and of which strength will you use to fill this order? What auxiliary label(s) will you need to apply if any? What side effects will the pharmacist probably inform the patient about?

BIBLIOGRAPHY

Clayton BD, Stock YN: *Basic pharmacology for nurses* ed 12, St Louis, 2001, Mosby.

Drug facts and comparisons 1999, St Louis, 1999, Facts and Comparisons.

Hardman JG, Limbird LE, eds: *Goodman & Gilman's the pharmaceutical basis of therapeutics*, ed 8, New York, 1990, Pergamon.

Koda-Kimble MA, Guglielmo BJ, Young LY: *Applied therapeutics: the clinical use of drugs*, ed 7, Baltimore, 2001, Lippincott.

Mosby's Drug Consult, St Louis, 2004, Elsevier.

Rang HP, et al: *Pharmacology*, ed 4, Philadelphia, 2001, Churchill Livingstone.

Stedman's concise medical dictionary of the health professions, ed 3, Baltimore, 1997, Williams & Wilkins.

Shargel L et al: *Comprehensive pharmacy review*, ed 4, Baltimore, 2001, Lippincott.

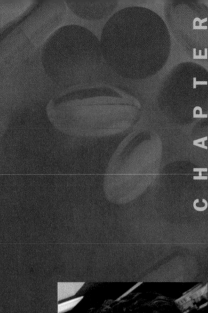

26

Vitamins and Minerals

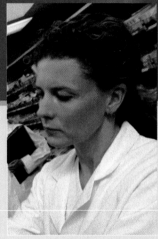

Objectives

- List the conditions that can occur from a deficiency of the vitamins covered in this chapter.

- Explain the functions of vitamins and minerals.

- Describe the difference between water-soluble and fat-soluble vitamins.

- List the recommended daily allowance (RDA) of each vitamin.

- List the trace elements and the importance of each.

- List the most common minerals.

- Write the chemical symbol for the most commonly used minerals.

- Describe the adverse effects if vitamins and minerals are overused.

- List the foods in which these common elements can be found.

TERMS AND DEFINITIONS

Anemia *A deficiency of circulating red blood cells; a symptom of disease, not itself a disease*

Avitaminosis *Vitamin deficiency*

Coenzyme *A compound that activates an enzyme*

Cofactor *A factor that must be present for other factors to be active. All coenzymes are cofactors but not all cofactors are coenzymes.*

Electrolytes *Charged elements called cations (which have positive charges) and anions (which have negative charges)*

Enzyme *A protein that speeds up a reaction by reducing the amount of energy required to initiate a reaction; also called a biological catalyst*

Fat-soluble vitamins *Vitamins that are soluble in fat and therefore are stored in the body fat. Vitamins A, D, E, and K are fat-soluble.*

Hemoglobin *The iron-containing blood cell that carries oxygen to the tissues*

Hypervitaminosis *A condition caused by the presence of too many vitamins; more common with fat-soluble vitamins.*

Intrinsic factor *A naturally produced protein that is necessary for the absorption of vitamin B_{12}*

Molecular biosynthesis *The making of chemical compounds within a living organism*

Trace elements *Elements that are needed by the body in very small amounts*

Water-soluble vitamins *Vitamins that are soluble in water and are not readily stored by the body; continually excreted in the urine and must be constantly replaced.*

VITAMINS

A	Retinol
B_1	Thiamine
B_2	Riboflavin
B_3	Nicotinic acid, niacin
B_5	Pantothenic acid
B_6	Pyridoxine
B_9	Folic acid
B_{12}	Cyanocobalamin
C	Ascorbic acid
D_2	Ergocalciferol
D_3	Cholecalciferol
E	Alpha-tocopherol
K	Phytonadione

MINERALS

Name	Chemical Symbol (Example of Form Found in Drug Preparations)	Name	Chemical Symbol (Example of Form Found in Drug Preparations)
Major Minerals		**Trace Mineral Elements (10 Currently Known To Be Essential in Humans)**	
Calcium	Ca (calcium carbonate, calcium acetate, many others)	Chromium	Cr
Chlorine	Cl (available as a mineral chloride)	Cobalt	Co
Magnesium	Mg (magnesium sulfate, magnesium chloride)	Copper	Cu (cupric sulfate)
		Fluorine	F
Phosphorous	P (dibasic calcium phosphate, tricalcium phosphate, others)	Iodine	I (iodized table salt)
		Iron	Fe (ferrous sulfate, ferrous fumarate, ferrous gluconate, iron dextran, and iron sucrose)
Potassium	K (potassium chloride, salt substitute, others)	Manganese	Mn
Sodium	Na (NaCl, table salt)	Molybdenum	Mo (not currently available as a separate supplement because of its toxicity)
Sulfur	S (available as a mineral sulfate)	Selenium	Se
		Zinc	Zn (zinc sulfate, zinc acetate)

Introduction

Like herbals, most vitamins and minerals in small quantities are considered supplements and do not require a prescription. They are sold over-the-counter (OTC) in pharmacies, grocery markets, and in herbal stores across America. The Food and Drug Administration (FDA) regulates all drugs that are sold OTC to ensure proper manufacturing and labeling. Vitamins and minerals are termed "essential" if disorders occur if they are not present in large enough amounts. There are many essential vitamins such as A, B, C, D, and E. Examples of the important essential minerals found in the body include calcium, chlorine, magnesium, potassium, phosphorous, and sodium. Trace elements are agents that the body requires to run various enzymatic reactions; however, they are only needed in extremely small amounts. Examples of trace elements include cobalt, copper, iodine, selenium, manganese, and zinc.

Vitamins and minerals are necessary for proper growth and development. Most of these supplements are contained in everyday foods. If one has a well-balanced diet, then all the daily nutritional requirements are normally met. These include the larger quantities of various vitamins and the necessary mineral elements and trace mineral elements. This chapter covers three main types of supplements: vitamins, mineral elements, and trace mineral elements. Each type differs in its function in the body. All water-soluble vitamins function as coenzymes causing important reactions to occur in the body.

Fat-soluble vitamins act in several ways. Vitamin D acts on the nucleus of the cell to cause a normal physiological change in the cell. Vitamin K acts as a coenzyme to produce four factors that enable the blood to clot. Vitamin A becomes incorporated in the rod cells of the eyes, enabling us to see at night. Vitamin E (and other vitamins) bind to free radicals that would otherwise damage cells.

The mineral elements are usually called "minerals" and in the body are either found in very large or extremely small quantities. Most minerals found in the body in large quantities usually form structures in the body, such as the calcium and phosphate in bone, or comprise a large portion of essential ions in body fluids, such as sodium, chloride, and calcium.

When a major or trace mineral element combines with another molecule to enable that molecule to do something, the element is called a cofactor. For example, calcium also combines with several separate clotting factors that, when activated, enable the blood to clot. Many of the trace elements are cofactors for different enzymes.

Certain elements are needed by the body in only trace or very small amounts. Although vitamins and minerals are essential in keeping the body healthy, they should never be taken in excess. If this happens, toxicity called hypervitaminosis may occur.

In addition to hypervitaminosis, potential toxic problems can be caused if a person supplements his or her diet with various vitamins or minerals but neglects to ask the doctor or pharmacist about possible interactions between the prescription drugs taken and the vitamin or mineral supplement. Many of these vitamin and mineral supplements have interactions with medications and could affect the patient's health. Therefore it is important for the pharmacy technician to know the interactions of supplements. As always, if the pharmacy technician suspects a patient may be taking a vitamin or mineral supplement that might interact with the patient's prescription, he or she should alert the pharmacist.

Vitamins

When supplementing a diet with vitamins, an important distinction must be made between the fat-soluble and water-soluble types. Vitamin B (including all of the B complex) and vitamin C are water-soluble. Any excess B or C vitamins can usually be excreted in the urine. In contrast, fat-soluble vitamins such as A, D, E, and K may be stored by the body in the lipids of a cell. They accumulate instead of being excreted. As they accumulate in a cell, they may reach such a high level that they interfere with the cell's function. This makes fat-soluble vitamins a greater source of potential toxic effects when they are taken in excess.

The FDA considers all vitamins, minerals, herbs, amino acids, and extracts as dietary supplements. There are guidelines that manufacturers must meet, which are listed in Box 26.1.

Although the FDA has limited control over supplements, these supplements are classified as a food ingredient. Therefore the FDA's Center for Food Safety and Applied Nutrition (CFSAN) is responsible for the safety of any food including these food supplements. When an illness or accident concerning a supplement is reported to the FDA, an inspection of the manufacturing plant, formulation, or processing method may be done. This is the only time that a supplement may be inspected. All of this information obtained by the FDA is available to consumers.

In addition to ensuring that all regulatory requirements are met, the FDA also regulates the recommended daily allowance (RDA) of vitamins and minerals. This regulatory guideline is used to inform consumers of the necessary requirements of average healthy adults and to make certain that overdosing resulting from lack of supplement information does not occur. The FDA has a Med Watch hotline (1-800-FDA-1088, or e-mail at http://www.fda.gov/medwatch/report/consumer/consumer.htm) where all health care providers or consumers can report problems concerning supplements, medical foods, devices, and drugs. All information regarding who reported the information is kept confidential.

Examples of the most common vitamins are listed in Table 26.1 along with their RDA and possible toxic side effects.

FAT-SOLUBLE VITAMINS (A, D, E, AND K)

Vitamin A

Vitamin A is also called beta-carotene or retinol. Vitamin A has four primary functions. First, it is an important part of the visual pigment for rods in the retina of the eye. Rods enable us to see in dim light. Because rods have no color pigment,

BOX 26.1 FOOD AND DRUG ADMINISTRATION (FDA) REGULATORY REQUIREMENTS FOR DIETARY SUPPLEMENTS AND NONREGULATED ITEMS

Regulatory Requirements

Manufacturers must notify FDA of any "new" dietary ingredient that is not already present in a food substance

Label Information

The agent is a food supplement

The name and address of the manufacturer (packer or distributor)

A complete list of all ingredients

The net contents of the package

A "supplement facts" panel listing each ingredient within the package or ingredient may be listed in the "other ingredient" area below the panel

The statement "This statement has not been evaluated by the FDA. This product is not intended to diagnose, treat, cure, or prevent any disease." This is to ensure that consumers do not believe it is a medication approved by the FDA.

Not Regulated by FDA

The safety of the ingredients within the container (FDA only regulates the safety of prescription medications)

Specific quantity of supplement in a tablet or capsule

Disclosure of proprietary information pertaining to the supplement (such as the formulation used to make a vitamin tablet). Proprietary information would include the filler used in making a tablet or capsule, the chemical coating on a tablet, and so forth.

TABLE 26.1 Drug Interactions of Fat- and Water-Soluble Vitamins

Vitamin	Solubility	Chemical Name	Overdose	Drug Interactions
A	Fat	Retinol, beta-carotene	Nausea, vomiting, diarrhea,	Mineral oil (interferes with vitamin A absorption)
B vitamins	Water	See Table 26.2	B_1: none	B_1: none
			B_2: none	B_2: none
			B_3: liver damage, heartburn, nausea, vomiting, diarrhea	B_3: inhibits the effects of sulfinpyrazone
				B_5: none
				B_6: none
			B_5: none	B_{12}: none
			B_6: ataxia, neuropathy	
			B_{12}: none	
C	Water	Ascorbic acid	Damage to heart and kidneys, fatigue, nausea	Warfarin (decreases effects); iron (increases absorption)
D	Fat	Ergocalciferol (vitamin D_2); cholecalciferol (vitamin D_3)	Weakness, nausea, vomiting, headache, dry mouth	Digoxin (increase D_2 toxicity); mineral oil (decrease oral absorption)
E	Fat	Alpha-tocopherol	Anemia	May decrease iron intake in children; may increase bleeding if patient on anticoagulants or vitamin K
K	Fat	Phytonadione		Mineral oil (interferes with vitamin A and K absorption) Decreases warfarin effectiveness

there is no color perception in dim light. Without an adequate intake of vitamin A, people have night blindness and cannot see well or at all in dim light. Severe deficiency of vitamin A over a long period of time can result in blindness. The second function of vitamin A is to protect against cancer in the skin and other epithelial (surface) cell types in the respiratory and digestive tracts, urinary bladder, and breast. Patients who are deficient in vitamin A may be more susceptible to these types of cancer. A third major function is to stimulate the immune system so that bacterial, viral, and parasitic infections are efficiently dealt with and the organisms are eventually destroyed. The final, most important, function is that vitamin A acts as an antioxidant, soaking up free radicals that could be dangerous to cells. The full extent of damage that free radicals can cause is unknown, but they have been implicated in cancer, Alzheimer's disease, and aging.

Vitamin A also has several functions that are not as important. It is necessary for proper bone growth, renal function, and digestive activity, and vitamin A is associated with normal reproductive function in both sexes.

Sources of Vitamin A. Vitamin A sources include dairy products (whole milk, butter, cheese, and egg yolks), liver, and fish. It is also present in yellow and green fruits and vegetables. Many dairy products, such as butter substitutes and all forms of milk, are fortified with vitamin A.

Hypervitaminosis A. Symptoms of hypervitaminosis A include headaches, vomiting, skin peeling, loss of appetite, irritability, and a wasting away of bone mass and, in fatal cases, destruction of the liver. Birth defects can also occur in children whose mothers ingested large amounts of vitamin A during the first 3 months of pregnancy.

Vitamin D

There are two precursors of vitamin D: cholecalciferol and ergocalciferol. Cholecalciferol (vitamin D_3) is produced by the skin in the presence of ultraviolet (UV) light. The UV light changes modified cholesterol present in the skin to vitamin D_3. Ergocalciferol (vitamin D_2) is the result of UV radiation on a yeast product called ergosterol found in bread and milk. This is the form of vitamin D that is added to dairy products and bread. Ingested ergocalciferol or cholecalciferol absorbed through the skin are both transported to the liver where the hormone calciferol is formed. Calciferol is then transported to the kidney where the final product, a hormone called calcitriol (also called vitamin D hormone), is produced.

Calcitriol increases phosphorus absorption and calcium intake. It is also necessary for providing adequate calcium and phosphate to mother and child during pregnancy and during breast-feeding.

Sources of Vitamin D. Dairy foods such as milk, eggs, and cheeses contain vitamin D in the form of ergocalciferol. Natural and artificial sunlight provide UV radiation that makes vitamin D in the skin.

Deficiency of Vitamin D. A deficiency of vitamin D can cause bone weakness and deformities called rickets in children, and in adults it can cause a similar weakened bone structure called osteomalacia. In osteomalacia there is also a reduction in bone mass called osteoporosis. Osteoporosis can also occur in postmenopausal women and in older men if vitamin D and calcium intake is not sufficiently high.

Hypervitaminosis D. Vitamin D excess may cause hypercalcemia (higher than normal calcium blood levels). Toxic effects of vitamin D can cause calcium deposits in various areas, such as in soft tissue and joints, causing muscle weakness or pain. In severe cases convulsions or even death can occur.

Drug Interactions. Interactions between vitamin D and digitalis may cause arrhythmias. Thiazide diuretics and vitamin D can cause hypercalcemia, and mineral oil may antagonize the absorption of vitamin D.

Vitamin E

Vitamin E has been promoted extensively over the past decade as a potent antioxidant. It is essential for normal metabolism and protection of the skin, eyes, tissues, and muscles. It also seems to protect red blood cells from damage.

Source of Vitamin E. Vitamin E can be found in whole grains such as wheat and rice germ, nuts, corn, vegetables, and dairy products (eggs and butter).

Deficiency of Vitamin E. A vitamin E deficiency may cause anemia and cardiovascular disease.

Hypervitaminosis E. Fully documented cases of hypervitaminosis E have not been reported in the literature.

Drug Interactions. The use of mineral oil may decrease the absorption of vitamin E.

Vitamin K (Phytonadione)

Vitamin K is responsible for the formation of blood coagulation factors.

Source of Vitamin K. Vitamin K can be found in wheat, legumes, egg yolks, milk, and vegetables such as broccoli and spinach. Certain bacteria in the intestine also produce vitamin K as a byproduct of their metabolism.

Deficiency of Vitamin K. Deficiency of vitamin K can cause an increased tendency to bleed. The bleeding may be manifested as repeated nosebleeds, blood in the sputum without coughing, spontaneous bruising (i.e., bruising not caused by injury) in several parts of the body, or blood in the urine. Excess bleeding may also be a sign that the patient is taking an excess of drugs that prevent the clotting of blood: for example, if a patient misses a dose or doses of warfarin (an oral anticoagulant) and takes double or triple the normal dose to make up for it, or if a patient takes lots of aspirin for a headache or cold and is also taking warfarin (because aspirin behaves similarly to an anticoagulant).

Hypervitaminosis K. Hypervitaminosis K has not been reported.

WATER-SOLUBLE VITAMINS (B AND C)

All of the B complex vitamins are water-soluble. This includes B_1 (thiamine), B_2 (riboflavin), B_3 (nicotinic acid [niacin]), B_5 (pantothenic acid), B_6 (pyridoxine), B_9 (folic acid), and B_{12} (cyanocobalamin).

Sources of B Vitamins

B vitamins can be found in foods such as peas, beans, red meats, flour, and yeasts. See Table 26.2 for the list of common B vitamins and their sources. Depending on which B vitamin is deficient, different side effects can occur. These are discussed in the following section.

Deficiencies of B Vitamins

People at high risk of vitamin B deficiencies include older adults, if they have poor diets, and pregnant or lactating (breast-feeding) women, because of the additional requirements of the fetus. The four major B deficiencies are listed in Table 26.3. Anyone who suffers from a poor diet is prone to be deficient in many other vitamins and minerals.

People who may be more susceptible to vitamin B deficiencies, as well as a wide variety of other vitamin deficiencies, include alcoholics, smokers, and those persons with any disease that may affect intake or processing of necessary vitamins and/or minerals. Deficiencies may go unnoticed for several years until illness occurs. Fortunately, there are many medications that can be taken to replace the necessary amounts of the B vitamins.

TABLE 26.2 B Vitamins—Sources, Function, and Deficiency States

Vitamin	Chemical Name	Food Sources	Function	Deficiency
B_1	Thiamine	Grains, cereals, beans, pork, and liver	Metabolism	Beriberi (wet and/or dry forms)
B_2	Riboflavin	Cereals, eggs, dark green vegetables, milk, liver	Maintains mucous membranes, metabolic energy pathways	Discolored tongue and dry scaling and fissuring of the lips
B_3	Nicotinic acid	Nuts, beans, pea, wheat, rice, grains	Fat synthesis, protein metabolism and electron transport	Diarrhea, dementia, depression, skin discoloration
B_5	Pantothenic acid	Vegetables, cereals, yeast, liver	Coenzyme	Fatigue, headaches, nausea, muscle spasms
B_6	Pyridoxine	Meat, liver, chicken, salmon, trout, beans, rice, whole grains	Amino acid and fatty acid metabolism	Skin disorders, depression, nausea, impaired vision and nerve function
B_9	Folic Acid	Green vegetables and liver	Production of red blood cells	Nerve damage
B_{12}	Cyanocobalamin	Meats, liver, chicken, dairy products	Formation of red blood cells	Pernicious anemia, megaloblastic anemia

TABLE 26.3 Four Major Deficiency Diseases Resulting from a Lack of B Vitamins

Disorder	Vitamin Deficiency
Pernicious anemia	Cyanocobalamin (B_{12})
Megaloblastic anemia	Folic acid (B_9)
Pellagra	Nicotinic acid (niacin), nicotinamide
Beriberi	Thiamine (B_1)

B vitamins enable proper cellular functioning of the body system. They do this by acting as coenzymes that combine with the protein portions of enzymes to form the complete enzymes. The enzymes cause important reactions to occur within the cell. If the body becomes vitamin B deficient, the enzymes will not work and the cells will not function properly. Some of the important enzymatic reactions that fail to occur include those involved in the immune system, carbohydrate metabolism, protein synthesis, neurotransmission, and blood formation. For the current RDA of all B vitamins as well as other vitamins covered in this chapter see Table 26.4.

The B Vitamins in Greater Detail

Vitamin B_1 (Coenzyme). Thiamine has three major functions that help maintain the body system. It is important for proper carbohydrate metabolism so that energy can be produced from ingested carbohydrates. In this process, the carbohydrates are broken down and energy in the form of adenosine triphosphate (ATP) is produced; this energy is transferred by carrier molecules to the mitochondria of the cell. Water is a by-product of this process, and some of this water is excreted

TABLE 26.4 Recommended Daily Allowances (RDA) of Vitamins for Men and Women

Vitamin (Common Name)	RDA* (Women/Men)	Solubility
Vitamin A	800 mcg/1000 mcg	Fat
Vitamin B_1 (thiamine)	1000 mcg/1200 mcg	Water
Vitamin B_2 (riboflavin)	1200 mcg/1500 mcg	Water
Vitamin B_3 (nicotinic acid)	14 mg/15 mg	Water
Vitamin B_5 (pantothenic acid)	No RDA, but 5 mg/day is the accepted amount	Water
Vitamin B_6 (pyridoxine)	1.5 mg/1.7 mg	Water
Vitamin B_9 (folic acid)	150 mcg/150 mcg	Water
Vitamin B_{12} (cyanocobalamin)	2 mcg/2 mcg	Water
Vitamin C (ascorbic acid)	50 mg/50 mg	Water
Vitamin D	5 mcg/5 mcg	Fat
Vitamin E	8 mcg/10 mcg	Fat
Vitamin K	50 mcg/45 mcg	Fat

*In some cases these amounts are based on the lowest end of the range. For information regarding the full range, refer to the FDA website at http://www.fda.gov/medwatch/report/consumer.htm

as urine or perspiration. Another role thiamine plays is in the well-being of the nervous and cardiovascular system.

Deficiency of Vitamin B_1. A deficiency in vitamin B_1 can cause a condition known as beriberi. The symptoms include wasting of the muscles and the malfunctioning of the nervous system. Other signs of a deficiency include anorexia, constipation, nausea, mental confusion, and depression.

Vitamin B_2 (Coenzyme). Riboflavin is another important component for proper enzymatic activity in the metabolism of carbohydrates and its production of energy for the body system. It is necessary for proper growth and maintenance of the body.

Deficiency of Vitamin B_2. A deficiency of vitamin B_2 can cause anemia and affect the nervous system and cause depression. In addition, because of its part in the maintenance of healthy mucous membranes, the tongue, mouth, eyes, and skin may be adversely affected by drying out or soreness. Headaches, burning sensations of the skin (especially the feet), cracking of the corners of the mouth, and seborrheic dermatitis are other symptoms of vitamin B deficiency.

TECH NOTE! Riboflavin is generally taken orally on a daily basis. It may turn the urine a yellow to orange color.

Vitamin B_3 (Coenzyme). Nicotinic acid is also known as niacin. This vitamin is used in tissue respiration and metabolism. Although there are two related compounds, nicotinic acid and nicotinamide, they are used in much the same way in the body because nicotinic acid is eventually converted to nicotinamide. However, when nicotinic acid and nicotinamide are taken orally, they do behave differently shortly after ingestion. Nicotinic acid has been found to reduce low-density lipoprotein (LDL) (the bad cholesterol). It also releases histamine and causes peripheral vasodilation. Its counterpart, nicotinamide, does not have these effects. However, nicotinamide may help prevent insulin dependant diabetes mellitus (IDDM) in high-risk patients. Nicotinic acid and nicotinamide are also necessary for lipid metabolism, proper nerve functioning, and overall maintenance of cells.

Deficiency of Vitamin B_3. A deficiency of niacin can cause a condition known as pellagra. The symptoms include diarrhea, weakness, lethargy, dermatitis, dementia, sores in the mouth, and gastrointestinal (GI) problems.

TECH NOTE! One of the most common side effects of taking niacin is red flushing of the face. In addition, a fall in blood pressure may cause dizziness.

Vitamin B₅ (Coenzyme). Pantothenic acid is another compound that is a coenzyme and thus affects body metabolism. It is incorporated either into a coenzyme or into the enzyme itself where it is used to synthesize important compounds in the body such as fatty acids, steroid hormones, and other molecules necessary for protein and carbohydrate metabolic processes. Pantothenic acid is produced by bacteria within the GI tract of many animals and can also be found in plant cells.

Deficiency of Vitamin B₅. Symptoms of B₅ deficiency include headache, sleep disturbances, muscle cramps, and fatigue. The medication used to replace pantothenic acid is calcium pantothenate.

Vitamin B₆ (Coenzyme). Pyridoxine functions in the metabolism of carbohydrates, proteins, and fats in the diet. The increased metabolism that is an effect of B₆ is the main reason this vitamin is added to diet preparation. Increased metabolism reduces the breakdown of carbohydrates so that they are not absorbed by the body. It also helps in the absorption of B₁₂ and is a component needed for the production of many different amino acids, including a major amino acid neurotransmitter found in the brain and spinal cord.

Deficiency of Vitamin B₆. A B₆ deficiency causes skin problems such as seborrheic type lesions, stomatitis, and even seizures depending on the severity. It can cause dwarfism, blindness, dementia, depression, and osteoporosis.

Drug Interactions with Vitamin B₆. Pyridoxine may antagonize the effect of a medication called levodopa (L-DOPA) used to treat Parkinson's disease.

Vitamin B₉ (Coenzyme). Folic acid is an essential vitamin for DNA synthesis and the creation of cells in areas that have high growth turnover. These areas include the bone marrow where red and white blood cells are formed and the GI tract. Folic acid can be found in green vegetables such as broccoli, avocado, and beets. Other sources include orange juice and meats such as liver. It is metabolized in the liver and then goes to the bone marrow cells where it can be used.

Deficiency of Vitamin B₉. Vitamin B₉ deficiencies include diarrhea, weight loss, weakness, sore mouth, irritability, and behavior disorders. Interactions may occur with phenytoin, estrogen, or nitrofurantoin.

Vitamin B₁₂ (Coenzyme). Cyanocobalamin is mainly obtained from dietary intake. It is required by the body for red blood cell production, myelin sheath production (myelin speeds the conduction of nerve impulses in the nervous system), and the synthesis of nucleic acids. Smokers have an increased need for vitamin B₁₂.

Deficiency of Vitamin B₁₂. Persons deficient in Vitamin B₁₂ may experience anemia, dementia, depression, hair loss, poor growth rate in children, and loss of appetite. The specific type of red cell anemia that is seen in pernicious anemia is called megaloblastic anemia. The term *pernicious* means "serious" or "severe" and does not relate to a particular cell type. *Megaloblastic* means that the red cells are abnormally formed. Pernicious anemia results from the loss of intrinsic factor, a protein produced by the same stomach cells that produce hydrochloric acid. Normally, vitamin B₁₂ is bound to intrinsic factor, enabling vitamin B₁₂ to be absorbed into the blood. If there is no intrinsic factor produced, vitamin B₁₂ is not absorbed. Persons suffering from disorders of the stomach or those who have had gastric surgery such as gastrectomies (removal of the stomach) may develop B₁₂ deficiency. Most cases of pernicious anemia are autoimmune in which the body develops antibodies against the cells that produce intrinsic factor. As a result, the cells are destroyed and not replaced. After a period of time, there are too few cells left to produce intrinsic factor and pernicious anemia develops. People who have no vitamin B₁₂ absorption at all will require vitamin B₁₂ injections for the rest of their lives. If there are some stomach cells left that produce intrinsic factor, there may be limited absorption; in those cases, a larger than normal oral dose would be required to ensure that some of the vitamin is absorbed. Vitamin B_{12} is available OTC in an oral form and by prescription for the injectable form.

> **TECH NOTE!** Before the 1900s pernicious anemia was a fatal disease often affecting older adults. By the early 1900s patients were being treated by feeding them large amounts of liver to build up red blood cells. It was not until 1948 that vitamin B_{12} was isolated and not until the 1950s that supplements were available.

Vitamin C

Vitamin C is also known as ascorbic acid and is also well-known as another antioxidant. Its main function is the formation of the connective tissue that is found in bones, teeth, and gums. It also aids in healing wounds.

Deficiency of Vitamin C. Vitamin C cannot be synthesized by the body, so this vitamin must be consumed on a daily basis. Vitamin C deficiency results in the disease known as scurvy, which causes excessive bleeding in the skin and gums and causes the teeth to become loose. Vitamin C is important for the proper nutrition of cells and their permeability (how easily molecules can penetrate the membrane). A deficiency can decrease the immune system's ability to produce T cells. These cells aid in fighting infection. Vitamin C is found in citrus fruits and a wide variety of vegetables. The RDAs of vitamin C for adults are listed in Table 26.4.

> **TECH NOTE!** If you overcook vegetables the vitamin C can be lost. It is recommended that vegetables be cooked as little as possible to reduce the destruction of vitamin C and all other vitamins.

ANTIOXIDANTS

Many of the vitamins that are popular are advertised as being antioxidants. Although there has been much research on antioxidants, there are still many debates regarding whether antioxidants can actually increase the lifespan. Nevertheless they do bind to free radicals that are responsible for damage to the cells and tissues inside the body. The main antioxidant vitamins are vitamins A, C, and E.

Minerals

Minerals are inorganic elements (i.e., they do not contain carbon) and are the ingredients of the earth's crust. Only small amounts are necessary for proper functioning of many metabolic steps within the body. For instance, zinc sulfate is important for normal growth, for the sense of smell and taste, and for skin hydration. It also helps heal wounds. The normal recommended dose for an adult is 15 mg per day. See Table 26.5 for common minerals and trace elements.

ZINC EXCESS

If zinc is taken in excess, side effects can range from nausea, vomiting, and diarrhea to pulmonary edema, hypotension, and tachycardia.

Drug Interactions

Penacillamine, a chelator, is a drug that binds to metals and is used to treat metal toxicity. It binds to zinc and increases its renal excretion.

TABLE 26.5 Common Minerals and Trace Elements (TE), Their Actions, and Deficiencies

Mineral/TE	Indication	Deficiency	Overdosage
Calcium	Bone formation, cell transport, nerve and muscle functions	Osteoporosis, rickets	Kidney stones or damage
Copper	Iron utilization, skin pigmentation, nervous system functions	Poor bone growth, nausea, nervous system disorders, poor response of immune system	Jaundice
Magnesium	Normal muscle and heart function; necessary for vitamin C and calcium metabolism	High blood pressure, kidney and heart problems, mental confusion	
Phosphorous	Necessary for healthy bones and teeth; component of phospholipids*	Muscle weakness, defective bone function, arthritis	
Potassium	Cellular transport, normal muscle, heart, kidney and nervous system functions	Muscle weakness, lethargy, poor growth, and cardiac disturbance	Cardiac arrhythmias; cardiac arrest
Iron	Hemoglobin/oxygen transport	Anemia, poor growth, confusion, loss of appetite	GI disturbance, black stools
Selenium	Proper immune functioning and growth	Heart and bone disease	GI disturbance, liver damage
Manganese	Necessary for bone formation and for metabolism of amino acids, lipids, cholesterol	Poor hair growth, nails, and osteoporosis	None known
Zinc	Proper growth and reproduction; helps heal wounds	Decreased vitamin D absorption, nausea, hair loss, birth defects, decreased immune response, decreased sperm count	Blurred vision, decreased consciousness, tachycardia

GI, Gastrointestinal.
*Phospholipids are required for the formation of cell membranes.

IRON

Iron (ferrous sulfate, ferrous fumarate, ferrous gluconate) is also an important mineral that plays a role in the transport of oxygen within the blood. Within the red blood cell, iron in hemoglobin binds tightly to the oxygen molecule, thus allowing oxygen to be transported throughout the body. Iron gives blood its red color. Much of the iron within the body is found in hemoglobin. Iron is used in other metabolic body functions, and iron is also found in all muscles (it gives muscles their red color). Iron is also stored in the liver, giving that organ its color.

Iron Deficiency

Iron deficiency anemia is one of the most common types of anemia, and it affects more than 30% of the world's population. Iron deficiency can occur for many reasons:

- Lack of iron in the diet
- Pregnancy: typically, pregnant women require 12 mg more per day than nonpregnant women

TABLE 26.6 Recommended Daily Allowance for Iron

Age	Amount
7-12 mo	11 mg
1-3 yr	7 mg
4-8 yr	10 mg
9-13 yr	8 mg
14-18 yr	11-15 mg
19-50 yr	8-18 mg
>50 yr	8 mg

- Inadequate intestinal absorption
- Excessive blood loss
- Certain forms of kidney failure in which the kidneys fail to produce erythropoietin*
- Alcoholism
- Blood loss in women during menstruation

Symptoms of iron deficiency include hair loss, shortness of breath, lethargy, and even heart palpitations. The toxic effects of an overdose are severe and include acidosis, liver and kidney impairment, and coma. See Table 26.6 for recommended daily allowance for iron.

DO YOU REMEMBER THESE KEY POINTS?

- The main vitamins required by the body and their functions
- Water-soluble vitamins
- Fat-soluble vitamins
- The main minerals required by the body and their functions
- The cause of pernicious anemia
- The RDA for vitamins
- How iron is used in the body
- Causes of iron deficiencies
- The supposed effects of free radicals and how antioxidants are used to limit the damage from them

REVIEW QUESTIONS:

Multiple Choice

1. All of the following vitamins are water-soluble except
   A. Vitamin C
   B. Vitamin E
   C. Vitamin B
   D. Ascorbic acid

2. Cyanocobalamin is the chemical term for _____ and is important in avoiding _____ .
   A. Vitamin B_{12}, pernicious anemia
   B. Vitamin K, anemia
   C. Vitamin C, free radicals
   D. Vitamin E, immunity problems

3. Two important minerals that humans require are
   A. Ascorbic acid and pyridoxine
   B. Zinc sulfate and phytonadione
   C. Folic acid and calcitriol
   D. Ferrous and zinc sulfate

---

* Erythropoietin is a hormone necessary to make red blood cells. Epoetin is available in injectable form and is normally given to dialysis patients but can also be given to patients with severe anemia.

4. All of the following vitamins have antioxidant properties except
    A. Vitamin A
    B. Vitamin C
    C. Vitamin E
    D. Vitamin D

5. The FDA considers all the following substances as food ingredients except
    A. Amino acids
    B. Vitamins
    C. Minerals
    D. Aspirin

6. All of the following statements are true concerning retinol except
    A. It is also called vitamin A
    B. It is an antioxidant
    C. Aids in the absorption of vitamin D
    D. Can be found in several dairy products, fruits, and vegetables

7. The vitamin most associated with proper blood clotting is
    A. Phytonadione
    B. Niacin
    C. Thiamine
    D. Vitamin A

8. Of the statements listed, which is not true concerning the condition pernicious anemia?
    A. It can be caused by a lack of vitamin B
    B. It is commonly experienced by individuals with a deficiency of intrinsic factor
    C. Intrinsic factor is caused by hydrochloric acid
    D. It is a fatal disease

9. Iron deficiency can be caused by the following reasons except
    A. Alcoholism
    B. Pregnancy
    C. Coffee
    D. Kidney failure

10. Calcium deficiency can cause which of the following condition(s)?
    A. Rickets
    B. Osteoporosis
    C. Osteomalacia
    D. All of the above

True/False
*If the statement is false, then change it to make it true.

1. All minerals are natural and do not have to be taken through supplements if a proper diet is eaten.

2. All vitamins are water-soluble; therefore all can be taken as often as needed or wanted.

3. The initials "FDA" stand for the "Federal Department of Agriculture."

4. The FDA considers all over-the-counter vitamins and minerals as food supplements.

5. Iron is a main component of hemoglobin and is responsible for oxygen content.

6. A deficiency of vitamin D can cause rickets.

7. Goiter can be caused by too much iodine.

8. Antioxidants are agents that combine with and reduce free radicals.

9. Vitamin A is responsible for normal metabolism.

10. Nicotinic acid is believed to be active in lowering cholesterol.

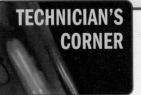

TECHNICIAN'S CORNER

An elderly female patient presents herself at the pharmacy window with the following questions: She is currently taking vitamins A, B, C, D, and E. She would like to know if that is okay.

#1 What do you know about these vitamins?
#2 What would you tell her?

BIBLIOGRAPHY

Hillman RS: Hematopoietic agents: growth factors, minerals, and vitamins. In Harman JG, Gilman AG, Limbird LE, editors: *Goodman and Gilman's the pharmacological basis of therapeutics*, New York, 2001, McGraw-Hill.

Marcus R: Agents affecting calcification and bone turnover: calcium, phosphate, parathyroid hormone, vitamin D, calcitonin, and other compounds. In Harman JG, Gilman AG, Limbird LE: *Goodman and Gilman's the pharmacological basis of therapeutics*, New York, 2001, McGraw-Hill.

Marcus R, Coulston AM: The vitamins: introduction. In Harman JG, Gilman AG, Limbird LE, editors: *Goodman and Gilman's the pharmacological basis of therapeutics*, New York, 2001, McGraw-Hill.

Marcus R, Coulston AM: The water-soluble vitamins: the vitamin B complex and ascorbic acid. In Harman JG, Gilman AG, Limbird LE, editors: *Goodman and Gilman's the pharmacological basis of therapeutics*, New York, 2001, McGraw-Hill.

Marcus R, Coulston AM: The fat-soluble vitamins: vitamins A, K, and E. In Harman JG, Gilman AG, Limbird LE, editors: *Goodman and Gilman's the pharmacological basis of therapeutics*, New York, 2001, McGraw-Hill.

Mason JB: Consequences of altered micronutrient status. In Goldman L, Bennett JC, editors: *Cecil textbook of medicine*, ed 21, Philadelphia, 2000, WB Saunders.

McKenry LM, Salerno E: *Mosby's pharmacology in nursing*, ed 21, St Louis, 2001, Mosby.

Salerno E: *Pharmacology for health professionals*, St Louis, 1999, Mosby.

Williams SR: *Essentials of nutrition and diet therapy*, ed 7, St Louis, 1999, Mosby.

National Institutes of Health (NIH) Bethesda, MD (website: www.fda.gov)

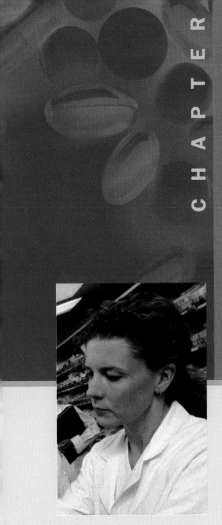

CHAPTER 27

Vaccines

Objectives

- Describe the importance of vaccines.

- Explain how vaccines are produced.

- List the most common vaccines.

- Explain how the body builds up immunity against diseases.

- Describe where immune cells are produced and what their function is.

- Differentiate between active and passive immunity.

- List the schedule for administering vaccines.

- Explain why some vaccines need boosters, whereas others do not.

- Explain under which circumstances adults should receive vaccines.

TYPES OF VACCINES

Immune Globulins	Antitoxins/Antivenins	Viral Vaccines
Cytomegalovirus immune globulin	Black widow spider	Hepatitis A
Gamma globulin	Diptheria	Hepatitis B
Hepatitis B immune globulin	Rabies	Influenza virus
Tetanus immune globulin		Measles, mumps, rubella (MMR)
Varicella-zoster immune globulin	**Toxoids**	Poliovirus
	Tetanus	Varicella (chicken pox)
	Diphtheria	Yellow fever

Introduction

Humans have always been plagued by both bacterial and viral microbes that have caused disease and even death. In addition to outside invaders, the body may need to deal with cancer cells or a misdirected attack from the immune system (autoimmune disease). Fortunately, there are highly organized defense mechanisms that work specifically on eliminating unwanted entities.

There are several factors that contribute to the overall wellness of a person. The development of vaccines to prevent infections has directly contributed to the current longevity of humans. However, there are still specific regions of the earth, such as third-world countries, where there is a higher risk of contracting bacterial and viral infections.

This chapter describes the major functions of the immune system and then focuses on the various types of bacteria and viruses that can affect the body. It also explains the timetable for immunizations. In addition, the immunological malfunctions of the body and the agents given to treat them are discussed.

The Lymphatic System

The body has a built-in defense mechanism that helps protect it from invading organisms. From birth, one of the most important functions of the body is to defend against invasion. The lymphatic system is a primary source of immune cell production and is commonly referred to as the immune system. The lymph nodes produce our natural arsenal of weapons. There are many lymph nodes that serve the body by destroying bacteria and cancer cells, using various methods to stop them from entering the bloodstream. Although there are many lymphoid tissues and small vessels located throughout the body, there are a few main production centers that are responsible for much of the arsenal of the body's army. The thymus, tonsils, and spleen are larger organs of the lymphatic system, each having specific functions.

THYMUS

The thymus is an important organ located in the upper chest and in the middle of the neck region as shown in Figure 27.1. The primary function of the thymus is to produce lymphocytes, which ultimately circulate through lymph nodes and lymphatic tissues and help provide immunity. The thymus begins producing these lymphocytes before birth and the organ is much larger in childhood than adulthood.

TONSILS

Other important lymphoid tissues are the tonsils and the adenoids, located in the throat and nose, respectively. The tonsils help fight off infection by filtering bacteria and other infective material.

SPLEEN

The spleen is located in left side of the upper abdomen (Figure 27.1). It is also the largest lymphatic organ in the body. The function of the spleen is to filter large amounts of blood cells as they reach the end of their life cycle. Macrophages within the spleen help in the removal of cellular debris. The result is the destruction of old blood cells, bacteria, and any foreign bodies.

TYPES OF IMMUNE CELLS

The many nodes and tissues located throughout the body produce some of the fighting cells of the immune system. When first contact is made with a foreign body (antigen), antibodies are formed. Then, certain immune system cells remember that specific antigen until the next time contact is made and more antibodies can be formed quickly. The body, having built up its arsenal, has the necessary forces to then fight off that antigen invader.

Lymphocytes make up a major portion of the body's fighting cells. They patrol the body circulating through the bloodstream. Many reside in lymph nodes and tissues waiting to attack foreign bodies. There are two types of lymphocytes—B cells and T lymphocytes. B cells are smaller cells that have antibodies imbedded into their cell walls. They mainly reside in the lymph nodes and can multiply into many thousands of the same type cells. When activated they become plasma cells that initiate an antibody response to invading antigens. T lymphocytes are also located in the lymph nodes and remains there until an antigen attaches to its surface protein at specific receptor sites. These T cells then perform a cell-mediated immune response. This response can be a direct killing of the attached cell and antigen or the T cells can release a chemical signal that calls in macrophages

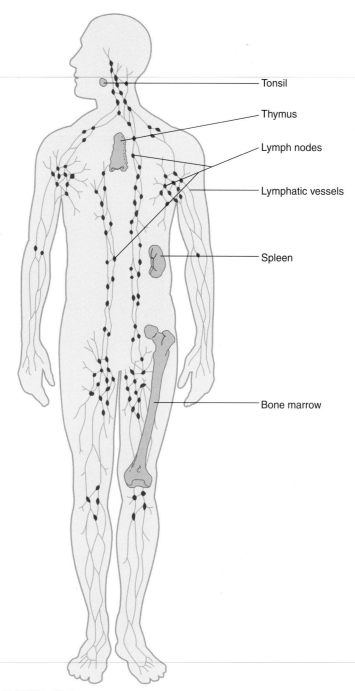

FIGURE 27.1 Overview of the major lymphatic organs within the body.

that destroy the invading cells. Table 27.1 lists major immune cells along with their location and primary function.

Immunizations

For diseases such as whooping cough, tetanus, and polio, a weakened form of the agent (which acts as an antigen in the body) is given as an immunization to stimulate the production of antibodies, which protect the body from the disease. It is important that children receive the course of vaccinations recommended by the

TABLE 27.1 Major Immune Response Cells

Major Cell Types	Origin of Production	Location in Body	Function
T lymphocytes	Lymph nodes	Lymph nodes	Produces more T lymphocytes that are sensitized to specific antigens
B lymphocytes	Bone marrow (prenatal, produced in liver)	Lymph nodes	Produces specific antibodies
Plasma cells	Lymph from B cells	Bloodstream	Antibodies
Memory cells	Lymph from B cells	Lymph nodes	Creates a memory antibody
T cells	Thymus gland	Bloodstream, lymph nodes	Binds to a specific antigen

Centers for Disease Control and Prevention because they are at risk for contracting diseases such as measles, mumps, rubella, chicken pox, whooping cough, and polio. Without the benefit of immunizations, many children may contract these childhood diseases. Historically thousands of children have died from diseases such as measles and mumps or have been physically scarred by the effects of polio. Although children still can contract these diseases today, they are seen less commonly, and death is rare because of the widespread use of immunizations.

By immunizing children and adults, society is better protected against diseases such as chicken pox, measles, and influenza. Those persons with weakened immune systems, such as older adults, chemotherapy patients, transplant recipients, and persons with AIDS, are also at higher risk than most to catch and succumb to these diseases. Another high-risk group is people from countries where immunizations are not given. In addition, many diseases can be transmitted through blood or other body fluids. Therefore anyone sharing needles or having unprotected sex with an infected person is at risk. Unfortunately not all conditions may be detected. Many newly infected persons do not know that they are infected or how they contracted the disease.

TYPES OF IMMUNITY

There are two types of immunity—active and passive.

Active Immunity

Active natural immunity occurs when the body is exposed to a disease and actively produces antibodies to respond to the disease the next time that the body comes in contact with it.

Active acquired immunity occurs when a vaccine is administered. Vaccines are of two types—live or inactive. Live vaccines must be attenuated or weakened. With these vaccines, there is a small risk of developing a full-blown infection. However, once the body builds antibodies against the injected antigen, the body has a long-lasting immunity. For vaccines that are made from killed or inactive antigens, the risk of infection is lower. The disadvantage is that booster shots are needed to keep the antibodies at a high enough level.

Passive Immunity

Passive immunity does not require any work on the part of the body. It receives protection from outside sources, such as by administration of immune globulin in passive acquired immunity, or from mother to child in passive natural immunity.

TECH NOTE! Did you know that vaccines are always kept in the refrigerator at the pharmacy?

HOW VACCINES ARE PREPARED

Viral Vaccines

Live virus vaccines must be attenuated before they are given to patients. The virions taken are weakened or defused so that they do not cause the full-blown disease. This is achieved by treating the virions with various chemicals that destroy the interior components—the disease causing portion of the virus. A virus, or any foreign substance that causes a disease or allergy, can be referred to as an antigen. When injected into the body, the body's immune system responds by making antibodies. Millions of antibodies overcome the small number of antigens injected in the vaccine. Examples of major types of viral vaccines are given in Table 27.2.

For those vaccines that need to be given in a series or as boosters, the outer shell of the virus is used as an antigen. Because the capsule or outer shell of the antigen may not invoke the response needed for the body to fight off further attacks, boosters must be given to remind the body and build up antibodies within the immune system. Some bacterial antigens, such as those from cholera and typhoid, may require boosters.

Bacterial Vaccines

Toxoids. Some vaccines are referred to as toxoids. These are inactivated bacterial toxins. Although the bacterial cell has been altered so that it cannot cause disease, it still can induce an antibody response within the body. Major toxoids are listed in Table 27.3.

Many people believe that after they are 18 years old they never need immunizations again. However, there are vaccines, such as the tetanus vaccine, that should also be given to adults. Although tetanus immunizations are given to children combined with diphtheria and pertussis, tetanus immunizations should be

TABLE 27.2 Common Viral Vaccines, Diseases Treated, Route of Administration

Vaccine Agents	Disease Treated	Route of Administration
Havrix	Hepatitis A	Intramuscular (IM)
Recombivax HB	Hepatitis B	IM
Fluzone	Influenza	IM
MMR II	Measles, mumps, and rubella	Subcutaneous (SC)
Attenuvax	Measles	SC
Mumpsvax	Mumps	SC
Meruvax II	Rubella	SC
Orimune	Polio	Orally (PO)
Varivax	Chicken pox	SC
YF-Vax	Yellow fever	SC

TABLE 27.3 Common Toxoids and Route of Administration

Toxoid Agents	Type	Disease Treated	Route of Administration
Tetanus toxoid		Tetanus	SC
			IM
Diphtheria and tetanus	Diphtheria, tetanus		IM
DPT	Whole cell	Diphtheria, tetanus, pertussis	IM

DPT, Diphtheria, pertussis, and tetanus; *IM*, intramuscular; *SC*, subcutaneous.

BOX 27.1 THREE TYPES OF LESS COMMON VACCINES AND THEIR SPECIFIC CHARACTERISTICS

Antiidiotypic Vaccines
A newer type of vaccine based on using an antibody that is shaped like the antigen. When the antibody is administered to a person, the body will react as though it were the antigen. The immune system will create antibodies to fight off the disease. In effect, the body is making an antibody against the injected antibody. This second antibody can then be injected to act as the vaccine and will create a third antibody. In the future, this method may make it possible to kill deadly viruses such as human immunodeficiency virus (HIV).

Subunit Vaccines
These are small pieces of the genetic code that come from the disease microbe. These are injected into bacterium or yeast and are grown. They are then harvested and used as a vaccine to stimulate the body to produce an immune response. Because there are only pieces of the original virion or antigen, they do not carry the coverage of immunity that a complete antigen would. Hepatitis B is a subunit vaccine that is grown in yeast cells and then given as a vaccine.

Acellular and Conjugated Vaccines
When a vaccine is disassembled or fragmented to isolate specific antigens from entire cells, it is referred to as an acellular vaccine. Pertussis is one type of vaccine made in this manner. Bacterial cells that have been altered and mixed with toxoids to increase their overall effectiveness are called conjugated vaccines. Such is the case with tetanus or diphtheria.

given every 10 years throughout one's life. Tetanus is a disease caused by a bacterium that can be contracted through scrapes and cuts from dirty objects.

Miscellaneous Vaccines. Although the two most common vaccines are inactivated (killed) or attenuated (weakened), there are other less-common types of vaccines available as shown in Box 27.1. These are slightly different in their composition to the usual types.

Unfortunately, the only two types of vaccines that are available are those that protect against viruses and bacterial microbes. Immunizations for other diseases such as malaria (caused by a parasite) and fungal infections have not been developed.

DEVELOPMENT OF VACCINES

To develop a vaccine, researchers must collect a large number of contagious cells. Most vaccine development has come about through the use of laboratory animals. For instance, the rabies vaccine was first grown in the nervous systems of rabbits. Most vaccines, however, were created to protect against bacterial microbes or those viruses that could be grown in or on animal tissue. In the beginning of vaccine research, this was difficult to accomplish if the diseases only occurred in humans. Since then, scientists have discovered how to retrieve culture cells from humans. This paved the way for the development of vaccines against polio, mumps, and measles.

Currently, research is being done on a vaccine for the human immunodeficiency virus (HIV), the virus that causes acquired immunodeficiency syndrome (AIDS). Although the viral particles can be grown in monkey tissue, monkeys do not develop the disease. Even if researchers succeed in developing a vaccine, there is a danger with vaccine administration. If even a few virions are not killed before being used in a vaccine (i.e., the vaccine contains live virus particles), an epidemic could spread across the country. This scenario occurred in the 1950s when the first polio vaccine was produced and given to millions of people. There were a few batches containing live viruses that were accidentally injected into well persons who then contracted polio.

CHILDHOOD IMMUNIZATION

Because children are at a high risk for catching many airborne diseases, a series of immunizations has been recommended. In the United States, children cannot register for school unless they have proof of their immunizations. See Table 27.4 for a recommended schedule for immunizations for children through 18 years of age.

TECH NOTE! Many hospitals require proof of childhood immunizations before hiring technicians. Keeping your records available for proof will help you avoid having to get a blood test to check for previous immunizations.

Hepatitis Vaccine

Hepatitis B can cause many serious side effects including diarrhea, vomiting, jaundice, and lack of energy. It can lead to liver damage or even death if left untreated. This virus is contagious via blood and body fluids. It can be contracted through having unprotected sex, sharing syringes, or being stuck with an infected needle. It can also be transferred from the mother to the newborn at birth. The vaccine for Hepatitis B is given in a series of three to four doses depending on age at the initial dose. Newborns receive their first immunization soon after birth. The second dose is given about 1 month after the first. The third is given 4 four months, followed by the last dose when the child is approximately 6 months old.

Side Effects. Usual side effects of the hepatitis B vaccine include soreness at the injection site and sometimes a slight fever.

Diptheria, Pertussis, and Tetanus (DPT) Vaccine

Diptheria is a disease that causes breathing problems resulting from thick mucus covering the back of the throat.

Pertussis is also known as whooping cough because of the traumatic coughing spasms it can cause. Coughing can be so severe that it is hard to eat, drink, or even breathe. It may lead to pneumonia and possibly death.

Tetanus is commonly known as lockjaw because the victim's jaw locks in place; the person cannot eat or swallow food. It also causes painful muscle spasms all over the body.

Vaccines for diphtheria, pertussis, and tetanus can all be given together in five separate doses. These are spread out over several years. The first is given at 2 months of age, then at 4 months, 6 months, 15 to 18 months, and at 4 to 6 years.

TABLE 27.4 Childhood Immunization Schedule

Vaccine	1 mo	2 mo	4 mo	6 mo	12 mo	15 mo	1 1/2 yr	2 yr	4–6 yr	11–12 yr	13–18 yr
Hepatitis B	x	x	x	x	x	x	x				
DPT		x	x	x		x	x		x		
HiB		x	x	x	x	x					
Polio		x	x	x	x	x	x		x		
MMR					x	x			x	x	x
Varicella					x	x	x	x	x	x	x

DPT, Diphtheria, pertussis, tetanus; *HiB, Haemophilus influenzae; MMR,* measles mumps, rubella.

Side Effects. Side effects include fever and soreness at the injection site. Children older than the age of 7 years should not receive the combination DPT; they should receive the diphtheria and tetanus vaccine. Pertussis vaccine is only given to those younger than the age of 7 because pertussis is not seen in children after age 7.

Haemophilus Influenzae *Type B (HiB) Vaccine*

HiB Vaccine is given to prevent the bacterial infection *Haemophilus influenzae* type B. Children younger than 5 years can contract this bacterial infection from other children or adults. The symptoms can be mild if the infection remains in the nose or throat. However, the infection may spread into the lungs. Pneumonia, meningitis, brain damage, and entire body infections known as systemic infections can occur, and death can result. A series of four shots is given to children at 2, 4, and 6 months and between 12 to 15 months of age.

Side Effects. Common side effects include redness and swelling at the injection site and sometimes a fever.

Polio Vaccine

Polio was once a common disease, affecting many people in America. The main symptom of polio is paralysis of the muscles of the legs and respiratory system. Many children and adults who contracted this disease died. Some who survived had to wear leg braces to help them walk. The polio vaccine was developed in the mid-1950s and was soon given to all people free of charge in a sugar tablet. People went to nearby schools where the vaccine was given to all adults and children. Because of this effective vaccine, polio was totally eradicated from the United States. Unfortunately, we still must immunize against this disease because some countries have not had the same success in eradicating the disease as the United States has.

Until recently, oral polio vaccines were an option. But an oral dose can cause polio in 1 in 2.4 million people, so today only the injectable form is used because it has not caused any infection. Children should receive the series of four immunizations at 2 and 4 months, then between 6 and 18 months, and a booster between 4 to 6 years of age. Because all children have been given this vaccine since the mid-1950s, most adults do not need to receive it because they are already immunized.

Side Effects. Some soreness at the injection site is not uncommon.

Measles, Mumps, and Rubella (MMR) Vaccine

Measles is a very serious disease that begins with flulike symptoms and fever. If the symptoms are ignored, the disease can progress to a major infection, causing pneumonia, brain damage, or even death. Throughout history this disease has been responsible for thousands of deaths among children and adults alike.

Mumps is a disease that affects the parotid glands of the body. These glands become visibly enlarged, and the disease is accompanied by a fever. Mumps may also cause meningitis and deafness.

Rubella is also known as German measles. In pregnant women, this contagious disease can cause birth defects in the unborn child or even a miscarriage. For this reason, women should be given this vaccine three months before becoming pregnant if they have never had rubella. In children the main symptoms include rash and fever.

Immunization against measles, mumps, and rubella are given together as one vaccination. This is normally done twice; once between 12 and 15 months old and again between 4 to 6 years of age.

Side Effects. The most common side effects include fever and rash. In some cases allergic reactions can cause more serious problems; however, these are rare.

Chicken Pox Vaccine

Varicella vaccine is more commonly known as the chicken pox vaccine. This is a relatively new vaccine. Most children have contracted this disease from other children via air or by touching the fluid within the skin blisters of infected children. Although this is a very contagious disease, it rarely causes death. Symptoms include skin blisters, fever, and an itchy rash. Some people can experience more severe effects, such as brain damage, infection, or, rarely, even death.

Another disorder caused by the same virus that causes chicken pox (herpes zoster) is shingles, which may appear in adulthood in a person who had childhood chicken pox. After laying dormant for several years, the virus may become activated and cause acute inflammation of the dorsal root ganglia. Symptoms include painful lesions along the nerves. Treatment for shingles includes medications such as valacyclovir (Valtrex), which can be given orally or intravenously. Acyclovir (Zovirax) may also be used over a seven-day period to reduce pain and promote healing. There is no cure for shingles.

Side Effects. If the disease is contracted through immunization, only a mild form of disease results. After the injection there can be soreness at the injection site and mild fever.

Considerations. Although the vaccine is recommended between 12 and 18 months of age, anyone can get this vaccine. Persons who should not get this vaccine include pregnant mothers or those who are immunocompromised.

Pneumonia Vaccine

Pneumococcal conjugate vaccine is given for *Streptococcus pneumoniae* that causes meningitis. This is a very serious disease that still affects children, causing pneumonia, brain damage, and death. Children younger than the age of 5 years are at the highest risk for this bacterial infection. The vaccine results in immunity for 3 years, and it is given in three doses spaced at 2, 4, 6 months, then between 12 to 15 months of age. Older children who might be at high risk of infection can also be given the vaccine. The total number of doses may vary. Older children and adults can be given another type of vaccine to protect them from meningitis and pneumonia. This vaccine is called pneumococcal polysaccharide.

Side Effects. Side effects include redness or tenderness at the injection site, and some children have a slight fever. In very rare cases, all vaccines may cause an allergic reaction. Therefore it is important to watch for any severe reactions after the vaccine is given.

ADULT VACCINES

If a pregnant mother should contract hepatitis, there is a high risk of transmitting the disease to the fetus. Therefore doctors weigh the potential risk of the mother contracting the disease from the vaccine and causing damage to the fetus against the possibility of catching the disease if the vaccine is not given. Vaccines such as diphtheria and tetanus (DT), hepatitis B, and influenza may be given to high-risk women. If a mother has not previously been given the rubella vaccine, she must wait until the child is born before receiving the vaccine because of the risk of getting a mild case of rubella, which could be harmful to the fetus.

Immune globulins are different from vaccines because they are not prepared in a laboratory, but must be attained from a human or animal donor. Gamma globulins contain antibodies that can be passed to the recipient, giving them passive immunity. Immune globulins are given for immediate protection against a specific virus. Because the immunity is passive, the protection does not last long. Examples of common globulins are given here:

- Cytomegalovirus Immune Globulin
- Gamma Globulin
- Hepatitis B Immune Globulin
- Tetanus Immune Globulin
- Varicella-Zoster Immune Globulin

Adults primarily receive immunizations when they are planning to travel outside of the United States. The U.S. military immunizes all troops against 12 top contagions that exist across the world. On a smaller scale, persons who are traveling to foreign countries often get specific vaccines to guard against contagions. Other persons who may need a specific vaccine are scientists; researchers; or those who work in close contact with a disease, such as those caring for laboratory animals; or those who live in regions that have an epidemic outbreak. Listed in Table 27.5 are the types of vaccines available and when they should be administered.

TECH NOTE! Tuberculosis (TB) vaccine is routinely given by many countries such as the Philippines. As a health care worker, pharmacy technicians will have a yearly TB test to test for exposure to TB. Although there is a vaccine for TB, we do not use it here in the United States. A TB vaccine does not guarantee immunity, which is why the United States does not use it. If a vaccine is given, antibodies are developed against the antigen; therefore all TB tests would show positive results and a chest x-ray film would be necessary to rule out TB. Chapter 18 discusses the microbe that causes TB.

Antitoxins and antivenins are yet another type of passive immunity system that can give short-term immediate protection from serious symptoms. These agents contain antibodies that can neutralize dangerous toxins. For example, stepping on a rusty nail may allow the pathogen *Clostridium tetani* to enter through the wound and into the bloodstream where it may cause poisoning. The tetanus antitoxin can be given to the victim against this life-threatening condition. Antivenins are given to counteract poison from creatures such as snakes and spiders. Common antitoxins include those for diphtheria, rabies, and botulism. Common antivenins include antivenin (*Latrodectus mactans*) for black widow spider venom, and crotalidae polyvalent for rattlesnake venom.

TECH NOTE! Remember that in all cases it is far worse to contract the disease than to risk the chance of adverse reactions from a vaccine.

TABLE 27.5 Example of Vaccines

Vaccine	Disease or Organism	Recommendation
Cholera	*Vibrio cholerae*	Persons living or traveling to endemic areas where the disease occurs; military
Plague	*Yersinia pestis*	Persons protecting against wild rodents in endemic areas; military
Yellow fever	Endemic areas	Persons living in or traveling to endemic areas; military
Anthrax	Anthrax	Military only at this time

- The various types of immunity
- How vaccines work
- The common childhood diseases
- Which diseases each immunization covers
- The major types of adult immunizations that are given and why
- Where most vaccines are kept in the pharmacy

REVIEW QUESTIONS:

Multiple Choice

1. The most common side effects from vaccinations is(are)
   A. Fever
   B. Soreness a the injection site
   C. Vomiting
   D. Both A and B

2. The vaccine given to protect against *Streptococcus pneumoniae* is
   A. HiB vaccine
   B. Varicella zoster
   C. Pneumococcal conjugate vaccine
   D. None of the above

3. Shingles is related to the childhood disease
   A. Measles
   B. Mumps
   C. Rubella
   D. Chicken pox

4. Vaccines can protect humans against all of the following diseases except
   A. Viruses
   B. Fungus
   C. Bacteria
   D. All of the above

5. The two basic types of immunity are
   A. Bacterial and viral
   B. Live and inactive
   C. Active and inactive
   D. Active and passive

6. Vaccines can be altered by which of the following ways?
   A. Attenuated or weakened
   B. Inactivated or killed
   C. Attenuated or activated
   D. A and B

7. When the body comes into contact with a contagious disease, it causes
   A. Antibodies to be produced
   B. Antigens to be produced
   C. A body rash
   D. No reaction

8. Which of the statements is true concerning toxoids?
   A. Toxoids are bacterial toxins that have been inactivated
   B. All bacterial vaccines are toxoids
   C. Both A and B
   D. None of the above

9. Vaccines that are composed of small pieces of genetic code harvested from bacterium or yeast are
   A. Acellular vaccines
   B. Conjugated vaccines
   C. Subunit vaccines
   D. Toxoid vaccines

10. Most adults need vaccines for all of these reasons, except
    A. They never got them as children
    B. They are in the military
    C. They are health care workers
    D. Adults need vaccines for all of the above

True/False

*If the statement is false, then change it to make it true.

1. The thymus helps provide immunity.

2. Most vaccinations have no side effects.

3. Hospital technicians must have an annual tuberculosis test.

4. Polio vaccine is routinely given in an oral form rather than by injection.

5. Hepatitis B is a serious condition affecting the kidneys.

6. Pertussis vaccine is normally combined with diphtheria and tetanus vaccines.

7. Attenuated vaccines can often give protection for a lifetime.

8. Tetanus vaccine should be given every five years.

9. When vaccines are injected antibodies are produced by the body to fight off antigens injected.

10. Many third world countries do not immunize children.

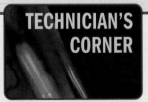

TECHNICIAN'S CORNER

Visit the website of the Centers for Disease Control at www.cdc.gov and print out the most recent list of suggested immunizations for children.

BIBLIOGRAPHY

Tortora et al: *Microbiology: An introduction,* ed 4, Redwood City, Calif, 1992, Benjamin/Cummings.

McKenry L, Salerno E: *Pharmacology in nursing,* St Louis, 2001, Mosby.

Centers for Disease Control (CDC) website at www.cdc.gov

28

Oncology Agents

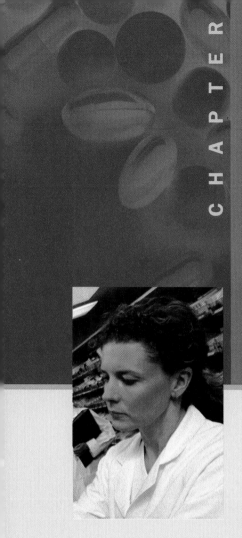

Objectives

- List common types of cancer.

- List four causes of cancer.

- Describe how cancer spreads.

- Describe the methods used to diagnose cancer.

- Explain the method of action for the classification of drugs listed in this chapter.

- Define oncology terms.

- Describe the stages of normal cell reproduction.

- List the types of agents that are vesicant and the precautions technicians need to take when preparing them.

- Describe the most common side effects of chemotherapy.

- List the treatments used in the fighting cancer.

- Differentiate between acute lymphocytic and myelogenous leukemia.

- Describe how nuclear medicine is used in oncology.

Antineoplastic *An agent used to prevent the development, proliferation, or growth of neoplastic cells; a medication used in treatment of abnormal cells*

Benign *A nonmalignant neoplasm*

Biopsy *A procedure in which a piece of tissue is removed from a patient for examination and diagnosis; the tissue is a sample of the whole*

Cancer *A general term used to describe malignant neoplasms*

Carcinogen *A substance or chemical that can increase the risk of developing cancer*

Chemotherapy *The treatment of a disease with toxic chemical substances to slow the progress of the disease or to kill cells*

Deoxyribonucleic acid (DNA) *The complex nucleic acids that are bases for genetic continuance*

Invasive *The tendency for a tumor or mass to move into tissues and / or organs in close proximity*

Leukemia *A progressive disease marked by malignancy of the blood forming cells found in the hemopoietic tissues, organs, and bloodstream, causing the circulation of abnormal blood cells*

Lymphoma *A term used to describe a malignant disorder of lymphoid tissue*

Malignant *An invasive and destructive pattern of rapid, abnormal cell growth; often fatal*

Melanoma *A malignant neoplasm of the pigmented cells of skin; may metastasize to other organs*

Metastasis *The movement or spread of cancerous cells through the body to organs in distant areas*

Mitosis *Cellular reproduction that creates two identical daughter cells from the parent cell's DNA*

Morphology *The appearance of an organism such as size, shape, and characteristics*

Mutation *An unexpected change in the molecular structure within the DNA, causing a permanant change in cells*

Neoplasm *An abnormal tissue growth*

Oncogene *A previously normal gene that may be adversely affected by an infection such as a retrovirus, which causes a mutation and may produce cancer*

Remission *The span of time during which a disease, such as concer, is not spreading, this may be permanent or temporary*

Sarcoma *A malignant neoplastic growth arising from the connective tissue*

CHEMOTHERAPEUTIC DRUGS

Trade	Generic	Pronunciation	Trade	Generic	Pronunciation
Adriamycin	doxorubicin	dox-oh-**ru**-bi-sin	Gemzar	gemcitabine	gem-**sit**-ah-been
Blenoxane	bleomycin	blee-oh-**my**-sin	Hydrea	hydroxyurea	hye-droxy-you-**re**-ah
Myleran	busulfan	byoo-**sul**-fan	Idamycin	idarubicin	eye-da-**roo**-bi-sin
Paraplatin	carboplatin	**car**-bow-pla-tin	Ifex	ifosfamide	i-**fos**-fa-myde
BiCNU	carmustine	kar-**mus**-teen	Mustargen	mechlorethamine	me-klor-**eth**-ah-meen
Leukeran	chlorambucil	klor-**am**-byoo-sil	Alkeran	melphalan	**mel**-fa-lan
Platinol	cisplatin	**sis**-pla-tin	Methotrex	methotrexate	meth-oh-**trex**-ate
Cytoxan	cyclophosphamide	sye-kloe-**fos**-fa-mide	Taxol	paclitaxel	pack-li-**tax**-el
Cytosar-U	cytarabine	sye-**tare**-ah-been	Zanosar	streptozocin	strep-toe-**zoe**-sin
DTIC-Dome	dacarbazine	da-**kar**-ba-zeen	Vumon	teniposide	ten-nye-**poe**-side
Cosmegen	dactinomycin	dak-tin-oh-**my**-sin	Hycamtin	topotecan	toe-po-**tee**-can
VePesid	etoposide	e-teh-**poh**-side	Velban	vinblastine	vin-**blas**-teen
Fludara	fludarabine	flew-**dare**-ah-been	Oncovin	vincristine	vin-**kris**-teen
Adrucil	fluorouracil	flure-oh-**your**-a-sil	Navelbine	vinorelbine	vin-**nor**-ell-been

Introduction

Not long ago, the diagnosis of cancer meant certain death. The lack of knowledge pertaining to this life-changing disease led most people to feel hopelessness. As the scientific community began to attain more knowledge about the etiology (causes) of cancer, its early diagnosis, and various treatments, the diagnosis of cancer resulted in less invasive changes in everyday life. Today, the chances of getting cancer can be decreased, and many cancers can be cured. Because of early detection and more advanced treatments, more people are cancer survivors today than ever before.

This chapter covers the process by which cancer arises, how it spreads, and the medications used to treat some of the most common cancers. There are many different types of cancer that can strike different areas of the body. The incidence of some cancers, such as skin cancer, may be decreased. The chances of acquiring skin cancer increase the longer the skin is exposed to direct sunlight. If precautionary measures are taken, such as wearing sunscreen, the chances of skin cancer may decrease. Unfortunately the prevention of cancer is not an exact science.

One of the frustrating aspects of headline news stories regarding cancer is the continuous inference that every conceivable food product or eating habit may lead to cancer. In reality, everything in life should be done in moderation. Even then, there is the genetic factor that none of us can alter. Although there is much research and testing being done by geneticists to alter genes, it is not a treatment for cancer at this time. In the meantime, the most effective way to fight cancer is to lessen the risk by treating the body in a responsible manner and by making routine visits to the doctor.

In this chapter we define cancer and its nature and introduce some of the more common medications used in its treatment. Common side effects from antineoplastics are also covered. Much of the information pertaining to the preparation of chemotherapeutic agents is in Chapter 13.

What is Cancer?

Under normal circumstances, cells within the body proliferate, especially in the intestinal epithelium and within the bone marrow. Our body constantly replicates

BOX 28.1 TYPES OF CANCER AND THEIR POSSIBLE OUTCOMES

Types of Cancer

Carcinomas	These originate in the epithelial tissues of organs such as the lungs and intestines.
Leukemias	Originate in the bone marrow and spleen. These are areas that produce a large amount of blood cells. Leukemia often strikes children.
Lymphoma	A general term used for malignant tumors within the lymphatic tissues.
Sarcomas	A term used to describe cancers of the muscle and bone. It stems from the connective tissue within these areas.

Possible Outcomes of Tumor Growth

There is a possibility that the growth of benign cells is limited to a specific location and may cause no problems for the individual.

The benign cell growth may get large enough to affect an organ's or tissue's normal functioning.

Cancerous cells may break off and travel to other parts of the body where they grow in an uncontrolled manner.

Cancerous cells may become invasive, moving into adjoining tissue and/or organs and becoming life-threatening.

cells to replace old cells or damaged cells or to increase the cell population. The normal cycle of life for cells is required if the body is to remain in homeostasis. There is a set of steps that cells normally follow. An important step, in addition to replication of new cells, is their eventual death. If the cell controls malfunction and the cells grow much faster than normal and do not stop proliferating, tumors may form. Benign tumors are non-cancerous and may include moles, warts, and other lesions. Malignant tumors or cancers continuously produce cells that can move and colonize at new sites within the body. However, malignant or cancerous tumors can also begin as moles, warts, or lesions. Only proper diagnosis can determine the nature of the growth.

There are four main types of cancer based on their location as well as four possible outcomes, covered in Box 28.1. The outcome of cancer treatments is determined by early diagnosis, type of treatment, genetics, and finally attitude of the patient.

What Causes Cancer?

There are three different causes of cancer (in addition to genetics): environmental contaminants, radiation, and viruses. There are many different environmental contaminants, known as carcinogens, that can cause cancer. For example, cigarette smoking may cause cancer. This is due to the many additives contained in tobacco that have been isolated, tested, and proven to cause cancer in laboratory animals. Another causative agent of cancer is radiation. Any type of radiation that breaks the bonds of the DNA can lead to mutations in the DNA that can result in cancer. For example, radiation in the form of the sun rays or through x-rays may lead to mutations if the body is exposed long enough. Other types of cancer-causing agents include radioactive materials, coal, soot, and certain dyes. Viruses can also cause certain types of cancers. Viruses replicate by using their host's components. The host is the person who has contracted the virus. The virus inserts itself into human DNA and creates proteins from the host's DNA to build new virions. The normal genes are affected by the virus, and the newly mutated genes are referred to as oncogenes. Oncogenes are small bits of genes that are normally present in cells but are not dangerous unless they are not "turned off"

BOX 28.2   CHARACTERISTICS OF CANCER GROWTH AND TREATMENT

Morphology: The morphology of a cell or organism is its shape characteristics. Most cancerous cells have rigid edges or edges that are not smooth, unlike noncancerous cells that tend to be smooth and round. Cells can also form large masses or may remain as small cells. Normal cells tend to have an appearance of flattened cells, whereas cancer cells tend to be more round.

Growth pattern: There are different characteristics that cell types have. Whether they will grow quickly or slowly and how fast they may travel to different parts of the body are some of the patterns that identify types of cancer. When cancer cells are grown in a culture dish they tend to form multilayers because they do not following the same growth pattern as normal cells. Normal cells will form a single layer.

Karyotype: The actual mutation that a cancer cell has is contained in the karyotype (see Figure 28.1). Within the DNA of the cell is the mutation or cancer gene that initiates uncontrollable growth. Included in the DNA are also various components that can help speed up the growth. Normal cells have the capability to divide between 20 to 60 times before they are too old to continue; however, cancer cells have been observed to divide thousands of times furthering their out-of-control nature. This may decrease the effectiveness of the medication or treatment given to kill the cancer cells.

Response to therapy: Because different cancers have different morphologies, growth patterns, and karyotype, they may or may not be responsive to treatment. Many times multiple agents are used to treat the growth of cancer cells.

through normal reactions. Another possible cause of cancer under investigation is genetics. Although there is no clear evidence that certain cancer-causing genes are inherited, this possible cause remains a theory.

Diagnosis of Cancer

Although cancer can strike any area of the body, this chapter covers the most common types of cancers and their progression. Through the use of x-ray examinations, magnetic resonance imaging (MRI), sonograms, biopsies, and radiopharmaceuticals, many cancers can be identified and treated. A pathologist will determine the level or grade of the tumor based on its appearance when observed under a microscope. As the diagnosis is being made, several aspects of the cancer must be considered, such as the morphology, growth pattern, karyotype, and response to chemotherapy agents. An explanation of each consideration is given in Box 28.2.

Ordinarily, if a cancer is diagnosed in the early stages it may be surgically removed. If there is no reoccurrence within 5 years, it is normally considered cured. With new advancements in the treatment of cancers, some can be cured even if they are discovered in later stages. For example, many leukemias are curable—especially in children. Other cancers are being detected in the early stages because of new types of diagnosis and early detection. This can be attributed to public education. For example, breast cancer and prostate cancer are cured more often because people are having checkups that detect cancerous masses in time.

Types of Cancer

There are more than 100 known cancers of the human body. The following cancers have multiple agents that can be used to treat them. They are a sample of the types of diseases that can strike most age groups.

Hodgkin's lymphoma, or Hodgkin's disease, is a cancer of the lymphatic cells that are located in the lymph nodes. This disease was named after Thomas Hodgkin who was the doctor who first described its features.

Non-Hodgkin's lymphoma is not Hodgkin's disease but is named after Hodgkin because it also affects the lymphatic system. It may have a nodular or diffuse pattern that spreads; non-Hodgkin's lymphoma may have a low, moderate, or high rate of malignancy. Its morphology is different than that of Hodgkin's disease.

Kaposi's sarcoma is a type of cancer that affects the skin and is marked by brownish-purplish colored skin lesions that can spread to internal organs. Persons who are most likely to acquire this type of cancer are those who suffer from acquired immunodeficiency syndrome (AIDS). Because the immune system is compromised the body is more susceptible to a variety of diseases.

Leukemia arises in the bone marrow and lymphatic system. A malfunctioning bone marrow produces abnormal leukocytes (white blood cells [WBCs]). These leukocytes can crowd out normal blood cell production; the disease is often fatal. There are two major groups of leukemias—lymphocytic leukemia and myelogenous leukemia. Each group is subdivided into many different types of cancer.

- Acute lymphocytic leukemia: The cure rate of this type of leukemia is more than 90%. This type of leukemia usually affects children, although adults can also get it. Approximately 75% of those with the disease will go into remission.
- Acute myelogenous leukemia: This type of leukemia is the most common among adults, with 10 to 20% of those affected being children. The increase of WBCs, in addition to a decreased production of red blood cells (RBCs), makes the body more susceptible to infection. In fact, the cause of death is usually an invading microorganism rather than the disease itself. It is a rapidly progressing disease, and a person can succumb to it in less than 6 months.

Most treatments for cancer include more than one agent and may also be followed by or preceded by radiation therapy.

Treatments for Cancer

There are four standard types of treatments that are used to treat cancer—surgery, radiation therapy, implanted radioactive isotopes, and chemotherapy. Nuclear medicine is another advancing treatment that is discussed later in the chapter. There have been new advancements in each type of treatment that lessen the risk of recurrence and side effects. Age is an important factor that must be considered in patients who have been diagnosed with cancer. The risk of cancer increases in individuals older than 65 years. Age can make treatment difficult because older adults usually have other illnesses that can make treatment more dangerous. In children, cancer can grow quickly because they are growing rapidly. However, children tend to respond to chemotherapy and recuperate more quickly than older patients.

For many types of cancer, oncologists (doctors that specialized in the treatment of cancer) refer to a protocol (a set of guidelines) that recommends multiple agents used simultaneously to treat cancer. Examples of combination therapy are listed in Table 28.1.

SURGERY

Surgery, usually one of the first courses of treatments, can quickly and effectively eliminate tumors. When a mass or tissue is removed, a large area of surrounding normal tissue is also taken to ensure that all cancer cells have been removed.

TABLE 28.1 Sample of Combination Therapies

Disease	Drug Set	Agents
Ovarian cancer	CC	Carboplatin, cyclophosphamide
Breast cancer	CFM	Cyclophosphamide, fluorouracil, mitoxantrone
Lung cancer	CAV	Cyclophosphamide, doxorubicin, vincristine
Testicular cancer	BEP	Bleomycin, etoposide, cisplatin
Hodgkin's lymphoma (pediatric)	COMP	Cyclophosphamide, vincristine, methotrexate, prednisone
Sarcoma	DI	Doxorubicin, ifosfamide, mesna
Non-Hodgkin's lymphoma	MIV	Mitoxantrone, ifosfamide, etoposide

Although the procedure may be a success, an oncologist normally follows up with either radiation or chemotherapy to ensure that all the cancerous cells are gone.

RADIATION

Radiation can be used to diagnose or treat certain diseases. For example, x-ray imaging, computed tomography (CT) scans, and radioisotope scans all use electromagnetic waves to project images as the waves pass through the body. Although radiation is also known to be a carcinogen, if used correctly it can kill cancer cells. In cancer treatment, radiation is categorized by the intensity of the rays. These are alpha, beta, and gamma rays. Both alpha and beta rays are normally used to treat superficial lesions, whereas gamma rays are stronger and can treat deeper lesions.

RADIOACTIVE ISOTOPES

There are certain cancers that may require alternative types of treatment because of their location or nature. In this case, implants can be placed directly into the cancer site. This may be effective in cancers of the tongue or the cervix. The implants may be left in from hours to a few days.

CHEMOTHERAPY

There are many different types of medications that are used to treat cancers, some of these agents are listed in Table 28.2. Often, these agents are very effective at eradicating cancer cells. The disruption caused by interfering with the normal metabolism of cancer cells causes them to die. The different routes of administration of chemotherapeutics are listed in Table 28.3. Other agents commonly given during the treatment of cancer are those that relieve symptoms of cancer or the side effects of chemotherapeutic agents, such as the loss of hair, emesis, loss of energy, loss of weight, and pain.

TECH NOTE! A bone marrow transplant has a much greater chance of curing both adults and children with leukemia who do not respond to traditional treatments. The bone marrow is transplanted by intravenous (IV) infusion. The new bone marrow naturally attaches to the patient's bones and alters the defective bone marrow by making healthy red and white blood cells.

Agents Used in the Treatment of Neoplastic Diseases

Antimetabolite Agents. The building blocks of DNA are formed by nucleic acids often referred to as bases. These bases form the fundamental configuration of DNA. The structure of antimetabolites is similar to the bases that form the

TABLE 28.2 Common Types of Chemotherapeutic Agents

Generic	Trade	Classification	Indication	Route of Administration
Doxorubicin	Adriamycin	Antibiotic	Leukemias, tumors	IV
Carboplatin	Paraplatin	Alkylating agent	Ovarian tumor	IV
Bleomycin	Blenoxane	Antibiotic	Lymphomas, squamous cell carcinomas	IV
Busulfan	Myleran	Alkylating agent	Leukemia	PO, IV
Carboplatin	Paraplatin	Alkylating agent	Ovarian cancer	IV
Carmustine	BiCNU	Alkylating agent	Brain tumors, Hodgkin's and non-Hodgkin's lymphomas	IV, wafer
Chlorambucil	Leukeran	Alkylating agent	Leukemia, lymphomas	PO
Cisplatin	Platinol	Alkylating agent	Ovarian/testes tumor	IV
Cyclophosphamide	Cytoxan	Alkylating agent	leukemias, Hodgkin's disease, lymphomas	PO, IV
Cytarabine	Cytosar-U	Antimetabolites	Myclocytic leukemias	IV
Dacarbazine	DTIC-Dome	Alkylating agent	Melanoma, Hodgkin's	IV
Dactinomycin	Cosmegen	Antibiotic	Wilms' tumor	IV
Etoposide	VePesid	Plant extract	Lung and testicular cancer	PO, IV
Fludarabine phosphate	Fludara	Antimetabolites	Leukemia	IV
Fluorouracil	Adrucil	Antimetabolites	Cancer of the colon, rectum, breast, stomach, pancreas	IV
Gemcitabine	Gemzar	Miscellaneous antineoplastics	Adenocarcinoma of the pancreas; antimetabolite	IV
Hydroxyurea	Hydrea	Miscellaneous antineoplastics	Leukemia, recurrant cancer of the ovary	PO
Idarubicin	Idamycin	Antibiotic	Adult leukemias	IV
Ifosfamide	Ifex	Alkylating agent	Sarcoma, cancer of testes	IV
Mechlorethamine	Mustargen	Alkylating agent	Hodgkin's disease, lymphomas	IV
Melphalan	Alkeran	Alkylating agent	Multiple myelomas	PO, IV
Methotrexate	Methotrex	Antimetabolites	Leukemia, psoriasis, rheumatoid arthritis	PO, IV
Paclitaxel	Taxol	Antimitotic	Ovarian/breast cancer	PO, IV
Streptozocin	Zanosar	Alkylating agent	Cancer of the pancreas	IV
Teniposide	Vumon	Plant extract	Childhood leukemia	IV
Topotecan	Hycamtin	Hormone	Ovarian cancer	IV
Vinblastine	Velban	Antimitotic	Hodgkin's disease, tumors	IV
Vincristine	Oncovin	Antimitotic	Leukemia, tumors	IV
Vinorelbine	Navelbine	Antimitotic	Lung cancer	IV

IV, Intravenous; *po*, orally.

DNA strands, but because they are not identical they do not allow the process of mitosis to finish. Therefore the cells into which these substances are introduced are not able to replicate. Antimetabolites are often used in the treatment of leukemia. The most common side effects include nausea, vomiting, fever, anorexia, bone marrow depression, and jaundice. Antimetabolites include the following:

Cytarabine
Fluorouracil
Floxuridine
Fludarabine
Mercaptopurine
Methotrexate
Thioguanine

TABLE 28.3 Routes of Administration of Chemotherapeutic Agents

Abbreviation	Definition	Specifics of Use
Traditional		
PO	By mouth	Tablets, capsules taken orally
IM	Intramuscularly	Into the muscle
IT	Intrathecal	Into a sheath
IV	Intravenous	Into the vein
Newer Routes		
Infusion pumps	Syringe pump	A portable pump worn by the patient that administers a preset amount of drug through a catheter inserted into the tumor
Implants	Tablet/capsules	Implanted into the cancerous area where the medication can be dispersed over a set period of time

Antibiotics. The antibiotics that are used to treat certain types of cancers are not in the same category as those that are used to treat infections. They are specific to tumors that cause cancer. They bind directly to the cancer cells' DNA and prevent the synthesis of any new cells. These agents are not used in the treatment of infections because of their toxic effects. Instead they are used to destroy newly forming cancer cells. Because they also destroy normal cells along with the cancer cells, they produce side effects that include severe emesis (vomiting), nausea, diarrhea, red urine, and a loss of hair. Agents of this type include the following:

Bleomycin
Dactinomycin
Daunorubicin
Doxorubicin
Idarubicin
Mitomycin
Mitoxantrone
Pentostatin
Plicamycin

Mitotic Inhibitors. Mitotic inhibitors prevent mitosis at the metaphase stage. Mitosis is the process of cell division that all cells (Figure 28.1) must perform. The agents used to prevent this synthesis are a group of alkaloids derived from plants. Diseases such as Hodgkin's disease and various cancers that may not respond to other treatment are often treated with these types of agents. Side effects of these agents are common side effects of chemotherapy. These agents include the following:

Etoposide
Teniposide
Vinblastine
Vincristine
Vinorelbine

Each cell that produces the next generation of cells leaves a part its genetic makeup behind. Genes are contained within the chromosomes of the DNA, located in the cell's nucleus. The process of producing new cells is referred to as replication. When a cell replicates, it copies all the chromosomes (all of the genes of the cell are replicated). As the chromosomes are duplicated, they are evenly divided into two daughter cells or new cells and are contained within the new nuclei.

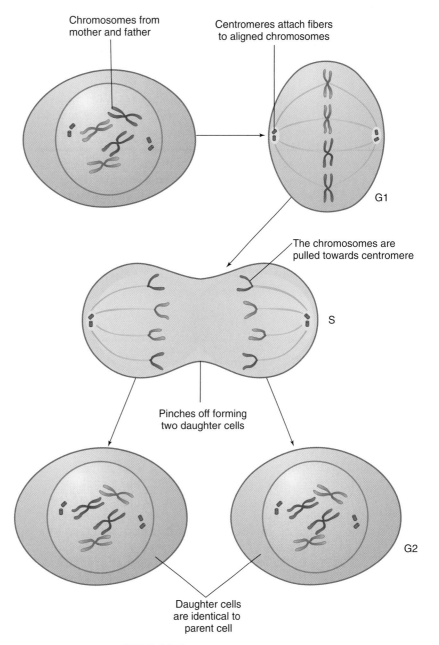

Chromosomes from mother and father

Centromeres attach fibers to aligned chromosomes

G1

The chromosomes are pulled towards centromere

S

Pinches off forming two daughter cells

G2

Daughter cells are identical to parent cell

FIGURE 28.1 Cell reproduction: mitosis.

Mitosis is the process by which the cell's nucleus is divided. The entire process of mitosis starts with prophase, followed by metaphase, anaphase, and then telophase. This process is sometimes abbreviated as the "M" phase for mitosis. Each part of the process is specific and lasts a certain period of time. The last stage, called cytokinesis, is the separation of the daughter cells. The mitotic phase and cytokinesis are the end processes of the cell's lifespan. After cytokinesis takes place, the new cell enters a much longer phase referred to as interphase. There are three parts of the interphase process, the first of which is called G1 (Fig. 28.1). The replication process begins in this stage as the centrioles pull apart chromosomes preparing for mitosis once again. Centrioles anchor to the chromosomes at opposite ends of the cell and separate them. The second part of interphase is the S phase in which DNA replication starts. Lastly, the G2 phase of interphase prepares the cells for the mitotic phase, and the process begins over again.

Alkylating Agents. There are two major types of alkylating agents—the nitrogen mustards and nitrosoureas. Although their structures are similar, their methods of action and side effects are somewhat different. Because alkylation is a normal reaction that takes place in the DNA between chemical compounds, these agents are able to bind to certain bases of the DNA. New bonds (created by alkylation) are made between components; when this happens, the rapidly dividing cancer cells are damaged and are unable to proliferate any further. Diseases most often treated with these agents include Hodgkin's disease, retinoblastoma, lymphocytic leukemia, and inoperable cancers. Side effects are the same as the chemotherapeutic agents' common effects.

Nitrogen Mustards. Nitrogen mustards were some of the first agents used to treat cancer in addition to radiation or surgery. These agents were used in chemical warfare in World War I. On examination of soldiers exposed to these agents, it was discovered that nitrogen mustards decreased the WBCs. Because of this effect on WBCs, they were used to treat leukemia, which is marked by a high WBC count. Although effective, the first nitrogen mustards had severe side effects and have since been replaced with agents that are derived from the same chemical structure but are better tolerated. These agents are the following:

> Chlorambucil
> Cyclophosphamide
> Ifosfamide
> Mechlorethamine
> Melphalan
> Uracil mustard

Nitrosoureas. These agents cross the blood-brain barrier that surrounds the central nervous system. Because of this ability, they can be used to treat cancers within the brain. The following drugs are nitrosoureas:

> Carmustine
> Lomustine
> Streptozocin

Miscellaneous Agents. Various other agents are commonly used to treat cancer. One group, hormones, includes the corticosteroids, androgens, and antiandrogens. Most hormone agents are indicated for cancers that are influenced by hormonal control. Corticosteroids can be useful in treating leukemia and lymphomas. They also work to decrease inflammation and edema in vital areas. Both estrogen and androgens can be used to treat breast cancer. Antiandrogens are used to treat prostate cancer.

There are other agents that do not fall neatly into the categories previously discussed. One such agent is interferon, a natural protein found in the body. When used in treatment, it boosts immune cells, which are then better able to attack cancerous cells. It also changes the structure of the cells making them less "cancerlike" and more normal in their behavior. Interferon is used for a special form of leukemia known as hairy cell leukemia. The specific actions of other miscellaneous agents used to treat cancer are listed in Table 28.4 along with the types of cancers for which they are used.

Side Effects of Chemotherapy

Because cancer is caused by a malfunction of our own cells, it is hard to differentiate between defective cells and normal cells. The components are the same in both. This is not the problem for antibiotics used to treat infections caused by microbes because the cell of microbes are not the same as humans. Therefore medications can be made that will attack microbial cells and not our own. When fighting off cancerous cells, the only way to ensure a full remission is to kill off the cells. Unfortunately good cells are killed off along with them, especially

TABLE 28.4 Miscellaneous Cancer Treatment Agents

Agent	MOA	Types of Cancer
Asparaginase	Depletes asparagine (necessary for cell survival)	Lymphocytic leukemia
Dacarbazine	Inhibits synthesis in the G2 phase	Hodgkins disease
Docetaxel	Inhibits activity of microtubules in the G1 phase	Breast cancer
Gemcitabine	Inhibits synthesis in S phase	Adenocarcinoma of pancreas
Hydroxyurea	Inhibits specific DNA synthesis	Head, neck, and ovarian cancer; melanomas.
Paclitaxel	Antimicrotubule agent in the G2 phase	Metastatic ovarian cancer
Procarbazine	Inhibitor in the S phase	Hodgkins disease

fast-growing cells such as those responsible for hair growth. As the cancer cells are killed off, the cells of the hair are too. Fortunately, hair will grow back in time.

TECH NOTE! Various agents are classified as vesicant. These agents must be handled very carefully because any contact with exposed skin can cause irritation and sloughing of the skin. When preparing chemotherapy, either special chemotherapy gloves must be worn or the technician must double glove to protect the skin. If a chemotherapeutic agent spills on the gloves, the top glove can be removed and discarded into an appropriate container, and a new pair of gloves can be worn. All agents that are vesicant have special auxiliary labels adhered to the container. The auxiliary label alerts the nurse who will be handling and administering the agent.

Biological Response Modifiers

Chemotherapeutic agents may destroy not only cancer cells but also the cells of the body's immune system. Patients treated with chemotherapeutics often become anemic or, because of a reduction of WBCs, they develop leukopenia. Because WBCs are essential in protecting the body from various infections, special medications are used to boost the immune cells. Two main agents used to treat chemotherapy side effects are erythropoietin and filgrastim. Both agents are used to stimulate specific bone marrow production of blood cells; erythropoietin stimulates RBC production and filgrastim stimulates WBC production. The patient's blood serum must be monitored to dose these medications properly. The manufacturer's storage instructions require them to be stored in the refrigerator between 2°C and 8°C. They must not be shaken or frozen.

Erythropoietin. Erythropoietin is primarily used to treat anemia in patients with malignant neoplasms who acquire anemia during chemotherapy. It may also be used to treat persons with human immunodeficiency virus (HIV) or end-stage renal disease. Normal doses of erythropoietin range from 2000 to 10,000 units/mL. A normal dosing regimen is 150 units/kg three times a week.

Filgrastim. Filgrastim binds to bone marrow cells and stimulates growth of neutrophils. Neutrophils are key players in the immune system. They are part of the WBC defense mechanisms and are often destroyed by the chemotherapy treatment. When this happens, a condition known as leukopenia may occur, increasing the risk of infection to the patient.

Normal dosage of filgrastim is 5 mcg per kilogram per day (5 mcg/kg/day). It is given when WBCs decrease below a certain level and may be given on a daily basis until the WBC levels increase to a normal level. Dosage strength is 300 mcg/mL.

BOX 28.3 EXAMPLES OF RADIOPHARMACEUTICALS AND THEIR USE

Chromioum-51 sodium chromate	For labeling red blood cells for examination
Indium-111 Capromab	For prostate cancer imaging
I-131 sodium iodide	For thyroid imaging
Strontium-89	Treatment of pain from bone cancer
Technetium Tc99m	Used as a diagnostic tool to determine coronary artery disease (CAD) See Chapter 22
Gallium scan	To evaluate infections of the kidney and certain tumors; used in brain, gastrointestinal bleed, bone, liver, gall bladder, thyroid, lung, and heart scans

Cytoprotective Agents

Mesna is a cytoprotective agent used to treat the side effect of hemorrhagic cystitis caused by ifosfamide. It is given IV at a concentration of no more than 20% of the ifosfamide dose. Another agent used to lessen side effects is amifostine. This agent is given along with the chemotherapy agent cisplatin to prevent its toxic effects.

Nuclear Pharmacy Technician

Nuclear pharmacy is a new area of pharmacy that technicians may be exposed to and therefore must be educated about. The agents used in nuclear pharmacy are referred to as radiopharmaceuticals. These agents are used as diagnostic tools, as well as for treatments, and may be administered to the patient in oral, IV, or inhaled forms. Just as chemotherapy agents must be handled carefully when being prepared in the pharmacy, so must nuclear medications. Radiopharmaceuticals are isotopes that can be seen on radiographs as small specs as they participate in the cell activity within the body system. Types of nuclear medicine scans are listed in Box 28.3.

A nuclear pharmacy technician is expected to help prepare the medications, label them, and perform quality control testing under the direction of a licensed pharmacist. For safety purposes, each person in the nuclear pharmacy must wear a meter that gives a reading of the radioactive levels that he or she is exposed to. In addition, each medication package is labeled with a monitor that gives a reading of radioactive level. If the contents are damaged somehow, the meter will reflect the level of exposure. It is imperative that all personnel comply with the proper handling of the radioisotopes both during preparation and disposal. All medications are prepared in a vertical flow hood (see Chapter 13) and are disposed of in a special lead container. The half-life of the radioisotope determines how long it takes for the isotope to decay.

DO YOU REMEMBER THESE KEY POINTS?

- What types of elements may cause cancer
- How to decrease the possibility of acquiring certain cancers
- What are the diagnostic tools used to determine the type and stage of cancer
- What is leukemia and what are the various types
- How cancer grows
- What are the types of treatments available to cancer patients
- What are the main types of chemotherapy treatments
- Why side effects of chemotherapy are similar
- How is nuclear pharmacy used in the diagnosis and treatment of cancer

■ The method of action for each of the chemotherapeutic agents covered

■ Terminology used to describe cancer and its treatments

REVIEW QUESTIONS:

Multiple Choice

1. Which of the following cell processes are not normally seen in cells?
A. Replication
B. Mitosis
C. Death
D. Metastasis

2. The term used to define the spread of cancer cells into other areas of the body is
A. Melanoma
B. Cancerous
C. Malignant
D. Metastasis

3. Factors that are taken into account when diagnosing cancer include
A. Etiology
B. Karyotype
C. Morphology
D. All of the above

4. The small sections of a gene that usually perform normally within a cell but when altered by a retrovirus can produce cancerous cells are referred to as
A. Oncogenes
B. Tumors
C. Neoplasms
D. None of the above

5. A type of cancer that affects the lymphatic system and may or may not have a high grade of malignancy is referred to as
A. Leukemia
B. Hodgkin's disease
C. Non-Hodgkin's disease
D. Kaposi's sarcoma

6. Which of the following chemotherapeutic agent is NOT used to treat cancer?
A. Antimetabolites
B. Mitotic inhibitors
C. Nitrogen mustards
D. Filgrastim

7. The process of mitosis is a set of stages that begins with
A. G2 phase
B. Cytokinesis
C. S phase
D. G1 phase

8. When preparing radiopharmaceuticals guidelines require
A. The use of radioactive meter
B. Specialized containers for disposal
C. Preparation within a vertical flow hood
D. All of the above

9. Which of the following person(s) may be at higher risk for acquiring cancer?
A. Persons older than 65 years
B. Children
C. Smokers
D. All of the above

10. Which of the following side effects are most commonly seen after chemotherapy treatment?
A. Nausea and vomiting
B. Diarrhea
C. Immunosuppression or anemia
D. All of the above

True/False

*If the statement is false, then change it to make it true.

1. Cancer can be caused by a virus.

2. There are preventative measures that can eliminate any chance of acquiring cancer.

3. Only pharmacists can prepare radiopharmaceuticals.

4. Surgery does not necessarily eliminate cancers and is normally followed with radiology and or chemotherapy.

5. Radioactive isotopes are often implanted directly into the cancer site for treatment.

6. Anticancer agents that alter normal hormone levels include corticosteroids.

7. Vesicant agents must be prepared by a pharmacist.

8. Chemotherapy drugs are administered IV or IM only.

9. Erythropoietin is used to promote growth of neutrophils.

10. Traditional antibiotics can be used to treat cancer.

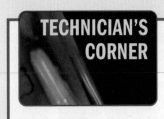

TECHNICIAN'S CORNER

Using a comprehensive drug textbook, such as *Facts and Comparisons* or *Mosby's Drug Consult*, look up the following chemotherapy agents and list their brand name, ROA, and preparation guidelines:

Idarubicin
Doxorubicin
Mitomycin

BIBLIOGRAPHY

Stedman's Concise Medical Dictionary for Health Professionals, ed 3, Baltimore, 1997, Williams & Wilkins.

Drug facts and comparisons, ed 53, St Louis, 1999, Wolters Kluwer.

Fremgen B, Frucht S: *Medical terminology*, ed 2, Upper Saddle River, NJ, 2002, Prentice Hall.

Harman JG, Gilman AG, Limbird LE, editors: *Goodman and Gilman's the pharmacological basis of therapeutics*, New York, 2001, McGraw-Hill.

Malarkey LM, McMorrow ME: *Nurse's manual of laboratory tests and diagnostic procedures*, ed 2, Philadelphia, 2000, Saunders.

Mosby's Drug Consult, St Louis, 2004, Elsevier.

Basic Sciences for the
Pharmacy Technician

29 *Microbiology*

30 *Chemistry*

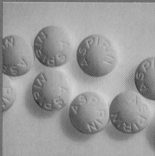

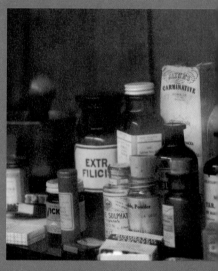

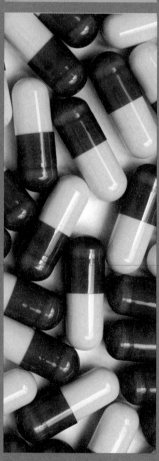

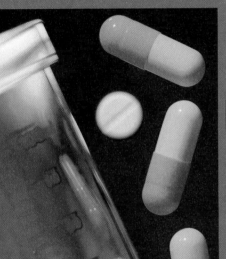

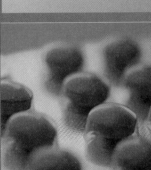

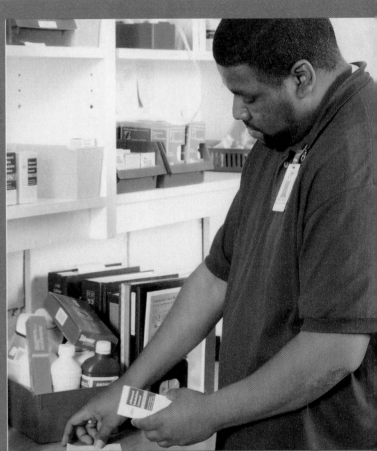

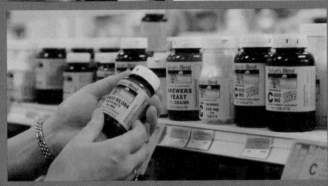

29

Microbiology

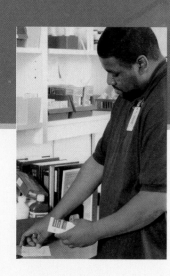

Objectives

- Describe the Golden Age of Microbiology and its importance in the medical field.

- List the five kingdoms.

- List at least two different types of organisms within each kingdom.

- Differentiate between prokaryotic and eukaryotic cells.

- List the major components of the eukaryotic cell.

- Describe the functions of the major components of eukaryotic cells.

- List the steps required to perform a Gram stain.

- Describe the characteristics of bacterial cell walls of gram-positive and gram-negative microbes.

- Differentiate between gram-positive and gram-negative results.

- Describe the differences between microbes and viruses.

- List some of the most common conditions caused by species within each kingdom.

- Explain how and why bacteriophages are used to protect against viruses.

TERMS AND DEFINITIONS

Aerobic *Organisms that need oxygen to survive*

Anaerobic *Organisms that live in the absence of oxygen*

Binary fission *The method of reproduction by which a single cell divides into two separate cells*

Biology *The study of life*

Catalyst *A molecule that allows chemical reactions to take place rapidly but is not altered in the reaction*

Enzyme *A protein that causes chemical changes to take place*

Facultative anaerobe *A microorganism that can live with or without oxygen*

Heterotrophic *The ability to reproduce asexually*

Microbial *Refers to micro- (very small) organisms not visible without a microscope*

Microbiology *The study of microscopic organisms*

Morphology *The study of characteristics of organisms*

Peptidoglycan *The substance that comprises bacterial cell walls, specifically of gram-negative and gram-positive microbes*

Species *Of Latin origin meaning "kind"*

Taxonomy *The science of classification and nomenclature of organisms*

Vectors *The host that carries the disease; does not need to be living*

Virology *The study of viruses*

Virus *An organism that replicates by using the host's cell parts, including deoxyribonucleic acid (DNA), ribosomes, and proteins*

ORGANISMS AND DISEASES THEY CAUSE

Organisms	Species	Condition	Organisms	Species	Condition
Protozoa	*Plasmodium falciparum*	Malaria	Helminths	Helminths	
Fungi	*Candida albicans*	Multiple conditions		Roundworms	
	Tinea	Athlete's foot		Flatworms	
Bacteria	*Borrelia burgdorferi*	Lyme disease		Flukes	
	Clostridium botulinum	Botulism		Tapeworms	
	Clostridium tetani	Tetanus	Virus	Human immunodeficiency virus (HIV) retrovirus	AIDS
	Helicobacter pylori	Stomach ulcers			
	Haemophilus influenzae	Meningitis		Herpesvirus	Herpes
	Mycobacterium leprae	Leprosy		Poliovirus	Polio
	Mycobacterium tuberculosis	Tuberculosis		Poxvirus	Chicken pox
	Neisseria gonorrhoeae	Gonorrhea		Rabies virus	Rabies
	Staphylococcus aureus	Meningitis		Rhinovirus	Common cold
	Streptococcus pneumoniae	Meningitis			
	Streptococcus pyrogenes	Scarlet fever			

Introduction

Biology is the study of life. Some forms of life cannot be seen without the aid of a microscope. Microbiology is the study of very small microorganisms. This includes bacteria, some forms of fungus, and protists. Viruses are even smaller than bacteria. Virology is the study of viruses. Special microscopes and techniques are needed to view viruses because they are so small. It is important to have an understanding of how microbes work in order to appreciate how antibiotics and other agents fight off infections and other conditions that affect the human species. To look into the world of microbes, we must first have some background on how life has been explained scientifically. From the dawn of mankind, humans have tried to define what life is. To understand life, we must understand life forms and how they interact with each other.

As scientific techniques advance so does our insight into the mysterious world of microbial life forms. Because of the strange and bizarre life forms that have been discovered on this planet, scientists believe now, more than ever, that life may exist on other planets. Microbes have been found in fossils dating back over 3 billion years before the beginning of mankind. They have adapted to the drastic and harsh changes in the environment since the beginning of their existence. Microbes can live regardless of adverse conditions. Bacteria and other life forms have been a part of human evolution. Humans benefit from bacteria in many ways. This chapter explores both the positive and negative effects of bacteria on humans.

Charles Darwin (Evolution)

In 1831, Charles Darwin traveled to the Galapagos Islands. There he studied the various species on each island. He discovered that evolution plays a key role in the survival of the fittest. It was his observations of the animals on the Galapagos Islands that made him question the theories of how species inhabited islands far from the mainland. The theories at the time considered one or two possibilities.

1. Island species came from the mainland at some point; thus they where exactly the same species
2. Island species were created on the islands and were totally different than their counterparts on the mainland

Darwin found that the species were not totally different nor were they the same as the species on the mainland. His research led him in another direction. From all his recorded notes and from previous research by animal researchers, Darwin found that tortoises, birds, insects, and even plants living on the many islands were similar to one another. However, even though they lived in close proximity to one another, the species were different from one island to another. The reason for this major difference, Darwin believed, was that each species followed a different evolutionary path. The various animals and organisms living on each island developed into different species altogether. Only those species that survived the changes on each island would reproduce. Therefore only the fittest survived. Darwin formed taxonomic categories based on the phylogenetic relationship between offspring from previous generations.

The Golden Age of Microbiology

Until the discovery of the microscope in the 1600s, scientists did not know that organisms were made of cells nor did they know about microscopic organisms (see Chapter 1). An English eyeglass maker by the name of Robert Hooke invented the first microscope. His first observations, made with a crude type of microscope, were the cells of a simple cork. He described them as tiny boxes or cells. This was the beginning of the study of microscopic organisms. In 1674, Anton van Leeuwenhoek invented a more sophisticated microscope and documented the observation of tiny microbes in a drop of water and teeth scrapings. He referred to these small organisms as "animalcules." Although many microbes were now being discovered, there were many debates in the scientific world as to their origins.

In the beginning of microbiology most scientists believed in spontaneous generation. The idea was that some organisms were generated from other organisms or their byproducts. For example, it was believed that flies came from manure; maggots came from decaying corpses; and mice and snakes came from common soil. In the 100 years after the invention of the microscope, these inaccurate beliefs were disproved by scientific methods. They were replaced by the understanding that new life arises from preexisting living organisms. Scientific methods were set in place, and these methods are still used today to prove or disprove hypothesis.

A timeline of major advances in the field of microbiology is listed in Figure 29.1.

LOUIS PASTEUR

Louis Pasteur was a French scientist who devised experiments that would set the standards for scientific research in the future. He proved that unseen microorganisms exist in the air and in nonliving material such as broth. By using broth-filled glass beakers that were made to trap airborne microbes he proved that the broth could be kept from contamination. The steps he followed to test his hypothesis are shown in Box 29.1.

Many advances in scientific knowledge took place—from newly discovered bacteria to understanding the theory of evolution. It is no wonder that this time period was called the Golden Age of Microbiology. Most of the discoveries made during this time extended human life. With the knowledge of bacteria and other microbes, scientists and doctors were able to fight infection. The average lifespan of an adult in the 1600s was 40 years; in contrast, midlife today is 40 years and many people live into their 80s and 90s.

Classifications of Organisms (Taxonomy)

Scientists have classified organisms into seven different groups. These groups are based on structural similarities and clarify how different organisms survive and interact with each other. This knowledge serves to aid scientists in understanding evolutionary changes. The study of naming and classifying organisms is called taxonomy. Taxonomy is a difficult area of study because it can be hard to classify new organisms in a specific group when they may have similarities to more than one group.

ROBERT WHITTAKER (THE FIVE KINGDOMS)

The five kingdoms—plant, animal, fungi, protist, and Monera—were conceived by a scientist by the name of Robert Whittaker and are still in use today (Table 29.1). Four of the five kingdoms consist of eukaryotic organisms. Within each

(Text continued on 544)

1900s	1953	Watson, Crick Discovered the form of DNA
	1944	Avery, MacLeod, McCarty Discovered that DNA is the genetic material
	1943	Delbruck, Luria Discovered that bacteria could become infected with viruses
	1935	Stanley, Northrup, Summer Gained the ability to crystallize viruses
	1928	Fleming, Chain, Florey Credited with the discovery of penicillin
	1910	Ehrlich Discovered Syphilis
	1890	Ehrlich Proved the theory of immunity
	1887	Petri Created the Petri dish used for isolation of bacteria
	1884	Escherich Discovered the bacteria *Escherichia coli*
	1884	Gram Created the Gram staining process to determine bacterial cell wall
	1883	Koch Discovered the bacteria *Vibrio cholerae*
	1882	Koch Discovered the bacteria *Mycobaterium tuberculosis*
	1881	Koch Created pure cultures
	1880	Pasteur Began immunization techniques
	1879	Neisser Found the microbe (named after him) *Neisseria gonorrhoeae* also known as gonorrhea
	1876	Koch Discovered the germ theory of disease
	1867	Lister Proved that cleaning the hands between surgeries decreased the spread of infection from patient to patient
	1864	Pasteur Created pasteurization
	1861	Pasteur Proved spontaneous generation as described in previous figure
1800s	1857	Pasteur Discovered fermentation

FIGURE 29.1 The Golden Age of Microbiology.

TABLE 29.1 Kingdoms, Cell Characteristics, and Examples

Kingdoms	Characteristics	Examples
Plantae	Eukaryote	Pine tree, green algae, ferns, flowers
Animalia	Eukaryote	Sponges, worms, apes, starfish, humans
Protista	Eukaryote	Algae, water molds, amoebae
Fungi	Eukaryote	Molds, yeasts, fungi
Monera	Prokaryote	Gram-positive and gram-negative bacteria

BOX 29.1 LOUIS PASTEUR'S EXPERIMENT

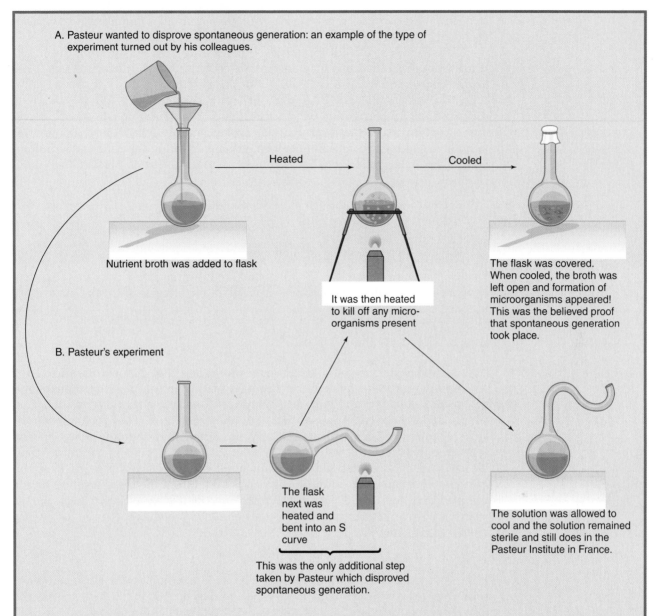

A. Pasteur wanted to disprove spontaneous generation: an example of the type of experiment turned out by his colleagues.

Nutrient broth was added to flask

Heated

Cooled

It was then heated to kill off any micro-organisms present

The flask was covered. When cooled, the broth was left open and formation of microorganisms appeared! This was the believed proof that spontaneous generation took place.

B. Pasteur's experiment

The flask next was heated and bent into an S curve

This was the only additional step taken by Pasteur which disproved spontaneous generation.

The solution was allowed to cool and the solution remained sterile and still does in the Pasteur Institute in France.

Step 1: He filled several short-necked flasks with beef broth and boiled them. Some were left open and allowed to cool; they later became contaminated. The flasks that had been sealed were not contaminated.

Step 2: He filled the boiled broth into long-necked flasks that had been bent into an S-shaped curve. After cooling they showed no signs of contamination. Although the air could get to the broth, the microbes could not (because of the unique shape of the necks of the flasks).

Conclusions: From step 1 he concluded that microbes present in the air had contaminated the broth. From step 2 he proved that it was not air but the microbes in the air that actually contaminated the broth. He also proved that heat could kill the airborne contaminants. These basic steps were the beginning of aseptic technique that we now use in preparing medications.

kingdom, the organisms are next divided into different phylum, followed by classes, orders, family, genus, and then finally species. These seven different classifications are used to organize all the known living organisms on planet Earth. Each kingdom, of course, contains many different types of organisms.

Viruses are not included in the five kingdoms. Scientists differ on the classification of viruses because they do not fit nicely into the characteristics of a "life form." Viruses are discussed at the end of this chapter.

Eukaryotes and prokaryotes have different characteristics. The most obvious difference that eukaryotes have a nucleus and prokaryotes do not. Also, eukaryotes do not have a cell wall structure as prokaryotes do. This difference makes it possible for antibiotics to kill microbes without harming the cells of the human body. Each eukaryotic kingdom is differentiated from the others by four main criteria:

1. Their individual pattern of development
2. Nutritional requirements
3. Tissue differentiation
4. Possession of flagella (form of locomotion)

We briefly review each of the five kingdoms, isolating specific organisms that may have an adverse affect on humans—from plants to eukaryotes to the prokaryote kingdom, Monera.

PLANTAE

This kingdom includes both land (terrestrial) and water plants (aquatic). They are mainly multicellular and are classified further on the basis of their photosynthetic pigmentation. Plants are eukaryotic organisms that obtain their food supply and energy from the sun through photosynthesis. They include mosses, ferns, flowers, conifers, and an array of other organisms. Humans have a special relationship with plants; we need them for nutrition and protection from weather. We use parts of plants to build homes and make clothing as well as to treat various medical conditions. For example, digoxin is taken from the plant foxglove and is used to treat heart conditions. The bark from the ash tree *(Taxus brevitolia)* is used to treat ovarian cancer. More recently, *Ginkgo biloba* has been used to increase memory (see Chapter 10).

Plant Cell Structure

Plant cells contain many of the same structures as animal cells. However, plant cells acquire energy very differently than animals do. Figure 29.2 illustrates the differences between animal and plant cells. Plants have chloroplasts that are used to convert sunlight into energy, which is then stored. In addition plants have a cell wall that is composed of cellulose that maintains cell shape. The vacuole of a plant cell also is much larger than those found in animal cells. Luckily, there are not many diseases that are easily transmitted by plants. Because plants are linked in many ways to animal cells, we have benefited from many plants, using them for food, flavorings, and colorings and to treat various conditions.

Medically Relevant Conditions

Poison ivy and poison oak can cause a skin reaction when touched. There are many plants that can cause gastrointestinal (GI) upset or worse if eaten by people or animals, and a few, such as digitalis, can cause death. Thus it is wise to never ingest plants if you are not sure of the consequence. Many plants are used medicinally for treating various conditions that affect humans. Some of these are discussed in Chapter 10. In addition to use as a medicinal product, plants also have nutritional and industrial value. Both animals and humans depend on plants for food.

ANIMALIA

The kingdom Animalia contains more species than any of the other kingdoms. Species in this kingdom are more complex physiologically than other species and rely on many motor skills and sensory organs. Ingested food must be broken down through a series of complicated steps before it can be used. More complex nervous systems may be necessary depending on the species of animal. The animal kingdom includes the more simplistic sponges, jellyfish, and clams and more complex organisms such as spiders, frogs, reptiles, marsupials, and mammals.

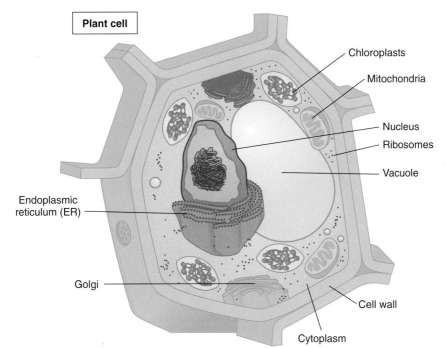

Plant cell

Chloroplasts

Mitochondria

Nucleus

Ribosomes

Vacuole

Endoplasmic reticulum (ER)

Golgi

Cell wall

Cytoplasm

Plant and Animal Cells

Same structures

Nucleus
Ribosomes
Smooth ER
Rough ER
Golgi
Vacuoles
Mitochondria
Cell membrane

Differences

Animal cells:
No cell wall
No chloroplasts
Small vacuoles

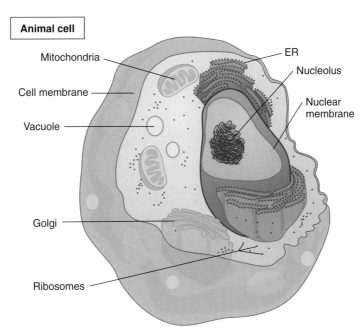

Animal cell

Mitochondria

Cell membrane

Vacuole

Golgi

Ribosomes

ER

Nucleolus

Nuclear membrane

FIGURE 29.2 Major components of a plant cell **(A)**, an animal cell **(B)**, and a bacterial cell **(C)**. Animal cells do not have a cell wall, whereas bacterial cells are surrounded by either a thin or thick wall of peptidoglycan. *Continued*

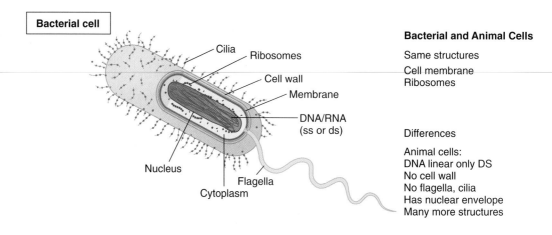

Bacterial cell

Cilia
Ribosomes
Cell wall
Membrane
DNA/RNA
(ss or ds)

Nucleus
Flagella
Cytoplasm

Bacterial and Animal Cells

Same structures
Cell membrane
Ribosomes

Differences

Animal cells:
DNA linear only DS
No cell wall
No flagella, cilia
Has nuclear envelope
Many more structures

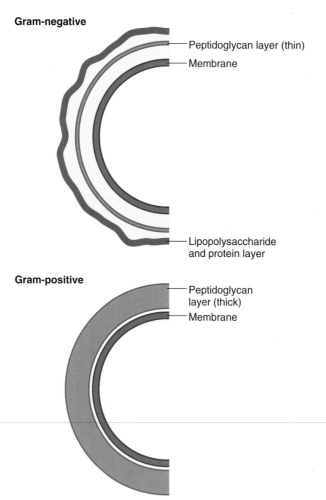

Gram-negative

Peptidoglycan layer (thin)
Membrane

Lipopolysaccharide
and protein layer

Gram-positive

Peptidoglycan
layer (thick)
Membrane

FIGURE 29.2 cont'd

Animal: Eukaryotic Cell Structure

Animal cells contain different structures than cells from plants and prokaryotes. The most obvious difference between animal cells and bacterial and plant cells is the lack of a cell wall. The cell composition for animal cells is shown in Figure 29.2.

Animal cells also lack the chloroplast that plant cells use to store energy from the sun. Animal cells get their energy from food rather than from the sun. Inside

TABLE 29.2 Characteristics and Structure of an Animal (Eukaryotic) Cell

Cell Component	Structure	Description
DNA	Double helix	Genetic code responsible for many characteristics
RNA	Chain	A messenger for coding proteins
Nucleus	Envelope containing DNA	Contains DNA and nucleolus. The nucleolus manufactures substances (such as ribosomes) used in the cytoplasm
Endoplasmic reticulum (ER)	Membranous network	Contained throughout the cytoplasm. Contains many cells used to produce and transport products
Ribosomes	Small dotlike structures	ER that contains ribosomes is referred to as rough ER. It produces proteins such as enzymes
Smooth ER	Membranous network	Produces various lipid substances; has no ribosomes
Golgi	Flat membranous stacks of sacs	Serves as a transport system for enzymes and proteins and adds onto some products produced before they are sent out of the cell
Lysosomes	A single sac filled with digestive juices	Digestive sacs that dispose of unwanted particles within the cell. They are then emptied outside of the cell
Mitochondria	Cell-like structure with membranous material	Responsible for making adenosine triphosphate (ATP) that is then carried to places within the cell where energy is needed to produce enzymes and so forth. Cells contain many mitochondria that are located near production areas such as ER
Centrosomes	Rodlike structures	These contain centrioles, which are symmetrical in design. They are needed at the beginning of reproduction

each animal cell are many structures that all work in unison. The nucleus contains the DNA of the cell. This is the genetic code of the animal. Other structures in the cell include ribosomes, mitochondrion, Golgi, plasma membrane, cytoplasm, vesicles, and rough and smooth endoplasmic reticulum. The functions of each are outlined in Table 29.2.

Because four of the five kingdoms are made up of eukaryotic organisms, there are many types of species that can cause human diseases. Various organisms in the animal kingdom can be transmitted to humans from various vectors. Vectors are the carriers of disease organisms. How the organism moves through various environments throughout its life cycle ultimately reveals ways to avoid contact as explained in the following.

Medically Relevant Conditions

The amoeba *Entamoeba histolytica* is a parasitic organism that feeds on red blood cells. Its mode of transportation is from human to human via ingestion of cysts that are excreted in the feces. The vector or carrier of these disease-causing microorganisms includes humans and mosquitoes.

Trichomonas vaginalis is another protozoan that causes infections in the male urinary tract and in the vagina of females. It is transferred mostly by sexual intercourse.

Dysentery is caused by another protozoa ciliate *Balantidium coli* and is transferred by feces to the mouth in a cyst form. When they are ingested, they travel to the colon where they replicate.

Sporozoa, such as *Plasmodium vivax*, are responsible for the disease malaria. Their life cycle involves an infected female mosquito. The sporozoa in the salivary glands of the mosquito easily move into the human bloodstream once the mosquito bites the human. From there the sporozoa move to the liver where they replicate and move into the bloodstream. As the parasites are released into the bloodstream, their toxic by-products cause the host to become sick. When an uninfected mosquito bites an infected human, the cycle repeats (Figure 29.3).

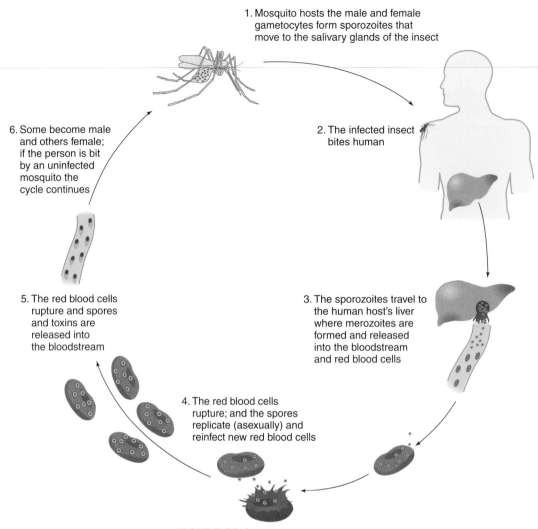

1. Mosquito hosts the male and female gametocytes form sporozoites that move to the salivary glands of the insect

2. The infected insect bites human

3. The sporozoites travel to the human host's liver where merozoites are formed and released into the bloodstream and red blood cells

4. The red blood cells rupture; and the spores replicate (asexually) and reinfect new red blood cells

5. The red blood cells rupture and spores and toxins are released into the bloodstream

6. Some become male and others female; if the person is bit by an uninfected mosquito the cycle continues

FIGURE 29.3 Life cycle of *Plasmodium vivax*.

Helminths (worms) are also protists but are categorized under different phyla (heading) than protozoa (single-celled organisms). They are either Platyhelminthes (flatworms) or Aschelminthes (roundworms). These worms are multicellular eukaryotic organisms that have many of the same organs that humans do. They have digestive, circulatory, nervous, excretory, and reproductive systems. These types of helminths live in soil, feed on organic material, and are free living. Those that lack a digestive system remain parasitic. They must absorb digested nutrients from a host. Other differences between free living and parasitic helminths are that the parasitic helminths may lack means of locomotion and their nervous system is simple, because they do not have to be sensitive to their environment. The parasitic helminth life cycle is complex, which requires a more sophisticated reproductive system. The human parasitic diseases are listed in Table 29.3. All forms of these parasites can be avoided by using a few precautions:

- Always cook meat thoroughly
- Wear shoes when walking outside on soil
- Never drink from stream water because it may be contaminated with feces from animals upstream
- Wash your hands after playing with animals or after cleaning cat litter boxes

TABLE 29.3 Parasitic Diseases Contracted by Humans

Organism	Species	Life Cycle
Phylum: Platyhelminthes		
Trematoes (flukes)	*Paragonimus westermani*	Miracidium swims and imbeds in a snail and develop into the next form cercariae that invades lobster. Man eats lobster and contracts the adult fluke. Defecation into water continues the cycle
Cestodes (tapeworms)	*Taenia saginata*	Proglottids containing eggs are found in feces defecated onto grass. Cattle ingest proglottids containing eggs. They hatch and bore into muscle and form a cyst. These are ingested by humans in uncooked meat where the cycle continues
	Echinococcus granulosus	Humans ingest eggs excreted in feces. Eggs hatch within the small intestine, larvae migrates to liver or lungs. A cyst is formed. In the wild the host may be eaten by another animal where the cycle continues
Phylum: Aschelminthes		
Nematodes (roundworms)	*Enterobius vermicularis*	This species spends its entire life in the human host. Adult pinworms deposit eggs around the perianal region where it can be transferred via exposure to contaminated clothing
	Ascaris lumbricoides	Adult form lives in small intestines of human host. Eggs are excreted and can survive in soil until another host ingests it. Eggs hatch in intestines, travel to lungs to mature stage, then migrate to intestine to continue cycle
	Necator americanus	Lives in small intestines of humans, eggs are excreted and live in soil. Infects host by penetrating through the skin of the feet where it gets carried to the lungs via blood. It is coughed up then ingested into the stomach where it enters the intestine
	Trichinella spiralis	Undercooked pork or beef containing cyst form enters the human digestive tract where they reproduce live nematodes. They migrate to various muscles and tissues and remain to be parasites of the host

PROTISTA

Most of the organisms in the kingdom Protista are unicellular, and all are eukaryotic. They are made up of five different plantlike and animal-like organisms. All are heterotrophic, which means they reproduce asexually. Some cause diseases in other organisms.

Protists include algae, water molds, amoebae, and protozoans. Algae and water molds can be found in and around coastal waters. Certain forms of algae are macroscopic reaching lengths from a few meters up to 50 m. From large brown kelp beds off the coast to algae found growing in trees, algae prefer moist to wet areas and need light to survive. They produce chlorophyll, which they use as a food source. Some protists, such as brown algae or lichens, anchor themselves to a surface. Other organisms like euglenoids and green algae propel themselves by means of a flagellum or whiplike structure that moves them through water.

Protozoans can live in water or soil, and they live off of bacteria and other organic particles. Protozoans can be a part of an animal's "normal flora" and most do not cause disease. Their three modes of locomotion are listed in Figure 29.4.

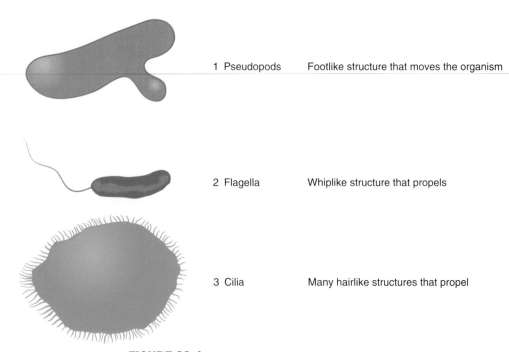

1	Pseudopods	Footlike structure that moves the organism
2	Flagella	Whiplike structure that propels
3	Cilia	Many hairlike structures that propel

FIGURE 29.4 Three forms of locomotion in protozoa.

FUNGI

The Fungi kingdom is divided into true fungi and slime molds. Many have a complex reproductive cycle. Lichens are specialized type of fungi that can grow in the most inhospitable environments.

Fungi are different from bacteria. The DNA of a fungus is contained within a nuclear membrane. Some of the organisms that belong in the fungi kingdom include fleshy-type fungi, such as mushrooms, and also yeasts and certain types of molds. Fungi are either anaerobes (need air) or facultative anaerobes (partial air). Yeasts are the only fungi that are not multicellular, but they too absorb nutrients from plants. They are round or oval in shape and may be found on leaves of plants. They multiply by budding as seen in Figure 29.5.

TECH NOTE! Yeast (facultative anaerobe) is usually associated with baking bread and making beer. As the species *Saccharomyces cerevisiae* (baker's yeast) buds off, it expands and the bread dough rises. The yeast in beer gives off CO_2 as a byproduct and gives beer its unique taste.

Molds may have long filaments called hyphae and may form a mass large enough to be seen by the naked eye. Molds can infect and ultimately destroy (spoil) plants and food. Fungi play an important role in the environment, because they are responsible for decomposing plant organisms. They use dead plants as a food source while cleaning the environment. Plants are more susceptible to fungal infections than humans. Many fungi do not cause illness; however, there are some infections that humans get from specific species.

Medically Relevant Conditions

The species *Candida albicans* is a yeastlike organism that is part of the normal flora in the mouth and genitourinary tract of humans. It is kept in check by the bacterial flora also present in the mouth and genitourinary areas. When antibiotics are taken that kill off the normal bacterial flora of these areas, the fungus *C. albicans* can proliferate and cause an infection. Other conditions caused by

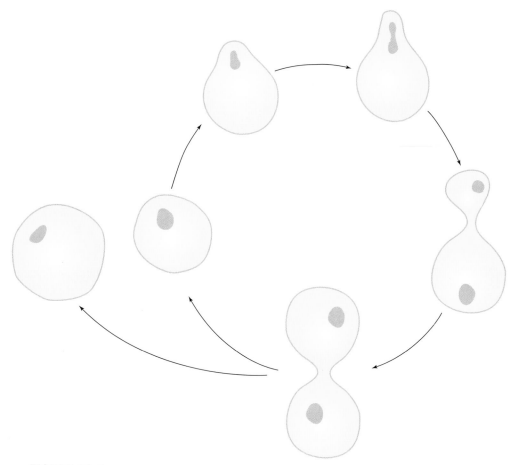

FIGURE 29.5 Budding process of replication of yeast cells. Yeast multiplies asexually by budding or spouting a new cell that then breaks away from the mother cell.

BOX 29.2 CONDITIONS CAUSED BY FUNGI

Candida albicans	Multiple conditions
Tinea pedis	Athlete's foot
Pneumocystis carinii	Pneumonia
Tinea cruris	Jock itch
Tinea unguium	Cutaneous infection
Tinea capitis	Ringworm

fungi are athlete's foot lung infections, vaginal infections, and even sepsis. Fungus prefers warm moist environments; however, some species of fungi can grow under low moisture conditions. A disease caused by a fungus is called mycosis. The types of agents used to kill fungi are referred to as antifungal agents (see Chapter 24). There are many conditions caused by fungi as shown in Box 29.2.

The next section describes the characteristics of prokaryotic cells, the conditions caused by these organisms, and how antibiotics are used to treat them. Please refer to Chapter 24 for specific antimicrobial actions of antibiotics and their side effects.

MONERA

Monera, the smallest organisms (in size) of the seven kingdoms, may be the simplest in physiology but are the most abundant worldwide. Fossils of bacteria have

Procaryotic cell size	Description of basic form		Description of basic cocci or bacilli shapes	
Coccus	oval or round	1. 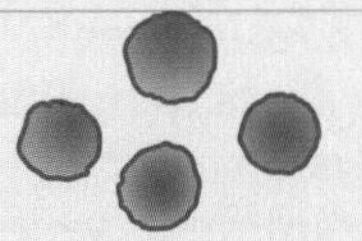	diplococcus diplobacilli	5. 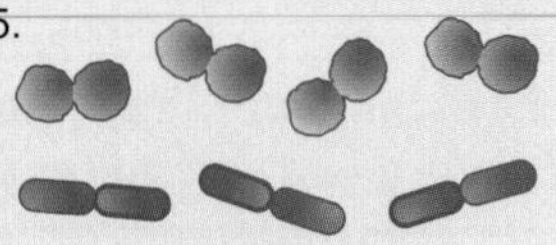
Bacillus	rectangular, rod shaped	2. 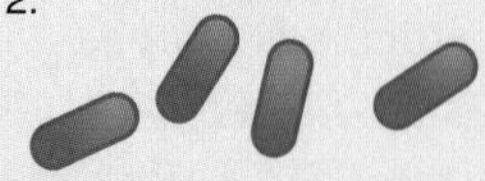	streptococcus streptobacilli	6. 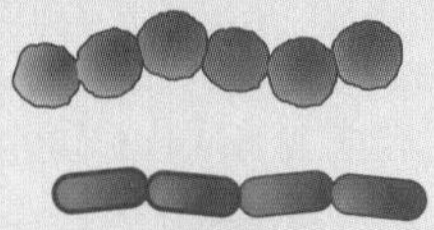
Spirilla	twisted, helical, corkscrew, spiral	3. 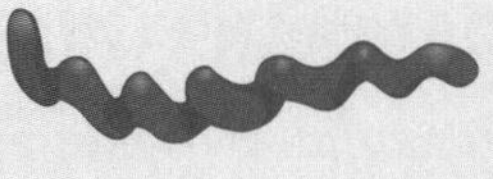	staphylococci staphlobacilli	7. 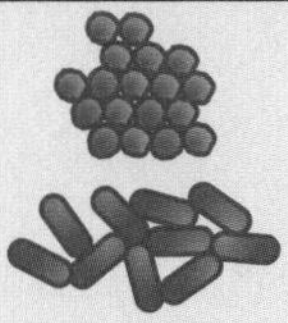
	vibrios	4. 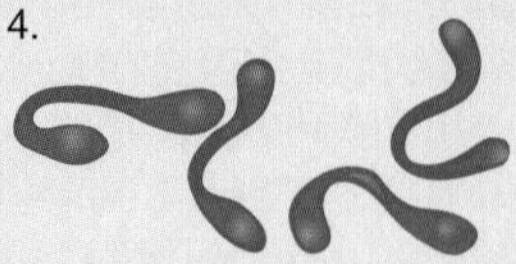		

FIGURE 29.6 Morphology of prokaryotic organisms. Pictures 1 through 6 show the various morphologies or shapes of microbes. The most common shapes include 1, coccus; 2, bacilli; 3, spirilla; 4, vibrios. Picture 5 shows cocci microbes that are found in sets of two, called diplococci or diplobacilli. Those microbes found in strips are shown in picture 6, streptococci or streptobacilli. Picture 7 shows staphylococci and staphlobacilli, which are found in clusters.

been dated back 3.5 billion years; in contrast, eukaryotic cells date back only 1.5 billion years. The cell structure of prokaryotes is less complicated than that of eukaryotic cells. Bacteria are further classified depending on how they derive their energy, as well as other characteristics.

Characteristics and Structure of Prokaryotes

Until now, we have explored a few of the many different types of eukaryotic cell organisms. There are many basic differences between prokaryotic and eukaryotic cell structures. The visual characteristics of bacteria and other microbial organisms are used to describe an organism's morphology or appearance (Figure 29.6).

Other characteristics specific to prokaryotes are that they can reproduce by binary fission (divide in two), they do not have a nuclear envelope, and, most amazingly, they have the ability to live in the most inhospitable environments, which adds to their prevalence. Prokaryotes may be anaerobic or aerobic. Before the discovery of these minute life forms, the effects of bacteria were attributed to other causes such as evil spirits.

Brief History of Antibiotics

In 1928, Alexander Fleming, a scientist who was studying crops plagued by infections, noticed that one of his agar plates was contaminated with a mold. This mold, later named *Penicillium notatum*, had a zone of clearance around it where no bacteria were growing because the mold had lysed the bacteria being grown on the agar plate. It took many years to isolate the active component within the mold—penicillin. Penicillin destroys bacteria by interacting with enzymes that are present within the bacterial cell wall.

TABLE 29.4 Classes of Microorganisms within the Kingdom Prokaryote

Common Name	Class	Characteristics
Wall-less prokaryotes	Mycoplasmas	Smallest known bacteria that can live outside host cells. Lipid-type barrier helps protect them
Typical gram-positive cell wall	Rods, cocci	Thick walls made of peptidoglycan
	Actinomycetes	Thick walls made of peptidoglycan
Typical gram-negative cell wall	Anaerobic photosynthetic bacteria	Thin walls made of peptidoglycan
	Cyanobacteria	Thin walls made of peptidoglycan
	Nonphotosynthetic bacteria	Thin walls made of peptidoglycan
Altered cell wall type	Archaebacteria	Walls not composed of peptidoglycan but polysaccharides or proteins

STRUCTURE OF THE BACTERIAL CELL WALL

Because bacteria have many characteristics that are different from human body cells, certain drugs can be used to attack and kill bacteria without harming human cells. The bacteria cell has a wall that protects it in the same way that our skin protects us from damage and intrusion (see Figure 29.2). Bacterial cell walls are made of a finely woven network of two forms of peptidoglycan molecules, which form a semirigid protective barrier around the internal parts and is referred to as a NAG-NAM formation. Sugar linkages are sandwiched between the inner membrane and outer membrane.

Penicillin disrupts NAG-NAM links and causes the bacteria to lyse or break open. Because human cells have a different type of membrane, and not a wall, surrounding them, they are not harmed.

In gram-positive bacterial walls there are many layers of peptidoglycan between the membranes. The cell walls also contain teichoic acids (alcohol base), either lipoteichoic acid or wall teichoic acid. The negative charge of this alcohol base plays a part in the overall growth and regulation of the cell. In contrast, gram-negative cell walls have only one layer of peptidoglycan and no teichoic acid. They do contain various proteins and sugars on the outer membrane and can withstand certain antibiotics, such as penicillin, as well as detergents, digestive enzymes, and certain dyes. In addition, gram-negative cell walls contain a lipid that becomes toxic when in the bloodstream of the host. There are openings on the surface of the gram-negative cell's outer cell membrane that allows some chemicals to penetrate the cell. These openings are responsible for the difference shown between gram-negative and gram-positive bacteria on Gram stain; thus laboratory technicians can differentiate between the two types of organisms (Table 29.4).

Exterior of Bacterial Cell Walls

Glycocalyx is a sticky substance that surrounds many different types of bacteria. This viscous layer is composed of different material depending on the species. Its purpose is to protect the bacteria from phagocytosis by the host's immune system cells. Bacteria can adhere better to surfaces with help from the sticky polysaccharide or polypeptide slime layer. This increases the chance of bacteria survival.

ANTIBIOTIC SPECTRUM AND RESISTANCE

Antibiotics destroy bacteria by breaking down the cell walls of bacteria. To choose the right drug to destroy a specific bacteria, the type of microbe must be determined. The first step in this process is to determine if the bacteria are gram positive or gram negative.

Most penicillins are very effective at breaking down the cell walls of gram-positive microbes. However, many forms of bacteria are not destroyed by penicillin because they secrete another type of enzyme that cleaves (cuts) the bond within the penicillin structure, thus rendering it useless against the bacteria. The name for this bacterial enzyme is penicillinase. Special additives can be added to penicillin-type agents to stop their destruction. Additives such as sulbactam added to ampicillin (Unasyn) allow the antibiotic to break the bacterial bonds, allowing lysis to occur.

TECH NOTE! When a word ends in –ase, it means that it is an enzyme.

As the antibiotic spectrum broadens, so does the effectiveness against microbes; thus broad-spectrum antibiotics are effective against more microbes than narrow-spectrum antibiotics are. Narrow-spectrum antibiotics normally affect gram-positive microbes, whereas broad-spectrum antibiotics may affect gram-negative microbes. Broad-spectrum agents such as aminoglycosides are much more effective against gram-negative bacteria. Another important aspect of bacterial organisms is their ability to live with or without oxygen.

Some agents are very specific, killing one type of bacteria. This is why it is important to choose the correct antibiotic. (See Table 29.5 for an example of common types of conditions caused by bacteria.)

Bacteria reside just about everywhere in the world. Environments that house bacteria include hot springs, the bottom of the ocean, deep in the earth's crust, and the mouths and intestinal systems of humans. Bacteria that can live in the presence of air are called aerobic, whereas those that grow only in the absence of air are called anaerobic. Some bacteria called facultative anaerobes can live with

TABLE 29.5 Commonly Caused Bacterial Conditions

Organism	Disease	Morphology
Borrelia burgdorferi	Lyme disease	*Difficult to Gram stain
Clostridium botulinum	Botulism	Anaerobic, gram-positive rods
Clostridium tetani	Tetanus	Anaerobic, gram-positive rods
Escherichia coli	Cystitis (an opportunistic bacteria from the GI tract)	Gram-negative rods
Helicobacter pylori	Stomach ulcers	Aerobic, gram-negative rods
Haemophilus influenzae	Meningitis, respiratory infections, septicemia	Aerobic, gram-negative rods
Mycobacterium leprae	Leprosy	*Difficult to Gram stain
Mycobacterium tuberculosis	Tuberculosis	*Difficult to Gram stain
Neisseria gonorrhoeae	Gonorrhea	Aerobic, gram-negative cocci
Staphylococcus aureus	Boils, carbuncles, abcesses	Aerobic, gram-positive cocci
Streptococcus pneumoniae	Pneumonia	Aerobic, gram-positive cocci
Streptococcus pyrogenes group A beta hemolytic	Scarlet fever	Aerobic, gram-positive cocci

*For those microbial organisms that cannot be grown on artificial media agar plates, other means are used, such as acid-fast staining or an immunological test to determine if the disease is present.

a small amount of air or in airless environments. The relationship that some bacteria have with animals is mutually beneficial. This means that both organisms benefit from one another. For instance, various bacteria reside within the human gut, including *Escherichia coli* and *Lactobacillus*, which help break down food that can be absorbed into the body. The bacteria benefit by the nutrient-rich environment.

Viruses

One of the major disagreements in the scientific community is how to classify viruses. They do not fit nicely into any of the kingdoms outlined previously. In fact, viruses have their own field of study called virology (the study of viruses). Viruses not only infect animals but also infect plants and even bacteria. Plant viruses are responsible for destroying many food crops to the detriment of both people and livestock.

CLASSIFICATION OF VIRUSES

Viruses can be categorized into three types:

1. Animal viruses
2. Plant viruses
3. Bacterial viruses

MORPHOLOGY AND CHARACTERISTICS OF VIRUSES

Viruses may have a double or single strand of DNA. They are different from other organisms because they can also have a double or single strand of RNA.

Basic classification of viruses includes determining their outer covering and any additional coating that they may contain as shown in Figure 29.7.

Unenveloped viruses are covered by capsids; capsids are protective coverings made of proteins called capsomeres. Enveloped viruses have a capsid plus a covering of proteins, fats, and carbohydrates. Different viruses have different appearances; sometimes they resemble small space capsules.

There are other ways to classify viruses or virions, such as determining their method of replication. This is probably one of the characteristics that is most different from the characteristics of organisms in any of the five kingdoms. As shown in Figure 29.8, viruses do not seem to replicate in any of the previously described methods; instead, they assemble themselves just as cars are assembled in a processing plant. In all living organisms except viruses, DNA is double stranded. RNA is replicated from the DNA information. Viruses invade a host cell and take over this replication to make more viral DNA.

Other differences between viruses and organisms of the other kingdoms include the way that viruses survive. Most organisms obtain nutrition from organic means or from the sun by photosynthesis and replicate by fission (splitting into two), sexual, or asexual means. Viruses do not fit any of these categories. They are closer to parasites, although most parasites do not kill their hosts as viruses do. Viruses assemble new virions by using the cell parts from their hosts. Some viruses can travel from host to host by way of blood, body fluids, or even the air. Thus, although they do have some similarities with other organisms, they do not behave as entities that can replicate without the components of the cells that they invade. All viruses are so small that they cannot be seen with a light microscope. To isolate and identify viruses, different methods must be used.

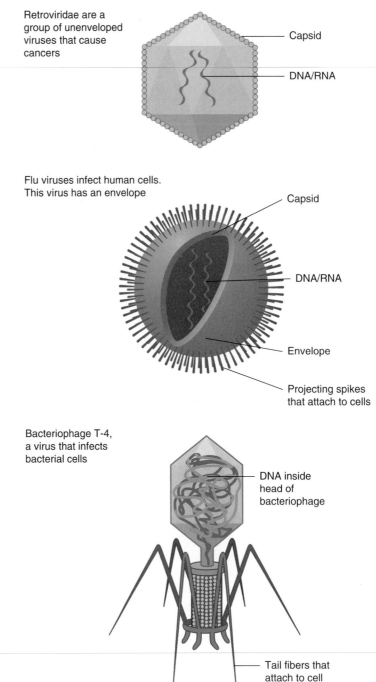

Retroviridae are a group of unenveloped viruses that cause cancers

Capsid

DNA/RNA

Flu viruses infect human cells. This virus has an envelope

Capsid

DNA/RNA

Envelope

Projecting spikes that attach to cells

Bacteriophage T-4, a virus that infects bacterial cells

DNA inside head of bacteriophage

Tail fibers that attach to cell

FIGURE 29.7 Viral composition. **A,** Unenveloped (capsomeres). **B,** Enveloped virus. **C,** Bacteriophage.

ANALYSIS OF VIRIONS

Viruses that infect bacteria (such as bacteriophages) can be grown on agar plates. However, those that cannot be grown on agar plates must be grown in animals, such as mice, rabbits, or other laboratory animals, to observe their presence. Once the animal is infected, the tissue can be analyzed. To view the morphology of a virus an electron microscope (a very high-powered microscope) is used. The most common way to identify viruses is by their reaction with antibodies. When the human body comes into contact with a foreign substance it makes antibodies in response to the antigen (foreign body) as shown in an experiment aimed at determining antibody formation in Figure 29.9.

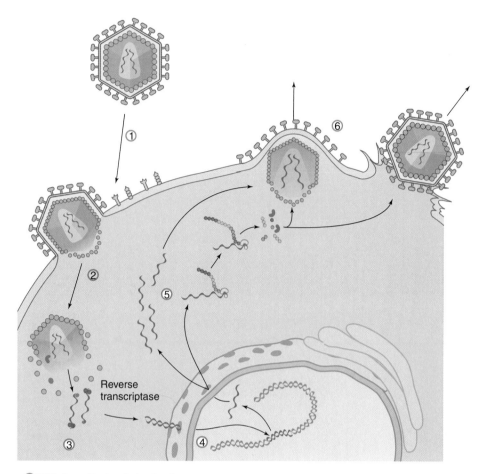

① HIV virus attaches to host cell

② The capsid releases viral RNA into cytoplasm

③ The host's enzyme is used to replicate viral RNA into DNA

④ During latency period the viral DNA stays in the host cell's DNA

⑤ The virus's DNA is activated where it codes for proteins and RNA
strands to be assembled

⑥ The newly formed viral cells either bud off or lyse out of the host
cell releasing free HIV

FIGURE 29.8 HIV Viral replication. Diagram of the replication process of viruses. Each component is made independently inside the host cell. All materials are made from the host cell. Once the parts are made, they are assembled.

There are human viral diseases, such as human immunodeficiency virus (HIV), that cannot be grown in laboratory animals. Although chimpanzees can be infected with one strain of HIV, they do not show any symptoms. Thus, viruses such as HIV are more difficult to learn about or perform tests on.

Another problem with the study of viruses is that viruses are made of the same components as their host. This means that they are more difficult to kill because the antibiotic will kill the healthy cells too, although researchers have discovered that viruses can be manipulated to work for them rather than against them. Examples of well known viral diseases include the following:

Virus	Human Disease
HIV Retrovirus	Acquired immunodeficiency syndrome (AIDS)
Herpesvirus	Herpes
Poliovirus	Polio
Poxvirus	Chicken pox
Rabies virus	Rabies
Rhinovirus	Common cold

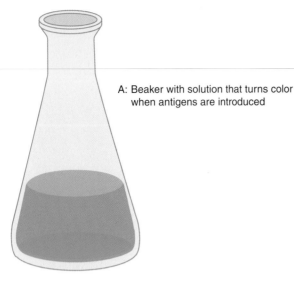

A: Beaker with solution that turns color
when antigens are introduced

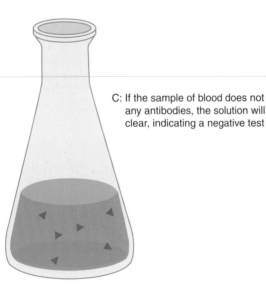

B: A sample of blood (containing
antibodies) is placed in beaker

Add 1. Antigen
        2. Compound that turns color when/
            if antigen binds to antibodies

Result: Positive: As the the antigens ▲
              bind to antibodies Y
              the solution turns color

C: If the sample of blood does not contain
any antibodies, the solution will remain
clear, indicating a negative test

FIGURE 29.9 Determination of antibody formation: antibody test using bacteriophages. This proves whether a person has formed antibodies against a certain antigen. A sample of blood (containing an antibody) (O) is placed in a beaker **(A)**. To this, two components are added: a complement (color when bound to both antigen and antibody) and the antigen (A) to the antibody. The result would be that O and A bind together resulting in a color that makes this test positive **(B)**. A sample of blood (with no antibody) is placed in a beaker. To this the two components are added. The result in this case is negative because there is no antibody present to complete the color change **(C)**. Thus the blood has not come into contact with that specific antigen before.

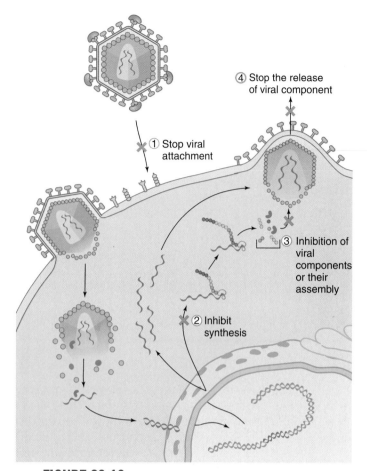

FIGURE 29.10 The four ways to stop viral infections.

HOW VIRAL INFECTIONS ARE STOPPED

With the use of a variety of medications, many viral infections can be halted or delayed. Although more is being discovered concerning viruses, there are only a handful of agents that are currently being used to treat various conditions caused by viruses. Each drug must be very specific in its mechanism of action to lessen the adverse effects on normal human cells. The antivirals can succeed through one of four main mechanisms of action in overcoming viral synthesis and eventual spread. These are shown in Figure 29.10 and listed in Box 29.3. Most agents are aimed at disruption of the DNA of the virus or a closely related component of the newly synthesized DNA viral strand. Drugs such as zidovudine cause inhibition of the viral replication of HIV. This drug moves into the DNA where it halts continued synthesis of new viral DNA. Other agents such as acyclovir inhibit viral DNA polymerase, which ultimately halts the synthesis of new viral DNA; acyclovir is used against herpes simplex and varicella-zoster viruses. Nonnucleoside reverse transcriptase inhibitors (NNRTIs) cause the premature termination of the growing viral DNA strand by interfering with specific enzymes of the virus.

BOX 29.3 METHODS OF VIRAL INHIBITION

1. Inhibit the ability of the virus to attach to the hosts' cell. If an antibody can be made to fit the viral coating then it may be possible to inhibit the attachment of the virion to a host cell
2. Inhibit replication by suppressing synthesis of viral DNA/RNA. By interjecting an antiviral agent that attaches itself to the DNA of the host cell, it may disrupt the replication process that codes for important proteins and enzymes used by the virion. Other components include disruption of specific nucleic acids, DNA polymerase, and other critical enzymes necessary to the formation of viral DNA/RNA strands.
3. Inhibit the ability of the virus to assemble itself properly: If protein synthesis is disrupted, the virion may not be able to build a necessary component that is needed to continue infecting new hosts.
4. Inhibit the ability of the virus to breakout of the host cell. If the assembly process is disrupted or altered, it may be possible to inhibit the virion from assembling its components in the proper order or manner. This faulty virion cannot attach itself to the host's cell wall to move out of the cell where it continues to reinfect new host cells.

DNA, Deoxyribonucleic acid; *RNA*, ribonucleic acid.

USING VIRUSES TO FIGHT DISEASE

One of the most studied types of viruses is the bacteriophage. These viruses can be loaded with a vaccine and then used to immunize humans. For example, by removing the DNA inside the capsid (head) of the bacteriophage, a nondisease causing strain of poxvirus can be inserted. The virus is then injected into the human bloodstream where the virus vaccine can easily attach to human cells and stimulate immunity to the poxvirus.

DO YOU REMEMBER THESE KEY POINTS?

- The names of the five kingdoms
- How the kingdoms are broken down
- Who was responsible for the theory of evolution
- The contributions of Louis Pasteur to microbiology
- How the Golden Age of Microbiology changed history
- The characteristics of and differences between animal, plant, and bacterial cells
- The components of an animal cell and their functions
- The types of diseases/conditions spread by the organisms discussed in this chapter
- What morphological characteristics are used to distinguish between organisms
- The importance of the Gram stain in determining morphology of bacteria
- The composition of bacterial cell walls and how antibiotics affect them
- The types of environments that bacteria can be found in
- The differences between microorganisms and viruses
- How viruses replicate
- How viruses can be stopped from replicating and spreading
- The components of viruses

REVIEW QUESTIONS:

Multiple Choice

1. Charles Darwin is best know for
- A. Evolution
- B. Genetics
- C. Taxonomy
- D. Classification

2. Of the groups of organisms listed, which one is not eukaryotic?
- A. Fungi
- B. Bacteria
- C. Animalia
- D. Plants

3. Of the five-kingdom classification system, which of those listed include bacteria?
- A. Plantae
- B. Animalia
- C. Protista
- D. Monera

4. Viruses can contain which of the following types of nucleic acids?
- A. Double-stranded DNA
- B. Single-stranded DNA
- C. Double- or single-stranded RNA
- D. All of the above

5. Which of the microbe(s) listed is(are) part of a persons "normal flora"?
- A. *Candida albicans*
- B. *Borrelia burgdorferi*
- C. *Streptococcus pyrogenes*
- D. Both A and C

6. Alexander Fleming is best known for the
- A. Discovery of viruses
- B. Discovery of penicillin
- C. Classification of drugs
- D. Scientific method

7. The disease malaria is caused by the microbe
- A. *Entamoeba histolytica*
- B. *Plasmodium vivax*
- C. *Trichomonas vaginalis*
- D. *Balantidium coli*

8. The function of the Golgi is to
- A. Transport proteins through the cell membrane
- B. Tag proteins to aid them reach their final destination
- C. Produce ATP; the power source for the cell
- D. Produce proteins

9. The main types of locomotion of protozoa are
- A. Pseudopods
- B. Flagella
- C. Cilia
- D. All of the above

10. Some microbes can resist antibiotics because of specific enzymes that are called
- A. Antimicrobials
- B. Penicillinase
- C. Antienzymes
- D. Antibiotics

True/False

*If the statement is false, then change it to make it true.

1. Only animals can catch viruses.

2. All cells have the same components.

3. The mitochondria within each cell are analogous to a powerhouse.

4. Gram-negative bacteria has a thicker layer of polypeptide bonds.

5. The primary difference between smooth endoplasmic reticulum (ER) and rough ER is the absence of ribosomes on smooth ER.

6. Protists include algae, water molds, and amoebae.

7. Plants use chloroplasts for the same purpose that animals use mitochondria.

8. Spontaneous generation was believed to explain how life begins.

9. Cocci, bacilli, and spirilla are the three main morphologies of bacteria.

10. Both animal and plant cells multiply by binary fission.

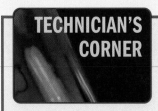

TECHNICIAN'S CORNER

Following the steps outlined in the workbook, perform a Gram stain of the cheek cells from inside of your mouth. Locate and describe the morphology of the cells.

Compare your cells to those bacterial cells listed in the lab book.

To learn more about microbiology check out these websites:

www.cellsalive.com

BIBLIOGRAPHY

Campbell N, *Biology*, ed 2, Redwood City, Calif, 1991 Benjamin/Cummings.

Greulach V, Chiappetta V: *Biology: The science of life*, Morristown, NJ, 1977, Silver Burdett.

Malarkey LM, McMorrow ME: *Nurse's manual of laboratory tests and diagnostic procedures*, ed 2, Philadelphia, 2000, Saunders.

Tortora G, Case CL, Funke BR: *Microbiology: An introduction*, ed 4, Redwood City, Calif, 1991 Benjamin/Cummings.

Voet D, Voet J: *Biochemistry*, 1990, John Wiley & Sons.

30
Chemistry

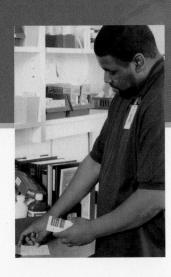

Objectives

■ Name the 10 basic ions necessary for proper electrolyte balance and what each one contributes to the body.

■ Define the terms atom, molecule, proton, neutron, and electron.

■ Distinguish between ionic and covalent bonds.

■ List the types of molecules that are formed from various nucleic acids.

■ List the 20 amino acids necessary in a balanced diet.

■ Distinguish between acids and bases.

■ Be able to convert temperature from Fahrenheit to Celsius.

■ Distinguish between anions and cations.

■ Describe how sodium bicarbonate balances pH.

■ Explain how chemistry plays an important part in the action and reactions of drugs.

■ Describe how enzymes and proteins are used in the body.

■ Define the terms inorganic and organic as related to chemistry, giving an example of each.

■ Explain the components of an amino acid and how chains are formed.

■ Define metabolism in terms of anabolism and catabolism.

■ Explain how mitochondria powers the body with adenosine triphosphate (ATP).

Amino acids *Macromolecules that make up proteins*

Anabolism *To build up; the construction phase of metabolism*

Atom *The smallest unit of an element*

Atomic mass *The mass (mostly referred to as weight) of an atom expressed in the units of 1.660×10^{-24}*

Catabolism *To break down; the destruction phase of metabolism*

Covalent bond *The sharing of electrons between two atoms*

Electron *The smallest subset of an atom that contains a negative charge*

Enzyme *A protein that helps a reaction take place in a living organism without chemical enzyme changing*

Gram *A basic unit of weight (mass) of the metric system equal to the weight of a cubic centimeter (cc) or a milliliter (ml) of water*

Kcal *A measurement of energy or heat expended or used up in a chemical activity; the amount of heat needed to change the temperature of 1 kg of water*

Ion *An atom or a group of atoms with a leftover unbalanced charge*

Ionic bond *The transfer of electrons between two atoms*

Macro *Large*

Metabolism *The physical and chemical change that takes place within an organism*

Meter *Basic measurement of length in the metric system*

Micro *Small*

Micrograms *1000th of a milligram; metric unit of measure*

Milligrams *1000th of a gram; metric unit of measure*

Mole *Avogadro's number; 6.02×10^{23} atoms, molecules, or ions*

Molecule *The smallest particle of a compound*

Neutron *A subset of an atom that does not contain charge*

Nucleic acid *The bases contained within deoxyribonucleic acid (DNA)*

Orbit *The rotation of electrons around the atom*

Proton *A subatomic particle of an atom that holds a positive charge*

Valence *The number of electrons gained, lost, or shared when an atom bonds with another atom; determined by the electrons in the outer orbit*

Introduction

At first, it may not seem as though chemistry has much to do with the health care field. However, this is not true. Chemistry is at the heart of the discovery of new medicines and treatments and the understanding of chemical interactions in the body. It is important for pharmacy technicians to become acquainted with the chemical reactions and interactions in the body. The goal of this chapter is to present the basics of chemistry and answer questions concerning why drugs interact with one another and the importance of these reactions within the body system. Chemistry also uses many of the same metric terms as pharmacy; therefore knowledge of metric terms will not only increase your knowledge of chemistry terminology but also reinforce your knowledge of terms used in pharmacy.

Parts of an Atom

Atoms are made up of smaller particles called protons (positively charged), electrons (negatively charged), and neutrons (no charge). The center of the atom, the nucleus, contains the protons and neutrons. The electrons of a specific atom orbit around the nucleus in much the same way that the planets in our solar system orbit around the sun (Figure 30.1).

The nucleus of an atom is very small. Most of the atom is empty space. Most atoms have an equal number of positively charged protons (+) and negatively charged electrons (−), giving them a net charge of zero. If an atom has more or fewer electrons than protons, it becomes charged and is called an ion. The structure of each atom is determined by the number of electrons that it has in the outer orbit.

There are two types of bonding between atoms—ionic bonds and covalent bonds. When two atoms come into close contact with each other, the nucleus (positively charged) of the first atom is attracted to the other atom's electrons (negatively charged) and vice versa. These two atoms can either exchange or transfer electrons forming ionic bonds, or they can share the electrons forming covalent bonds. Covalent bonds are stronger than ionic bonds because the electrons are held in a tighter arrangement. The joining of two or more different types of atoms can create different molecules, such as carbohydrates (sugars), lipids (fats), proteins (meat), and nucleic acids (DNA). Sometimes, when two oppositely-charged ions come together, such as sodium (Na^+) and chloride (Cl^-), some of their charges are taken away because they form an ionic bond (NaCl). Not all charges are dropped when ions combine; in many cases there are charges left over, which are usually indicated at the right of the chemical name with plus or minus signs.

The periodic table of elements has all of the known elements strategically placed according to their properties (Figure 30.2). There are seven horizontal rows of elements. All of the elements are placed in a specific box next to other elements that are closely related to them—for example, across the top of the table are numbers 1 through 8.

Looking down the first column of the chart, there are three important alkali metals: lithium, sodium, and potassium. They are in the same column because of their similarities. They all have one electron in their outer shell and they all are white, soft, and very reactive metals.

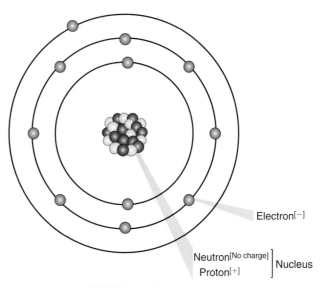

Electron[−]

Neutron[No charge]
Proton[+]
Nucleus

FIGURE 30.1 Electron orbit.

1	2	3	4	5	6	7	8	9	10	11	12	13	14	15	16	17	18
₁H																	₂He
₃Li	₄Be											₅B	₆C	₇N	₈O	₉F	₁₀Ne
₁₁Na	₁₂Mg											₁₃Al	₁₄Si	₁₅P	₁₆S	₁₇Cl	₁₈Ar
₁₉K	₂₀Ca	₂₁Sc	₂₂Ti	₂₃V	₂₄Cr	₂₅Mn	₂₆Fe	₂₇Co	₂₈Ni	₂₉Cu	₃₀Zn	₃₁Ga	₃₂Ge	₃₃As	₃₄Se	₃₅Br	₃₆Kr

FIGURE 30.2 Periodic table of elements. The elements K, Na, Cl, Mg, Se, and Cu are highlighted.

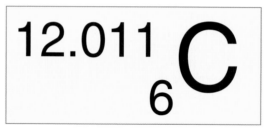

FIGURE 30.3 Carbon, represented by the letter *C*. Below the element is the atomic number. Above is the atomic weight.

TECH NOTE! A period refers to the row across the table, whereas a group indicates the vertical column. Each element is assigned a symbol; below the symbol is the atomic number.

Elements are also listed in order based on the chemical property and size. As you can see there are numbers assigned to each element. In Figure 30.3, carbon is the sixth element on the table, indicated with the number 6. Above the number 6 is 12.011, indicating the weight of the atom. The entire periodic table of elements categorizes elements by their elemental properties such as weight and types of bonds that they form. This makes it easier to learn their properties. Although the table lists each element by itself, in nature they are not found by themselves. For instance, the metal sodium (Na^+) by itself is highly reactive and would explode if it came into contact with oxygen. The same can be said of Cl^- (chloride). Even as a solid, chloride gives off deadly vapors when isolated. However, if you combine these two elements, you have NaCl, or sodium chloride (i.e., table salt). NaCl is also used in the hospital intravenous (IV) bags that antibiotics and other medications are placed into for administration to patients. Highlighted within the periodic table (Figure 30.2) are the elements most used in the pharmacy. They are the elements in the body that are measured in laboratory blood tests.

Charges are grouped in pairs, any excess electrons will appear as a − (negative sign), whereas any deficiency will appear as a + (positive sign). For example, in a molecule of water each hydrogen atom has one electron that can be shared or bonded. Oxygen has eight electrons. This number indicates the total number of electrons in oxygen. There are two electrons in the oxygen's inner shell and six in the outer shell. Oxygen is able to accept another two electrons in its outer shell. When joined with two hydrogen molecules, there is no overall charge (neutral) as shown in Figure 30.4.

There are some common atoms that form tight bonds with other atoms to make substances such as water (oxygen and hydrogen) and common table salt (sodium chloride). Some of these compounds are listed Table 30.1.

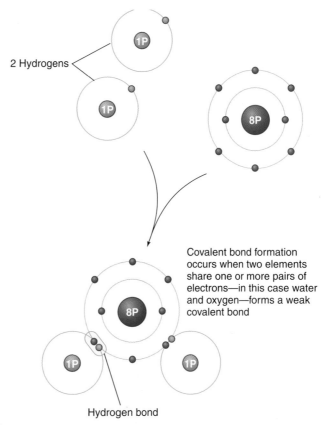

FIGURE 30.4 Water molecule formation. Water is one of the most important compounds on earth. It composes approximately 65% to 75% of all living cells.

TABLE 30.1 Chemical Charges of Compounds

Substance	+ Charge	− Charge	Chemical Symbol
Water	2 H	O^{-2}	H_2O
Ammonia	3 H	N^{-3}	NH_3
Acetate	2 C^{+4}, 3H	O_2^{-2}	$C_2H_3O_2^{-}$
Magnesium hydroxide	Mg^{+2}, H	O^{-2}	$MgOH$
Ferrous sulfate	Fe^{+2}, S^{+4}	O_4^{-2}	$FeSO_4^{-}$
Sodium chloride	Na+	Cl^{-}	$NaCl$
Potassium chloride	K^{+}	Cl^{-}	KCl
Bicarbonate	H^{+}, $1C^{+4}$	O_3^{-2}	HCO_3^{-}
Potassium phosphate	K+, P^{+4}	O_4^{-2}	KPO_4^{-3}
Hydrochloric acid	H^{+}	Cl^{-}	HCl
Sodium bicarbonate	Na^{+}, H^{+}, C^{+4}	O_3^{-2}	$NaHCO_3$

Molecules

There are two distinct areas of study in chemistry—inorganic chemistry and organic chemistry. Inorganic chemistry is the study of all types of molecules that do not contain carbon atoms. Examples include some metals and gases such as iron (Fe) and oxygen (O). Together, the molecule FeO_2 makes ferric oxide or rust. Organic chemistry is the study of substances that contain carbon as one of the components of a molecule. What contains the most important carbon-based substances? The human body.

TECH NOTE! If you look up the method of action of a specific drug and you read "unknown" it is because science still cannot answer the question of precisely how many drugs work.

The human body is composed of millions of molecules that form a complex series of actions and reactions within the body and with outside influences. Some of these influences are the food we eat, drugs we take, ambient temperature, stress, and even the air we breathe. The human body is so complex that scientists are still learning new things about the body and how it works. Chemical reactions make life happen; the types of bonds, charges, reactions, and molecules formed are important.

ENZYME ACTIVATORS AND INHIBITORS

Enzymes are proteins that can regulate the speed of reactions. They can be inactive until they come into contact with elements (called ions). For example, elements or ions such as chloride, zinc, iron, and magnesium can all serve as activators of the digestive enzyme pepsin. Once pepsin is activated, it helps break down food to be absorbed by the intestines. Another enzymatic reaction is the reaction of hydrogen peroxide on a cut or scrape. Pharmacology includes the study of these types of reactions.

TECH NOTE! Hydrogen peroxide (H_2O_2) is used as an antiseptic. Have you poured hydrogen peroxide over an open wound? When it comes into contact with an enzyme (called catalase) present in living tissue, a reaction occurs causing bubbles of oxygen to form. The oxygen helps remove foreign tissue debris.

Have you ever wondered how the human body can produce energy and perform other functions so quickly? It is because of catalysts (enzymes). These are protein molecules that speed up reactions by lowering the amount of energy needed to complete the reaction. Enzymatic reactions can speed up a reaction pathway.

Metabolism: Anabolism and Catabolism

The foods we eat must be broken down into usable molecules (catabolism) and built up into other new useful molecules (anabolism). All the processes that occur within the body are broken down into a series of steps such as those in the metabolic citric acid cycle, more commonly known as the Krebs cycle (Figure 30.5). This cycle is the step-by-step process of the transformation of molecules, such as fatty acids, amino acids, and carbohydrates, into other molecules necessary to the body. A series of reactions are possible because of the interactions between ions and enzymatic reactions. This allows the body to break down and/or build up substances as needed. Metabolism is necessary for the control of hormones, protein synthesis, pH (acid/base), lipid (fat) levels, glucose (sugar) levels, and more. This area of study is called biochemistry and plays an important role in the study of pharmacology.

ELECTROLYTE REPLACEMENT

The human body needs certain nutrients on a daily basis. These are essential for proper growth and overall maintenance of the body. Diagnostic blood tests can reveal to a doctor and a pharmacist (when done in a hospital) any deficiencies of essential nutrients that may effect the health of a patient. Laboratory tests may help ensure that the proper dosage of medication and/or replacement therapy is given.

There are specific values that a pharmacist will look for depending on the type of medication that the patient is taking. For instance, when a patient is placed on an aminoglycoside, such as gentamicin, he or she will have clearance levels

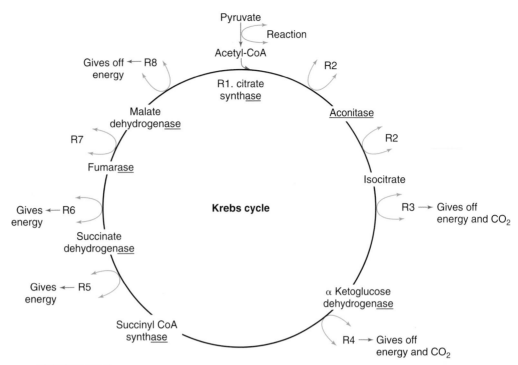

FIGURE 30.5 The Krebs cycle is a complex series of chemical reactions that releases energy.

drawn at a certain times after the gentamicin IV has been administered. The results will tell the pharmacist how fast the patient's body is clearing the drug (excretion). The condition of the patient's kidneys affects the amount of drug that should be given. If a patient is older, he or she will naturally have a decrease in drug clearance. If an aminoglycoside is dosed at too high a level, it can build up in the kidneys. This adds an additional strain on the body system. Patients that may be at high risk are those with kidney failure, older adults, children, and those with an existing medical problem.

Electrolyte levels are another type of laboratory test result that pharmacists will receive in the pharmacy daily. Certain patients must be placed on hyperalimentation, more commonly known as hyperal, total parenteral nutrition, or peripheral parenteral nutrition. An IV bag is hung daily as a nutritional supplement if the patient cannot eat food, is healing from a stomach or intestine operation, or is about to undergo surgery to the stomach or intestines. Ingredients of a hyperal bag include electrolyte, vitamin, and mineral replacement. This preparation is precalculated by the pharmacist after laboratory values have been sent to pharmacy. The technician is responsible for pulling all the parenteral medications to be placed in the hyperal and for preparation of the bag. The size of the bags can range anywhere from 1 L up to 3 L. Regardless of the size of the hyperal or the dosing, a new bag must be hung daily to ensure sterility. Electrolyte replacement consists of the ions potassium, sodium, chloride, phosphate, and magnesium. In addition, most hyperals include an assortment of vitamins added daily. A standard preformulated hyperal is usually given to the patients until their laboratory results are received by the pharmacy. Except for the bag on the first day, each daily bag of hyperal is usually tailor-made to the patient's specific needs.

There are two types of ions—cations (those with a positive charge) and anions (those with a negative charge). Many cations and anions form bonds between one another, forming various molecules such as proteins, amino acids, and many different types of enzymes. Remember, enzymes are proteins that regulate reactions. What follows is a closer look at the role some of these important ions have in the human body:

K: Potassium is found mostly inside the cell, as opposed to the outside (extracellular fluid) where many other ions are found. It is the principle cation intracellular fluid, and is necessary for homeostasis. It plays a major role in the maintenance of muscles, such as the heart, and nerve impulses. A deficiency can cause a wide range of side effects, including cardiac irregularities. An excess of K can cause lmpaired conduction of heat.

Na: Sodium is a key component in the transfer of water between areas of the body and is found mostly in the extracellular fluid of the body. Na is the most abundant cation in extracellular fluid.

Cl: Chloride is found both inside and outside the cells of the body. Chloride has a negative charge, which makes it an anion. Cl is the most abundant anion in extracellular fluid. It also contributes to osmotic pressure. The combination of sodium (cation) and chloride (anion) NaCl makes up more than 65% of the acidic ions of the blood. HCl (hydrogen and chloride) is another important combination in the body that works to help break down food in the stomach. Chloride is also important for the health of the heart muscle.

Mg: Magnesium is found in bones and the soft tissues of the body. It is used in the synthesis of adenosine triphosphate (ATP) and the release of energy from ATP. It plays a part in the overall maintenance of muscles of the heart and skeletal system and of the tissues of the nervous system. It is also a component, in combination with other ions, that helps proper bone growth.

Cu: Copper is a metal that the body uses in very minute amounts. This ion helps keep the blood vessels, hair, and skin in a healthy state. It also is believed to play a role, along with iron, as a component of hemoglobin. Copper deficiency can affect the number of white blood cells. Too much copper can cause diarrhea, destruction of the liver, and even death.

P: Phosphorus is found mainly in the bones. It participates in the making of certain enzymes, including ATP. This important enzyme is responsible for supplying the energy that human cells require. P is always found in combination with alkalies.

Fe: When you think of iron, you may think of cast iron or you may think of good, healthy blood. The iron in the body is the same type of iron used in construction but in very small amounts. Iron is necessary to help hemoglobin bind to oxygen molecules as we breathe. If iron is deficient, anemia (iron deficiency anemia) may result. The amount of hemoglobin decreases as well as the amount of oxygen carried by the blood. Iron is fat-soluble. Therefore an excessive iron intake can cause a toxic buildup leading to severe side effects, including brain damage, coma, or even death. This is especially true in children.

Ca: Calcium is important because it helps children grow big and strong, which is why it is important for children to drink enough milk. Calcium not only helps growing children's bones but also is important as we grow older. Ca must be activated by vitamin D to be absorbed. Calcium is necessary to keep an acid/base balance and is a factor in blood coagulation. A decrease in calcium can cause cramping or twitching of the muscles. As we age, the body decreases its production of many necessary vitamins and minerals. Some drugs increase the absorption of calcium, whereas other drugs may decrease the absorption. This is one of the details that a pharmacist looks for when giving a patient consultation. For example, tetracycline should not be taken with calcium supplements because they decrease the effectiveness of the antibiotic. Not enough calcium in the body will contribute to weak bones and muscles. This is especially true in the older adults. Many older citizens have osteoporosis, which is directly related to many years of calcium deficiency. Too much calcium can contribute to heart and kidney disease. In addition to proper bone growth, calcium helps the muscles by increasing electrical impulses.

Zn: Zinc is only needed in very minute amounts. It is a vital component of the enzyme carbonic anhydrase found in hemoglobin. This enzyme helps in the stabilization of the blood's pH. Zn can never stand alone, it must be in combination with other chemicals.

Mn: Manganese is another important component of enzymes active in the Krebs cycle. It is needed for proper growth, reproduction, and lactation. Mn is found in soft tissue, bone, and muscle.

I: Iodine is necessary for the proper functioning of the thyroid gland. A shortage of iodine can lead to goiter (enlargement of the thyroid gland).

ACID-BASE REACTIONS

Acid-base reactions within the body are some of the most important reactions because they can make the difference between life and death. The pH scale is a representation of the amount of hydrogen (H+) in water. It is a logarithmic function. This means that a 10-fold increase in hydrogen is represented by one unit. The pH ranges from 1 (the most acidic) to 14 (the most basic). The normal pH of a blood is 7.4 pH. If the pH of the blood changes by 0.4, such as to 7.8 or 7.0, life would end quickly for that person. The body works hard to maintain pH at a steady 7.4 by making buffers such as sodium bicarbonate. ($NaHCO_3$). Remember, the ions that form molecules (as described previously) drive reactions that can change pH balance.

TECH NOTE! Sodium bicarbonate is always kept on a crash cart for emergency situations, such as cardiac arrest. In cardiac arrest, the body is unable to keep the pH at 7.4 and becomes acidic (called acidosis), which can be fatal. Sodium bicarbonate is injected into the bloodstream where it can stabilize the blood pH.

Amino Acids

Molecules that form amino acids are made up of five basic parts shown in Figure 30.6. First, each amino acid is built from a central carbon atom. Second, a hydrogen is joined to all carbons. Third, a hydrogen makes an amino group off to one side. Fourth, a carboxyl group is created off the other side. The fifth part of the amino acid is the R group that represents a different amino acid because of its

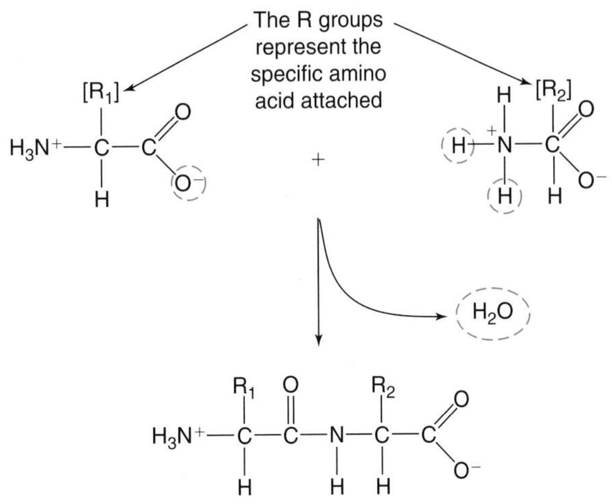

FIGURE 30.6 Amino acid structure.

different amino acid structure. By changing R group attachment, the entire amino acid is changed (see Figure 30.7). Therefore they perform different functions that include neurotransmitters (see Chapter 17) metabolic intermediates, and poisons. Each one of these amino acids can form long chains by linking the amino group of one to the carboxyl group of the next.

When this linking occurs, a reaction called dehydration takes place (the loss of a water molecule). When many amino acids join together, proteins are made. The overall molecule will not look like a straight chain, however, because the polarity of the molecules form different shapes. Amino acid chains can range from a few strung together to more than a thousand.

There are 547 individual amino acids in the 4 amino acid chains of a hemoglobin molecule. If one of those amino acids is in the wrong place or missing, a person may have sickle cell anemia. Amino acids play an important role in everyday life because they are the components of proteins, many of which are enzymes. Enzymes are necessary for reactions to occur. There are 20 main amino acids that make up almost every protein known in the animal kingdom. They also make up many nutrients that the human body needs (see Figure 30.7).

The rings (called benzene rings) are a shortcut representation of a specific chemical arrangement as shown in Figure 30.7. Each corner of the ring represents a carbon atom and its adjoining hydrogen atom. The way in which the body breaks down various amino acids allows the body to produce energy to run bodily functions, such as moving about, working, and playing. For instance, alanine, cysteine, glycine, serine, and threonine are turned into pyruvate. Pyruvate then enters the mitochondria (the cells' powerhouse) where it goes through the Krebs cycle. It is then converted many times with the end result of three molecules of ATP, which powers further reactions. Mitochondria are the human body's powerhouses; they produce power much the same way that a hydroelectric plant produce energy with the use of turbines and generators. The mitochondria (see Chapter 29) are contained within human cells and produce much of the power we use.

Measurements

The metric system is used in chemistry for quantitative measurements. Length is defined in terms of meters and volume in cubic centimeters (cc), milliliters (ml), and liters (L). Weight is written in kilograms (kg), milligrams (mg), and micrograms (mcg). Temperature is written as degrees Celsius.

Mass is often referred to as weight in pharmacy although its meaning is defined differently. Mass includes area or space taken up by an object based on gravity, whereas weight leaves out the pull of gravity. The mole is the same as the gram atomic weight. For example, if you want to know how much one mole of a chemical weighs, such as penicillin (PCN) $C_{16}H_{18}O_4N_2S$, refer to the periodic chart of elements for the gram number of each element. Looking at the table of elements, we see that the mass of one mole of PCN is as follows:

$$16(12 \text{ gm}) + 18(1 \text{ gm}) + 4(16 \text{ gm}) + 2(14 \text{ gm}) + 32 = 334 \text{ gm}$$

So, if we want to determine how many moles are in 218 grams of PCN, we would do it this way:

$$\text{moles of penicillin} = 218 \text{ gm PCN} \times \frac{1 \text{ mole PCN}}{334 \text{ gm PCN}} = 0.653 \text{ mole PCN}$$

The numbers come from the table of elements; for instance, carbon has the mass of 12.011 g, which we can round off to 12 g. This is then multiplied by the number of carbon atoms in the chemical (in this case penicillin). You would repeat the process for each of the remaining elements.

Amino acid base 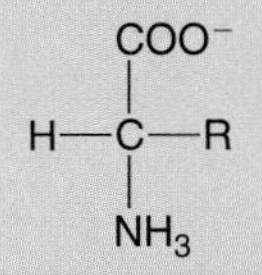	R-side chain
$$\begin{array}{c} COO^- \\ | \\ H-C-R \\ | \\ NH_3 \end{array}$$	R-side chain
Basic Amino Acids	
Arginine	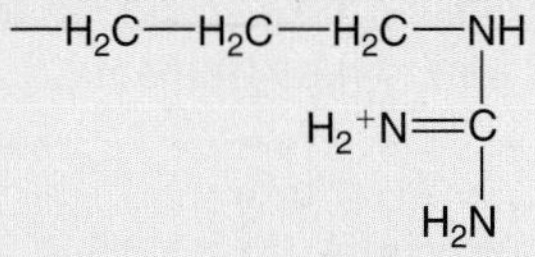 $-H_2C-H_2C-H_2C-NH$; $H_2{}^+N=C$; H_2N
Lysine	$-(H_2C)_3-H_2C-NH_3$
Histidine	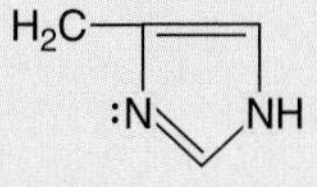 H_2C ; $:N \quad NH$ (imidazole ring)
Amino Acids with Aromatic Rings	
Phenylalanine	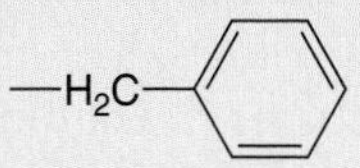 $-H_2C-$ (benzene ring)
Tyrosine	$HO-$ (benzene ring) $-CH_2$
Tryptophan	(indole ring) $-CH_2$; N-H
Acidic Amino Acids and their Amides	
Aspartic Acid	$-H_2C-COO^-$
Asparagine	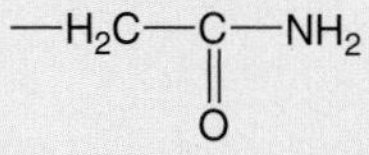 $-H_2C-\underset{O}{\overset{}{C}}-NH_2$
Glutamic acid	$-H_2C-H_2C-COO^-$
Glutamine	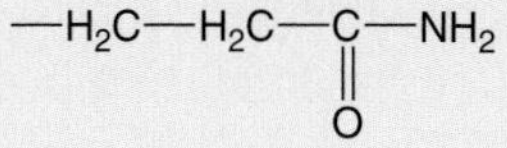 $-H_2C-H_2C-\underset{O}{\overset{}{C}}-NH_2$

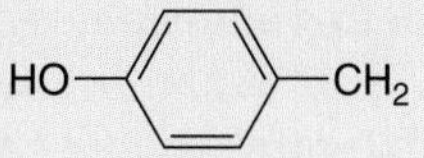

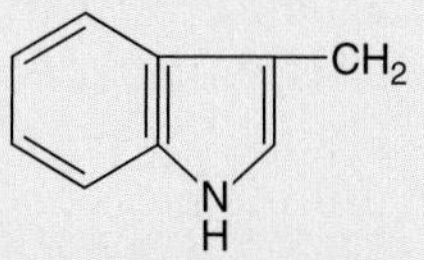

Amino acid	R-side chain
Amino Acids with Aliphatic R-Groups	
Glycine	$-H$
Alanine	$-CH_3$
Valine	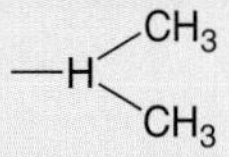 $-H \big\langle \begin{array}{c} CH_3 \\ CH_3 \end{array}$
Leucine	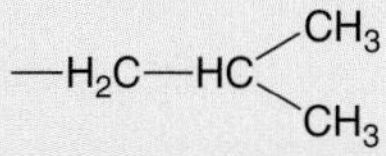 $-H_2C-HC \big\langle \begin{array}{c} CH_3 \\ CH_3 \end{array}$
Isoleucine	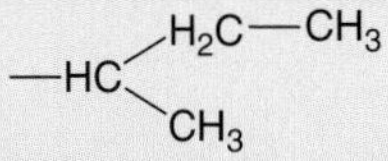 $-HC \big\langle \begin{array}{c} H_2C-CH_3 \\ CH_3 \end{array}$
Non-Aromatic Amino Acids with Hydroxyl R-Groups	
Serine	$-H_2C-OH$
Threonine	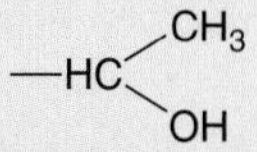 $-HC \big\langle \begin{array}{c} CH_3 \\ OH \end{array}$
Amino Acid with Sulfur-Containing R-Groups	
Cysteine	$-H_2C-SH$
Methionine	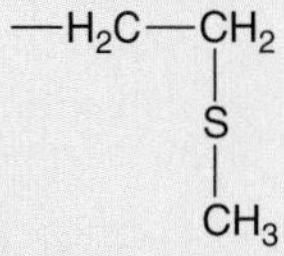 $-H_2C-CH_2$; S ; CH_3
Imino Acids	
Proline	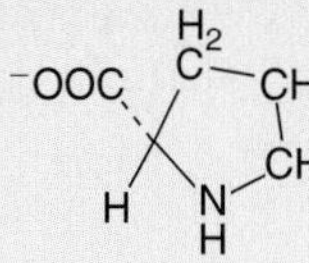 ^-OOC ... $\underset{H}{\overset{C}{C}}$; $\begin{array}{c} H_2 \\ C-CH_2 \\ CH_2 \\ N-H \end{array}$ (ring)

FIGURE 30.7 Essential amino acids.

TECH NOTE! When you work with certain chemicals, you will see the term millimoles. This is where the term comes from: 1 millimole is equal to 1/1000 mole. Phosphate is written in millimoles; the abbreviation is mM.

Another measurement used is temperature. When taking a patient's temperature, the readout in the metric system is measured in Celsius degrees rather than the standard Fahrenheit degrees. In the 1700s, a Swedish astronomer, Anders

Celsius, began to use a scale that represented "0" as the freezing point of water and 100 as the boiling point of water. All degrees between these two settings are divided into 100 equal parts, each representing a Celsius degree. The more commonly used Fahrenheit scale is credited to Daniel Fahrenheit in the 1700s in the United States. He was a German instrument maker who was the first to use mercury in a glass thermometer. He set the freezing of water as 32 degrees and the boiling of water as 212 degrees Fahrenheit.

To convert from Fahrenheit to Celsius, plug the numbers into an easy to remember formula where F is the degree in Fahrenheit, a is 1.8, and C is 32. Remember to use algebra when solving for C (just like solving for X).

$$C = \frac{F - 32}{1.8} \qquad F = 1.8(C) + 32$$

$$C = \frac{98.6 - 32}{1.8} \qquad F = 1.8(37) + 32$$

$$C = \frac{66}{1.8} \qquad F = 66.6 + 32$$

$$C = 37.0 \qquad F = 98.6$$

Volume and length in science have been based on the metric system for many decades, although in the United States, schools have resisted converting because of the large population already using the English system of measurement. However, in chemistry and pharmacy, it is used exclusively; therefore the metric system must be learned by all health care workers. The metric system units are always in multiples of 10, making it easier to learn than most mathematic units. Learning the prefix and suffix of each type of unit is the simplest way to memorize the metric system (Table 30.2).

For volume, the term "milli" means one-thousandth; therefore milliliter means one thousandth of a liter or 1 ml. Another unit that is equal to ml is a cubic centimeter (cc). A cubic centimeter is equal to one-thousandth of a liter. The most common volume measurements and English equivalents are listed in Table 30.3.

The metric length is based on meters, again 10 is the base number. A centimeter is one-hundredth of a meter or 0.01 meter. A standard inch is equivalent to 2.54 centimeters. A person who stands 5 feet tall is both 60 inches or (60 × 2.54 meters) 152.40 centimeters tall. A millimeter is one-thousandth of a meter; a kilometer is one thousand meters. There are about 30 centimeters per foot or approximately 90 centimeters per yard. By this number you can picture a meter next to a yard stick and see that it is about 10 centimeters different.

TABLE 30.2 Metric Terms

	Meaning	Unit Value
Prefix		
Micro	1 millionth	0.000001
Milli	1 thousandth	0.001
Centi	1 hundredth	0.01
Kilo	1 thousand	1000
Bases		
Liter	Volume	
Meter	Length	
Gram	weight	
Combined	**Terms**	
Microgram	1 mcg	0.000001 gram
Milliliter	1 ml	0.001 liter
Centimeter	1 cm	0.001 meter
Kilogram	1 kg	1000 grams

TABLE 30.3 Metric Measurements

ml or cc	Liters	Standard English Measurement
1	0.001	1/5 teaspoon (tsp)
5	0.005	1 tsp
15	0.015	1 tablespoon (tbsp)
*30 (29.57)	0.03	1 ounce
*240 (236)	0.24	1 cup
*500 (473)	1/2 liter or 0.5	1 pint
*1000 (946)	1 liter	1 quart

*Rounded.

DO YOU REMEMBER THESE KEY POINTS?

- The major chemical elements that are essential to humans
- The difference between ionic and covalent bonds
- The difference between an anion and a cation
- What makes up an element
- What makes up a molecule
- What an enzyme is and the importance of enzymatic reactions
- The measurements used in chemistry and in pharmacy
- The pH of the blood that is necessary for human life
- What makes a base or an acid

REVIEW QUESTIONS:

Multiple Choice

1. If the temperature is 100 degrees Fahrenheit, how many degrees Celsius is it?
   A. 37° Celsius
   B. 37.7° Celsius
   C. 73.3° Celsius
   D. None of the above

2. Which of the following statements is true concerning the parts of an atom?
   A. Protons are negatively charged, electrons are positively charged, and neutrons are neutral in charge
   B. Neutrons are negatively charged, electrons are positively charged, and protons are neutral in charge
   C. Protons are positively charged, neutrons are negatively charged, and electrons are neutral in charge
   D. Protons are positively charged, electrons are negatively charged, and neutrons are neutral in charge

3. Which of the following molecules is not essential to life?
   A. Carbohydrates
   B. Lipids
   C. Proteins
   D. All are important

4. The elements in the periodic table of elements are listed in order of all of the following criteria except
   A. According to properties and number of protons
   B. According to size
   C. According to their shapes
   D. According to weight of the atoms

5. Which of the chemicals listed has no charge when combined into a compound?
   A. Sodium chloride
   B. Sodium bicarbonate
   C. Ferrous sulfate
   D. Both A and B

6. The best definition to the distinction between organic and inorganic chemistry is
   A. Organic is about people, whereas inorganic is about all other life
   B. Organic is about carbon, whereas inorganic is not
   C. Organic is about humans, whereas inorganic is about bacterial components
   D. Organic explains reactions, whereas inorganic does not

7. Of the elements listed which is not monitored by the pharmacy when preparing hyperals for patients?
   A. Potassium   C. Magnesium
   B. Sodium   D. Hydrogen

8. Which chemical listed is a component of the enzyme adenosine triphosphate?
   A. Fe   C. P
   B. K   D. Both B and C

9. A blood pH of 7.9 is considered
   A. Acidic   C. Normal
   B. Basic   D. Buffered

10. Pyruvate is a key component is the making of
   A. Amino acids   C. The citric acid cycle
   B. The Krebs cycle   D. ATP

True/False
*If the statement is false, then change it to make it true.

1. Proteins are made up of amino acids.

2. Dehydration is the loss of a water molecule when amino acids combine.

3. Sodium chloride is a buffer.

4. Iron and zinc play key roles in the blood's hemoglobin count.

5. A peripheral parenteral nutrition may be ordered for a person who is unable to eat.

6. Most IV solutions are placed into isotonic solutions such as NaCl.

7. Anions are positive, whereas cations are negative.

8. Enzymes always make reactions move forward.

9. Metabolism is the making of molecules.

10. Ionic and covalent refer to the two types of bonds that atoms form.

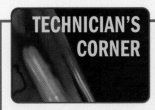

TECHNICIAN'S CORNER

A customer comes into the pharmacy to get a prescription for ferrous sulfate tablets filled. She is on the following drugs:

Tetracycline
Milk of Magnesia
Cimetidine

The pharmacist will give a consultation to the patient, letting her know if there is any problem, but you want to know for yourself if there is any contraindication. What, if any, interactions are there between ferrous sulfate and the patient's current medications?

Look up the answer in the *Mosby's Drug Consult*.

Starting Your
Career as a
Pharmacy Technician

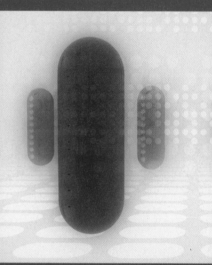

31 *Pharmacy Organizations and the Future of Technicians*

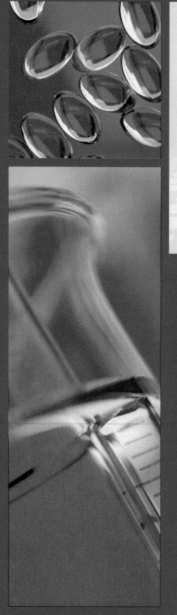

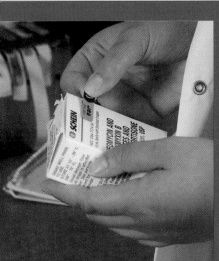

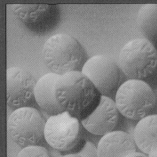

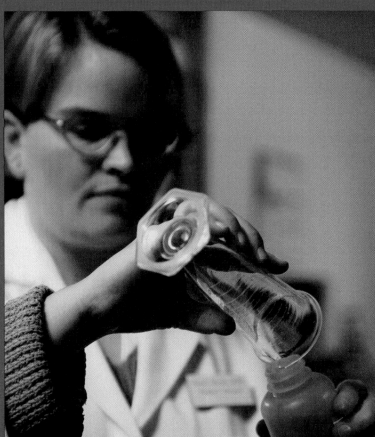

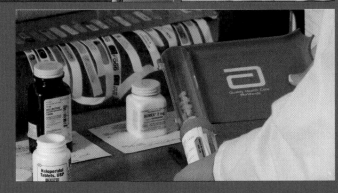

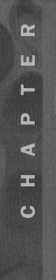

CHAPTER

31

Pharmacy Organizations and the Future of Technicians

Objectives

- List the most common organizations available to technicians.
- Determine which attributes each pharmacy organization has that are important to technicians.
- List the positive attributes of joining a pharmacy association.
- Demonstrate how to find a specific state's requirements for pharmacy technicians.
- Describe the changing trends in pharmacy technology as they pertain to technicians.
- Describe the various aspects of the National Certification Examination.
- List the various methods that pharmacy technicians can use to learn more about pharmacy.
- Explain how networking may be important in the search for a pharmacy technician position.
- How to approach job searching.
- How to use the Internet for research and information.

Introduction

Throughout this book, the role of technicians in pharmacy practice has been emphasized. As outlined in the History of Pharmacy (Chapter 1), the roles of pharmacy technicians have changed drastically over time. The primary role of technicians will continue to change in the foreseeable future. Among the changes are increased responsibility, a wider range of jobs available, bonuses, raises in pay, and better benefits. However, along with these changes comes the need for higher education, more legal responsibility, and continuing education. This trend can be seen across the United States as more states require a high school diploma in order for a person to become a registered technician, and more states have accepted the National Certification Board as their measure of the knowledge base of pharmacy technicians. This chapter is dedicated to the awareness of the future pharmacy technician—to learn about organizations and how they can best serve the technician and to know what there is to strive for in addition to the basic skill level. This will help the student technician determine the best road to follow. We begin with the basic information concerning the national organizations, then the benefits of certification and the importance of preparing to search for a job, and finally a look into the possible future roles of the pharmacy technician.

Organizations

There are four main associations that are concerned with the practice of pharmacy:

> American Society of Health-System Pharmacist (ASHP)
> American Association of Pharmacy Technicians (AAPT)
> National Pharmacy Technician Association (NPTA)
> American Pharmaceutical Association (APHA)

Each association has a state-run organization that can be accessed through its website. The only way to determine whether the organization in your state has the benefits that you require is to visit the website and learn about its resource areas for technicians. There are many different resources that will benefit the career-oriented technician, they are as follows:

- Continuing education
- Legislative movement toward promoting technicians
- A pharmacy technician division
- Journals, books, and other educational references
- Seminars for continuing education and networking capabilities
- Message boards for communicating with other technicians
- A good website that has links to other important technician sites

Table 31.1 lists the websites for each of the organizations. It would be good to visit each site and read the mission statement to find out the level at which pharmacy technicians participate in the association. Each individual state chapter may operate differently than another state's chapter. Therefore, it is important to check out your specific state's chapter to find the differences. As pharmacy technology increases in qualifications, responsibilities, and benefits, it is necessary to join an association that will provide continuing education specific to technicians and advocate for the profession.

TABLE 31.1 National Organizations of Pharmacy

Organization	History	Benefits	Resource Areas	Specific to Technicians	Miscellaneous	Fees*
ASHP www.ashp.org	Founded in 1925 to meet the needs of hospital pharmacy. Changed name in mid 90s from hospital pharmacy to health-system pharmacy to expand information and services to a wider range of pharmacies	Monthly journal includes continuing education Biannual seminar meetings Influences laws concerning pharmacy practice Other benefits: credit card, insurance coverage, member loan program, has product line for sales	Info on: Acute care, practice management, ambulatory care, clinical, home care, long-term care, managed care, students, technicians, patient safety	Accreditation process for pharmacy technician training programs provides course curriculum, aseptic technique videos, books, and links to other websites of interest	Each state has its own association headed by pharmacists Many have technician divisions, 30,000 members nationally	$57 annually (no journal)$ 148.00 includes journal No student rates available
AAPT www.pharmacy technician.com	Annual seminars include continuing education units, possible networking capabilities	Message board on Internet (to communicate with others), pharmacy technician products such as books, patches, bags, miscellaneous items	Links to websites	Promotes pharmacy technicians, provides continuing education specific to technicians	This organization is run by pharmacists and technicians. It has all seminar meetings in Midwest to East coast only, no West coast coverage	Active $50 annually Student $25 annually
NPTA www.pharmacy technician. org	Founded in 1992 by Mike Johnston; based in Houston TX	Journal: *Today's Technician* includes continuing education annual seminar meetings that includes continuing education for technicians and possible networking capabilities	Links to websites	Promotes pharmacy technicians, provides continuing education specific to technicians	This organization is run by and promotes only technicians. It is the newest organization of pharmacy technicians and has more than 25,000 members	$36 annually (no journal) $54 includes journal (includes free continuing education No student rates available
APHA www.apha net.org	Founded in 1852. First established pharmacy group in United States	Journal: *Pharmacy Today,* provides various insurance to members, discounts on cars, phones, and so forth	Links to websites	Some state branches allow technicians to join. Most do not have technician divisions and do not stress the vocation of technicians	N/A	$55 annually

*Fees are current at the time of this book's printing.

National Certification

In the infancy of any profession, a lack of regular guidelines and standards, or continuity, exists. Pharmacy technicians work across the United States and in all types of pharmacy settings under different rules determined by the individual states, which makes this profession challenging. At some point in the near future a national minimum standard for the profession must be met and agreed on across the United States. Although there will always be some variations from state to state, the overall skill level of a pharmacy technician should be a well-known standard. Currently there is a wide range of skill levels, experience, pay, and belief systems. One of the most basic aspects is the lack of a common title. Pharmacy technicians are also known as pharmacy clerks and pharmacy assistants. Other variances from state to state include pay, benefits, job description, and latitude of skill range.

The Pharmacy Technician Certification Board (PTCB) is an organization founded in 1995 by four organizations (listed in Box 31.1) with the intent to implement an examination, which would certify that a technician had met a basic skill level. The PTCB examination is given three times per year on the same days nationwide and at many different locations. There are different versions of the examination; therefore the results are weighted differently. The scoring is done by an independent group that grades the various areas of pharmacy knowledge based on the difficulty of the question. Because of the variance in examinations, the examination is described as being very easy to very hard. The passing score is 70%, and the results are sent out several weeks after the end of the examination. The types of pharmacy knowledge that are tested include the following:

- Pharmacy math
- Pharmacy law (federal only)
- Pharmacy operations
- Drug names (trade/generic)
- Drug classifications

Once certification is attained, technicians are required to obtain 20 hours of continuing education every 2 years. Continuing education can be obtained through pharmacy organizations that offer free continuing education to members, journals that include continuing edcation units, or seminars. Technicians who meet these requirements may use the initials CPhT on their identification tag, indicating that they are a certified pharmacy technician. Continuing edcation is less expensive for association members, although many drug companies give free continuing education units to pharmacists. Technicians can use the same continuing education units as pharmacists, although certain courses can be rather difficult

BOX 31.1 HISTORY OF THE PHARMACY TECHNICIAN CERTIFICATION BOARD (PTCB)

Founding Associations
American Society of Health-System Pharmacists (ASHP)
American Pharmaceutical Association (APHA)
Illinois Council of Health-System Pharmacists (ICHP)
Michigan Pharmacists Association (MPA)

Goals
To work more effectively with pharmacists
To give greater patient care and service
To create a minimum standard of knowledge of pharmacy technicians
To help employers determine knowledge base of pharmacy technicians

to understand. Independent pharmacists and other small businesses offer low-cost continuing education credit on the Internet.

Many pharmacy technicians receive a raise in pay after completion of the PTCB examination, although some pharmacies do not recognize the examination possibly to keep technician wages low. As time passes and federal and state regulations stiffen with respect to qualified personnel, the necessity of skilled technicians will undoubtedly rise to the top of pharmacy issues, and the examination will be accepted as a basic requirement (for further information, see Box 31.1 for the history of the examination).

Two Sides of the Story

If pharmacy technicians are not required to have a more in-depth knowledge of pharmacology and other aspects of pharmacy, then wages, benefits, and variety of skills will not increase. However, errors in pharmacy are increasing partially due to the shortage of pharmacists. Because of this shortage, pharmacists cannot perform all the tasks necessary, including overseeing technicians. If this continues, errors will continue to increase and pharmacies will be in direct noncompliance with the new laws requiring a decrease in error rate.

On the other hand, if the minimum requirement should include national certification or college degrees, then the current supply of pharmacy technicians would be in jeopardy because most seasoned technicians do not want to return to school to continue performing their jobs. In which case, a national pharmacy technician shortage could rival the current pharmacist shortage. Wages would rise sharply and errors again would become a problem with a shortage in workforce. What is the answer to this problem? The answer lies somewhere in the middle. Each state is researching the levels of training that it will require of its technicians and will allow a transition period for their current technicians. When the state of Texas required national certification, it allowed more than 1 year for all technicians to become certified. In addition, many pharmacies subsidized the cost of the examination if the technician passed and small raises have been given to technicians who were willing to reach the higher level of knowledge. However, many states do not require any type of skill level or even registration for their technicians.

The Professional Technician

Many websites are available to learn tips for preparing resumes and cover letters and about the interview process. Remember that as a student your work experience is not a strong point because this is a new vocation for you, instead you must focus on your educational background. It is important that the program you attend supply you with an adequate knowledge base to prepare you for this important vocation in pharmacy. The importance of attendance and punctuality in pharmacy cannot be stressed enough. It is best to arrive early for interviews and a few minutes early every day to work. This shows your dedication to your profession.

Less is More . . .

Pharmacy is predominantly a conservative profession. Dressing professionally includes proper clothing; shoes; hairstyle; and the lack of off-colored hair, facial jewelry, visible tattoos, or any other feature that detracts attention from your personality. Medical personnel should appear to be professional, knowledgeable, competent, and not scary looking to the patients. You will not find many doctors with strange haircuts or nurses with pierced noses popping bubble gum at the patient's bedside. It is just as important that the pharmacy technician show the public that he or she is professional and not view the vocation as just a job. This is shown directly and immediately by appearance and demeanor.

The Possibilities . . .

Although it is impossible to foresee the future of any profession, there are clear indications regarding the direction a profession is taking. Reviewing the history of pharmacy, a trend can be seen. The education requirements of pharmacists have increased from a BS degree in pharmacy (requiring 5 years of college) to a Pharm D degree (requiring 6 years) because of the necessary skill level needed in today's pharmacy practice. The pharmacist's role is more clinically oriented to patient consultation, as well as to providing information services to medical staff. The roles of pharmacy technicians are changing as well. The technician's role has evolved from a clerk, cashier, and shelf-stocker to a clinical technician, chemotherapy technician, nuclear medicine pharmacy technician, and inventory specialist technician. In addition to the change in duties are the changing guidelines that all states are researching to provide a base level of training for pharmacy technicians in the future.

Getting Involved

Each of the pharmacy organizations needs new pharmacy technician leaders and advocates who will promote the profession of pharmacy technicians.

TECH NOTE! The American Medical Association is one of the most well-known organizations that medical personnel reference for current information. Listed on its website are the most popular fast-growing new professions in the United States. It was no surprise that pharmacy technician was first on the list.

TECH NOTE! Each year pharmacy technicians celebrate the profession. National Pharmacy Week is held every October 20 to 26.

DO YOU REMEMBER THESE KEY POINTS?

- The new roles of pharmacists
- The new roles of pharmacy technicians
- The major pharmacy associations
- The types of resources that pharmacy associations offer technicians
- The importance of national certification and the benefits to technicians
- The requirements of national certification after passing the examination
- The type of information tested in the PTCB examination
- Why it is in the best interest of state pharmacy boards to either accept the PTCB or require their own examination for pharmacy technicians

REVIEW QUESTIONS:

Multiple Choice

1. The pharmacy association run for and solely by technicians is
   A. NPTA
   B. AAPT
   C. ASHP
   D. APHA

2. Certified technicians must meet which of the following PTCB standards?
   A. Continuing education
   B. State registration requirements
   C. Membership in a pharmacy association
   D. All of the above

3. All of the following statements are true concerning national certification except
   A. All 50 states have the examination the same day
   B. All 50 states have the examination three times per year
   C. All 50 states are aware of the certification examination results
   D. All 50 states give raises to technicians who pass the PTCB examination

4. All of the following statements are true concerning pharmacy technicians in general except
   A. Dressing professionally can increase chances of being hired
   B. Punctuality is extremely important in working in pharmacy
   C. It is not expected that pharmacy technicians take the PTCB examination
   D. Communication is an essential skill for pharmacy technicians

5. The following reasons to become involved in pharmacy organizations are true except
   A. For networking possibilities
   B. For new information on the future of pharmacy technicians
   C. To increase knowledge about new pharmaceuticals through CE
   D. For the tax deduction

True/False

*If the statement is false, then change it to make it true.

1. All technicians have the same level of knowledge and skills.

2. All states require registration and certification.

3. Pharmacy technicians can use continuing education units that are written for pharmacists.

4. Continuing education can be attained through pharmacy journals, seminars, and special presentations.

5. Technicians do not need to pay dues if they join a pharmacist's association.

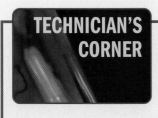

TECHNICIAN'S CORNER

Go to the following Internet sites and fill out the following questionnaire. This may be used to answer the questions at the end of this chapter.

www.ashp.org
www.aphanet.org
www.pharmacytechnician.org
www.pharmacytechnician.com

What is the current membership fee for a Pharmacy Tech Student?

Appendixes

A   *Abbreviations*

B   *200 Top-Selling Drugs for 2002*

C   *Top 30 Herbal Remedies*

D   *Math Review for Pharmacy Technicians*

E   *Health Insurance Portability and Accountability Act of 1996 (HIPAA)*

F   *Proper Hand Care for Medical Asepsis in Pharmacy*

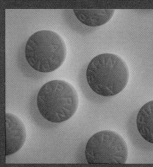

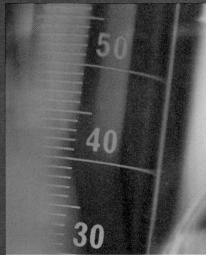

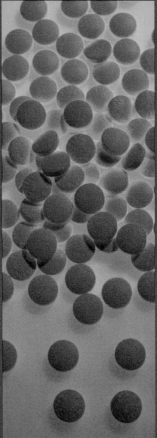

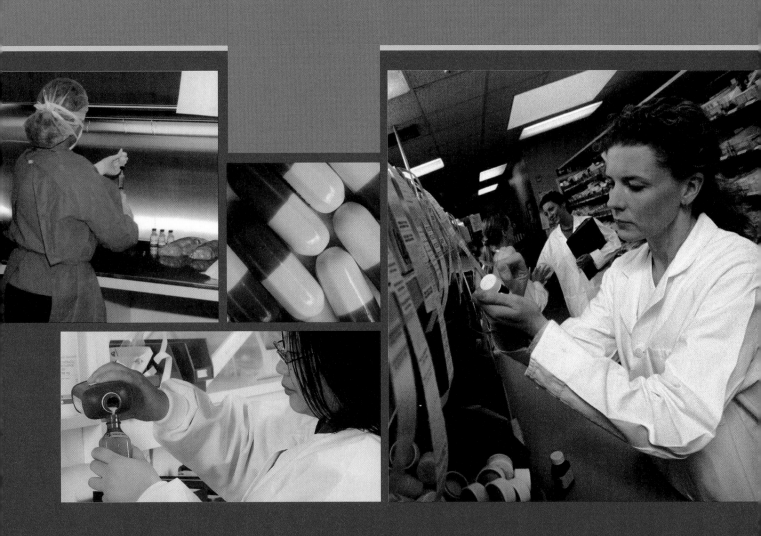

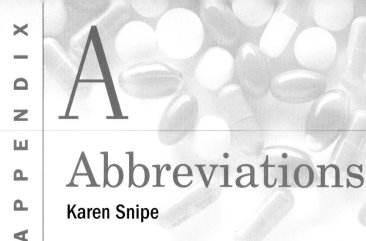

APPENDIX

A
Abbreviations

Karen Snipe

Common Abbreviations Used in Pharmacy

a̅a̅ *of each*

ac *before meals*

a.d. *right ear*

ad *up to*

ad lib *as needed or desired*

am *morning*

amp *ampule*

amt *amount*

a.s. *left ear*

asap *as soon as possible*

au *both ears*

aq *water*

bid *twice a day*

bm *bowel movement*

BP *blood pressure*

BSA *body surface area*

C *centigrade*

c̄ *with*

c *cup*

Ca *calcium*

cap *capsule*

CBC *complete blood count*

cc *cubic centimeter*

Cl *chlorine*

cm *centimeter*

CNS *central nervous system*

c/o *complaint of*

comp *compound*

CS *cesarian section*

CSF *cerebrospinal fluid*

CT *clotting time*

d *day*

D/C *discharge*

d/c *discontinue*

dict *as directed*

dil *dilute*

disp *dispense*

DNA *deoxyribonucleic acid*

DR, MD *doctor*

dr,℥ *dram*

Dx *diagnosis*

ECG, EKG *electrocardiogram*

EENT *eye, ear, nose, throat*

elix *elixir*

emul *emulsion*

Etoh *alcohol*

exp *expired*

ext *extract*

F *Fahrenheit*

Fe *iron*

FDA *Food and Drug Administration*

fl *fluid*

g *gram*

GI *gastrointestinal*

gr *grain*

gtt *drops*

H, hr *hour*

H_2O *water*

hs *bedtime, hour of sleep*

Hx *history*

IgG *immunoglobulin G*

IM *intramuscular*

inj *injection*

IT *intrathecal*

IU *International Unit*

IV *intravenous*

K *potassium*

kcal *kilocalorie*

kg *kilogram*

L *liter*

lb, # *pound*

liq *liquid*

m, ɱ *minim*

m *micron, microgram*

mcg *microgram*

mEq *milliequivalent*

Mg *magnesium*

mg *milligram*

min *minute*

mixt *mixture*

ml *milliliter*

mm *millimeter*

mo *month*

MRI *magnetic resonance imaging*

Na *sodium*

NaCl *sodium chloride*

neg *negative*

NF *National Formulary*

NKA *no known allergies*

NKDA *no known drug allergies*

non rep *do not repeat*

NS *normal saline*

N & V *nausea and vomiting*

no *number*

noc *in the night*

NPO *nothing by mouth*

NSAID *nonsteroidal antiinflammatory drug*

OD *right eye*

oint *ointment*

OR *operating room*

OS *left eye*

OTC *over the counter*

OU *each eye*

oz, ℥ *ounce*

p̄ *after*

pc *after meals*

per *by*

pm *afternoon*

po *by mouth*

pr *per rectum*

prn *whenever necessary*

pt *pint*

pt *patient*

pulv *powder*

q *every*

q2h *every 2 hours*

q4h *every 4 hours*

q6h *every 6 hours*

q8h *every 8 hours*

q12h *every 12 hours*

qam *every morning*

qd *every day*

qh *every hour*

qhs *every bedtime*

qid *four times a day*

qod *every other day*

qs *quantity sufficient*

qt *quart*

qty *quantity*

R/O *rule out*

RR *Recovery Room*

rep *repeat*

Rx *prescription, recipe*

s̄ *without*

sat *saturated*

SC, sq, subQ *subcutaneous*

Sig *label, let it be printed*

sl, subling *sublingual*

SOB *shortness of breath*

sol *solution*

solv *dissolve*

s̄s̄ *one-half*

stat *immediately*

supp *suppository*

SWI *sterile water for injection*

syr *syringe, syrup*

tabs *tablets*

tbsp *tablespoonful*

temp *temperature*

tid *three times a day*

tr, tinc *tincture*

trit *triturate*

tsp *teaspoonful*

u.d., u.dict *as directed*

ung *ointment*

USAN *United States adopted names*

USP *United States Pharmacopeia*

UTI *urinary tract infection*

vag *vaginal*

VO *verbal order*

vol *volume*

VS *vital signs*

wa *while awake*

x *times*

y *year*

> *greater than*

< *less than*

= *equal to*

↑ *increase*

↓ *decrease*

Drug and Chemical Abbreviations

ACE *angiotensin-converting enzyme*

APAP *acetaminophen*

ASA *aspirin, acetylsalicylic acid*

AZT *zidovudine*

Ca *calcium*

CCB *calcium channel blocker*

Cl *chlorine*

CO$_2$ *carbon dioxide*

DDAVP *desmopressin acetate*

DES *diethylstilbestrol*

DIG *digoxin*

D5 *5% dextrose*

D5/0.9 NS *5% dextrose and 0.9% sodium chloride*

Fe *iron*

FeSO$_4$ *ferrous sulfate*

HCl *hydrochloric acid*

HCTZ *hydrochlorothiazide*

H$_2$O *water*

INH *isoniazid*

K *potassium*

KCl *potassium chloride*

MAOI *monoamine oxidase inhibitors*

MgSO$_4$ *magnesium sulfate*

MOM *milk of magnesia*

MS, MSO$_4$ *morphine sulfate*

MVI *multivitamin*

NaCl *sodium chloride*

NaHCO$_3$ *sodium bicarbonate*

NPH *neutral protamine Hagedorn (insulin)*

NSAID *nonsteroidal antiinflammatory drug*

NTG *nitroglycerin*

O$_2$ *oxygen*

PB *phenobarbital*

PCA *patient-controlled analgesia*

PCN *penicillin*
PNV *prenatal vitamins*
T$_3$ *triiodothyronine*
T$_4$ *levothyroxine*
TCN *tetracycline*
TMP *trimethoprim*
TMP/SMX *trimethoprim / sulfamethoxazole*
t-PA *tissue plasminogen activator*
ZnO *zinc oxide*

Disease States

AIDS *acquired immunodeficiency syndrome*
CA *cancer*
CHF *congestive heart failure*
CVA *cerebrovascular accident*
DVT *deep vein thrombosis*
GERD *gastroesophageal reflux disease*
HIV *human immunodeficiency virus*
HTN *hypertension*
MI *myocardial infarction (heart attack)*
MS *multiple sclerosis*
URI *upper respiratory infection*
UTI *urinary tract infection*

Organizations

AAPT *American Association of Pharmacy Technicians*
APhA *American Pharmaceutical Association*
ASHP *American Society of Health-Systems Pharmacists*
CDC *Centers for Disease Control and Prevention*
DEA *Drug Enforcement Administration*
FDA *Food and Drug Administration*
HCFA *Health Care Financing Administration*
NHA *National Healthcareer Association*
JCAHO *Joint Commission on Accreditation of Healthcare Organizations*
NABP *National Association of the Boards of Pharmacy*
P&T *Pharmacy and Therapeutics Committee*
PTCB *Pharmacy Technician Certification Board*
PTEC *Pharmacy Technician Education Council*

B

200 Top-Selling Drugs for 2002

Karen Snipe

Trade Name	Generic Name	Indication
1. Premarin	Conjugated estrogens	Hormonal replacement
2. Synthroid, Levoxyl	Levothyroxine	Hormonal replacement
3. Lipitor	Atorvastatin	Lipid/cholesterol lowering
4. Prilosec	Omeprazole	Ulcers/GERD
5. Lortab, Vicodin	Hydrocodone/APAP	Narcotic analgesic
6. Proventil	Albuterol	Asthma/bronchodilator
7. Norvasc	Amlodipine	Hypertension/calcium channel blocker
8. Claritin	Loratadine	Antihistamine
9. Trimox, Amoxil	Amoxicillin	Antibiotic
10. Prozac	Fluoxetine	Antidepressant
11. Zoloft	Sertraline	Antidepressant
12. Glucophage	Metformin	Diabetes
13. Lanoxin	Digoxin	Cardiac glycoside/fibrillation
14. Prempro	Conjugated estrogen/medroxyprogesterone	Hormonal replacement
15. Paxil	Paroxetine	Antidepressant
16. Zithromax (Z-pack)	Azithromycin	Antibiotic
17. Zestril	Lisinopril	HBP/ACE inhibitor
18. Zocor	Simvastatin	Lipid/cholesterol lowering
19. Prevacid	Lansoprazole	Ulcers/GERD
20. Augmentin	Amoxicillin/clavulanate potassium	Antibiotic
21. Celebrex	Celecoxib	NSAID/COX2 inhibitor
22. Coumadin	Warfarin	Anticoagulant
23. Vasotec	Enalapril	HBP/ACE inhibitor
24. Lasix	Furosemide	CHF/loop diuretic
25. Cipro	Ciprofloxacin	Antibiotic
26. Keflex, Keftab	Cephalexin	Antibiotic
27. K-Dur	Potassium chloride	Potassium supplement
28. Deltasone	Prednisone	Antiinflammatory steroid
29. Pravachol	Pravastatin	Lipid/cholesterol lowering
30. Biaxin	Clarithromycin	Antibiotic
31. Ortho Tri-Cyclen	Norgestimate/ethinyl estradiol	Birth control
32. Tylenol #3	Acetaminophen/codeine	Narcotic analgesic
33. Tenormin	Atenolol	HBP, beta-blocker

Trade Name	Generic Name	Indication
34. Zyrtec	Cetirizine	Antihistamine
35. Ambien	Zolpidem	Hypnotic/insomnia
36. Darvocet N	Propoxyphene N/APAP	Narcotic analgesic
37. Xanax	Alprazolam	Anxiety/panic disorder
38. Ultram	Tramadol	Analgesic
39. Accupril	Quinapril	HBP, ACE inhibitor
40. Cardizem CD	Diltiazem	Angina/HBP, calcium channel blocker
41. Glucotrol XL	Glipizide	Diabetes
42. Allegra	Fexofenadine	Antihistamine
43. Toprol XL	Metoprolol	HBP/beta-blocker
44. Dyazide	Triamterene/HCTZ	CHF
45. Cardura	Doxazosin	HBP/alpha-blocker
46. Fosamax	Alendronate	Osteoporosis
47. Lotensin	Benazepril	HBP/ACE inhibitor
48. Procardia XL/Adalat CC	Nifedipine	Angina/calcium channel blocker
49. Viagra	Sildenafil citrate	Erectile dysfunction
50. Advil, Motrin, Nuprin	Ibuprofen	NSAID
51. Depakote	Valproate sodium	Seizures
52. Dilantin	Phenytoin	Anticonvulsant
53. Wellbutrin SR	Bupropion HCl	Antidepressant
54. Neurontin	Gabapentin	Anticonvulsant
55. Cozaar	Losartan	HBP/vasoconstrictor
56. Diflucan	Fluconazole	Antifungal
57. Claritin D	Loratadine/pseudoephedrine	Antihistamine/decongestant
58. Relafen	Nabumetone	NSAID/osteoarthritis
59. Avandia	Rosiglitazone maleate	Diabetes
60. Levaquin	Levofloxacin	Antibiotic
61. Risperdal	Risperidone	Antipsychotic
62. Xalatan	Latanoprost	Glaucoma
63. Cefzil	Cefprozil	Antibiotic
64. Triphasil, Trivora-28	L-norgestrel/ethinyl estradiol	Birth control
65. Ziac	Bisoprolol/HCTZ	HBP, beta-blocker
66. Serevent	Salmeterol	Asthma
67. Lescol	Fluvastatin	Lipid/cholesterol lowering
68. Ortho Novum 7/7/7	Norethindrone/ethinyl estradiol	Birth control
69. Imitrex	Sumatriptan	Migraines
70. Flovent	Fluticasone propionate	Asthma
71. Ceftin	Cefuroxime	Antibiotic
72. Celexa	Citalopram	Antidepressant
73. Effexor XR	Venlafaxine	Antidepressant
74. Septra, Bactrim	Trimethoprim/sulfamethoxazole	Antibiotic
75. Zyprexa	Olanzapine	Antipsychotic
76. Zantac	Ranitidine	Ulcer/H2 blocker
77. Singulair	Montelukast	Asthma
78. Vioxx	Rofecoxib	NSAID/COX2 inhibitor
79. Plavix	Clopidogrel	Atherosclerosis/antiplatelet
80. Diovan	Valsartan	HBP, angiotensin II receptor
81. Hyzaar	Losartan/HCTZ	HBP, diuretic
82. Serzone	Nefazodone	Antidepressant
83. Bactroban	Mupirocin	Topical antibiotic
84. Zestoretic	Lisinopril/HCTZ	HBP, ACE inhibitor
85. Evista	Raloxifene	Osteoporosis
86. Miacalcin	Calcitonin salmon	Paget's disease/osteoporosis

Trade Name	Generic Name	Indication
87. Prinivil	Lisinopril	HBP, ACE inhibitor
88. Adderall	Amphetamine mixed salts	CNS stimulant/ADHD
89. Detrol	Tolterodine	Urinary incontinence
90. Azmacort, Nasacort	Triamcinolone	Corticosteroid/allergies
91. Amaryl	Glimepiride	Diabetes type II
92. Combivent	Ipratropium/albuterol	Asthma
93. Lotrel	Amlodipine/benazepril	HBP, ACE inhibitor
94. Alesse	Levonorgestrel/eth. estradiol	Birth control
95. Calan, Isoptin	Verapamil	HBP, angina
96. Plendil	Felodipine	HBP/calcium channel blocker
97. OxyContin	Oxycodone	Narcotic analgesic
98. Concerta	Methylphenidate XR	ADD, ADHD, narcolepsy
99. Phenergan	Promethazine	Antihistamine/antinausea
100. Nolvadex	Tamoxifen	Breast cancer
101. Aricept	Donepezil	Alzheimer's disease/dementia
102. Tiazac, Cartia XT	Diltiazem	Angina/calcium channel blocker
103. Arthrotec	Diclofenac misoprostol	Arthritis
104. Tobradex	Tobramycin/dexamethasone	Ophthalmic agent
105. Elavil	Amitriptyline	Antidepressant
106. Alphagan	Brimonidine	Glaucoma
107. Altace	Ramipril	HBP, ACE inhibitor
108. Flomax	Tamsulosin	Benign prostatic hyperplasia
109. Accutane	Isotretinoin	Acne
110. Combivir	Zidovudine/lamivudine	Antiviral/AIDS
111. Humulin N	Insulin	Diabetes type I
112. Viracept	Nelfinavir	Antiviral/AIDS
113. Valtrex	Valacyclovir	Antiviral
114. Dynacin	Minocycline	Antibiotic
115. Ritalin	Methylphenidate	ADHD
116. Tagamet	Cimetidine	Ulcers/H2 antagonist
117. Zovirax	Acyclovir	Antiviral
118. Rheumatrex	Methotrexate	Antineoplastic/rheumatoid arthritis
119. Nexium	Esomeprazole	GERD
120. Inderal	Propanolol	HBP, myocardial infarction, migraines
121. Cleocin	Clindamycin	Antibiotic
122. Advair Diskus	Salmeterol/fluticasone	Asthma, bronchodilator
123. Zerit	Stavudine	Antiviral
124. Antivert	Meclizine	Motion sickness, vertigo
125. Mircette	Desogestrel/ethinyl estradiol	Birth control
126. Epivir	Lamivudine	Antiviral
127. Coreg	Carvedilol	HBP, beta-blocker
128. Skelaxin	Metaxalone	Muscle relaxant
129. Proscar	Finasteride	Benign prostatic hyperplasia
130. Vicoprofen	Hydrocodone/ibuprofen	Narcotic analgesic
131. Loestrin FE	Norethindrone/eth. estradiol	Birth control
132. Nasonex, Elocon	Mometasone furoate	Topical corticosteroid
133. Soma	Carisoprodol	Muscle relaxant
134. Cleocin	Clindamycin	Antibiotic
135. Vibramycin	Doxycycline	Antibiotic
136. Plaquenil	Hydroxychloroquine	Malaria
137. Glucotrol	Glipizide	Diabetes type II
138. Pamelor	Nortriptyline	Antidepressant
139. Lodine	Etodolac	NSAID/osteoarthritis

Trade Name	Generic Name	Indication
140. Naprosyn	Naproxen	NSAID
141. Tegretol	Carbamazepine	Seizures
142. Fiorinal	Butalbital/aspirin/caffeine	Analgesic
143. Compazine	Prochlorperazine	Antipsychotic
144. Tofranil	Imipramine	Antidepressant
145. Flagyl	Metronidazole	Antiprotozoal
146. Reglan	Metoclopramide	Antiemetic/nausea
147. Retin-A	Tretinoin	Acne
148. Avapro	Irbesartan	HBP, ACE inhibitor
149. Feldene	Piroxicam	NSAID/arthritis
150. Bentyl	Dicyclomine Chloride	Irritable bowel syndrome
151. Atarax	Hydroxyzine HCl	Anxiety, tension
152. Mycostatin	Nystatin	Antifungal
153. Atrofen	Baclofen	Muscle relaxant
154. Glucovance	Glyburide/metformin	Antidiabetic
155. Theo-Dur, Slo-bid	Theophylline	Bronchodilator
156. Lithonate	Lithium carbonate	Mania/antipsychotic
157. Fioricet	Butalbital/codeine/APAP	Narcotic analgesic
158. Sinemet	Carbidopa/levodopa	Parkinson's disease
159. Indocin	Indomethacin	NSAID
160. Betapace	Sotalol	Ventricular arrhythmias
161. DDAVP	Desmopressin	Diabetes/hemophilia
162. Nizoral	Ketoconazole	Antifungal
163. Nitrostat	Nitroglycerin	Angina
164. Haldol	Haloperidol	Antipsychotic
165. Luminal	Phenobarbital	Anticonvulsant
166. Dura-Tabs	Quinidine sulfate	Atrial arrhythmias
167. Lotrimin	Clotrimazole	Antifungal
168. Droxia, Hydrea	Hydroxyurea	Cancer/brain tumors
169. Duphalac	Lactulose	Laxative
170. Colchicine	Colchicine	Gout
171. Toradol	Ketorolac	NSAID
172. Cogentin	Benztropine	Parkinson's disease
173. Garamycin	Gentamycin	Antibiotic
174. Sumycin	Tetracycline	Antibiotic
175. Benemid	Probenecid	Gout
176. Estrace	Estradiol	Hormonal replacement
177. Asacol	Mesalamine	Antiinflammatory
178. Zofran	Ondansetron HCl	Antinausea (chemotherapy)
179. Baycol	Cerivastatin sodium	Cholesterol lowering
180. Neoral	Cyclosporine	Immunosuppressant
181. Neupogen	Filgrastim	Neutropenia
182. Luvox	Fluvoxamine maleate	Obsessive compulsive disorder/ antidepressant
183. Benzamycin	Erythromycin/benzoyl peroxide	Acne
184. Humalog	Insulin lispro	Diabetes type I
185. Accolate	Zafirlukast	Asthma
186. Crixivan	Indinavir sulfate	HIV/AIDS
187. Roxicet, Endocet	Oxycodone/APAP	Narcotic analgesic
188. Pulmicort Turbohaler	Budesonide	Allergies
189. Lupron Depot	Leuprolide acetate	Prostate cancer
190. Catapres	Clonidine HCl	HBP
191. Stadol NS	Butorphanol tartrate	Narcotic analgesic

Trade Name	Generic Name	Indication
192. Viramune	Nevirapine	Antiviral
193. Cosopt	Dorzolamide/timolol	Glaucoma
194. Prandin	Repaglinide	Diabetes type II
195. Remeron	Mirtazapine	Antidepressant
196. Humulin 70/30	Insulin	Diabetes type I
197. Ditropan XL	Oxybutynin Cl	Bladder instability
198. Tricor	Fenofibrate	Hyperlipidemia
199. Cortisporin	Neomycin/polymyxin/hydrocortisone	Topical antibiotic
200. Corgard	Nadolol	HBP/beta-blocker

ACE, angiotensin-converting enzyme; ADD, attention deficit disorder; ADHD, attention deficit and hyperactivity disorder; AIDS, acquired immunodeficiency syndrome; APAP, acetaminophen; CHF, congestive heart failure; CNS, central nervous system; GERD, gastroesophageal reflux disease; HBP, high blood pressure; HCTZ, hydrochlorothiazide; NSAID, nonsteroidal antiinflammatory drug.

C

Top 30 Herbal Remedies

Karen Snipe

Trade Name	Generic Name	Reported Uses
Aloe Vera (leaf)	*Aloe* spp.	Wound and burn healing
American Ginseng (root)	Ginseng	Energy, stress, immune system builder
Bilberry (berry)	*Vaccinium myrtillus*	Eye and vascular disorders
Cascara Sagrada (aged bark)	*Rhamnus persiana*	Laxative
Cat's Claw (root, bark)	*Uncaria tomantosa*	Antiinflammatory, antimicrobial, antioxidant, immunosupportive
Chondroitin	Nutriceutical	Osteoarthritis
Cranberry (berry)	*Vaccinium macrocarpon*	Urinary tract infection
Echinacea (flower, root)	*Echinacea purpurea* *Echinacea angustifolia*	Antiviral, arthritis, immunostimulant
Evening Primrose (seed oil)	*Oenothera biennis*	ADD, diabetes, skin disorders, endometriosis, hyperglycemia, MS, PMS, menopause, arthritis
Feverfew (leaf)	*Tanacetum parthenium*	Antiinflammatory, rheumatoid arthritis, migraines
Garlic (bulb)	*Allium sativum*	Antimicrobial, HBP, cholesterol
Ginger (root)	*Zingiber officinale*	Antiemetic, antiinflammatory, GI distress, dyspepsia
Ginkgo Biloba (root)	*Ginkgo biloba*	Memory, increased blood flow, dementia, asthma
Glucosamine	Nutriceutical	Osteoarthritis and rheumatoid arthritis
Goldenseal (root)	*Hydratis canadensis*	Antimicrobial, gastritis, bronchitis, cystitis
Grapeseed (seed, skin)	*Vitis vinifera*	Antioxidant, allergies, circulation, asthma
Green Tea (leaf)	*Camellia sinesis*	Anticancer, antioxidant, lower cholesterol
Isoflavones (Soy)	Nutriceutical	Cancer prevention, decreased bone loss, lower cholesterol, menopausal symptoms
Kava (root)	*Piper methysticum*	ADD, ADHD, anxiety, sedation
Milk Thistle (seed)	*Silybum marianum*	Antioxidant, liver diseases
Panax (Asian) (root)	*Panax ginseng*	Same as American ginseng
Saw Palmetto (berry)	*Serenoa repens*	Benign prostatic hyperplasia
Siberian Ginseng (root)	*Eleutherococcus senticosus*	Athletic performance, stress, immune builder
St. John's Wort (flowering buds)	*Hypericum perforatum*	Depression, anxiety, antiviral, antibacterial, antiinflammatory
Valerian (root)	*Valeriana officinalis*	Sedative, PMS, menopause, muscle spasms
Wild Yam (tuber)	*Dioscorea villosa*	Female vitality
Black Cohosh (root)	*Cimicifuga racemosa*	Menopause, PMS, mild depression, arthritis
Fish oils	Nutriceutical	Diabetes, dysmenorrhea, HBP, memory, psoriasis
Melatonin	Nutriceutical	Insomnia
Dong Quai (root)	*Angelica sinensis*	Anemia, HBP, energy (females), menopause, dysmenorrhea, PMS

ADD, attention deficit disorder; ADHD, attention deficit hyperactivity disorder; GI, gastrointestinal; HBP, high blood pressure; MS, multiple sclerosis; PMS, premenstrual syndrome.

D

Math Review for Pharmacy Technicians

James J. Mizner, Jr

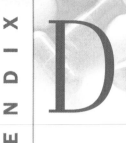

Proportions

A ratio is a relationship between two parts of a whole or between one part and the whole. A ratio can be written either as 1/2 or 1:2. A proportion is a relationship between two ratios. A proportion may be written as 1/2 = 2/4 or 1:2::2:4. Most pharmaceutical calculations performed in either retail or institutional settings can be accomplished by using proportions.

There are two ways to solve proportion problems. The first involves cross multiplying and dividing, and the second is described as comparing the means and extremes. Both methods will yield the same answer if set up correctly. The following problem is solved using both methods.

$$\frac{4}{7} = \frac{x}{28} \text{ where } x \text{ is the unknown}$$

METHOD 1: CROSS MULTIPLY AND DIVIDE

$$\frac{4}{7} = \frac{x}{28}$$

1. Multiply the numerator on the left hand side of the equation by the denominator on the right hand side

$$4 \times 28 = 112$$

2. Multiply the denominator of the left hand side of the equation by the numerator on the right hand side of the equation

$$7 \times x = 7x$$

3. Divide both sides of the equation by the denominator that is on the side where a number is multiplied by x.

$$\frac{112}{7} = \frac{7x}{7}$$

$$16 = x$$

4. Always make sure that measurement units (such as *mg* or *units*) in the numerators correspond with one another and the units in the denominators are the same with one another. If they are not, the likelihood of an incorrect answer increases.

METHOD 2: MEANS AND EXTREMES

1. $4:7::x:28$, where the first and last number in the series are considered the extremes and the two numbers in the middle are considered the means. In this situation the 4 and the 28 represent the extremes and the 7 and *x* represent the means. One multiplies the extremes (4×28) and then multiplies the means $(7 \times x)$.

$$4 \times 28 = 7 \times x$$
$$112 = 7x$$

2. Divide both sides of the equation by the number that is on the side where a number is multiplied by *x*.

$$112 \div 7 = 7x \div 7$$
$$16 = x$$

3. Always make sure that the measurement units (such as *mg* or *units*) in the first and third positions are the same and that the units in the second and fourth position are the same. If they are not, the likelihood of an incorrect answer increases.

QUESTIONS
1. If you have a cephalexin suspension of 250 mg/5 ml and need a dose of 375 mg, how many ml do you need?
2. If you have an albuterol liquid of 2 mg/5 ml and need a dose of 6 mg, how many ml do you need?
3. If you have atenolol 50 mg/tablet and need a dose of 25 mg, how many tablets do you need?
4. If you have Warfarin 5 mg/tablet and need a dose of 17.5 mg, how many tablets do you need?
5. If you have aspirin 5 gr/tablet and need a dose of 7.5 gr, how many tablets do you need?

Percents

Percents are another method of showing a relationship between parts and the whole. Percent means "parts per 100." A number less than 1 is considered less than 100%, and a number greater than 1 is greater than 100%. A percent can be calculated using ratios, fractions, or decimals.

RULES

1. To convert a decimal to percent, multiply the number by 100 and add a percent (%) sign.
2. To convert a percent to a decimal, remove the % sign and divide by 100.
3. To convert a fraction to a percent, divide the numerator by the denominator, multiply by 100, and add a % sign.
4. To convert a percent to a fraction, drop the % sign, write the value of the number as the numerator, place it over a denominator of 100, and reduce it to its lowest terms.
5. To convert a ratio to a percent, divide the first number by the second number, multiply by 100 and add a % sign.

Percents can be calculated by setting up a proportion. The numerator represents parts and the denominator wholes. The left hand side of the equation can be expressed as

$$\frac{\text{Parts of the whole}}{\text{Whole}}$$

The right hand side of the equation is expressed in a percent form, where the numerator is a percent of the whole (the denominator is considered 100%).

$$\frac{\text{Percent}}{100\%}$$

The equation would look like this:

$$\frac{\text{Parts of the whole}}{\text{Whole}} = \frac{\text{Percent}}{100\%}$$

To solve this type of problem, one must know two of the three variables: parts of the whole, the whole, or percent. One must identify the term as a part of the whole, the whole, or a percent. After identifying them and placing them in the equation, one cross multiplies and divides to find the missing term.

QUESTIONS
1. What is 25% of 60?
2. What is 9% of 70?
3. What percent is 14 of 30?
4. What percent is 17 of 85?
5. What number is 105% of 95?
6. What number is 75% of 75?

Metric, Household, and Apothecary Conversions

The practice of pharmacy uses the metric system, the household system, and the apothecary system for the calculation of dosage and doses. A pharmacy technician must be able to calculate doses of medication in any of these systems and to convert them from one system to another system. It is essential to memorize the basic conversions. By using proportions one can solve any conversion.

METRIC SYSTEM

Weight (gram)
1000 microgram (mcg) = 1 milligram (mg)
1000 mg = 1 gram (g)
1000 g = 1 kilogram (kg)
Volume (liter)
1000 ml = 1 liter (l)

HOUSEHOLD SYSTEM

Weight
2.2 lb = 1 kg
Volume
5 ml = 1 teaspoon (tsp)
3 tsp = 1 tablespoon (tbsp)
2 tbsp = 1 fluid ounce (fl oz)
8 fl oz = 1 cup

2 cups = 1 pint (pt)
2 pt = 1 quart (qt)
4 qt = 1 gallon (gal)

APOTHECARY SYSTEM

Weight
20 grains (gr) = 1 scruple
3 scruples = 1 dram
8 drams = 1 ounce
12 ounces = 1 pound
Volume
60 minims = 1 fluid dram
8 fluid dram = 1 fluid ounce

Apothecary	Metric
16.23 minims	= 1 ml
1 fl dram	= 4 ml
1 fl oz	= 29.57 ml (30 ml)
1 g	= 15.432 gr
1 gr	= 65 mg
1 lb (avoirdupois)	= 454 g
1 oz (apothecary)	= 31.1 g
1 oz (avoirdupois)	= 28.35 g

QUESTIONS

1. How many mg are in 25 g?
2. How many grams is 1.5 kg?
3. How many ml are in 2.5 fl oz?
4. How many teaspoons are in 4 fl oz?
5. How many tablespoons are in 1 fluid pint?
6. How many ml are in 1.75 liters?
7. How many mg are in 7.5 gr?
8. How many gr are in 200 mg?
9. How many g are in 4 oz (wt)?
10. How many mcg are in 0.5 mg?
11. How many pounds does a 60-kg person weigh?
12. You have a pint solution containing 5 mg/ml. How many mg does the pint contain?
13. A dose of an antacid is 1 tablespoon. How many doses are in an 8-oz bottle?
14. You are to prepare a dose containing 5 gr of active ingredient. How many 65-mg tablets will be used?
15. A physician orders diphenhydramine elixir 2 tsp four times a day. A 4-oz bottle containing 12.5 mg per teaspoon is supplied. How many mg will the patient receive in each dose?
16. You are told to dispense 1 cup of medication. The dose is 1 tablespoon and the concentration is 20 mg/ml. How many grams of medication are being dispensed?
17. If there are 25 mg in a tablespoon, how many grams are in 1 liter of solution?
18. A 6 fl oz bottle of cough syrup is given as 1 tsp four times a day. How many doses are in the bottle?
19. A patient is to receive one tablet of Nitrostat 1/200 gr. How many mg are in one tablet?
20. A medication has 150 mg in 480 ml. How many mg are in 1.5 fl oz?
21. How many gr are found in 0.4 mg?
22. There are 100 mg in a teaspoon. How many grams are in 1 gallon?

23. One pint of a product contains 500 mg. How many mg are found in 5 ml?

24. There are 250 mcg in 1 teaspoon. How many mg are in 4 fl oz?

25. How many grains are found in a teaspoon of medication if it contains 125 mg/teaspoon?

Units

Several pharmaceutical products made from biological products are expressed as "units" or International Units. Examples of these products include insulin, heparin, and vitamin E. Units represent an amount of activity within a particular system. Each pharmaceutical product is unique in determining the amount of activity of that product. Units represent a concentration and may be expressed as units/tablet or units/ml.

QUESTIONS

1. A patient is to receive Humulin insulin (100 units/ml) at a dose of 65 units at 7:30 am. How many ml should be drawn into the insulin syringe?

2. You are to prepare a minibag of intravenous fluids and must put 1000 units of heparin in 100 ml of normal saline. You have a multidose vial that has 10,000 units/10 ml. How many milliliters must be put in the intravenous minibag?

3. A physician's hospital medication order calls for isophane insulin suspension to be administered to a 150-lb patient on the basis of 1 unit/kg per 24 hours. How many units of isophane insulin suspension should be administered daily?

4. Pertussis vaccine contains 4 protective units per 0.5 ml. How many protective units would be contained in a 7.5-ml multiple dose vial?

5. If 1 mg of penicillin V represents 1520 penicillin V units, how many micrograms represent 1 unit?

Milliequivalents

Certain pharmaceutical products contain dissolved mineral salts and are capable of carrying an electrical charge through the solution. These substances are measured in milliequivalents (mEq) and are extremely important when working with intravenous fluids. Sodium chloride (NaCl) and potassium chloride (KCl) are two of the more common products expressed in mEq.

QUESTIONS

1. An order requires 30 mEq of potassium phosphate. You have available 4.4 mEq/ml of potassium. How many milliliters will you put in the intravenous bag? (Hint: 4.4 mEq : 1 ml :: 30 mEq : x)

2. A 20% KCl solution has a strength of 40 mEq in 15 ml. You receive an order for 20 mEq, how many milliliters are needed?

Pediatric Dosages

Children require different amounts of medication than adults. These doses are affected by the individual's age, weight, body surface area, organ development, sex, and disease state. Age in children is broken down into the following general categories:

Neonate: birth to 1 month
Infant: 1 month to 1 year

Early childhood: 1 year to 5 years
Late childhood: 6 years to 12 years
Adolescence: 13 years to 17 years

To calculate the appropriate dosage for children, one of several methods may be used. Young's rule uses age as a guide for children 1 to 12 years old; Clark's rule uses weight as the determining factor; mg/kg uses the patient's weight in kg; and body surface area uses both height and weight as the basis for choosing a dose.

$$\text{Young's rule} = \frac{\text{Age of child (expressed in years)}}{\text{Adult of child (in years)} + 12} \times \text{Adult dose}$$

$$\text{Clark's rule} = \frac{\text{Weight of child (expressed in pounds)}}{150 \text{ lbs}} \times \text{Adult dose}$$

All four of the previously mentioned methods require the use of the adult dose for drug calculation, and the given parameter desired by each method should be provided so that the practitioner can calculate the appropriate pediatric dose. The adult dose may be measured in mg, ml, units, mEq, gr, or tablets.

QUESTIONS

1. How much medication should be given to a 5-year-old child if the adult dose is 500 mg?

2. How much medication should be given to a child weighing 60 lbs if the adult dose is 100 mg?

3. How much medication should be give to a child weighing 40 lbs if the adult dose is 2 mg/kg/day?

4. How much medication should be given in one dose to a child weighing 70 lbs if the adult dose is 10 mg/kg/day and the patient is to receive four doses a day?

5. How much medication should be given to a child who is 30 months old if the adult dose is 100 mg?

Concentration/Dilution

A concentration is a strength. It can be expressed as a fraction (e.g., mg/ml, mEq/ml, units/ml), a ratio (e.g., 1:100, 1:1000, 1:10,000), or a percent (e.g., 10%, 25%, 50%). Percents are found in solids (%w/w) and in solutions (%w/v or %v/v).

The %w/w is the number of grams per 100 g, %w/v is the number of grams per 100 ml, and %v/v is the number of ml/100 ml.

More than 90% of all problems involving concentrations result in a dilution, or in compounding a final product in which the final concentration is less than the initial strength. In daily application, a pharmacist receives an order to prepare a product of a given strength and volume (weight). This is known as the final strength (FS) and final volume (FV). The pharmacist must go to the shelf, choose the product of a given strength [initial strength –(IS)], and determine the amount [initial volume (IV)] needed to prepare the compound. The same process is done in preparing solids, except an initial weight (IW) and final weight (FW) are substituted for initial and final volumes.

One can use the following equation for this situation:

$$\text{Initial Volume} \times \text{Initial Strength} = \text{Final Volume} \times \text{Final Strength}$$

or

$$\text{IV} \times \text{IS} = \text{FV} \times \text{FS}$$

THREE HINTS TO PREVENT ERRORS IN SOLVING DILUTION PROBLEMS

1. Initial Strength (IS) must be larger than Final Strength (FS).
2. Initial Volume (IV) must be less than Final Volume (FV).

3. Final Volume (FV) minus Initial Volume (IV) equals amount of diluent (inert substance) to be added to make the final volume.

QUESTIONS

1. A 20% solution has been diluted to 480 ml and is now a 5% solution. What was the initial volume?

2. A 12.5% (w/v) topical antiseptic is available to the pharmacy. The pharmacist receives an order for 100 ml of a 1:4000 solution. How much of the original solution is necessary to fill the order?

3. A pharmacy receives an order for 4 oz of 5% solution. How much active ingredient is required to make the solution?

4. A pharmacist has weighed out 3 g of coal tar and given it to the technician to compound a 1% ointment. What is the final weight of the correctly compounded prescription?

5. How many 600-mg ibuprofen tablets are needed to make 4 oz of a 15% ibuprofen ointment?

6. One tablespoon of 85% boric acid solution is diluted to 10%. How many 2-oz bottles can be prepared from the final solution?

7. A drug is supplied as a 40 mg/ml in a 50-ml vial. You have been asked to make 10 ml of a 10 mg/ml solution. How much concentrate and diluent are needed?

8. The pharmacy has 8 oz of a 40% solution, and 120 ml of water is added to decrease the concentration. What is the new concentration?

9. A technician is asked to weigh out 10 g of menthol and told to dissolve it in distilled water to make a 5% solution. An order is received from a physician and the technician is asked to make a 2.5% solution. What is the final volume?

10. How many milliliters of water must be added to make a 20% solution from 1 liter of a 50% solution?

Alligation

Alligations are used in pharmacy when a pharmacist or pharmacy technician is compounding either a solution or solid. The strength being prepared is different from what is available on the shelf. In this situation, there are at least two different concentrations on the shelf—one that is greater than the desired concentration and one that is less than the desired concentration.

For example a pharmacist receives an order to prepare 4 oz of a 10% solution using a 25% and 5% solution. How much of each these should the pharmacist use?

Step 1: Draw a tic-tac-toe table.

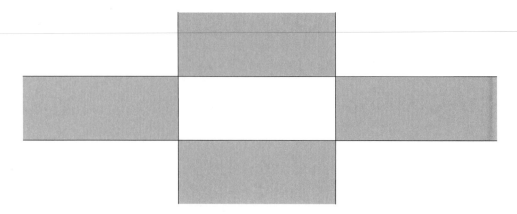

Step 2: Place the highest concentration in the upper left hand corner, the lowest concentration in the lower left hand corner, and the desired concentration in the middle.

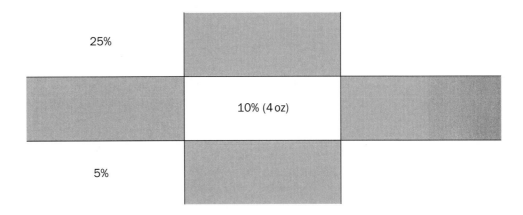

Step 3: Subtract the desired concentration from the highest concentration and place that number in the lower right hand corner and express the answer as parts. Next subtract the lowest concentration from the desired concentration and place that number in the upper right hand corner and label it as parts.

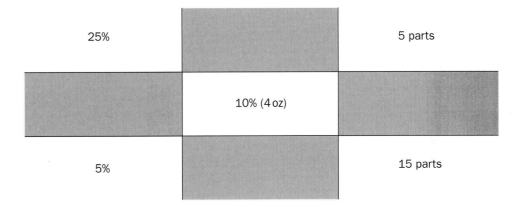

Step 4: Total the number of parts. 5 parts + 15 parts = 20 parts.

Step 5: Set up a proportion using the parts of the highest and lowest concentration and the total quantity to be prepared.

$$25\%: \frac{5 \text{ parts}}{20 \text{ parts}} \times 40 \text{ oz} = 1 \text{ oz of } 25\% \text{ needed}$$

$$25\%: \frac{15 \text{ parts}}{20 \text{ parts}} \times 4 \text{ oz} = 3 \text{ oz of } 5\% \text{ needed}$$

Step 6: Check your work by adding the amounts of each concentration to see if they equal the amount to be compounded.

QUESTIONS

1. You receive a prescription to make 4 oz of a 10% solution. On your shelf you find both 25% and 5% solutions. What proportions of each will you use?

2. The pharmacy receives a medication order to prepare a 15% ointment weighing 2 oz. Your pharmacy stocks a 50% ointment and a 10% ointment. How much of each are required to make this compound?

3. A physician telephones a prescription requiring 1 oz of a 1% ointment for a patient. The pharmacy carries only a 2.5% ointment. How much of the 2.5% ointment and an inert base must be incorporated to make this product?

4. A hospital pharmacy compounds a 25% soaking solution for patients. It is prepared by combining 10% and 30% solutions. How much of each is required to make 1 liter?

5. A pharmacy is to prepare a 500 ml of D5W. How much of D10W and SWFI are required to compound this solution?

6. A pharmacy is asked to make D7.5W using SWFI, D5W, D10W, and D20W. What are the possible combinations to make this product?

7. A pharmacy is to prepare 500 ml of D8W. The pharmacy stocks SWFI, D5W, and D10W. How much of these ingredients should be used to make this solution?

8. A physician orders a prescription of 4 oz of 1.5% hydrocortisone cream. The pharmacy stocks 0.5% and 2.5% cream. How much of each should be used to make this compound?

9. What proportions of a 10% ointment and 75% ointment should be used in preparing a 50% ointment?

10. What amounts of 90% alcohol and distilled water are needed to make 1 liter of 25% alcohol?

Flow Rates

Calculation of flow rates are used in the preparation of intravenous medications. A pharmacist may need to calculate the amount of fluid to be administered over a period of time, calculate the flow rate of intravenous fluids, and control the amount of medication that the patient is to receive. One of the variables a pharmacist may face is the number of drops of a medication in 1 ml. This is affected by the viscosity of the solution. Several intravenous sets are available including the following:

10 drops/ml
15 drops/ml
60 drops/ml (which is known as a mini-drip or micro-drip set)

A flow rate is the same as infusion rate and rate of infusion and can be calculated using the following equation:

$$\text{Rate of infusion} = \frac{\text{Volume of fluid (or amount of drug, i.e., mg, mEq, or units)}}{\text{Time of infusion}}$$

A pharmacist may need to determine when an intravenous bag may need to be changed. This can be calculated using the following equation:

$$\text{Time of infusion} = \frac{\text{Volume of fluid (or amount of drug)}}{\text{Rate of infusion}}$$

An infusion pump may be used to deliver an exact amount of medication to the patient. In this situation the pharmacist may need to know how many drops/minute are to be administered. This may be calculated by using the following equation:

$$\frac{\text{Drops}}{\text{min}} = \frac{\text{number of ml}}{\text{hour}} \times \frac{\text{number of drops}}{\text{ml}} \times \frac{1 \text{ hour}}{60}$$

1. How many ml would a patient receive in 1 hour if it takes 45 minutes for 100 ml to be infused?
2. If a patient is given 1 liter of an intravenous solution and the infusion rate is 125 ml/hour, how long will the intravenous bag last?
3. If a 1000-ml intravenous bag is hung at 9 am and the infusion rate is 100 ml/hour, when will the next bag need to be hung?

4. An intravenous is to flow at 100 ml/hour using a 10-drop set, how many drops per minute are administered?
5. A 1-liter intravenous is to flow at 75 ml/hour using a 15-drop set, how many drops per minute are administered?
6. If 250 ml at 30 drops/minute is administered using a mini-drip set, what is the flow rate in ml/hr?
7. If 2 g in 50 ml is administered over 60 minutes using a 10-drop set, how many drops per minute will the patient receive?
8. A 220-lb male is to receive 1 liter of a medication dosed at 10 mcg/kg/min. How many mg per hour will he receive?
9. A patient is to receive 100 ml over 45 minutes using a 10-drop set. How should the pump be set?
10. A patient is to receive 2 liters of normal saline infused over 24 hours using a 10-drop kit.
    a. How many ml/hour is this?
    b. How many ml/min is this?
    c. How many drops/min is this?

Temperature Conversions

To solve math problems converting Fahrenheit to Celsius or Celsius to Fahrenheit, the following formula can be used:

$$9C = 5F - 160$$

where C represents the temperature in Celsius and F represents the Fahrenheit temperature. Only one of the two variables must be known to solve this problem. For example, if one was given a temperature of 75 degrees F, one would multiply 75 degrees by 5, subtract 160 from the answer, and then divide it by 9. The answer would be 23.8 degrees C. On the other hand if one is told that the temperature was 20 degrees Celsius, one would multiply the 20 by 9, add 160 to it, and then divide it by 5, resulting in an answer of 68.

QUESTIONS

1. Convert the following temperatures to Celsius:
   a. 25 degrees F
   b. 35 degrees F
   c. 65 degrees F
   d. 50 degrees F

2. Convert the following temperatures to Fahrenheit:
   a. 45 degrees C
   b. 30 degrees C
   c. 25 degrees C
   d. 38 degrees C

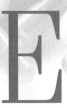

E

Health Insurance Portability and Accountability Act of 1996 (HIPAA)

Robert M. Fulcher and Eugenia M. Fulcher

THE Health Insurance Portability and Accountability Act of 1996 is better known as HIPAA. Although it was written in the later part of the 20th century, it was not placed in effect until April 14, 2003 because of problems encountered in setting rates and with computerizing parts of the system. HIPAA requires that all forms used in connection with medical information must be standardized. This means that all medical bills, laboratory reports, hospital records, and medication records must be formatted in the same manner. Every insurance company is required to use the same forms. More importantly for the pharmacy, it sets boundaries on the use and the disclosure of protected health information and requires that patients be informed on how their protected information will be used.

HIPAA legislation is divided into two sections. The first section, or Title I, protects insurance coverage for workers and their families when workers move from job to job or when terminated from a job. The second part of the legislation, or Title II, protects patient rights. The Department of Health and Human Services has established national standards for electronic health care transactions. Another provision is that all electronic patient information must be secured to protect the privacy of patients. The Centers for Disease Control and Prevention (CDC) has also joined into the act by stating that health information can be disclosed without authorization from the patient "for the purpose of preventing or controlling disease, injury, or disability," including "public health surveillance, investigation, and intervention."

When a patient is treated by a health care provider, a record is made of the treatment. The record will typically contain information about the diagnosis, treatment, and future plan of treatment for the patient. Statistical data or data taken without identification of the patient is not covered by the privacy rules of the HIPAA legislation. However, any disclosure that could be identified with the patient must have a signed consent form before it is released. The forms are provided to the patient in a hospital setting, in a physician's office, or when a prescription is filled in the pharmacy of his or her choice. Any provider that will use a third party in the treatment process must obtain the written consent of the patient before sharing any protected health information with the third party. This written consent must be obtained only once, but the consent form must be written in plain language and inform the patient that the information may be used and disclosed to the third party. Also, consent must state that the patient's right to review the privacy notice is available and that the patient has a right to request restrictions to or revoke consent. The form must be dated and signed by the individual, although the signature does not require verification.

The information that HIPAA protects includes the following:

1. Any information related to past, present, or future physical and mental health
2. Past, present, or future payments for health services received
3. Specific care the patient received, is receiving, or is willing to receive
4. Any information that can identify the patient as the individual receiving the care
5. Any information that someone could reasonably use to identify a patient as receiving care

This information is referred to as protected health information.

A limited number of scenarios do not require a specific authorization from the patient. Some of these special cases include local agencies, such as power, gas, and phone companies, or emergency medical assistance during an emergency, such as hurricanes or floods, when life-sustaining equipment is involved. When this scenario arises, the pharmacist should make the decision about whether to provide the information. If a patient designates a family member or another person for the release of information, the requirements of HIPAA do not apply. When law enforcement needs information to protect citizens or in response to court orders or subpoenas, the privacy of the information may be superseded by the need to protect the public.

Under the HIPAA statutes, a hospital is allowed to continue to give callers basic information about a patient, as long as the caller meets specific criteria. The caller must ask for a specific patient by name. The information relayed about the patient may be a one- or two-word description of the patient's condition, the patient's hospital phone number, and the patient's room number, unless the patient requests that this information not be released.

The rulings for the physician's office are stringent on identification of patients. The area for signing in for an appointment must be private, and the patient's name must be removed from the list immediately after signing in. This requirement is one reason that many physician's offices are using an electronic method of signature as a means of signing patients in for treatment. Under all conditions, the patient's privacy must be protected from other patients and visitors in the office.

Confidentiality is a major tenet of the HIPAA regulations. Because medical professionals and allied health professionals have dealings with patients, conversations with the patient must take place in an area where other patients cannot overhear what is being said. This tenet presents a major problem in pharmacy because in most states counseling of each patient is required by insurance companies. The patient counseling and education must be done in an area where privacy is ensured, such as a counseling room; but if this area is not available, the pharmacist must use professional judgment to ensure that the patients' rights are not violated.

Because patients with third-party payment obtain medication at check-out, the signature ledger should be protected. This means that the ledger should be out of sight except when a patient is signing, and the previous signatures should be covered before a new signature is obtained.

Handling medication bottles that have been brought back to the pharmacy for refills poses another problem. Any identification of the patient on the bottle, such as prescription number or name, must be obliterated either using a black marker or by stripping the label from the bottle before disposal. Some pharmacies are even separating old prescription bottles from other waste for special disposal. In addition, the label on any medication that is returned to the pharmacy for whatever reason must be removed from the bottle and the medication must be placed with damaged merchandise to be destroyed. The patient's privacy must always be protected.

HIPAA provides a set of standards for patient privacy and requires that all health care providers implement the policies and procedures to limit access to protected health information. In addition, health care professionals must remember that patients have rights. The rights of patients include the following:

- The right to obtain a written copy of the notice of privacy practices of the pharmacy where they obtain their medications
- The right to obtain a copy of their designated record set of protected health information (PHI)
- The right to request an amendment to their health record
- The right to obtain an accounting of any disclosures of their protected health information
- The right to file a complaint regarding the handling of their protected health information
- The right to authorize that protected health information be used or disclosed for purposes other than treatment, payment, or health care operation

Because we live in an electronic age, there is a growing need for the protection of patient privacy. With HIPAA, this privacy is protected and the patient has control of what medical information is relayed to entities, both in the medical field and out of the medical field.

F

Proper Hand Care for Medical Asepsis in Pharmacy

Robert M. Fulcher and Eugenia M. Fulcher

HAND cleansing is a routine procedure for medical asepsis in the medical arena, including pharmacy, whether in an inpatient or community pharmacy. Handwashing has long been the cornerstone of infection control, but compliance with this procedure has not always been easy. Beginning in the 1960s, the Centers for Disease Control and Prevention (CDC) issued guidelines for how health care workers should properly cleanse their hands to prevent transmission of transient flora found on the hands.

Resident flora live and grow in both the epidermis (outer layer of the skin) and the dermis (deeper layer of the skin). Resident flora are for the most part nonpathogenic. Transient flora live and grow only on the epidermis. These bacteria adhere to the skin during the daily activities of touching people, objects, and supplies. Transient flora tend to be more pathogenic and are easily passed to others through contact. On the other hand, these bacteria can be easily removed from the skin by washing hands. Therefore, it is of utmost importance for the pharmacy technician to adhere to the guidelines for hand sanitization as issued by the CDC.

Hands should be carefully washed each day on arrival in the pharmacy area, when the hands are obviously soiled, after using the rest room, and after eating. These are basically the times that were taught to us as children, but compliance is difficult. In 2002 the CDC changed the guidelines to call for medical aseptic hand sanitization during the day to keep bacteria to a minimum while handling medications. The new cleansing requirements still applied to those times listed previously, but hands may be sanitized with an alcohol-based handrub between handwashing. Using an alcohol-based handrub is faster, does not require rinsing, is more effective in removing transient flora, and prevents drying of the pharmacy technician's hands from constant handwashing. The drying of skin leads to chapped, irritated, and cracked skin that in turn leads to dermatitis. The procedure for sanitizing hands takes only 20 to 30 seconds, whereas handwashing requires 1 to 2 minutes.

The disadvantages of alcohol-based handrubs are the stinging sensation if the skin is cut or scraped, and they are more expensive than soap and water. Furthermore, if the hands are grossly contaminated or dirty, alcohol-based hand rubs are not effective.

The amount of handrub required depends on the manufacturer, and is indicated in the instructions for use. The appropriate amount of handrub should be placed in the center of the palm of the hand, and then the hands should be rubbed together, ensuring that the handrub reaches all parts of the hands, including between the fingers. The rubbing motion should continue until the entire rub is absorbed.

Because the handrub is alcohol-based, the fluid will be flammable and should be handled in the same manner as all flammable substances. The bottles should be safely placed to prevent spillage, and the hands should be rubbed together with enough friction to perform the task but should not be rubbed so vigorously that it may cause static electricity.

As with all medical personnel, the pharmacy technician should perform hand sanitization for medical asepsis and for prevention of transmission of transient flora. Keeping the hands clean is important for both the technician and for patients who are receiving medications. If the pharmacy technician is preparing intravenous fluids, the handwashing techniques are more stringent and should be followed according to the policies and procedures of the medical facility.

Glossary

Abortifacient   Any treatment that causes abortion of a fetus

Abortivo   Cualquier tratamiento que causa el aborto de un feto

Absorption   The taking in of nutrients from food and liquids

Absorción   La toma de nutrientes de alimentos y líquidos

Accommodation   The change that occurs in the ocular lens when it focuses at various distances

Acomodación   El cambio que ocurre en el lente del ojo cuando éste enfoca a varias distancias

Acidification   The conversion to an acid environment

Acidificación   La conversión a un ambiente ácido

Acidosis   The increase of acid content of the blood resulting from the accumulation of acid or loss of bicarbonate; the pH of blood is lowered

Acidosis   El aumento del contenido ácido en la sangre como resultado de la acumulación de ácido o de la pérdida de bicarbonato; la disminución del pH de la sangre

Acoustic nerve   The cranial nerve that controls the senses of hearing and equilibrium which eventually leads to the cerebellum and medulla

Nervio acústico   El nervio craneal que controla los sentidos del oído y del equilibrio y que eventualmente llega hasta el cerebelo y la médula

Acquired immunity   Immunity that has been acquired through exposure to an antigen or infectious agent

Inmunidad adquirida   Inmunidad que se adquiere por medio de la exposición a un antígeno o a un agente infeccioso

Addison's disease   Condition resulting in a decrease in adrenocortical hormones, such as mineralocorticoids and glucocorticoids, that causes symptoms including muscle weakness and weight loss

Enfermedad de Addison   Enfermedad que da como resultado una disminución de las hormonas adrenocorticoides, como mineralocorticoides y glucocorticoides, y que causa síntomas que incluyen debilidad muscular y pérdida de peso

Adjudication   Electronic insurance billing for medication payment

Adjudicación   Facturación electrónica del seguro para el pago de medicamentos

Aerobic   Organisms that need oxygen to survive

Aeróbico   Organismos que necesitan oxígeno para sobrevivir

Afferent   The direction of neuronal impulse from the body toward the central nervous system (CNS)

Aferente   La dirección del impulso neuronal desde el cuerpo hasta el sistema nervioso central (SNC)

Alkalosis   The increase of alkalinity of the blood resulting from the accumulation of alkali or reduction of acid content; the pH of blood is raised

Alcalosis   El aumento de la alcalinidad de la sangre como resultado de la acumulación de álcali o de la reducción del contenido ácido; el pH de la sangre es elevado

Alligation   A method of determining the needed amounts of two different concentrations to prepare a needed concentration

Aligación   Un método para determinar las cantidades necesarias de dos concentraciones diferentes para preparar una concentración dada

Amenorrhea   Absence or suppression of menses

Amenorrea   Ausencia o falta de menstruación

617

Amino acids Macromolecules that make up proteins

Aminoácidos Macromoléculas que forman las proteínas

Anabolism To build up; the constructive phase of metabolism

Anabolismo Acumular; la fase constructiva del metabolismo

Anaerobic Organisms that live in the absence of oxygen

Anaeróbico Organismos que viven en ausencia de oxígeno

Analgesic A drug that relieves pain by reducing the perception of pain

Analgésico Una medicina que alivia el dolor al reducir la percepción del dolor

Anaphylactic shock A severe allergic reaction that causes blood pressure to decrease rapidly, the heart to go into ventricular tachycardia, and airways to close; a medical emergency that will cause death if not treated immediately

Choque anafiláctico Una reacción alérgica severa que causa una rápida disminución de la presión sanguínea, taquicardia ventricular y cierre completo de las vías respiratorias; una emergencia médica que causa la muerte si no se trata inmediatamente

Androgen Male hormone

Andrógeno Hormona masculina

Anemia A deficiency of circulating red blood cells; a symptom of disease, not a disease

Anemia Una deficiencia de los glóbulos rojos en la sangre; un síntoma de enfermedad, no una enfermedad

Antibiotic spectrum The variety of microbes that a particular antibiotic can treat. Broad-spectrum agents can treat many different types of organisms, whereas narrow-spectrum agents treat only a select few.

Espectro de un antibiótico La variedad de microbios que un antibiótico específico puede tratar. Los agentes de espectro amplio pueden tratar muchos tipos de organismos diferentes, mientras que los agentes de espectro reducido pueden tratar sólo unos pocos.

Antibiotic Chemical agents produced by organisms used to treat infections

Antibióticos Agentes químicos producidos por organismos y que se utilizan para tratar infecciones

Antibodies Proteins contained within plasma cells that neutralize or destroy antigens; also known as immunoglobulins

Anticuerpos Proteínas que se hallan en las células plasmáticas que neutralizan o destruyen los antígenos; también conocidas como inmunoglobulinas

Antiemetic Agent that stops nausea and vomiting

Antiemético Agente que hace parar la náusea y el vómito

Antigen The marker on cell surfaces that marks the cell as a "self-cell"; stimulates the production of antibodies

Antígeno El marcador en la superficie celular que marca la célula como "auto-célula"; estimula la producción de anticuerpos

Antihypertensive Agent that decreases blood pressure

Antihipertensivo Agente que disminuye la presión sanguínea

Antiinflammatory A drug that reduces swelling, redness, and pain, and promotes healing

Antiinflamatorio Una medicina que reduce la hinchazón, el enrojecimiento y el dolor y facilita la curación

Antimicrobial Chemical agents produced by scientists to prevent growth of or kill microorganisms

Antimicrobiano Agentes químicos producidos por los científicos para impedir el crecimiento de microorganismos o para matarlos

Antineoplastic An agent used to prevent the development, proliferation, or growth of neoplastic cells; a medication used in treatment of abnormal cells

Antineoplástico Un agente que se usa para impedir el desarrollo, proliferación o crecimiento de las células neoplásticas; medicamento que se usa en el tratamiento de células anómalas

Antipruritic A drug that relieves itching, usually an antihistamine or an anti-inflammatory drug

Antipruriginoso Una medicina que alivia la picazón, por lo general un antihistamínico o un antiinflamatorio

Antiseptic A substance that slows or stops growth of microorganisms on surfaces such as skin

Antiséptico Una sustancia que retarda o detiene el crecimiento de microorganismos en superficies como la piel

Antitussive A drug that can decrease the coughing reflex of the central nervous system (CNS)

Antitusivo Una medicina que puede disminuir el reflejo tusígeno (de tos) del sistema nervioso central (SNC)

Anxiety Feelings of apprehension, dread, and fear, with characteristics including tension, restlessness, tachycardia, dyspnea, and a sense of hopelessness

Ansiedad   Sentimientos de aprensión, miedo y temor, con características que incluyen tensión, falta de descanso, taquicardia, disnea y una sensación de desesperanza

Apothecary   Latin term for pharmacist
Apotecario   Término latín para farmacéutico

Appendicitis   Inflammation of the appendix
Apendicitis   Inflamación del apéndice

Aqueous humor   A fluid that is found in the anterior and posterior chambers of the eye
Humor acuoso   Un fluido que se halla en las cámaras anterior y posterior del ojo

Arrhythmia   Irregular rhythm of the heart
Aritmia   Ritmo irregular del corazón

Artery   A vessel that carries oxygenated blood from the heart to the tissues of the body
Arteria   Un vaso sanguíneo que transporta sangre con oxígeno desde el corazón hasta los tejidos del cuerpo

ASA   Acetylsalicylic acid (aspirin)
ASA   Ácido acetilsalicílico (aspirina)

Aseptic technique   The procedures used to eliminate the possibility of a drug becoming contaminated with microbes or particles
Técnica aséptica   Los procedimientos que se usan para eliminar la posibilidad de que una medicina se contamine con microbios o partículas

Asthma   A condition in which narrowing of the airways impedes breathing
Asma   Una enfermedad en la cual el estrechamiento de las vías respiratorias impide el respirar

Atom   The smallest unit of an element
Átomo   La unidad más pequeña de un elemento

Atomic mass   The mass (mostly referred to as weight) of an atom expressed in the units 1660×10^{-24}
Masa atómica   La masa (la mayoría de las veces llamada peso) de un átomo expresada en unidades de 1660×10^{-24}

Attenuated   An altered or weakened live vaccine made from the disease organism that the vaccine protects against
Atenuado   Una vacuna de microorganismo vivo, modificado o debilitado, hecha del organismo de la enfermedad contra la cual protege dicha vacuna

Auditory canal   A 1-inch segment of tube that runs from the external ear to the middle ear

Canal auditivo   Segmento tubular de una pulgada de largo que va desde el oído externo hasta el oído medio

Auditory ossicles   The set of three small bony structures in the ear: malleus, incus, and stapes
Huesecillos del oído   La serie de tres pequeñas estructuras óseas en el oído: martillo, yunque y estribo

Autoimmune disease   Condition in which a person's tissues are attacked by his/her immune system; abnormal antigen-antibody reaction
Enfermedad autoinmunitaria   Enfermedad en la cual los tejidos de una persona son atacados por su propio sistema inmunológico; reacción anómala de antígeno-anticuerpo

Autonomic nervous system (ANS)   Division of the nervous system that controls the involuntary body functions; consists of sympathetic and parasympathetic divisions
Sistema nervioso autónomo (SNA)   Parte del sistema nervioso que controla las funciones corporales involuntarias, está formada del sistema simpático y del sistema parasimpático

Autonomic   Self-controlling or involuntary
Autónomo   Que se controla solo o de modo involuntario

Auxiliary label   An adhesive label that is attached to a container with specific instructions or information pertaining to the medication inside
Etiqueta auxiliar   Una etiqueta adhesiva que se pone en un envase con instrucciones específicas o información relativa al medicamento que hay en su interior

Avitaminosis   Vitamin deficiency
Avitaminosis   Deficiencia de vitaminas

Axon   The part of a nerve cell that conducts impulses away from a cell body
Axón   La parte de una célula nerviosa que conduce los impulsos nerviosos hacia el exterior de la célula

Ayurveda   A holistic medical system originating in India
Ayurveda   Un sistema de medicina holístico originario de India

Bacteria   Unicellular organisms
Bacterias   Organismos unicelulares

Bactericidal   Agents that kill bacteria
Bactericida   Agentes que matan bacterias

Bacteriostatic   Agents that prevent the growth of bacteria but do not kill the microbe
Bacteriostático   Agentes que impiden el crecimiento de las bacterias pero que no mata el microbio

Benign prostatic hypertrophy Nonmalignant enlargement of prostate gland
Hipertrofia prostática benigna Agrandamiento no maligno de la próstata

Benign A nonmalignant neoplasm
Benigno Un neoplasma no maligno

Binary fission The method of reproduction by which a single cell divides into two separate cells
División binaria El método de reproducción por el cual una célula simple se divide en dos células individuales

Biology The study of life
Biología El estudio de la vida

Biopsy A procedure in which a piece of tissue is removed from a patient for examination and diagnosis; the tissue is a sample of the whole
Biopsia Un procedimiento en el cual se extrae una porción de tejido del cuerpo de un paciente para analizarlo y hacer un diagnóstico; el tejido es una muestra del todo

Bipolar disorder Depressive psychosis, alternating between excessive phases of mania and depression; formerly known as manic-depressive
Trastorno bipolar Psicosis depresiva en la que se alternan fases exageradas de manía y de depresión; antes se conocía como psicosis maníaco-depresiva

Blister pack Container usually made of plastic that holds a single-dose tablet or capsule
Envase-ampolla Envase por lo general hecho de plástico que contiene una tableta o cápsula de una dosis unitaria

Blood urea nitrogen (BUN) A test that measures the nitrogen in the blood in the form of urea
Nitrógeno ureico en la sangre (BUN) Un análisis que mide el nitrógeno que hay en la sangre en forma de urea

Blood-brain barrier A barrier formed by special characteristics of capillaries to prevent certain chemicals from moving into the brain
Barrera hematoencefálica Una barrera formada por características especiales que poseen los capilares para impedir que ciertas sustancias químicas lleguen al cerebro

Board of Pharmacy State board that regulates pharmaceutical practice
Junta de Farmacia Junta estatal que regula la práctica farmacéutica

Bradykinins Chemicals produced by the body, responsible for inflammation and pain

Bradykinins Agentes químicos que produce el cuerpo y que originan inflamación y dolor

Brand/trade name Trademark of a drug or device created by the originating manufacturing company
Marca/denominación comercial Marca registrada de una medicina o de un aparato creado por la compañía fabricante original

Bulk compounding A larger quantity of medication that can fill a large order at one time or several smaller orders in the future
Compuesto al por mayor Una gran cantidad de medicamento que puede cubrir una cantidad grande de medicina recetada de una sola vez o varias cantidades pequeñas en el futuro

Bulk forming Fiber used as a stimulant to the intestines or to cause a feeling of fullness to decrease appetite
Formadores de masa Fibra que se utiliza como estimulante de los intestinos o para crear una sensación de saciedad a fin de disminuir el apetito

Calibration The markings on a measuring device
Calibración Las marcas (la escala) de un aparato de medida

Cancer A general term used to describe malignant neoplasms
Cáncer Un término general usado para describir neoplasmas malignos

Capillary Extremely small vessel that connects the ends of the smallest arteries (arterioles) to the smallest veins (venules), where exchanges of nutrients and wastes, O_2 and CO_2 can occur; blood vessels at cellular level
Capilar Vaso sanguíneo extremadamente pequeño que une las terminaciones de las arterias más pequeñas (arteriolas) a las venas más pequeñas (vénulas), en el que pueden producirse intercambios de nutrientes y sustancias de desecho, O_2 y CO_2 pueden ocurrir; vasos sanguíneos en los niveles celulares

Carbohydrates Chemical substances that include sugars, glycogen, starches, and cellulose with only carbon, hydrogen, and oxygen make up
Carbohidratos o hidratos de carbono Sustancias químicas en las que se incluyen azúcares, glucógenos, almidones y celulosas, y que están formadas sólo por carbono, hidrógeno y oxígeno.

Carcinogen A substance or chemical that can increase the risk of developing cancer
Carcinógeno Una sustancia o agente químico que puede aumentar el riesgo de desarrollar cáncer

Catabolism   To break down; the destructive phase of metabolism

Catabolismo   Descomponer; la fase destructiva del metabolismo

Catalyst   A molecule that allows chemical reactions to take place rapidly but is not altered in the reaction

Catalítico   Una molécula que permite que una reacción química se produzca con mayor rapidez pero sin que la molécula misma sufra modificaciones

Cataract   Loss of transparency of the lens of the eye

Catarata   Pérdida de transparencia del lente del ojo

Cell body   The main part of a neuron from which axons and dendrites extend

Cuerpo celular   La parte principal de una neurona de la cual se extienden los axones y las dendritas

Cerebrospinal fluid (CSF)   A fluid that fills the ventricles of the brain and also lies in the spaces of the brain or spinal cord and the arachnoid layer of the meninges

Fluido cerebroespinal (CSFO FCE)   Un fluido que llena los ventrículos del cerebro y que también se halla en los espacios de la capa aracnoidea de las meninges y del cerebro o de la médula espinal

Cervical   Neck region

Cervical   Región del cuello

Chemical structure   The shape of molecules and their location to one another

Estructura química   La forma de las moléculas y su ubicación respectiva

Chemotherapy   The treatment of a disease with toxic chemical substances to slow the disease process or to kill cells

Quimioterapia   El tratamiento de una enfermedad por medio del uso de sustancias químicas tóxicas para retardar el proceso de la enfermedad o matar ciertas células

Chiropractic   Manual manipulation of the joints and muscles

Quiropráctica   Manipulación manual de las articulaciones y los músculos

Chloasma   Hyperpigmentation of skin, limited or confined to a certain area

Cloasma   Hiperpigmentación de la piel, limitada o confinada a una cierta área

Chronic obstructive pulmonary disease (COPD)   A disease process where the lungs have decreased ability for gas exchange; also known as emphysema and chronic bronchitis

Enfermedad pulmonar obstructiva crónica (EPOC)   Proceso patológico en el cual disminuye la capacidad de los pulmones para inhalar y exhalar; también conocido como enfisema y bronquitis crónica

Chyme   The soupy consistency of food after mixing with stomach acids as it passes into small intestines

Quimo   La consistencia espesa en que se transforman los alimentos al mezclarse con los ácidos gástricos al pasar al intestino delgado

Clinical pharmacist   Pharmacist who monitors patient medications in inpatient and some retail settings

Farmacéutico clínico   Farmacéutico que controla los medicamentos de los pacientes en hospitales y algunas farmacias de venta al por menor

Coagulate   To solidify or change from a fluid state to a solid state

Coagular   Solidificar o cambiar del estado fluido al estado sólido

Code blue   A coded message to indicate an emergency in a hospital situation

Código azul   Un mensaje codificado para indicar una emergencia en un hospital

Coenzyme   A compound that activates an enzyme

Coenzima   Un compuesto que hace que se active una encima

Cofactor   A factor that must be present for other factors to be active

Cofactor   Un factor que debe estar presente para que otros factores sean activos

Communication   The ability to express oneself in such a way that one is readily and clearly understood

Comunicación   La capacidad de expresarse de modo que se produzca una comprensión clara e inmediata

Competency   The capability or proficiency to perform a function

Competencia   La capacidad o aptitud para cumplir una función

Compounding   The act of mixing, reconstituting, and packaging a drug

Composición   El acto de mezclar, reconstituir y empaquetar una medicina

Cones   Photoreceptors responsible for color (daylight vision)

Conos   Elementos fotorreceptores responsables de la visión en color (visión diurna)

Confidentiality To keep privileged customer information from being disclosed without the customer's consent
Confidencialidad Acto de no revelar información confidencial sobre un cliente o paciente sin el consentimiento del interesado

Congestive heart failure (CHF) Accumulation of blood in the circulatory system due to the heart's inability to pump efficiently
Insuficiencia cardiaca congestiva (ICC) Acumulación de sangre en el sistema circulatorio debido a la incapacidad del corazón de bombearla de manera eficaz

Constipation Dry, hard stools that may be decreased in frequency
Estreñimiento Deposiciones fecales secas y duras que pueden presentarse con menor frecuencia de la normal

Continuing Education (CE) Education beyond the basic technical education, usually required for license renewal
Educación continua (EC) Educación que va más allá de la educación técnica básica, usualmente necesaria para renovar una licencia

Cornea The transparent tissue covering the anterior portion of the eye
Córnea El tejido transparente que recubre la parte anterior del ojo

Cough reflex Response of the body to clear air passages of foreign substances and mucus by a forceful expiration
Tos refleja Respuesta del cuerpo para limpiar las vías respiratorias de sustancias extrañas y mucosidades por medio de una expiración vigorosa

Covalent bond The sharing of electrons between two atoms
Unión covalente El tipo de unión en el cual dos átomos comparten electrones

Cream A hydrophilic base
Crema Una base hidrófila

Cretinism Condition in which the development of the brain and body is inhibited by congenital lack of thyroid secretion
Cretinismo Enfermedad en la cual se inhibe el desarrollo cerebral y corporal debido a una carencia congénita de secreciones tiroideas

Cushing's disease Syndrome causing an increase in secretion of the adrenal cortex that includes symptoms such as a moon face and deposits of fat (buffalo hump)
Enfermedad de Cushing Síndrome que produce un incremento en la secreción de la corteza adrenal y que incluye síntomas como redondez del rostro y depósitos de grasa (joroba de búfalo)

Cycloplegia Paralysis of the ciliary muscle in the eye
Cicloplegia Parálisis del músculo ciliar en el ojo

Cystic fibrosis An inherited disorder that causes production of very thick mucus in the respiratory tract; affects the pancreas and sweat glands; patient experiences difficulty breathing and has frequent respiratory infections
Fibrosis quística Un trastorno hereditario que causa la producción de mucosidades muy espesas en el tracto respiratorio; afecta el páncreas y las glándulas sudoríparas; el paciente experimenta dificultad para respirar y padece infecciones respiratorias frecuentes

Debride To remove dead or damaged tissue
Desbridar Eliminar tejidos muertos o deteriorados

Decongestants Drugs that reduce swelling of the mucous membranes by constricting dilated blood vessels; reduced blood flow to nasal tissues, thus reducing nasal congestion
Descongestionantes Medicinas que reducen la hinchazón de las membranas mucosas al contraer los vasos sanguíneos dilatados; reduciendo el flujo sanguíneo a los tejidos nasales y la congestión nasal

Dendrite The part of a neuron that branches out to bring impulses to the cell body
Dendrita La parte de la neurona que se ramifica hacia el exterior para llevar los impulsos al cuerpo célula

Deoxyribonucleic acid (DNA) The complex nucleic acids that are base for genetic continuance
Ácido desoxirribonucleico (AND) Los ácidos nucleicos complejos que son la base de la continuidad genética

Depot An area of the body where a substance can accumulate or be stored for later distribution
Depósito Una área del cuerpo en la cual se puede acumular o almacenar una sustancia para su distribución posterior

Depression A mental state characterized by sadness, feelings of loss and grief, loss of appetite, and may include suicidal thoughts
Depresión Un estado mental caracterizado por tristeza, sentimientos de pérdida y pena, pérdida de apetito y puede incluir ideas de suicidio

Dermatitis   Inflammation of the skin associated with itching and burning
Dermatitis   Inflamación de la piel asociada con picazón y ardor

Desquamating   A normal process of shedding the top layer of the skin, also known as exfoliation
Descamación   Un proceso normal de desprendimiento de la capa superior de la piel, también se conoce como exfoliación

Diagnosis   A doctor's assessment of the cause of a condition
Diagnóstico   Una declaración de un médico sobre la causa de una enfermedad

Dialysis   The passage of a solute through a semipermeable membrane to remove toxic materials and to maintain fluid, electrolyte, and pH of the body system when the kidneys no longer work
Diálisis   El paso de un soluto a través de una membrana semipermeable para eliminar materiales tóxicos y para mantener el fluido, el electrolito y el pH del sistema corporal cuando los riñones no funcionan

Diarrhea   Frequent, watery, loose stools
Diarrea   Deposiciones fecales, frecuentes, aguadas y poco espesas

Digestion   The mechanical, chemical, and enzymatic action of breaking food into molecules that can be used in metabolism
Digestión   La descomposición mecánica, química y enzimática de los alimentos para convertirlos en moléculas utilizables en el metabolismo

Diuresis   The secretion and passage of large amounts of urine from the body
Diuresis   La secreción de grandes cantidades de orina y su expulsión del cuerpo

Diuretic   An agent that increases urine output and diuresis
Diurético   Un agente que aumenta la expulsión de orina y la diuresis

Dogma   Code of beliefs based on tradition rather than fact
Dogma   Código de creencias basado en tradiciones más bien que en hechos

Drug classification   Based on the action of a drug and its usage
Clasificación de medicinas   Se basa en el método de acción y en el uso de la medicina

Drug education coordinator (DEC)   Pharmacist who helps set protocol in a hospital setting

Coordinador de educación sobre medicinas (DEC)   Farmacéutico que ayuda a establecer un protocolo en el ámbito hospitalario

Drug Enforcement Agency (DEA)   Federal agency within the Department of Justice that regulates the misuse of controlled substances
Agencia para el cumplimiento de las leyes anti-droga (DEA)   Agencia federal del Departamento de Justicia que regula la mala utilización de las sustancias controladas

Dysmenorrhea   Painful menstruation
Dismenorrea   Menstruación dolorosa

Dystonia   Symptoms that include twisting, repeated jerking movements, and/or abnormal posture
Distonía   Síntomas que incluyen torsiones, contracciones involuntarias repetidas y/o posturas anómalas

Edema   A local or generalized condition in which body tissues retain an excessive amount of tissue fluid
Edema   Una enfermedad localizada o generalizada en la cual los tejidos corporales retienen una cantidad excesiva de fluido tisular

Efferent   The conduction of electrical impulses away from the CNS to the body
Eferencia   La conducción de impulsos eléctricos desde el SNC al resto del cuerpo

Electrolytes   Charged elements that called cations (which have positive charges) and anions (which have negative charges)
Electrolitos   Elementos cargados eléctricamente que se denominan cationes (con carga positiva) y aniones (con carga negativa)

Electron   The smallest subset of an atom that contains a negative charge
Electrón   La división más pequeña de un átomo que tiene carga negativa

Elixir   A base solution that is a mixture of alcohol and water
Elixir   Una solución de base que es una mezcla de alcohol y agua

Emesis   Vomiting
Emesis   Vómito

Endometriosis   Condition where tissue resembling endometrium is found outside the uterine cavity, usually in the pelvic area
Endometriosis   Enfermedad en la cual un tejido similar al endometrio se encuentra fuera de la cavidad uterina, usualmente en la región pélvica

Endometrium　Mucus membrane lining of the uterus
Endometrio　Membrana mucosa que recubre el útero

Enzyme　A protein that speeds up a reaction by reducing the amount of energy required to initiate a reaction; also called a biological catalysts
Enzima　Una proteína que acelera una reacción al reducir la cantidad de energía requerida para iniciar dicha reacción; se denomina también un catalítico biológico

Erythema　Redness of the skin resulting from capillary dilation
Eritrema　Enrojecimiento de la piel producido por la dilatación de los capilares sanguíneos

Ethics　The values and morals that are used within a profession
Ética　Los valores y principios morales vigentes en una profesión

Eustachian tube　A tubular structure within the middle ear that runs to the nasopharynx (throat)
Trompa de Eustaquio　Una estructura tubular en el interior del oído medio que llega hasta la nasofaringe (garganta)

Euthyroid　Normal functioning thyroid gland
Eutiroidismo　Funcionamiento normal de la glándula tiroides

Excretion　Elimination of waste products through stools and urine
Excreción　Eliminación de productos de desecho a través de las heces y la orina

Exophthalmos　Prominence of the eyeball due to increase thyroid hormone
Exoftalmos　Prominencia del globo ocular debido a un incremento de la hormona tiroidea

Expectorant　Chemical that causes the removal of mucous secretions from the respiratory system; loosens and thins sputum and bronchial secretions for ease of expectoration
Expectorante　Sustancia química que causa la expulsión de secreciones mucosas del sistema respiratorio; los expectorantes hacen menos espesos los esputos y secreciones bronquiales para facilitar su expulsión

Extrapyramidal　Symptoms of taking antipsychotic medications that include parkinsonism, dystonia, and tremors
Extrapiramidal　Síntomas de la toma de medicamentos antisicóticos, los cuales incluyen parkinsonismo, distonías y temblores

Facts and Comparisons　Reference book found in all pharmacies containing detailed information on all medications
"Facts and Comparisons"　Libro de referencia que se encuentra en todas las farmacias y que contiene información detallada sobre todos los medicamentos

Facultative anaerobe　A microorganism that can live with or without oxygen
Anaeróbico facultativo　Un microorganismo que puede vivir con o sin oxígeno

Fallopian tubes　Narrow passage between the ovary and the uterus
Trompas de Falopio　Pasaje estrecho entre los ovarios y el útero

Fat-soluble vitamin　Vitamin that is soluble in fat, and therefore is stored in body fat; vitamins A, D, E, and K are fat-soluble
Vitamina liposoluble　Vitamina que es soluble en grasa, y que por tanto se almacena en la grasa corporal; las vitaminas A, D, E y K son liposolubles

Fat-soluble　Drugs that are absorbed into the body's fat layer
Liposoluble　Medicinas que se absorben en la capa de grasa corporal

FDA　Food and Drug Administration
FDA　Administración de Drogas y Alimentos

Fertilization　The process by which the sperm unites with the ovum to create an new life
Fertilización　El proceso por medio de cual el espermatozoide se une con el óvulo para crear una nueva vida

Floor stock　Supplies kept on hand in different units of a hospital
Almacén de planta　Suministros que se tienen a mano en las distintas unidades de un hospital

Food and Drug Administration (FDA)　Federal agency within the Department of Health and Human Services that regulates the manufacture and safeguarding of medications
Administración de Drogas y Alimentos (FDA)　Agencia federal del Departamento de Salud y Servicios Humanos que regula la fabricación y el control de calidad de los medicamentos

Formulary　A list of preferred drugs to be stocked by the pharmacy; also a list of drugs covered by an insurance company
Formulario　Una lista de medicinas prioritarias para tener almacenadas en la farmacia; también, una lista de medicinas cubiertas por una compañía de seguros

Fungicide   Agents that kill fungus
Funguicida   Agentes que matan hongos

Gametes   Sex cells or ova and sperm
Gametos   Células sexuales; es decir, óvulos y espermatozoides

Gastritis   Inflammation of the stomach lining
Gastritis   Inflamación de los tejidos que recubren el estómago

Gauge   The size of the needle opening
Calibre   El tamaño de la abertura de la aguja

Generic name   Name assigned to a medication by the FDA; non-proprietary name of a drug
Nombre genérico   Nombre que la FDA le asigna a un medicamento; nombre común de una medicina

Globulin   Proteins that are insoluble in water; immune globulins protect against diseases
Globulina   Proteínas no solubles en agua; las inmunoglobulinas protegen contra las enfermedades

Glucose   Simple sugar
Glucosa   Azúcar simple

Goiter   Condition in which the thyroid is enlarged because of lack of iodine, known as simple goiter, or because of a tumor, known as toxic goiter
Bocio   Enfermedad en la cual la tiroides aumenta de tamaño debido a una carencia de yodo, se conoce como bocio simple; si es causado por un tumor, se conoce como bocio tóxico

Government insurance   Medicaid and Medicare
Seguro del gobierno   Medicaid y Medicare

Gram   A basic unit of weight (mass) of the metric system equal to the weight of a cubic centimeter (cc) or a milliliter (ml) of water
Gramo   Unidad básica de peso (masa) del sistema métrico y que es igual al peso de un centímetro cúbico (cc) o un mililitro (ml) de agua

Gram-negative bacteria   Bacteria that are unable to keep crystal violet stain when washed in acid alcohol
Bacteria gram negativa   Bacteria que no pueden mantener el colorante cristal violeta cuando se tratan con ácido alcohol

Gram-positive bacteria   Bacteria that are able to keep crystal violet stain when washed in acid alcohol
Bacteria gram positiva   Bacteria que mantienen el colorante cristal violeta cuando se tratan con ácido-alcohol

Graves' disease   Caused by hypersecretion of thyroid with diffuse goiter, exophthalmos, and skin changes
Enfermedad de Graves   Enfermedad originada por una secreción excesiva de la tiroides; esta enfermedad se presenta con bocio difuso, exoftalmos y cambios en la piel

Hard copy   The original prescription
Copia en papel   La receta original

Health Insurance Portability and Accountability Act of 1996 (HIPAA)   Federal act for protecting patients' rights
Ley de Responsabilidad y Transferibilidad del Seguro de Salud de 1996 (HIPAA)   Ley federal para proteger los derechos de los pacientes

Helminth   Multicellular worm
Helminto   Gusano pluricelular

Hemoglobin   The iron-containing pigment on red blood cells that carries oxygen to the tissues
Hemoglobina   El pigmento de los glóbulos rojos que contiene hierro y que transporta oxígeno a los tejidos

Herb   Any herbaceous plant consisting of fleshy stems
Hierba   Cualquier planta herbácea de tallos tiernos

Heterotrophic   The ability to reproduce asexually
Heterotrópica   La capacidad de reproducción asexual

Histamine   A substance that interacts with tissues, producing an allergic reaction
Histamina   Una sustancia que interactúa con los tejidos produciendo una reacción alérgica

HMO   Health Maintenance Organization
HMO   Organización para el mantenimiento de la salud

Homeopathy   A system of therapy based on the belief that medicinal substances that cause a specific symptom can be used to treat an illness that yields the same symptoms
Homeopatía   Un sistema terapéutico basado en la creencia de que las sustancias medicinales que causan un síntoma específico pueden usarse para tratar una enfermedad que presente los mismos síntomas

Homeostasis   The equilibrium pertaining to the balance of the body with respect to fluid levels, pH level, and chemicals
Homeóstasis   El equilibrio relativo al balance del cuerpo con respecto a los niveles de fluidos, pH y sustancias químicas

Horizontal flow hood   Environment for the preparation of sterile products that uses air originating from the back of the hood moving forward across the hood out into the room

Campana de flujo horizontal Medio para la preparación de productos estériles en el que se utiliza una corriente de aire que tiene su origen en la parte posterior de la campana y que continua hacia delante a través de la campana para después salir en la habitación

Hormone Chemical substances produced and secreted into the bloodstream or duct by an endocrine gland that result in a physiologic response at a specific target tissue

Hormonas Sustancias químicas producidas y secretadas en la corriente sanguínea o en los conductos por una glándula endocrina y que provocan una respuesta fisiológica en un tejido objetivo específico

Household system A system of measurement commonly used for weight, volume, and length in the United States

Sistema nacional Un sistema de medidas comúnmente usado para medir peso, volumen y largo en los Estados Unidos

Hydrophilic Water loving; any substance that easily goes into water

Hidrófilo Que le gusta el agua; cualquier sustancia que se disuelve fácilmente en agua

Hydrophobic Water hating; any substance that does not go into or mix in water

Hidrófobo Que rechaza el agua; cualquier sustancia que no se disuelve en el agua o que no se mezcla con ella

Hyperalimentation Parenteral nutrition for patients who are unable to eat solids or liquids

Hiperalimentación Nutrición parenteral para pacientes que no pueden ingerir alimentos sólidos o líquidos

Hypercalcemia Unusually high concentration of calcium in the blood

Hipercalcemia Concentración de calcio en la corriente sanguínea más alta de lo normal

Hyperglycemia Abnormally high glucose content circulating in the bloodstream

Hiperglicemia Contenido de glucosa en la sangre más alto de lo normal

Hypervitaminosis A disorder caused by the intake of too many vitamins; more common with fat-soluble vitamins

Hipervitaminosis Un trastorno causado por la toma de una cantidad excesiva de vitaminas; es más común con las vitaminas liposolubles

Hypocalcemia Low concentration of calcium in the blood

Hipocalcemia Baja concentración de calcio en la sangre

Hypoglycemia Abnormally low glucose content circulating in the bloodstream

Hipoglicemia Contenido de glucosa en la corriente sanguínea más bajo de lo normal

Immunity A type of resistance to infection resulting from an immune response from the body or from agents such as vaccinations

Inmunidad Un tipo de resistencia a una infección que es el resultado de una respuesta inmunológica del cuerpo o de agentes como las vacunas

Inert ingredient An ingredient that has little or no effect on body functions

Ingrediente inactivo Un ingrediente que tiene muy poco o ningún efecto en las funciones corporales

Influenza A respiratory tract infection caused by an influenza virus

Influenza Una infección del tracto respiratorio causada por un virus

Ingestion The act of taking in food or liquid

Ingestión Acto de tomar alimentos o líquidos

Inhibit To stop or hold back; to keep a reaction from taking place

Inhibir Detener o impedir una reacción; prevenir que ésta tenga lugar

Inpatient or in-house pharmacy Hospital pharmacy

Farmacia interna Farmacia de un hospital

Inpatient pharmacy A pharmacy in a hospital or institutional setting

Farmacia interna Una farmacia dentro de un hospital u otra institución

Inpatient A hospitalized patient

Interno Paciente hospitalizado

Insomnia Difficulty falling or staying asleep

Insomnio Dificultad para dormir o conciliar el sueño

International time A 24-hour method of keeping time in which hours are not distinguished between AM and PM, but are counted continuously and consecutively through the entire day

Tiempo internacional Un método de 24 horas para contar el tiempo en el cual las horas no se diferencian en a.m. y p.m., sino que se cuentan de forma continua y consecutiva a lo largo de todo el día

Intrinsic factor   A naturally produced protein that is necessary for the absorption of vitamin B_{12}

Factor intrínseco   Una proteína producida de forma natural y que es necesaria para la absorción de la vitamina B_{12}

Invasive   The tendency for a tumor or mass to move into tissues and/or organs in close proximity

Invasiva   La tendencia de un tumor o una masa a desplazarse hacia el interior de los tejidos y/o órganos que se hallan en sus proximidades inmediatas

Ion   An atom or a group of atom with a leftover unbalanced charge

Ión   Un átomo o un grupo de átomos con un resto de carga sin equilibrar

Ionic bond   The transfer of electrons between two atoms

Enlace iónico   La transferencia de electrones entre dos átomos

Kcal Kilocalorie   A measurement of energy or heat expended or used up in a chemical activity; the amount of heat needed to change the temperature of 1 Kg of water one degree Celsìus

Kcal Kilocaloría   Una medida de energía o calor que se desprende o se gasta durante una actividad química; la cantidad de calor que se necesita para cambiar la temperatura de 1 Kg de agua un grado Celsìus

Keratolytic   A drug that causes shedding of the outer layer of the skin

Queratolítico   Una medicina que ocasiona el desprendimiento de la capa externa de la piel

Labyrinth   A bony maze composed of the vestibule, cochlea, and semicircular canals of the inner ear

Laberinto   Un conjunto óseo formado por el vestíbulo, la clóquea y los canales semicirculares del oído interno

Laminar flow hood   Environment for the preparation of sterile products

Campana de flujo laminar   Medio para la preparación de productos estériles

Legend drug   Drug that requires a prescription for dispensing

Medicina de venta con receta   Medicina que no puede venderse sin una receta

Leukemia   A progressive disease marked by malignancy of the blood-forming cells found in the hemopoietic tissues, organs, and bloodstream, causing the circulation of abnormal blood cells

Leucemia   Una enfermedad progresiva caracterizada por la malignidad de las células sanguíneas que se hallan en los tejidos hemopoyéticos, en los órganos y en la corriente sanguínea, causando origen a la circulación de células sanguíneas anómalas

Lipids   Fats and fatty acids

Lípidos   Grasas y ácidos grasos

Lumbar   The region of the back that includes the area between the ribs and the pelvis; the area around the waist

Lumbar   La región de la espalda que incluye el área entre las costillas y la pelvis; la zona alrededor de la cintura

Lymphoma   A term used to describe a malignant disorder of lymphoid tissue

Linfoma   Un término que se usa para describir un trastorno maligno del tejido linfático

Macro   Large

Macro   Grande

Malignant   An invasive and destructive pattern of rapid, abnormal cell growth; often fatal

Maligno   Un patrón invasivo y destructivo de crecimiento celular rápido y anómalo; con frecuencia mortal

Mania   A form of psychosis characterized by excessive excitement, elevated mood, and exalted feelings

Manía   Una forma de psicosis que se caracteriza por una agitación excesiva, estado de ánimo elevado y sentimientos exaltados

MAR   Medication administration record

MAR   Registro de administración de medicación

Melanoma   A malignant neoplasm of the pigmented cells of skin; may metastasize to other organs

Melanoma   Un neoplasma maligno de las células pigmentadas de la piel; se puede metastatizar a otros órganos

Menopause   Cessation of menstruation; a natural phenomenon in which the woman passes from a reproductive state to a nonreproductive state

Menopausia   Cese de la menstruación; un fenómeno natural por el cual la mujer pasa de un estado reproductivo a otro no reproductivo

Metabolism   The physical and chemical changes that take place within an organism

Metabolismo   Los cambios físicos y químicos que tienen lugar dentro de un organismo

Metastasis   The movement or spread of cancerous cells through the body to organs in distant areas

Metástasis   El movimiento o la expansión de células cancerosas a través del cuerpo hasta órganos distantes

Meter   Basic measurement of length in the metric system
Metro   Medida básica de longitud del sistema métrico

Metered dose inhaler (MDI)   A method of supplying medications to the lungs through inhalation
Inhalador dosificador (MDI)   Un método de administración de medicamentos a los pulmones por medio de inhalación

Micro   Small
Micro   Pequeño

Microbial   Refers to microorganisms (very small) not visible without a microscope
Microbiano   Referente a microorganismos (muy pequeños) que no son visibles sin un microscopio

Microbiology   The study of microscopic organisms
Microbiología   El estudio de los organismos microscópicos

Microgram   1000th of a milligram; metric unit of measure
Microgramo   Milésima parte de un miligramo; unidad de medida métrica

Milligram   1000th of a gram; metric unit of measure
Miligramo   Milésima parte de un gramo; unidad de medida métrica

Miosis   Contraction of the pupil
Miosis   Contracción de la pupila

Mitosis   Cellular reproduction that creates two identical daughter cells from the parent cell's DNA
Mitosis   Reproducción celular que da origen a dos células hijas idénticas a partir del ADN de la célula madre

Mole   Avogadro's number: 6.02×10^{23} atoms, molecules, or ions
Mol   Número de Avogrado: 6.02×10^{23} átomos, moléculas o iones

Molecular biosynthesis   The making of chemical compounds within a living organism
Biosíntesis molecular   La producción de compuestos químicos en el interior de un organismo vivo

Molecule   The smallest particle of a compound
Molécula   La partícula más pequeña de un compuesto

Monoamine oxidase (MAO)   An enzyme (includes MAO-A and MAO-B) found in the nerve terminals, the neurons, and liver cells; inactivates chemicals such as tyramine, catecholamines, serotonin, and certain medications

Monoaminooxidosa (MAO)   Una enzima (incluye MAO-A y MAO-B) que se halla en las células de las terminales nerviosas, las neuronas y el hígado. esta enzima inactiva sustancias químicas como la tiramina, las catecolaminas, la serotonina y ciertos medicamentos

Monograph   Medication information sheet provided by the manufacturer that includes side effects, dosage forms, indications, and other important information
Monografía   Hoja de información sobre un medicamento proporcionada por el fabricante y que incluye efectos secundarios, formas de dosificación, indicaciones y otra información importante

Morals   Ethics; honorable beliefs
Moral   Ética; creencias honorables

Morphology   Appearance, including shape, size, structure, and gram stain characteristics of organisms; study of organisms without studying the function of organisms
Morfología   Apariencia de los organismos incluyendo características de forma, tamaño, estructura y coloración del gram de los organismos; estudio de los organismos sin estudiar sus funciones

Mortar and pestle   A bowl and rounded knob used to grind substances into fine powder
Mortero   Un tazón y mazo redondeado que se usan para moler sustancias hasta convertirlas en polvo fino

Mosby's Drug Consult   Reference book of medications

Mutation   An unexpected change in the molecular structure within the DNA, causing a permanent change in cells
Mutación   Un cambio inesperado en la estructura molecular del ADN que causa un cambio permanente en las células

Mycosis   Fungal disease
Micosis   Infección por hongos

Mydriasis   Dilation of the pupil
Midriasis   Dilatación de la pupila

Myopia   Nearsightedness
Miopía   Vista corta

Myxedema   Condition associated with the a decrease in overall thyroid function in adults; also known as hypothyroidism
Mixedema   Enfermedad relacionada con una disminución de la función tiroidea general en los adultos; se conoce también como hipotiroidismo

National Association of Boards of Pharmacy (NABP)   National organization for members of state boards of pharmacy

Asociación Nacional de Juntas Farmacéuticas (NABP) Organización nacional para miembros de juntas farmacéuticas estatales

Nationally Certified Technician Proficient in minimum standards set by the Pharmacy Technician Certification Board

Técnico con Certificación Nacional Individuo competente dentro de los estándares mínimos establecidos por la Junta de Certificación de Técnicos Farmacéuticos

Negative feedback A self-regulating mechanism in which the output of a system has input or control on the process; a factor within a system that causes a corrective action to return the system to normal range

Retrocontrol negativo Un mecanismo autorregulado en el cual el resultado de un sistema tiene entrada o control en el proceso; un factor dentro de un sistema que produce una acción correctiva para que el sistema vuelva a su ámbito normal

Neoplasm An abnormal tissue growth

Neoplasma Un crecimiento anómalo de un tejido

Nerve Terminal The end portion of the neuron where nerve impulses cause chemical to be released; these cross a small space, called a synaptic cleft, and carry the impulse to another neuron

Terminal nerviosa El extremo final de la neurona en donde los impulsos nerviosos causan que se liberen sustancias químicas; estas cruzan un espacio pequeño, denominado hendidura sináptica, y llevan el impulso a otra neurona

Neuron The functional unit of the nervous system, which included the cell body, dendrites, axon, and terminals

Neurona La unidad funcional del sistema nervioso, compuesta por el cuerpo celular, las dendritas, el axón y las terminales nerviosas

Neurosis Mental illness arising from stress or anxiety in the patient's environment without loss of contact with reality; phobias can be listed in this category

Neurosis Enfermedad mental que surge del estrés o la ansiedad en el entorno del paciente, sin que haya una pérdida de contacto con la realidad, las fobias pueden encuadrarse en esta categoría

Neutron A subset of an atom that does not contain a charge

Neutrón Una subdivisión de un átomo la cual no tiene carga

NKDA No known drug allergy

NKDA No se le conocen alergias a medicamentos

Nonproductive cough Cough that does not produce mucous secretions from respiratory tract

Tos improductiva Tos que no produce secreciones mucosas del tracto respiratorio (tos seca)

Normal flora Microorganisms that reside harmlessly in the body and do not cause disease but may aid the host organism

Flora normal Microorganismos que se hallan en el cuerpo y que no causan enfermedades, sino que pueden ser beneficiosos para el organismo en el que se encuentran

Nosocomial infection An infection acquired while hospitalized

Infección nosocomial Una infección adquirida durante una hospitalización

NSAIDs Nonsteroidal antiinflammatory drugs

NSAID Medicamentos antiinflamatorios no esteroides

Nucleic acid The bases contained within deoxyribonucleic acid (DNA)

Ácido nucleico Las bases que se hallan en el ácido desoxirribonucleico (ADN)

Ointment A hydrophobic product such as Vaseline

Ungüento Un producto hidrófobo como la vaselina

On-call A medication to be administered when directed, usually for preanesthesia

A petición Un medicina que se administra cuando se ordena, normalmente como preanestesia

Oncogene A previously normal gene that may be adversely affected by infection, such as a retrovirus, which causes a mutation and may produce cancer

Oncógeno Un gen que era normal pero que puede haber sido afectado de forma adversa por una infección, como un retrovirus, que causa una mutación y puede producir cáncer

Oocyte or ova The female reproductive germ cell

Oocito u óvulo La célula germinal femenina

Ophthalmic Pertaining to the eye

Oftálmico Perteneciente al ojo

Orbit The rotation of electrons around the nucleus

Órbita La rotación de los electrones alrededor del núcleo

Osteoporosis Condition associated with the decrease of bone mass and the softening of the bones, resulting in the increased possibility of bone fractures

Osteoporosis Enfermedad relacionada con una disminución de la densidad ósea y el ablandamiento de los huesos, que da como resultado un aumento en la posibilidad de fracturas óseas

OTC Over-the-counter
OTC De venta libre (sin receta)

Otic Pertaining to the ear
Ótico Perteneciente al oído

Outpatient pharmacy Pharmacies that serve patients in their communities; pharmacies that are not in inpatient facilities
Farmacia externa Farmacias que sirven a los pacientes en sus comunidades; farmacias que no están en instalaciones en la que hay pacientes internos

Over-the-counter (OTC) medication Medication that can be purchased without a prescription; non-legend medications
Medicamento de venta libre (OTC) Medicamento que se puede comprar sin receta; medicamentos de venta sin receta

Paget's disease Condition that affects older adults in which the density of the bones decreases, resulting in softening and weakening
Enfermedad de Paget Enfermedad que afecta a adultos de edad avanzada en la cual disminuye la densidad de los huesos, dando como resultado su ablandamiento y debilitamiento

Palliative Brings relief but does not cure
Paliativo Proporciona alivio, pero no cura

PAR Periodic automatic replacement
PAR Reemplazo automático periódico

Parasite Organism that requires a host for nourishment and reproduction
Parásito Organismo que necesita un organismo huésped para alimentarse y reproducirse

Parasympathetic nervous system Division of the autonomic nervous system that functions during restful situations; "breed or feed" part of ANS
Sistema nervioso parasimpático División del sistema nervioso autónomo que funciona durante los momentos de descanso; parte del SNA encargada de "criar o alimentar"

Parenteral Medication administered by injection, such as intravenously or intramuscularly
Parenteral Medicamento que se administra por inyección, como el que se administra por vía intravenosa o intramuscular

Passive immunity Resistance that has been acquired through a transfer of antibodies from another person or animal, or from mother to child
Inmunidad pasiva Resistencia que ha sido adquirida a través de una transferencia de anticuerpos de otra persona o animal, o de la madre al hijo

Peptic ulcer An ulcerative condition of the lower esophagus, stomach, or duodenum, usually resulting from the bacterium *Helicobacter pylori* (*H pylori*)
Úlcera péptica Enfermedad ulcerativa del esófago inferior, estómago o duodeno; por lo general, es producida por la bacteria *Helicobacter pylori* (*H pylori*)

Peptidoglycan The substance that comprises bacterial cell walls, specifically of gram-negative and gram-positive microbes
Peptidoglicano La sustancia que posee barreras de células bacterianas, específicamente de microbios gram negativos y gram positivos

Peripheral nervous system (PNS) The division of the nervous system outside the brain and spinal cord
Sistema nervioso periférico (SNP) La parte del sistema nervioso que está fuera del cerebro y la médula espinal

Peripheral parenteral Injection of a medication into the veins located on the periphery of the body system instead of a central vein or artery
Parenteral periférica Inyección de un medicamento en las venas localizadas en la periferia del sistema corporal, y no en una vena o arteria central

Peristalsis The contraction and relaxation of the tubular muscles of the esophagus and intestines that move food substances from the mouth to the anus
Peristalsis La contracción y relajación de los músculos tubulares del esófago y los intestinos que llevan las sustancias alimenticias desde la boca hasta el ano

Pharmacist Person who dispenses drugs and counsels patients
Farmacéutico Persona que dispensa medicamentos y aconseja a los pacientes

Pharmacology The study of drugs and their effects on the body
Farmacología El estudio de las medicinas, las drogas, y sus efectos en el cuerpo

Pharmacy clerk Person who assists the pharmacist at the front counter of the pharmacy; the person who accepts payment for medications
Dependiente de farmacia Persona que ayuda al farmacéutico en el mostrador de la farmacia; la persona que cobra por los medicamentos

Pharmacy Technician Certification Board National board for the certification of pharmacy technicians
Junta de Certificación de Técnicos Farmacéuticos Junta nacional para la certificación de técnicos de farmacia

Pharmacy technician Person who assists a pharmacist by filling prescriptions and performing other nondispensing tasks
Técnico farmacéutico Persona que ayuda al farmacéutico preparando recetas y realizando otras tareas, excepto despachar medicinas a los pacientes

Physician's Desk Reference (PDR) Reference book of medications
"Physicians' Desk Reference" (PDR) Libro de referencia sobre los medicamentos

Placebo Inert compound thought to be an active agent
Placebo Componente inactivo del que se piensa que puede ser un agente real

POS Point of sale
POS Punto de venta

PPO Preferred Provider Organization
PPO Organización de Proveedores Preferidos

Pre-op A drug ordered to be given before surgery
Pre-operatoria Una medicina que se receta para administrarla antes de una cirugía

Productive cough Cough that expectorates mucous secretions from respiratory tract
Tos productiva Tos que arrastra secreciones mucosas del tracto respiratorio

Professionalism Conforming to right principles of conduct (work ethics) as accepted by others in the profession
Profesionalismo Conducta que está en conformidad con los principios correctos (ética laboral) tal como los aceptan las otras personas de la profesión

Prophylaxis Treatment given before an event to prevent the event from happening
Profilaxis Tratamiento que se da antes de que ocurra un hecho para impedir que dicho hecho tenga lugar

Protectant A substance that acts as a barrier between the skin and an irritant
Protector Una sustancia que actúa como una barrera entre la piel y un agente irritante

Protocol A set of standards and guidelines within which a facility works

Protocolo Una serie de estándares y pautas de trabajo por las que se rige un establecimiento

Proton A subatomic particle of an atom that holds a positive charge
Protón Una partícula subatómica de un átomo que tiene carga positiva

Protozoa Kingdom Protista; unicellular organism that are parasites
Protozoos Reino Protista; organismo unicelulares parasitarios

Pruritis Itching
Prurito Picazón

Psychosis A mental illness characterized by loss of contact with reality
Psicosis Una enfermedad mental caracterizada por la pérdida de contacto con la realidad

Recall When a drug or device must be returned to the manufacturer due to failure to meet FDA standards
Devolución Cuando hay que devolver una medicina o un aparato al fabricante porque no cumple los estándares de la FDA

Reconstitution To mix a liquid and a powder to form a suspension or solution
Reconstitución Acción de mezclar un líquido con una sustancia en polvo para formar una suspensión o una solución

Remission The span of time during which a disease, such as cancer, is not spreading; this may be permanent or temporary
Remisión El lapso de tiempo durante el cual una enfermedad, como el cáncer, no se propaga; puede ser permanente o temporal

Repackaging The act of reducing the amount of medication taken from a bulk bottle; unit dosing is a form of repackaging
Re-envasado El acto de reducir la cantidad de medicamento que se toma de un envase grande; la dosis unitaria es una forma de re-envasado

Rhinitis Inflammation of the lining of the nose; runny nose
Rinitis Inflamación de los tejidos que recubren la nariz; nariz que gotea

ROA Route of administration
ROA Vía de administración

Rods Photoreceptors that respond to dim light and are responsible for black and white color (night vision)
Bastoncillos Elementos fotorreceptores que responden ante la luz atenuada y son

responsables para la visión en blanco y negro (visión nocturna)

RTS Return to stock

RTS Devolver al almacén

Rx Latin for "recipe," commonly used to mean "prescription"; legend drug; prescription drug

Rx Término latín para "receta", se usa con frecuencia para indicar "receta", medicina de venta con receta

Sarcoma A malignant, neoplastic growth arising from the connective tissue

Sarcoma Un crecimiento neoplástico maligno que surge del tejido connectivo

Schizophrenia A group of mental disorders characterized by inappropriate emotions and unrealistic thinking

Esquizofrenia Un grupo de trastornos mentales que se caracterizan por emociones inapropiadas y pensamientos irreales

Script A prescription

Escrito Una receta

Shaman Medicine person who holds a high place of honor in a tribe

Chamán Curandero que tiene un puesto de honor en una tribu

Sig Medication directions written in pharmacy terms on a prescription

Sig (Signatura) Instrucciones escritas para la medicación en términos farmacéuticos en una receta

Solute The ingredient that is dissolved into a solution

Soluto En una solución, el ingrediente que se disuelve

Solution A water base in which the ingredient(s) dissolve completely

Solución Una base de agua en la cual el ingrediente o los ingredientes se disuelven completamente

Solvent The greater part of a solution

Solvente La mayor parte de una solución

Somatic The motor neurons that control voluntary actions of the skeletal muscles

Somáticas Las neuronas motoras que controlan las acciones voluntarias de los músculos esqueletales

Species Of Latin origin meaning "kind"

Especies Palabra de origen latín que significa "tipo"

Sputum Fluid coughed up from the lungs and bronchial tissues

Esputo Fluido expulsado por la tos desde los pulmones y los tejidos bronquiales

STAT order A medication order that must be filled as soon as possible, usually within 5 to 15 minutes

Receta STAT Una receta que debe despacharse lo antes posible, por lo general en 5 a 15 minutos

Steroid Messenger chemical produced by the body that helps fight inflammation and pain

Esteroides Sustancias químicas que actúan como mensajeros y que son producidas por el cuerpo para ayudar a combatir la infamación y el dolor

Sunscreen A substance that protects the skin from ultraviolet (UV) light, which causes sunburns; skin protectant factor (SPF) rates effectiveness

Filtro solar Una sustancia que protege la piel de los rayos ultravioletas (UVA), los cuales causan quemaduras solares; el factor de protección de la piel (SPD) se usa para clasificar la eficacia de estos filtros

Suspension A solution is which the powder does not dissolve into the base and must be shaken before using

Suspensión Una solución en la cual el polvo no se disuelve en la base y debe agitarse antes de ser usada

Symbiotic A close relationship between two species

Simbiótica Una estrecha relación entre dos especies

Sympathetic nervous system Division of the autonomic nervous system that functions during stressful situations; "fight or flight" part of ANS

Sistema nervioso simpático División del sistema nervioso autónomo que funciona durante situaciones de estrés; la parte del SNA encargada de "luchar o huir"

Synthesis The formation of chemical components within the body system

Síntesis La formación de compuestos químicos dentro del sistema corporal

Synthetic Medication made in a laboratory

Sintético Medicamento hecho en un laboratorio

Syrup A sugar-based liquid

Jarabe Un líquido con base de azúcar

Systemic Pertaining to the entire body rather than to individual body parts

Sistémico Perteneciente a todo el cuerpo más bien que a partes individuales del mismo

Tardive dyskinesia Unwanted side effects of taking phenothiazines that include slow, rhythmical involuntary movements that are either generalized or specific to one muscle group

Discinesia tardía Efectos secundarios negativos de la toma de fenotiazinas y que incluyen movimientos involuntarios lentos y rítmicos que pueden ser generalizadores o afectar a un grupo muscular específico

Taxonomy The science of classification and nomenclature of organisms

Taxonomía La ciencia de la clasificación y nomenclatura de organismos

Therapeutic Curative, treatment that is effective

Terapéutico Curativo, tratamiento que es efectivo

Thoracic Relates to the thorax or the chest

Torácico Relativo al tórax o al pecho

Thrombin An enzyme that is formed in coagulating blood from prothrombin. This reacts with fibrinogen, converting it into fibrin, which is essential in the formation of blood clots. Tested by performing a prothrombin time (PT) or partial thromboplastin time (PTT) blood test

Trombina Una enzima que se forma a partir de la protombrina para coagular la sangre. Ésta reacciona con el fibrinógeno, que se convierte en fibrina, la cual es fundamental en la formación de los coágulos de sangre. Se analiza realizando análisis de sangre de tiempo de protrombina (TP) o de tiempo parcial de protrombina (TPP)

Thrombolytic Medication used to break up a thrombus or blood clot

Trombolítico Medicamento que se usa para deshacer un trombo o coágulo de sangre

Thyroxine Known as T_4; contains four ions of iodine

Tiroxina Conocida como T_4, tiene cuatro iones de yodo

Tincture A base solution of alcohol

Tintura Una solución con base de alcohol

Total parenteral nutrition Large-volume intravenous (IV) nutrition administered through the central vein (subclavian vein) in which allows for a higher concentration of solutions

Nutrición parenteral total Nutrición intravenosa (IV) de gran volumen administrada a través de la vena central (vena subclaviana), lo cual permite usar soluciones con concentraciones elevadas

Tourette's syndrome A disorder characterized by multiple motor tics, lack of muscle coordination, and involuntary purposeless movements that are accompanied by grunts and bark

Síndrome de Tourette Un trastorno que se caracteriza por múltiples tics motores,

incluyendo falta de coordinación muscular y movimientos involuntarios y sin sentido acompañados de gruñidos y rugidos

Toxoid A toxin that has been rendered harmless but still invokes an antigenic response

Anatoxina Una toxina que se ha vuelto inofensiva pero que todavía produce una respuesta antígena

Trace elements Elements that are needed by the body in very small amounts

Elementos traza Elementos que el cuerpo necesita en cantidades muy pequeñas

Trade name Brand name drug; the company that first applies for a patent on the chemical structure of a medication or generic name is allowed to name the product with a patented name

Denominación comercial Medicamento de marca; la compañía que primero solicita una patente de la estructura química de un medicamento o un nombre genérico se le permite darle un nombre a ese producto con una marca patentada

Triiodothyronine Known as T_3; contains three ions of iodine

Triodotironina Conocida como T_3, tiene tres iones de yodo

Tympanic membrane A membranous skin that separates the external ear from the middle ear

Membrana del tímpano Una piel membranosa que separa el oído externo del oído medio

Ulcer A stomach lesion on a mucous surface of the gastrointestinal (GI) tract

Úlcera Una lesión estomacal en la superficie mucosa del tracto gastrointestinal (TG)

Unit dose A single dose of a drug

Dosis unitaria Una sola dosis de una medicina

Universal precautions A set of standards that lowers the possibility of contamination; used to prepare medications

Precauciones universales Una serie de estándares que reducen la posibilidad de contaminación; se usan en la preparación de medicamentos

Urticaria A skin eruption of itching wheals

Urticaria Erupción cutánea de ampollas que producen picazón

Vaccine Toxoids or attenuated viral components that are given to create a response from the body that results in immunity

Vacunas Toxides o componentes virales atenuados que se administran para crear una respuesta del cuerpo que tiene como resultado la inmunidad

Valence   The number of electrons gained, lost, or shared when an atom bonds with another atom; determined by the electrons in the outer orbit

Valencia   El número de electrones que un átomo gana, pierde o comparte cuando se une con otro átomo; está determinada por los electrones que hay en la órbita más externa.

Vasodilation   Widening of the blood vessels that allows for increased blood flow

Vasodilatación   Ensanchamiento de los vasos sanguíneos que permite una mayor circulación de sangre

Vector   An entity by which infections are transferred, but the entity of transference does not have the disease; does not need to be living. For example, a mosquito bite transfers malaria. In this case, the mosquito is the vector

Vector   Una entidad que transmite infecciones, pero la entidad transmisora no padece la enfermedad. Por ejemplo, la picadura de un mosquito transmite la malaria. En este caso, el mosquito es el vector

Vein   A vessel that carries deoxygenated blood to or toward the heart

Vena   Un vaso sanguíneo que transporta la sangre sin oxígeno hasta el corazón

Vertical flow hood   Environment for preparation of chemotherapy treatments that uses air originating from the roof of the hood moving downward that is captured in a vent located on the floor of the hood

Campana de flujo vertical   Medio para la preparación de tratamientos de quimioterapia en el que se utiliza una corriente de aire que parte del techo de la campana y que se mueve hacia abajo, hasta entrar en un hueco de ventilación que se halla en el suelo de la campana

Villus   A projection from the surface of a mucous membrane; in the gastric tract, these projections increase the surface area for absorption of nutrients and liquids in the small intestines

Vellosidad   Una proyección de la superficie de una membrana mucosa en el tracto gástrico, estas proyecciones aumentan el área de superficie para la absorción de nutrientes y líquidos en el intestino delgado

Virology   The study of viruses

Virología   El estudio de los virus

Virus   An organism that replicates by using the host's cell parts, including deoxyribonucleic acid (DNA), ribosomes, and proteins

Virus   Un organismo que se reproduce utilizando partes de las células del organismo huésped, incluyendo el ácido desoxirribonucleico (ADN), ribosomas y proteínas

Viscosity   The thickness of a solution or fluid (e.g., corn syrup is very viscous)

Viscosidad   El espesor de una solución o fluido (ej.: el jarabe de maíz es muy viscoso)

Volume   The amount of liquid enclosed within a container

Volumen   La cantidad de liquido que puede contener un envase

Water-soluble vitamin   Vitamin that is soluble in water and is not readily stored by the body; continually excreted in the urine and must be constantly replaced

Vitamina soluble en agua   Vitamina que se disuelve en el agua y que por lo tanto no se almacena fácilmente en el cuerpo; se excreta continuamente en la orina, por lo cual tiene que reemplazarse constantemente.

Worker's compensation   A government-required and enforced coverage for workers injured on the job

Compensación laboral   Una cobertura de seguro que el gobierno exige y hace cumplir, destinada a trabajadores que se lesionan en el trabajo

Credits

Chapter 4

p. 47. Cleocin. Courtesy of Pfizer.

p. 50. Cimetidine. Courtesy of Zenith-Ivax Goldline Pharmaceuticals.

p. 51. Tegretol. Courtesy of Basel Pharmaceuticals.

p. 53. Amoxil. Courtesy of GlaxoSmithKline.

p. 55. Potassium Chloride. Courtesy of American Pharmaceutical Partners.

p. 56. From Potter PA, Perry AG: *Fundamentals of nursing: concepts, process, and practice*, ed 3, St Louis, 1993, Mosby.

Chapter 5

p. 76. Figure 5.6. **A.** From Brown M, Mulholland JL: *Drug Calculations Process and Problems for clinical practice*, ed 6, St Louis, 2000, Mosby. **B.** From Elkin M, Perry A, Potter P: *Nursing interventions and clinical skills*, ed 2, St Louis, 2000, Mosby.

p. 78. Figure 5.8. From Elkin M, Perry A, Potter P: *Nursing interventions and clinical skills*, ed 2, St Louis, 2000, Mosby.

Chapter 8

p. 124. Figure 8.4. From Potter PA, Perry AG: *Fundamentals of Nursing*, ed 5, St Louis, 2001, Mosby.

Chapter 13

p. 207. Figure 13.1. **A.** Courtesy of SIMS Deltec, Inc., St Paul, MN. **B.** From Elkin M, Perry A, Potter P: *Nursing interventions and clinical skills*, St Louis, 1996, Mosby.

p. 211. Figure 13.3. Courtesy of ESI Lederle, Division of American Home Products Corporation, St Davids, PA.

Chapter 15

pp. 246–249, 251–258. All illustrations of pills from *Mosby's Drug Consult*, St Louis, 2004, Mosby.

Chapter 16

pp. 273, 276. All illustrations of pills from *Mosby's Drug Consult*, St Louis, 2004, Mosby.

Chapter 17

pp. 298, 299, 301–305, 307–309. All illustrations of pills from *Mosby's Drug Consult*, St Louis, 2004, Mosby.

Chapter 18

pp. 324, 326, 327. All illustrations of pills from *Mosby's Drug Consult*, St Louis, 2004, Mosby.

Chapter 20

pp. 365, 366, 369, 373, 374. All illustrations of pills from *Mosby's Drug Consult*, St Louis, 2004, Mosby.

Chapter 21

pp. 388–391. All illustrations of pills from *Mosby's Drug Consult*, St Louis, 2004, Mosby.

Chapter 22

pp. 405–407, 409, 410, 412–415. All illustrations of pills from *Mosby's Drug Consult*, St Louis, 2004, Mosby.

Chapter 23

p. 440. Table 23.1. Modified from Beare FG, Myers JL: *Adult health nursing*, ed 3, St Louis, 1998, Mosby; and *Mosby's Medical, Nursing, and Allied Health Dictionary*, ed 5, St Louis, 1998, Mosby.

p. 425. Figure 23.1. From Frazier MS, Drzymkowski JW: *Essentials of human diseases and conditions*, ed 2, Philadelphia, 2000, W.B. Saunders.

p. 426. Figure 23.2. From Applegate E: *The anatomy and physiology learning system*, 2/e. W.B. Saunders, Philadelphia, 2000.

p. 427. Figure 23.3. From Frazier MS, Drzymkowski JW: *Essentials of human diseases and conditions*, ed 2, Philadelphia, 2000, W.B. Saunders.

p. 428. Figure 23.4. From Applegate E: *The anatomy and physiology learning system*, ed 2, Philadelphia, 2000, W.B. Saunders.

p. 435. Figure 23.5. From *Mosby's medical, nursing, and allied health dictionary*, ed 6, St Louis, 2002, Mosby; originally from Edge V, Miller M: *Women's health care*, St Louis, 1994, Mosby.

p. 435. Figure 23.6. From McKinney ES, Ashwill JW, Murray SS, et al: *Maternal-child Nursing*, Philadelphia, 2000, W.B. Saunders.

p. 435. Figure 23.7. From Leifer G: *Introduction to maternity-pediatric nursing*, Philadelphia, 2003, W.B. Saunders.

p. 439. Figure 23.8. **A.** From *Mosby's medical, nursing, and allied health dictionary*, ed 6, St Louis, 2002, Mosby; originally from Edge V, Miller M: *Women's health care*, St Louis, 1994, Mosby; **B.** From Leifer G: *Introduction to maternity-pediatric nursing*, Philadelphia, 2003, Saunders.

p. 439. Figure 23.9. From *Mosby's medical, nursing, and allied health dictionary*, ed 6, St Louis, 2002, Mosby; originally from Edge V, Miller M: *Women's health care*, St Louis, 1994, Mosby.

Chapter 24

pp. 436, 437, 447. All illustrations of pills from *Mosby's Drug Consult*, St Louis, 2004, Mosby.

Chapter 25

pp. 462, 463, 465. All illustrations of pills from *Mosby's Drug Consult*, St Louis, 2004, Mosby.

Index

Page numbers followed by f indicate figures; t, tables; b, boxes.

A

Abbreviations, 65
  dosage forms, 64
  in Drug Topics Red Book, 91t
  parenterals, 208b
  routes of administration, 64
Abortifacients, 423
"Abortion" pill, 439, 440
Absinthe, 7
Absorption, 64, 79
  GI system, 356, 360–361
Acarbose, 278
Accolate, 327
Accommodation, 333
Acebutolol, 414
Acellular vaccines, 513b
Acetaminophen, 254–255
  codeine and, 323
Acetazolamide, 391, 410
Acetohexamide, 278t
Acetylcholine HCL, 341
Acetylcysteine, 325
Acetylsalicylic acid. *See* Aspirin
Acid-base reactions, 571
Acidification, 378
Acidosis, 378
  excess iron, 504
Acne development, 145–146, 146
Acne treatments, 146
Acoustic nerve, 333
Acquired immunity, 508
Acromegaly, 270
ACTH, 268t
Active immunity, 511
Actos, 278
Acular, 344
Acupressure, 153, 155, 156t

Acupuncture, 153, 155, 156t
Acyclovir, 467
Adalat, 414
Addison's disease, 263, 275
  treatment of, 275–276
Additives, 81, 82t
ADH, 267, 268t
Adjudication, 227
Adrenal cortex conditions/diseases, 275–276
Adrenal effects of steroid agents, 482–483
Adrenal glands, 265, 269
  conditions and their treatment, 275–276
Adrenal medulla conditions/diseases, 276–277
Adrenalin, 326
Adrenocorticotropic hormone (ACTH), 268t
Adrenogenital syndrome, 275t
Adroid-25, 430
Adult immunizations, 516–517
Adverse medication reactions
  FDA reporting process, 16
  monographs, 20
Aerobic organisms, 539
AeroBid, 328, 485
Aerosols, 70
Aesculapius, 3, 5
Afferent, 283
Afferent neurons, 290
Afrin, 325
AIDS/HIV, 469, 557
  vaccine for, 513
AK-Pred (solution), 344
Albuterol, 326
Alcohol, historical use of, 7
Alcohol Anonymous, 245
Aldactazide, 390t
Aldactone, 390, 410
Aldosterone, 269t

Alendronate, 274
Alesse-28, 437
Algae, 549
Alkalosis, 378
Alkylating agents, 530
Allergies, 320
  agents/medications for, 323–325
    over-the-counter, 138
  no known drug allergy, 170
Alligation, 39, 56–58
Aloe vera, 152, 162
Alpha-adrenergic blockers, 430–431
Alprazolam, 256
ALS. *See* Amyotrophic lateral sclerosis (ALS)
Alternative medicine. *See* Complementary
    alternative medicine (CAM)
Aluminum hydroxide, 364
Aluminum magnesium hydroxide, 364t
Alupent, 326
Alu-Tab, 364
Alzheimer's disease, 302–303, 309t
Amantadine, 306
Amaryl, 278t
Ambien, 257
Amen, 434
Amenorrhea, 423
American Association of Pharmacy
    Technicians (AAPT), 96, 581, 582t
American history
  alcohol, use of, 7
  Colonial America, 6–7
  current trends, 8–10
  early pharmacists, 7
  early pharmacy technicians, 8, 29
  opium, use of, 7
  remedies of the 1800's, 7b
*American Hospital Formulary Service Drug
    Information* (AHFS DI), 92, 93t
American Pharmaceutical Association
    (APHA), 581, 582t
American Pharmacist Association (APA), 96
American Society of Health-Systems
    Pharmacists (ASHP), 96, 581, 582t
Amikacin, 460
Amikin, 460
Amiloride, 390
Amiloride/HCTZ, 390t
Amino acids, 356, 564, 571–572
Aminoglycosides, 346, 459–460
Aminophylline, 327, 485
Amitriptyline, 251
Amlodipine, 415
Amoebae, 549
  Entamoeba histolytica, 463, 547
Amoxicillin, 367t
Amphogel, 364

Ampicillin, 456
Ampules, 76f
Amyotrophic lateral sclerosis (ALS), 308
  drug treatment, 308
Anabolic Steroids Control Act (1990), 15
Anabolism, 564, 568
Anaerobic organisms, 539
Anafranil, 251
Analgesics, 131, 136, 137. *See also specific
    analgesic*
  controlled analgesia devices, 210
  intravenous preparations, 218–219
Anaphylactic shock, 474
Ancient beliefs/treatments, 3–5
  herbal remedies, 6
Ancient Chinese medicine, 155–157
Androderm, 429
AndroGel, 429
Androgens, 269t, 279, 423, 425–426, 427–430
Anectine, 310
Anemia, 493
  iron deficiency, 503–504
  and vitamin B_2 deficiencies, 500
  and vitamin B_{12} deficiencies, 501–502
Angina pectoris, 400b, 403
  treatment of, 415–416
Angiotensin converting enzyme agents, 412
Angiotensin II receptor antagonists, 413
Animal cells, 545f, 546–547
Animalia kingdom, 542t, 545–548, 549t
Anorexia, 500
ANS (autonomic nervous system), 283, 293
Antacids
  for GERD, 364, 364t
  for hyperacidity, 364
  OTC antacids, 141t, 363t
Anthrax vaccine, 517t
Antiandrogen, 430
Antianxiety agents, 244, 254–258
Antiarrhythmic agents, 407–408
Antibiotics, 447, 448. *See also specific
    antibiotic*
  aseptic technique for, 216, 218t
  for cancer, 528
  history of, 449, 552
  mechanism of action, 553
  modern, 450
  reference tables, 455t, 458t, 461t
  spectrum and resistance, 554–555
  topical, 148
Antibodies, 508
Anticholinergic agents, 328
Anticoagulants, 417
Antidepressants, 244, 250
  alternative, 253–254
  monoamine oxidase inhibitors, 251–252

Antidepressants *(Continued)*
  selective serotonin reuptake inhibitors, 252–253
  tricyclic, 250–251
Antidiuretic hormone (ADH), 267, 268t
Antiemetic, 152
Antiemetic medications, 373–374
Antiestrogen, 440
Antifungals, 462t
  eye infections, 347
Antigens, 474, 488t, 508
Antiglaucoma agents, 338–342
Antihelminthic agents, 466t
Antihistamines, 138–139, 320, 345, 486, 489t
  allergic mechanism, 486–488
  allergic reactions, blocking of, 488–489
  drug interactions, 488
Antihyperlipidemics, 405–406
Antihypertensive agents, 152
Antiidiotypic vaccines, 513b
Antiinfectives. *See also specific antiinfective*
  for eyes, 344–346
  list of, 447–448
Antiinflammatories. *See also specific antinflammatory agent*
  for eye conditions, 343–345
  list of, 474
  NSAIDS. *See* Nonsteroidal antiinflammatory drugs (NSAIDS)
  OTC medications, 131, 137–138
  for skin conditions, 147, 147t
Antimanics, 249–250
Antimicrobial agents, 447, 448
Antineoplastic, 521
Antioxidants, 502
  vitamin E, 498
Antiplatelet agents, 418
Antipruritic drugs, 131
Antipsychotic agents, 244, 246–249
Antipyretic agents, 137
Antiseptics, 131
Antitoxins, 517
Antitussive drugs, 131, 314, 323–324
Antivenins, 517
Antivert, 374
Anusol-HC, 483
Anxiety, 244
  antianxiety agents, 244, 254–258
Apothecary, 3
Apothecary system, 39, 40–41, 43
Appearance, 106
Appendicitis, 356
Aqueous humor, 333
Aredia, 274
Aricept, 303
Aristocort (po), 276

Aristocort (topical), 483
Aristospan (IV), 276
Aristotle, 3
Armour Thyroid, 273
Aromatherapy, 156t
Arrhythmia, 396, 400b, 403–404
  treatment of, 407–408
Art therapy, 156t, 157
Artane, 308
Artemisia absinthium, 7
Arteries, 396, 397
Arteriosclerosis, 400b
Artificial tears products, 348t
ASA. *See* Aspirin
ASAP orders, 174, 185
Aseptic technique, 170, 175, 206–207, 213, 214b
  for antibiotics, 216, 218t
  clean-up, 216
  errors in, 103
  hand placement, 216, 217f
  hood cleaning/maintenance, 213–216
Ash tree bark, 544
Asparaginase, 531t
Aspiration, 323t
Aspirin, 131, 137, 418t
  drug interactions, 139, 140t
  history of, 477
  strengths, 478t
  uses of, 477–478
Associations, 95–96, 581, 582t, 585
Asthma, 314, 322, 483
  treatment of, 483–486, 489
Atarax, 258
Atenolol, 413
Atherosclerosis, 400b, 402
Athlete's foot, 147, 462, 551
Ativan, 256
Atomic mass, 564
Atoms, 564, 565–566
Atrovastatin, 406
Atrovent, 328
Attenuated, 508
Auditory canal, 333
Auditory ossicles, 333
Autocrine hormones, 266
Autoimmune disease, 263, 272
Automated dispensing systems, 123–124, 183
  and inventory control, 236
Autonomic nervous system (ANS), 283, 293
Auxiliary labels, 114, 122–123, 123t
  compounded products, nonsterile, 196, 197b
  ear preparations, 352
Avandia, 278
Avitaminosis, 493
Avodart, 430

Avoirdupois system, 39, 41, 43
Avoirdupois weights, 42t
Avonex, 304
Axetil (Susp), 457
Axid Pulvules, 365
Axons, 283, 287, 288
Ayurveda medicine, 152, 153, 156t, 157
Azmacort, 328, 483, 485
Azopt, 340
AZT, 467

B

B cells, 509, 511t
Baclofen, 297, 304
Bacon, Roger, 3, 5
Bacteria, 447, 539. *See also* Infections
Bacterial cells, 546f
  cell wall, 553
Bacterial vaccines, 512–513. *See also*
    Vaccines
Bactericidal agents, 447, 449. *See also specific*
    agent
Bacteriostatic agents, 447, 449. *See also*
    specific agent
Baker Cell System, 236
Balances, 192, 193f, 198–199, 200
Balantidium coli, 547
Barbiturates, 255
Barrier devices, 438–439
Bayer, 418t
BBB, 283
Beclomethasone, 327, 485
Beclovent, 327, 485
Beconase AQ, 327
Benadryl, 139, 254, 324
Benazepril, 412
Benign, 521
Benign prostatic hypertrophy, 423
  medications for, 430–431
Benzocaine/menthol, 321
Benzodiazepine-like, 257
Benzodiazepines, 255–257
Benztropine, 308
Beriberi, 500
Beta-adrenergics, 338–340
  for asthma, 483–484
Beta-blockers, 89, 413–414
Betagan, 340
Betaseron, 305
Betaxolol, 339
Betoptic, 339
Betoptic S, 339
Biguanides, 278t
Billing, 227
  HMOs, 229–230
  insurance companies, 232–235

Billing *(Continued)*
  Medicaid, 231
  Medicare, 231
  PPOs, 230–231
  for prescriptions, 127
  third-party, 229–234
  workers' compensation, 231
Binary fission, 539
Bioavailability, 64, 81
  OTC medications, 134–135
Bioequivalence, 64, 81
Biofeedback, 156t, 157–158
Biological response modifiers, 531
Biology, 539, 540
  classification of organisms. *See* Taxonomy
Biopsies, 521
Biphasic medications, 437
Bipolar disorder, 244
Birth control, 434–440
Bisacodyl (OTC), 371
Bismuth, 367t
Bismuth subsalicylate (BSS), 369
Black cohosh, 152, 162
"Black humor," 5
Black sampson, 161
Bladder worm, 465t
Bleeding, and vitamin K, 498
Bleomycin, 528
Bleph-10 (solution, ointment), 346
Blindness, 338
  and vitamin B_6 deficiencies, 501
Blister packs, 188, 192
Blood clots, 400b, 404
  treatment of, 416–418
Blood glucose meters, 278–279
Blood pressure
  high, 401. *See also* Hypertension
  measurements, classification of, 403b
  readings, 402
Blood urea nitrogen (BUN), 378
Blood-brain barrier (BBB), 283
Boards of Pharmacy (BOPs), 13, 30
Body language, 105
  negative, 106b
Bonine Antiver, 374
Bradykinins, 474
Brain, 288–290
Brand name drugs, 88, 227
  versus generic, 229
Breathing, 318–319
Breathing dysfunctions, 320t
Brevicon, 436
Brinzolamide, 340
Bromocriptine, 441
Bronchiectasis, 321
Bronchitis, 321

Bronchodilators, 326–327
Buccal agents, 73
Bulk compounding, 188
Bulk forming, 131
Bumetanide, 410
Bumetidine, 389
Bumex, 389, 410
BUN, 378
Bupropion, 253
Buspar, 257
Buspirone, 257
Butabarbital, 255t
Butisol, 255t

C
C-II narcotics, 18t. *See also* Controlled
    substances
C-III narcotics, 18t. *See also* Controlled
    substances
C-IV narcotics, 18t. *See also* Controlled
    substances
C-V narcotics, 18t. *See also* Controlled
    substances
CAD. *See* Coronary artery disease (CAD)
CADs, 210
Calan, 414
Calciferol, 497
Calcimar, 274
Calcitonin, 268
Calcitonin-salmon, 274
Calcitriol, 497
Calcium acetate, 274
Calcium blocking agents, 414–415
Calcium carbonate, 274, 365
Calcium chloride, 274
Calcium citrate, 274
Calcium gluconate, 274
Calibration, 188
CAM. *See* Complementary alternative
    medicine (CAM)
Cancer, 522
  causes of, 523–524
  defined, 521, 522–522
  diagnosis of, 524
  growth characteristics, 524b
  leukemia, 521, 525
  lung, 322
  lymphoma, 521
    Hodgkin's, 525
    non-Hodgkin's, 525
  oncology agents. *See* Chemotherapeutic
    agents
  sarcoma, 521
    Kaposi's, 525
  terminology, 521
  treatments for, 525

Cancer (*Continued*)
  characteristics, 524b
  chemotherapy. *See* Chemotherapeutic
    agents
  combination therapies, 526t
  radiation, 526
  radioactive isotopes, 526
  surgery, 525–526
  tumors growth, outcomes of, 523b
  types of, 523b, 524–525
  what is, 522–523
Candida infections, 461–462, 550–551
Canker sores, 147
  and vitamin B_3 deficiencies, 500
Capillaries, 396, 397
Caplets, 67–68
Capoten, 412
Capsules, 67–68
  compounded products, nonsterile, 197,
    201–202
  sizes/types, 73
Captopril, 412
Carbachol, 341
Carbamazepine, 301
Carbidopa, 307
Carbohydrates, 356
Carbonic anhydrase inhibitors (CAIs), 339t,
    340, 390–391
  for CHF-related edema, 410
Carcinogens, 521
Cardioglycosides, 408
Cardiopulmonary resuscitation (CPR),
    322–323
Cardiovascular system, 397
  anatomy, 397
  cardiac cycle, 398–399
  conditions affecting, 399–404. *See also*
    specific condition
  conduction system, 398, 400f
  drugs for. *See also specific drug*
    angiotensin converting enzyme agents, 412
    angiotensin II receptor antagonists, 413
    beta blocking agents, 413–414
    calcium blocking agents, 414–415
    list of, 396–397
  oxygenation, 397–398, 399f
  terminology, 396
Cardizem CD, 414
Cardura, 431
Career opportunities, 34–35
Carisoprodol, 297
Carisoprodol/aspirin, 299
Carisoprodol/aspirin/codeine, 299
Carmustine, 530
Carpine, 341
Carteolol, 340

Catabolism, 564
Catalysts, 539
Cataracts, 333
Cefepime, 457
Cefixime, 457
Ceftin (Tab), 457
Cefuroxime, 457
Celexa, 252
Cell body, 283, 287, 288
Cell reproduction, 521, 529f
Central nervous system (CNS). *See* Nervous
    system
Cephalexin, 457
Cephalosporins, 456–457, 459
Cephulac, 370t
Cerebrospinal fluid (CSF), 283
Cerebyx, 300
Certification, 33–34, 101
  national certification, 100, 583–584
Cerumen buildup, 351
Cervical, 283
Cervical caps, 439
Chamomile, 152, 162
Characteristics, 34b
Chemical structure, 88
Chemistry, 564
  acid-base reactions, 571
  amino acids, 356, 571–572
  atoms, 564, 565–566
  electrolytes, 493, 568–571
  enzyme activators and inhibitors, 568
  measurements, 572–575
  metabolism, 80, 564, 568–571
  molecules, 564, 567–569
  periodic table, 566f
  terminology, 564
Chemotherapeutic agents. *See also* Parenteral
    agents/medications
  alkylating agents, 530
  antibiotics, 528
  antimetabolite agents, 526–527
  biological response modifiers, 531
  cytoprotective agents, 532
  disposal of, 219
  list of, 522, 527t
  miscellaneous agents, 530, 531t
  mitotic inhibitors, 528–529
  nausea and vomiting from, 372
  nitrogen mustards, 530
  nitrosoureas, 530
  preparation of, 176. *See also* Aseptic
    technique
    vertical flow hood, 213, 215
  routes of administration, 528t
  side effects of, 530–531
Chemotherapeutic supplies, disposal of, 219

Chemotherapy, 521. *See also*
    Chemotherapeutic agents
CHF. *See* Congestive heart failure (CHF)
Chicken pox vaccine, 516
Childhood immunizations, 514–516
Childproof caps, 22–23, 120
  exceptions, 121t
  nonresistant bottles, use of, 22–23, 23t
  waiver of, 120–121
Chinese medicine, 153, 156t
  ancient, 155–157
Chiropractic, 152, 156t, 158
Chlamydia, 452t
Chloasma, 423
Chlorambucil, 530
Chlordiazepoxide, 257
Chlorothiazide, 388, 409
Chlorotrianisene, 433
Chlorpheniramine, 139
Chlorpromazine, 248
Chlorpropamide, 278t
Chlor-Trimeton, 139
Chlorzoxazone, 298
Cholecalciferol, 498
Cholera vaccine, 517t
Cholestyramine, 405
Chronic bronchitis, 321, 326. *See also* Chronic
    obstructive pulmonary disease (COPD)
Chronic obstructive pulmonary disease
    (COPD), 314, 321
  medications for, 326–328
  mucolytics, 325
Chyme, 356
Cimetidine, 365
Cipro, 392t
Ciprofloxacin, 392t
Citalopram, 252
Citracal, 274
Civil War, 7
Clarithromycin, 367t
Classification of organisms. *See* Taxonomy
Climara, 432
Clinical pharmacists, 3
Clomid, 440
Clomiphene, 440
Clomipramine, 251
Clonazepam, 302
Clorazepate, 257
Clothing, 106
CNS (central nervous system). *See* Nervous
    system
Coagulate, 396
Code blue, 170
Codeine, 323
  and acetaminophen, 323
  with promethazine, 323

Coenzymes, 493
Cofactors, 493, 494
Cogentin, 308
Cognex, 303
Colace, 371
Cold agents/medications, 323–325, 467
  over-the-counter, 138, 320–321
Colds, 320
Colestid, 405
Colestipol, 405
Colonial America, 6–7
Color blindness, 338
Colostomies, 367
Common cold remedies, 320–321
Communication, 100
Communication skills, 8, 104–105, 107
  and appearance, 106
  body language, 105, 106b
  listening, 105–106
  phone etiquette, 106
  written, 107–108
Compazine, 247
Competencies, 100
  certification. *See* Certification
  communication. *See* Communication
    skills
  computer, 109
  laws, knowledge of, 101
  protocol, 101
  registration, 100–101
  reports, 109
  supplies, ordering of, 109–110
  typing, 109
Complementary alternative medicine (CAM),
    155, 156t
  acupressure, 153, 155, 156t
  acupuncture, 153, 155, 156t
  aromatherapy, 156t
  art therapy, 156t, 157
  Ayurveda medicine, 152, 153, 156t, 157
  biofeedback, 156t, 157–158
  Chinese medicine. *See* Chinese medicine
  chiropractic, 152, 156t, 158
  crystal healing, 156t, 158–159
  herbal remedies. *See* Herbal remedies
  pharmacist's perspective, 159–161
  placebo effect, 155
  trends toward, 154
  what is, 153
Compounding, 8, 188
  nonsterile, 192, 193f
    additives commonly used, 196b
    balances, 192, 193f, 198–199, 200
    capsules, 197, 201–202
    containers used, 196–197
    equipment used, 192, 194, 195f

Compounding *(Continued)*
    expiration dates, 198
    graduates, 195f, 201
    labels, 196
    mortar and pestle, 188, 194, 195f, 201
    preparation, 196
    records, 198
    solutions, 202
    techniques, 199, 201–202
    weighing and measuring, 198–199
  sterile. *See* Aseptic technique
Comprehensive Drug Abuse Prevention and
    Control Act of 1970, 15
Computer dispensing systems, 123–124,
    183
Computer skills, 109
Computer users, 88
Condoms, 438–439
Cones, 333
Confidentiality, 100, 108–109
Congestive heart failure (CHF), 378, 400b
  and edema, 384–385, 404
    diuretics for, 408–411 kd kld dllad akl kl
      akl klkld
  treatment of, 408–411
Conjugated estrogens, 433
Conjugated vaccines, 513b
Conjunctivitis, 337, 453
  antiinfective agents for, 345–347
Conn's syndrome, 275t
Constipation, 356, 362, 369–371
  treatment of, 369–371
  and vitamin B$_1$ deficiencies, 500
Consulting with patient. *See* Patient
    counseling
Continuing education, 29, 33, 96
Contraceptives, 434–440
Controlled analgesia devices (CADs), 210
Controlled substances, 17
  hospital pharmacies, 179
  ordering, 17
  prescriptions, 21
  ratings (scheduled substances), 17–18
  record keeping, 17
  refilling, 19
  registration forms, 17
Controlled-release infusion system (CRIS),
    211
Conversion(s)
  of fractions, 44–45
  metric, 43–44
  of percentages, 45
  ratio/proportion, 45–50
  weight, 52–53
COPD. *See* Chronic obstructive pulmonary
    disease (COPD)

Cornea, 333
Coronary artery disease (CAD), 400b, 401
  angina pectoris. *See* Angina pectoris
  arrhythmia. *See* Arrhythmia
  congestive heart failure. *See* Congestive
    heart failure (CHF)
  hyperlipidemia. *See* Hyperlipidemia
  hypertension. *See* Hypertension
  myocardial infarction. *See* Myocardial
    infarction (MI)
  thrombosis, 400b, 404
Corpus Hippocraticum, 4
Cortef, 276, 483
Cortenema, 483
Corticosteroids
  for asthma, 485
  for eye inflammations, 344–345
  for respiratory problems, 327–328
Cortisol, 269t
Coryza, 320
Cough
  nonproductive, 314
  productive, 314
  whooping, 323t
Cough medications, 140
  expectorants, 131, 140, 314, 324
  suppressants, 131, 314, 323–324
Cough reflex, 314
Counting the medication, 120
Covalent bond, 564
COX-1, 480–481
COX-2, 480–481
Cozaar, 413
Creams, 71, 188
Cretinism, 263, 272
Criminal liability, 25
Crinone, 434
CRIS, 211
Crohn's disease, 362
Cromolyn, 328
Cromolyn sodium, 486
Croup, 323t
Crystal healing, 156t, 158–159
CSF, 283
Current trends, 8–10
  in prescription processing, 127
Cushing's disease/syndrome, 263, 275
Cutivate, 328
Cyanocobalamin, 501–502
Cyclobenzaprine, 298
Cyclooxygenase, 480–481
Cyclophosphamide, 530
Cycloplegia, 333
Cycrin, 434
Cystic fibrosis, 314
  mucolytics, 325

Cytarabine, 527
Cytomel, 273
Cytoprotective agents, 532

D
Dacarbazine, 531t
Dactinomycin, 528
Danazol, 430
Danocrine, 430
Dantrium, 304
Dantrolene, 304
Darwin, Charles, 540
Databases, prescription, 118–119
Daunorubicin, 528
DEA (Drug Enforcement Agency), 13, 15, 16
DEA verification, 22
Deafness, 350
Deathly ill patients, 110
Decadron, 276
Decadron Phosphate (solution and ointment),
    345
Decongestants, 138, 139, 314, 320, 325, 345, 345t
DECs (drug education coordinators), 3, 9
Delestrogen, 432
Deltasone, 276, 482
Demadex, 389
Demecarium bromide, 342
Dementia, 303
  Alzheimer's disease, 302–303, 309t
  and vitamin B_3 deficiencies, 500
  and vitamin B_6 deficiencies, 501
  and vitamin B_{12} deficiencies, 501–502
Demulen, 437
Dendrites, 283, 287
Deoxyribonucleic acid. *See* DNA
    (deoxyribonucleic acid)
Depacon, 301
Depakene, 301
Depakote, 301
Depo-Estradiol, 432
Depogen, 432
Depolarizing agents, 310
Depo-Medrol, 276, 483
Depo-Provera, 434, 438
Depot, 423
Depot medications, 431
Depotest, 429
Depo-Testosterone, 429
Depression, 244
  antidepressants. *See* Antidepressants
  psychotic, antipsychotic agents for, 244,
    246–249
  and vitamin B_1 deficiencies, 500
  and vitamin B_2 deficiencies, 500
  and vitamin B_6 deficiencies, 501
  and vitamin B_{12} deficiencies, 501–502

Dermatitis, 474
and vitamin B_3 deficiencies, 500
DES (diethylstilbestrol), 433
Desogen, 437
Desquamating, 131
Desyrel, 253
Dexamethasone, 276, 345
Dextromethorphan/guaifenesin, 324
Diabetes insipidus, 271
Diabetes mellitus, 277
type 1, 277
type 2, 277–278
blood glucose meters, 278–279
Diabinese, 278t
Diagnosis, 152
Dialysis, 378, 386–387
replacement therapy for, 387–388
Diamox, 391, 410
Diaper rash, 462
Diaphragms, 439
Diarrhea, 356, 362
treatment of, 367–369
and vitamin B_3 deficiencies, 500
and vitamin B_9 deficiencies, 501
zinc excess, 502
Diasorb, 368t
Diazepam, 256, 302
Diclofenac, 344
Didronel, 274
Diethylstilbestrol (DES), 433
Digestion, 356
Digestive system. *See* Gastrointestinal (GI)
system
Digoxin, 153, 408, 544
Dilantin, 300
Diltiazem, 414
Dimenhydrinate, 374
Diovan, 413
Diphenhydramine, 139, 254, 324
Diphenoxylate w/atropine, 369
Dipivefrin, 342
Diptheria, pertussis and tetanus (DPT)
vaccine, 514–515
Diptheria vaccine, 516
Dipyridamole, 418t
Discharge pharmacies, 180
Disopyramide, 407
Disposal
of chemotherapeutic agents/supplies,
219
of nonreturnable drugs, 239
Distribution, 64, 79–80
Diuresis, 378
Diuretics, 378, 396
for CHF-related edema, 408–411
Diuril, 388, 409

DNA (deoxyribonucleic acid), 521
of a fungus, 550
Docetaxel, 531t
Doctor's orders
errors in, 102–103
hospital pharmacies, 172–174
translation of, 117–118
Docusate sodium (OTC), 371
Dogma, 3, 4
Donepezil, 303
Donnagel, 368t
Dorzolamide, 340
Dosage forms
abbreviations, 64
administration, routes of, 73–78
asthma treatment, 489
capsules and caplets, 67–68
creams, 71
description of, 82t
elixirs, 69
emulsions, 70
enemas, 71
gels, 72
implants, 69
inhalents and aerosols, 70
liquids, 69–71
list of, 64
lotions, 71–72
lozenges/troches, 68
ointments, 72
pastes, 72
patches, 69
powders, 72
repackaged medications, 189
semisolids, 71–73
solids, 66–69
sprays, 69–70
suppositories, 72
suspensions, 70–71
syrups, 69
tablets, 66–67
types of, 65–73
Doxazosin, 431
Doxepin, 251
Doxorubicin, 528
DPT vaccine, 514–515
Dramamine, 374
Dress, 106
Drip rates, 53–56
Drospirenone, 436
Drug classification, 88
Drug education coordinators (DECs), 3, 9, 172
Drug Enforcement Agency, 13, 15, 16
Drug Topics Red Book, 90–92, 93t
Ducolax, 371
Durabolin, 430

Dura-Estrin, 432
Durham-Humphrey Amendment (1951), 14
Dutasteride, 430
Duties
  of certified technicians, 33b
  nondiscretionary, 30
Dwarfism, 271, 272
  and vitamin B$_6$ deficiencies, 501
Dyazide, 390t
Dymelor, 278t
Dyrenium, 390, 410
Dysentery, 547
Dysmenorrhea, 423
Dysrhythmias, 396, 400b, 403
  treatment of, 407–408
Dystonia, 244

E

Early pharmacists, 7
Early pharmacy technicians, 8, 29
Ears, 348
  agents/medications for, 352, 454t. *See also
    specific agent / medication*
  list of, 334
  conditions affecting, 350–351. *See also
    specific condition*
  external ear, 349
  inner ear, 349–350, 351f
  middle ear, 349
  terminology, 333
Earwax, 351
Eastern medicine, 153, 154
Echinacea, 161
Echothiophate iodide, 342
ECPs, 439–440
Edema, 378, 384–384, 396
  carbonic anhydrase inhibitors, 390–391
  congestive heart failure and, 384–385,
    404
  diuretics for, 408–411
  loop diuretics, 389
  osmotics, 391
  potassium-sparing agents, 390
  thiazides and thiazide-like agents,
    388–389
Education, 8, 584
  continuing education, 29, 33, 96
Educational programs, 34
EEGs, 300
Efferent (motor) system, 283, 290–291, 292f,
  293f
Efferent neurons, 290–291
Effexor, 254
Eighteenth century medicine, 6
Elavil, 251
Eldepryl, 306

Electroencephalograms (EEGs), 300
Electrolytes, 493, 568–571
Electrons, 564
Elixirs, 69, 188
Emergency contraceptives (ECPs), 439–440
Emesis, 356, 372
  treatment of, 373–374
Emotional health, 245
  medication therapy. *See* Psychotherapeutic
    medications
  nondrug treatments, 245–246
  and vitamin B$_1$ deficiencies, 500
Emphysema, 321. *See also* Chronic obstructive
  pulmonary disease (COPD)
Employee incentive programs, 35
Emulsions, 70
Enalapril, 412
Endocrine system
  conditions/disorders, 270–279. *See also
    specific condition*
  drugs for. *See also specific drug*
    glandular conditions, 270–279
    list of, 263–264
  glands, 264–265. *See also specific gland*
    conditions/disorders, 270–279
    functions of, 267–270
  hormones, 266. *See also specific hormone*
  mechanism of action, 266–267
  terminology, 263
Endometriosis, 423, 429
Endometrium, 423
End-stage renal disease (ESRD), 384, 385t
  dialysis, 378, 386–388
Enemas, 71
Enoxacin, 392t
Entamoeba histolytica, 463, 547
Enzymes, 396, 493, 539, 564
  chemistry of, 568
  coenzymes, 493
E-pharmacies, 32
Epifrin, 342
Epilepsy, 300–302, 309t
Epinephrine, 326, 342
Epogen, 388
Equanil, 258
Ergocalciferol, 498
Ergot alkaloid, 441
Error. *See* Mistake or error
Erythema, 474
Erythromycin, 347
Erythropoietin, 388, 531
Eserine sulfate, 341
Esidrix, 388
Eskalith, 250
Esomeprazole magnesium, 366
ESRD. *See* End-stage renal disease (ESRD)

Esterified estrogen, 432
Esterified estrogen with
    medroxyprogesterone, 433
Esterified estrogen with methyltestosterone,
    432
Estinyl estradiol, 437
Estrace, 432
Estraderm, 432
Estradiol, 431, 432
Estradiol cypionate, 432
Estradiol valerate, 432
Estratab, 432
Estratest, 432
Estring, 432
Estrogen, 265, 269, 270, 279
Estrogen replacement therapy, 431
Estrogens, 431, 432, 437
Estrophasic medications, 438
Estropipate, 433
Estrostep, 438
Ethambutol, 329t, 330
Ethics, 25, 100, 108
    confidentiality, 100, 108–109
    pharmacist's perspective, 107
Ethinyl estradiol, 436, 437, 438
Ethynodiol diacetate, 437
Etidronate sodium, 274
Etoposide, 528
Eukaryotic organisms, 541, 544
Eustachian tubes, 333
Euthroid, 273
Euthyroid, 263
Evil spirits, 3–4, 6
Evolution, 540
Excretion, 64, 80, 356, 361, 378
Ex-Lax, 370, 370t
Exophthalmos, 263
Expectorants, 131, 140, 314, 324
Extrapyramidal, 244
Eye inserts, 83
Eyes, 334
    agents/medications for, 338, 454t. *See also*
        specific agent/medication
      antifungals, 347
      antiglaucoma agents, 338–342
      antiinfective agents, 344–346
      antiinflammatory agents, 343–345
      antivirals, 347–348
      artificial tears products, 348
      list of, 333–334
      over-the-counter, 76–77, 348
    anatomy of, 334–337
    artificial tears products, 348t
    conditions/disorders, 337–338. *See also*
        specific condition/disorder
    congestion/infections, 337

Eyes *(Continued)*
    antiinfection/antiinflammatory agents,
        343–348
    terminology, 333
    vision, 337
    and vitamin A, 495, 497
    and vitamin B$_2$ deficiencies, 500

F

Facts and Comparisons (F&C), 89–90, 93t
Facultative anaerobe, 539
Faith healing, 4, 156t, 166
Fallopian tubes, 423, 426–427
Famotidine, 365
Fat soluble drugs, 152
Fat soluble vitamins. *See* Vitamins
Faxing prescriptions, 115b
    in hospital settings, 173
FDA. *See* Food and Drug Administration
    (FDA)
Federal Food and Drug Act of 1906, 14
Federal laws, 13–15, 101b
Felodipine, 415
Female reproductive system, 426–427
Feosol, 387
Ferrous sulfate, 387, 503
Fertilization, 423
Feverfew, 152, 162
FiberCon, 369, 370t
Filgrastim, 531
Filling prescriptions. *See* Prescriptions
Filters
    HEPA filter, 216
    parenteral agents/medications, 212–213
Finasteride, 430
Flatulance, 374
    antiflatulance agents/medications, 363t, 374
Flatworms, 464, 465t, 539, 548
Fleet Bisacodyl, 370t
Fleet mineral oil, 370t
Fleet Prep Kit 1, 370t
Flexeril, 298
Flomax, 430
Flonase, 328
Floor stock, 170, 181
Florinef, 275
Flovent, 328
Floxin, 392t
Floxuridine, 527
Flu, 314, 320, 467, 469
    Haemophilus influenza type B vaccine, 515,
        516
Fludarabine, 527
Fludrocortisone, 275
Flukes, 465t, 539, 549t
Flunisolide, 328, 485

Fluoroquinolones, 392t
Fluorouracil, 527
Fluoxetine, 253
Fluoxymesterone, 429
Fluphenazine, 248
Fluphenazine deconate, 246
Flurbiprofen, 344
Fluticasone, 328
Folic acid, 501
Follicle-stimulating hormone (FSH), 268t, 425, 427, 428, 431
Follicle-stimulating hormone (FSH) stimulants, 441
Food, Drug and Cosmetic Act of 1938, 14
Food and Drug Administration (FDA), 13, 14, 188
   OTC medications. *See* OTC medications
   vitamins, regulation of, 495, 496t
Formulary, 88, 227, 229. *See also* Stock
   automated dispensing systems. *See* Automated dispensing systems
   inventory control. *See* Inventory control
   pharmacist's perspective, 228
Fosamax, 274
Fosinopril, 412
Fosphenytoin, 300
Fourteenth century medicine, 6
Foxglove, 153, 544
Fractions, 44–45
FSH, 268t, 425, 427, 428, 431
Fungi, 461, 539, 550. *See also* Parasites
   antifungals, 462t
     eye infections, 347
   Candida infections, 461–462
   malaria, 465
   Tinea infections, 462
Fungi kingdom, 542t, 550–551
Fungicides, 447
Furosemide, 390, 409
Future trends, 581, 585

G

Gabapentin, 301
Galen, 3, 5
Gametes, 423
Ganglions, 288
Gantanol, 392t
Gantrisin, 392t
Garamycin (IV), 460
Garamycin (ophthalmic ointment), 346
Garlic, 152, 162
Gastritis, 356
Gastroesophageal reflux disease (GERD), 362, 364
   antacids for, 364, 364t
   medications for

Gastroesophageal reflux disease (GERD) *(Continued)*
   H₂ antagonists, 365
   proton pump inhibitors, 366
Gastrointestinal (GI) system, 350
   absorption, 356, 360–361
   anatomy of, 357–361
   auxiliary organ functions, 361–362
   conditions affecting, 362. *See also specific disorder/condition*
   emesis, 356, 372
   flatulance, 374
   intestinal conditions, 367–371
   mouth and throat conditions, 362
   stomach conditions, 362–367
   vitamin B₃ deficiencies, 500
   drugs for. *See also specific drug*
     list of, 356
   excretion, 64, 80, 356, 361
   functions of, 357
   infections, 451–452
   ingestion, 356, 357–360
   terminology, 356
Gas-X, 374
Gauge, 206
Gels, 72
Gemcitabine, 531t
Gemfibrozil, 406
Generic drugs, 88, 89, 227. *See also specific drug*
   trade name *versus*, 229
Genetics
   DNA. *See* DNA (deoxyribonucleic acid)
   Mendel, Gregor, 3, 6
Genital herpes, 452t
Genoptic (ophthalmic), 460
Genoptic (solution), 346
Genora, 436
Genora !/50, 437
Gentamicin, 346, 460
GERD. *See* Gastroesophageal reflux disease (GERD)
Geriatric Handbook, 93t
German measles, 515
Gesterol, 434
GH, 268t
GI system. *See* Gastrointestinal (GI) system
Giantism, 270–271
Ginger, 152, 162–163
Gingko biloba, 152, 163, 544
Ginseng, 152, 163
Glaucoma, 337, 338t, 339t
   antiglaucoma agents, 338–342
Glaucon, 342
Glaxo Wellcome, 467
Glimepiride, 278t

Glipizide, 278t
Globulins, 508, 516, 517
Glucagon, 265, 269–270, 278t
Glucocorticoids, 269, 481–483
Glucophage, 278t
Glucose, 263
Glucotrol, 278t
Glyburide, 278t
Glycerin, 371, 391t, 411
GMP. *See* Good manufacturing process (GMP)
G-myticin (topical), 460
Goiter, 263, 272
Goldenseal, 152, 163
Golytely, 370t
Gonadotropin releasing hormone (GnRH), 425, 427, 431
Gonorrhea, 452t
Good manufacturing process (GMP), 13, 14, 136, 189
Goodman & Gilman's The Pharmacological Basis of Therapeutics, 93t
Government-run insurance programs, 227, 231
Graduates, 194, 195f, 201
Gram stain procedure, 450
Gram-negative bacteria, 447, 455t
Gram-positive bacteria, 447, 455t
Grams, 564
Grand mal seizures, 300, 301
Graves' disease, 263, 272
Grooming, 106
Growth hormone (GH), 268t
Growth rate, and vitamin B$_{12}$ deficiencies, 501–502
Guaifenesin, 323, 324
Gynogen-LA, 432

H

Haemophilus influenza type B vaccine, 515, 516
Haldol, 246
Half-life, 64, 81
Halls Zinc Defense, 320
Haloperidol deconate, 246
Halotestin, 429
Hansen's disease, 457, 459
Hard copy, 114, 126
Harrison Narcotic Act of 1914, 14
Hawthorn, 152, 163
HBP, 401. *See also* Hypertension
Headache products, 139
Health Insurance Portability and Accountability Act of 1996 (HIPAA), 13, 16
Health maintenance organizations (HMOs), 227
Heart. *See* Cardiovascular system

Helminths, 447, 464, 465t, 539, 548. *See also specific type of worm*
  antihelminthic agents, 466t
Hemodialysis, 386
Hemoglobin, 493
Hemothorax, 322
HEPA filter, 216
Heparin, 417
Hepatitis vaccine, 514, 516
Herbal remedies, 152, 153, 161–164, 164t. *See also specific herb*
  ancient, 6
  list of, 152
  preparations, 165
Herpes viruses, 469–470
Herpes zoster, 516
Herplex, 347
Heterotrophic, 539
High blood pressure (HBP), 401. *See also* Hypertension
HIPAA, 13, 16
Hippocrates, 3, 4
Hippocratic oath, 5
Histamine-2 antagonists, 365
Histamines, 474, 486, 488
  antihistamines. *See* Antihistamines
HIV/AIDS, 469, 557
  vaccine for, 513
HMOs, 227, 229–230
Hoarseness, 320
Hodgkin's lymphoma, 525
Home health pharmacies, 32
Homeopathy, 152, 156t, 165–166
Homeostasis, 283
Hookworms, 464, 465t
Horizontal flow hood, 206, 213, 216
Hormones, 263
  adrenocorticotropic hormone, 268t
  aldosterone, 269t
  androgens, 269t, 279, 423, 425–426, 427–430
  antidiuretic hormone, 267, 268t
  autocrine, 266
  calcitonin, 268
  cortisol, 269t
  description of, 266
  endocrine, 266
  estrogen, 265, 269, 270, 279
  estrogens, 431, 432, 437
  follicle-stimulating hormone, 268t, 425, 427, 428, 431
  function of, 266
  glucagon, 265, 269–270
  gonadotropin releasing hormone, 425, 427, 431
  growth hormone, 268t
  insulin, 265, 269, 270

Hormones (Continued)
  luteinizing hormone, 268t, 425, 427, 428, 431
  melatonin, 267
  oxytocin, 267, 268t, 271
  paracrine, 266
  parathyroid hormone, 268, 269
  progesterone, 265, 270, 279, 431, 434, 438
  progestins, 433–434, 437
  prolactin, 268t
  somatostatin, 269, 270
  structure of, 266
  testosterone, 265, 270, 279, 425, 427, 429
  thyroid-stimulating hormone, 268t
  thyroxine, 263, 268
  triiodothyronine, 263, 268
Hospital pharmacies, 170
  ASAP orders, 174, 185
  automated dispensing systems, 183
    inpatient pharmacies, 124–125
    outpatient pharmacies, 124
  chemotherapy preparations, 176
  clinics/units in need of medications from, 182
  controlled substances, 179
  discharge pharmacies, 180
  doctor's orders, 172–174
  inpatient pharmacies, 3, 29, 114, 170
    computer dispensing systems, 124–125
    prescriptions, taking in, 116–117, 119
    skills and tasks, 8, 30–31, 174–175
  intravenous technicians, 176
  intravenous therapy preparation, 176, 178
  inventory control technicians, 180–181
  nursing staff, relationship with, 184
  outpatient pharmacies, 3, 29, 114
    computer dispensing systems, 124
    prescriptions, taking in, 115–116, 118
    skills and tasks, 8, 31–32
  patient medication filling, 183–184
  policies and procedures handbooks, 171
  protocol, 171–172
  satellite pharmacies, 179–180
  specialty areas/departments stocked by, 181–182, 182b, 183b
  specialty tasks of technicians, 185
  standards, 172
  STAT orders, 170, 174, 184
Hospital-acquired infections, 447, 453
Hospitals
  floor stock, 170, 181
  pharmacies. See Hospital pharmacies
  protocol, 171–172
  sizes and types of, 170–171
  standards, 172
Household measurements, 40
Household system, 39

HTN. See Hypertension (HTN)
Humegon, 441
Humorsol, 342
Hycomine, 324
Hydorxyurea, 531t
Hydralazine/hydroxyzine, 103–104
Hydrochlorothiazide, 388
Hydrocodone, 323
Hydrocodone/chlorphreniramine, 324
Hydrocodone/phenylpropanolamine, 324
Hydrocortisone, 276, 483
Hydrophilic, 188
Hydrophobic, 188
Hydroxyprogesterone, 434
Hydroxyzine HCI, 258
Hydroxyzine pamoate, 258
Hylutin, 434
Hyperacidity, 364
  antacids for, 364
Hyperaldosteronism, 275t
Hyperalimentation, 29, 206, 220
Hypercalcemia, 263, 271, 273
Hypercortisolism, 275t
Hyperglycemia, 263, 271, 277
Hyperkalemia, 378
Hyperlipidemia, 400b, 401–402
  treatment of, 404–406
Hyperparathyroidism, 273–274
Hypertension (HTN), 400b, 401, 402
  and edema, 385
  treatment of, 411
Hyperthyroidism, 271–272
Hypervitaminosis, 493, 495
  vitamin A, 497
  vitamin D, 497
  vitamin E, 498
  vitamin K, 498
Hypnotic/sedative agents, 254–257
Hypocalcemia, 263, 274
Hypoglycemia, 263
Hypokalemia, 378
Hypoparathyroidism, 274
Hypotension, 404
  zinc excess, 502
Hypothalamus, 264–265, 267
  conditions and their treatment, 270–272
Hypothyroidism, 272–273
Hytone, 483
Hytrin, 430

I

ICSH, 268t, 425, 427, 428, 431
Idarubicin, 528
Ident-A-Drug, 92
Idoxuridine (IDU), 347
IDU, 347

Ifosfamide, 530
Ilotycin, 347
Imipramine, 251
Immune cells, 509–510, 511t
  injury response(s), 476t
Immune system, 509–510
Immunity, 508, 511
Immunizations, 510–517. *See also* Vaccines
  adult, 516–517
  antivenins and antitoxins, 517
  childhood, 514–516
  tetanus, 516, 517
Imodium AD (OTC), 369
Imodium (Rx), 369
Implants, 69
Impotence, 441
Incentive programs, 35
Incontinence, 378, 391
  treatment of, 392
Indapamide, 388
Inderal, 413
Inert ingredient, 423
Infections, 451
  ears, 453, 454t
  eyes, 453, 454t
  gastrointestinal, 451–452
  mouth, 453
  nose, 453
  nosocomial, 447, 453
  respiratory, 452–453
  sexually transmitted diseases, 451, 452t
  skin, 146, 453
Infertility medications, 440–441
Inflammation, 475–476
  antiinflammatories. *See* Antiinflammatories
  pain from, 477
  pain medications. *See* Pain
Influenza, 314, 320, 467, 469
  Haemophilus influenza type B vaccine, 515,
    516
Ingestion, 356, 357–360
Inhale, 64
Inhalents, 70, 78
Inhibit, 447
Injectable Drug Handbook, The, 92–93
Inpatient pharmacies. *See* Hospital
    pharmacies
Inpatients, 170
Insomnia, 244
  and vitamin B₅ deficiencies, 501
Insomnia products
  over-the-counter, 140
  sedative/hypnotic agents, 254–257
Instill, 64
Insulin, 265, 269, 270
  diabetes treatment, 277

Insurance, 227
  billing the carrier, 232–235
  claims processing, 233
    information required, 231–232
    problems, 233–235
  Health Insurance Portability and
      Accountability Act of 1996, 13, 16
  health maintenance organizations, 227,
      229–230
  Medicaid, 227, 231
  Medicare, 227, 231
  patient profiles, 232
  preferred provider organizations, 227,
      230–231
  types of, 229
  variances in, 232
  workers' compensation, 227, 231
Intal, 328, 486
Intentional torts, 24, 25
Interferon beta-1a, 304
Interferon beta-1b, 305
International time, 39, 59
Internet, 95
Interstitial cell stimulating hormone (ICSH),
      268t, 425, 427, 428, 431
Intestinal remedies, 142
Intramuscular medications. *See*
      Intravenous/intramuscular medications
Intrauterine devices (IUDs), 434, 435f
Intravenous technicians, 176
Intravenous/intramuscular medications. *See
      also* Parenteral agents/medications
  administration of, 76–77
    with cassettes, 210
    IV chambers, 210
    piggyback administrations, 77, 78f, 178,
        209, 211
  labels, 178, 223–224
  preparation of, 176, 178. *See also* Aseptic
      technique
  stock levels, 213
  supplies commonly used, 209b
  "syringe" medications, 216–218
    analgesic intravenous preparations,
        218–219
    chemotherapeutic agents, 219
    electrolytes and additives, 220, 222
    hyperalimentation, 29, 206, 220
Intrinsic factors, 493
Invasive tumors, 521
Inventory control, 235
  automated dispensing systems, 236
  bar coding, 236
  manual ordering, 236–237
  new stock, 237–238
  recalled drugs, 238

Inventory control *(Continued)*
  returns
    to manufacturer or warehouse, 238–239
    nonreturnable drugs and their disposal, 239
  special ordering considerations, 240
  suppliers, 239
  systems, 235–236
Inventory control technicians, 180–181
Iodoquinol, 463
Ionic bond, 564
Ions, 564
Ipratropium bromide, 328
Iron, 387, 503–504
Iron deficiency, 503–504
ISMO, 416t
Ismotic, 391t
Isoniazid, 329, 329t
Isoptin, 414
Isopto, 341
Isordil, 416t
Isosorbide, 391t
IUDs, 434, 435f

J
Job opportunities, 34–35
Journals, 94–95

K
Kaopectate, 369
Kaposi's sarcoma, 525
Kcal, 564
Kefauver-Harris Amendments (1962), 14–15
Keflex, 457
Kenalog (aerosol), 483
Kenalog-40 (IV), 276
Keratolytic drugs, 131
Ketorolac, 344
Kidney stones, 385, 386t
Kidneys, 379. *See also* Urinary system
  function of, 380–383
  nephron functions, 381–382
    tubular reabsorption, 382–383
    tubular secretion, 383
  renal failure, 384
    dialysis, 378, 386–388
Klonopin, 302
Krebs cycle, 568, 569f

L
Labels
  auxiliary. *See* Auxiliary labels
  compounded products, nonsterile, 196
  intravenous therapy preparations, 178,
    223–224
  prescription. *See* Prescriptions
  repackaged medications, 189

Labyrinth, inner ear, 333
Laminar flow hood, 206
Laniazid, injectable, 329
Lanoxin, 408
Lansoprazole, 366
Laryngitis, 320
Lasix, 390, 409
Latanoprost, 343
Laudanum, 5, 7
Laws
  federal laws, 13–15, 101b
  knowledge of, 101
  liability laws, 24–25
  state laws, 24
Laxatives, 370, 371
Legend drugs, 13, 152. *See also specific drug*
  prescriptions. *See* Prescriptions
Leprosy, 457, 459
Leukemia, 521, 525
Leukopenia, 531
Leukotrienes, 327, 485
Levlen, 437
Levobunolol, 340
Levodopa, 307
Levongestrel, 437
Levothroid, 273
Levothyroxine sodium, 273
LH, 268t, 425, 427, 428, 431
Liability laws, 24–25
Librium, 257
Lichens, 550
Lidocaine, 407, 408
Lids, 120–121. *See also* Childproof caps
Lioresal, 297, 304
Liothyronine sodium, 273
Liotrix, 273
Lipids, 356
Lipitor, 406
Liquaemin, 417
Lisinopril, 412
Listening skills, 105–106
Lithium, 250
Loestrin, 436
Lomotil, 369
Lomustine, 530
Look alike/sound alike drugs, 103–104
Loop diuretics, 389
  for CHF-related edema, 409
Lo-Ovral, 437
Loperamide, 369
Lopid, 406
Lopressor, 413
Lorazepam, 256
Losartan, 413
Lotensin, 412
Lotions, 71–72

Lou Gehrig's disease, 308
Lovastatin, 405
Loxapine, 249
Loxitane, 249
Lozenges, 68
Lozol, 388
Lumbar, 283
Luminal, 255t, 301
Lung cancer, 322
Luteinizing hormone (LH), 268t, 425, 427, 428, 431
Luteinizing hormone (LH) stimulants, 441
Lymphatic system, 509–510
Lymphocytes, 509–510, 511t
Lymphoma, 521
  Hodgkin's, 525
  non-Hodgkin's, 525

M

Maalox, 365
Macro, 564
Macrodantin, 392t
Magnesium hydroxide, 364
Magnesium salicylate, 254–255
Mail order pharmacies, 32
Mailing prescription medications, 23
Malaria, 465
  Plasmodiumvivax, 547, 548f
Male reproductive system, 425–426
Malignant, 521
Mandelamine, 392t
Mania, 244
  antimanics, 249–250
Mannitol, 391t, 410
Manufactured products, 81–83
MAOIs, 251–252
MAR, 170
Maxidex (suspension), 344
Maxipime, 457
Maxzide, 390t
Maxzide-25, 390t
MDI (metered dose inhaler), 64, 314
Measles, mumps and rubella (MMR) vaccine, 515
Measurements, 39. *See also* Conversion(s)
  apothecary system, 39, 40–41, 43
  avoirdupois system, 39, 41, 43
  avoirdupois weights, 42t
  chemistry, 572–575
  differences between systems, 42
  drip rates, 53–56
  household, 40
  household system, 39
  metric system. *See* Metric system
  pediatric dosing, 50–52
Mebaral, 255t, 302

Mechlorethamine, 530
Meclizine, 374
"Med Watch," 102
Medicaid, 227, 231
Medical information sheets provided by the manufacturer. *See* Monographs
Medicare, 227, 231
Medication administration record (MAR), 170
Medication errors, 101–104
Medication pick-up, 127
Medication reactions
  FDA reporting process, 16
  monographs, 20
Medicine men/women, 3–4
Medrol, 483
Medroxyprogesterone, 434, 438
Melanoma, 521
Melatonin, 267
Mellaril, 247
Melphalan, 530
Mendel, Gregor, 3, 6
Menest, 432
Meningitis, 516
Menopause, 423
Menotropin, 441
Mental health/illness
  medication therapy. *See* Psychotherapeutic medications
  nondrug treatments, 245–246
  and vitamin B_1 deficiencies, 500
Mephobarbital, 255t, 302
Meprobamate CIV, 258
Mercaptopurine, 527
Mestinon, 300
Mestranol, 437
Metabolism, 64, 80, 564, 568–571
Metamucil, 371
Metaproterenol, 326
Metastasis, 521
Metered dose inhaler, 64, 314
Meters, 564
Metformin, 278t
Methazolamide, 341
Methenamine, 392t
Methimazole, 272
Methocarbamol, 298
Methotrexate, 527
Methylprednisolone sodium succinate, 276, 483
Methyltestosterone, 430
Metoclopramide, 373
Metolazone, 389, 409
"Me-too" drugs, 228
Metoprolol, 413
Metric system, 40
  measurements, 42–43, 572–575
  slide, 43–44

Metripranolol, 340
Metrodin, 441
Metronidazole, 367t
Mevacor, 405
MG. *See* Myasthenia gravis (MG)
MI. *See* Myocardial infarction (MI)
Micrette, 437
Micro, 564
Microbial, 539
Microbiology, 540
  classification of organisms. *See* Taxonomy
  defined, 539
  golden age of, 541, 542f
  terminology, 539
Micrograms, 564
Micronase, 278t
Micronor, 434, 438
Microorganisms, 451b, 539
  classification of. *See* Taxonomy
Micturition, 378
Midamore, 390
Midodrine, 404
Mifepristone, 440
Military time, 39, 59
Milk of Magnesium, 364, 370t
Milk thistle, 152, 163
Milligrams, 564
Miltown, 258
Mineralocorticoids, 269
Minerals, 494–495, 502, 503t
  iron, 503–504
  list of, 494, 503t
  terminology, 493
  trace elements, 493, 494, 495, 503t
  zinc excess, 502
"Minipills," 436
Miochol-E, 341
Miosis, 333
Miostat, 341
Miotics, 339t, 341–342
Mistake or error
  medication errors, 101–104
  negligence, 24
Mitomycin, 528
Mitosis, 521, 529f
Mitoxantrone, 528
MMR vaccine, 515
Moduretic, 390t
Molds
  slime, 550
  water, 549
Mole, 564
Molecular biosynthesis, 493
Molecules, 564, 567–569
Monera kingdom, 542t, 551–552, 553t
Monoamine oxidase, 283

Monoamine oxidase inhibitors (MAOIs), 251–252
Monographs, 13, 19–20, 88, 89
Monoket, 416t
Monopril, 412
Montelukast, 327, 485
Morals, 25, 100. *See also* Ethics
"Morning-after pills," 439
Morphology, 447, 521
Mortar and pestle, 188, 194, 195f, 201
Motor neurons, 290–291
Mouth infections, 362, 453
  canker sores, 147, 500
  and vitamin B_2 deficiencies, 500
  and vitamin B_3 deficiencies, 500
  and vitamin B_9 deficiencies, 501
MS. *See* Multiple sclerosis (MS)
Mucolytics, 325
Mucomyst, 325
Multiple dose vials, 213
Multiple sclerosis (MS), 303–305, 309t
Multiple trace elements (MTE), 493
Muscle cramps, and vitamin B_5 deficiencies, 501
Mutations, 521
Myambutol, 330
Myasthenia gravis (MG), 299–300, 309t
Mycobacterial treatment, 459
Mycobacterium, 459
Mycosis, 447
Mydriasis, 333
Myelin sheath, 287
Mylanta, 365
Mylecon, 374
Myocardial infarction (MI), 400b, 401, 403
  non-pharmacological treatment for, 418
Myopia, 333
Mysoline, 301
Myxedema, 263, 272

N

Nandrolone, 430
Narcotics. *See* Controlled substances
Nardil, 252
Narrow leafed purple coneflower, 161
Nasacort, 483
NasalCrom, ophthalmic, 328
Nasalide, 328
Natacyn (suspension), 347
Natamycin, 347
National Association of Boards of Pharmacy (NABP), 29, 30
National Center for Complementary and Alternative Medicine (NCCAM), 154
National certification, 100, 583–584
National Pharmacy Technicians Association (NPTA), 96, 581, 582t

Nationally certified technicians, 100
Nausea. *See also* Vomiting
  and vitamin B$_1$ deficiencies, 500
  zinc excess, 502
Navane, 248
Nearsightedness, 333
Nebcin (IV), 460
Nebulizer asthma treatments, 486
Necon 1/35, 437
Necon 10/11, 437
Needles, 212
Negative feedback, 423
Negligence, 24
Nembutal, 255t
Neoplasms, 521. *See also* Cancer
  sarcoma, 521
Neostigmine, 299
Neo-synephrine, 325
Neptuzane, 341
Nerve terminals, 283, 287
Nerve transmission, 288
Nervous system, 245, 284–287
  acoustic nerve, 333
  autonomic system, 283, 293
  brain, 288–290
  central nervous system, 245
    brain, 288–290
    drug list, 283–284. *See also specific drug*
    efferent (motor) system, 283, 290–291, 292f,
      293f
    function of, 284–285
    spinal cord, 290
  conditions and their treatment
    Alzheimer's disease, 302–303, 309t
    amyotrophic lateral sclerosis, 308
    epilepsy, 300–302, 309t
    general nervous disorders, 297–299
    miscellaneous muscle agents, 309–310
    multiple sclerosis, 303–305, 309t
    myasthenia gravis, 299–300, 309t
    Parkinson's disease, 306–308, 309t
  drugs for. *See also specific drug*
    Alzheimer's disease, 302–303, 309t
    amyotrophic lateral sclerosis, 308
    epilepsy, 301–303, 309t
    general nervous disorders, 297–299
    list of, 283–284
    miscellaneous muscle agents, 309–310
    multiple sclerosis, 303–305, 309t
    myasthenia gravis, 299–300, 309t
    Parkinson's disease, 306–308, 309t
  efferent (motor) system, 290–291, 292f, 293f
  general nervous disorders, 297–299
  miscellaneous muscle agents, 309–310
  neurons, 283, 287–288, 290–291
  parasympathetic system, 283, 295–296

Nervous system *(Continued)*
  GI system, control of, 357
  peripheral nervous system, 285
    autonomic system, 283
    parasympathetic system, 283, 295–296, 357
    somatic system, 283, 293
    sympathetic system, 283, 293–295
  somatic system, 283, 293
  spinal cord, 290
  sympathetic system, 283, 293–295
  terminology, 283
Neuroblastomas, 276
Neuromuscular blockers, 309
Neurons, 283, 287–288, 290–291
Neurontin, 301
Neurosis, 244
Neurotransmitters, 288
Neutrons, 564
Newsmagazines, 94–95
Nexium, 366
Niacin, 500
Niacin OTC, 406
Niaspan RX, 406
Nicotinic acid, 406
Nifedipine, 414
Nitrobid, 416t
Nitro-Bid, 416t
Nitro-Dur, 416t
Nitrofurantion, 392t
Nitrogard, 416t
Nitrogen mustards, 530
Nitroglycerin, 415, 416
Nitrong, 416t
Nitrosoureas, 530
Nitrostat, 416t
Nizatidine, 365
NKDA, 170
No known drug allergy (NKDA), 170
Nocturia, 378
Nocturnal dialysis, 386–387
Nondiscretionary duties, 30
Non-Hodgkin's lymphoma, 525
Nonproductive cough, 314
Nonresistant bottles, use of, 22–23, 23t
Nonsteroidal antiinflammatory drugs
    (NSAIDS), 474, 478–480
  for eye disorders, 343–344
  over-the-counter, 137–138
Nordette, 437
Norelgestromin, 437
Norethindrone, 434, 436, 437, 438
Norflex, 298
Norfloxacin, 392t
Norgesic, 299
Norgestimate, 437, 438
Norgestrel, 437, 438

Norinyl, 436, 437
Norlutin, 434
Normal flora, 447, 448–449, 549
Noroxin, 392t
Norpace, 407
Nor-QD, 438
Norvasc, 415
Nose infections, 320, 453, 474
Nosocomial infections, 447, 453
NSAIDS. *See* Nonsteroidal antiinflammatory drugs (NSAIDS)
Ntg in D5W, 416t
Nuclear pharmacy technicians, 532
Nucleic acid, 564
Nydrazid, 329

O

Occupress, 340
Ocufen, 344
Ocular. *See* Eyes
Ofloxacin, 392t
Ogen, 433
Ointments, 72, 188
Olanzapine, 249
Omeprazole, 366, 367t
Omnibus Budget Reconciliation Act (OBRA 90), 15
OMNICELL, 236
Omnipen, 456
On-call medications, 170
Oncogene, 521
Oncology agents. *See* Chemotherapeutic agents
Ondansetron Hydrochloride, 374
Oocytes, 423
Ophthalmic. *See* Eyes
Opium, 16. *See also* Controlled substances
    historical use of, 7
Oral, 432, 434
Oral contraceptives, 434–440
Oral medications, 73
Orap, 249
Orbit, 564
Oreton, 430
Organizations, 95–96, 581, 582t, 585
Orinase, 278t
Orphan Drug Act (1983), 15
Orphenadrine, 298
Orphenadrine/aspirin/caffeine, 299
Ortho-Cept, 437
Ortho-Est, 433
Ortho-Evra, 437
Ortho-Novum, 436, 437
Ortho-Novum 1/35, 437
Ortho-Novum 7/7/7, 437
Ortho-Novum 10/11, 437

Ortho-TriCyclen, 438
Orvette, 438
Os-Cal, 274
Osmitrol, 391t, 410
Osmoglyn, 391t, 411
Osmotics, 391
    for CHF-related edema, 410–411
Osteoporosis, 263, 273
    and vitamin B_6 deficiencies, 501
    and vitamin D, 498
OTC medications, 13, 64, 114, 131, 132, 152, 474
    acne treatments, 146
    allergy agents, 138
    analgesics and antipyretic agents, 131, 136, 137
    antacids, 141t, 363t
    antihistamines, 138–139
    antiinflammatory drugs, 131, 137–138
    aspirin. *See* Aspirin
    for athlete's foot, 147
    bioavailability, 134–135
    for canker sores, 147
    categories of, 133–134
    cold agents/remedies, 138, 320–321
    common preparations, 131t–132t
    conditions treated with, 136–137
    considerations, 133
    cough medications, 140
    decongestants, 139
    for diarrhea, 367–369
    efficacy, 135
    eye products, 77–78, 348
    FDA approval process, 135–136
    FDA regulations, 134–135
    FDA reporting process, 16
    for flatulance, 363t, 374
    good manufacturing process, 136
    headache products, 139
    increase in, 132
    intestinal remedies, 142
    laxatives, 370, 371
    minerals. *See* Minerals
    patient counseling, 132
    potency, 134
    purity, 134
    recalls, 136
    safety and toxicity, 135
    for skin conditions, 143t
        acne treatments, 146
        athlete's foot, 147
        canker sores, 147
        inflammation products, 147, 147t
        sunscreen, 131, 144
        topical antibiotics, 148
        warts, 147

OTC medications *(Continued)*
  sleep aids, 140
  sore throat products, 141, 320–321
  stomach remedies, 141–142, 362–363, 363, 364–365
  sunscreen, 131, 144, 145t
  topical antibiotics, 148
  vitamins. *See* Vitamins
  for vomiting, 374
  warts, 147
Otic. *See* Ears
Otitis media, 350–351, 453
Ototoxicity, 351
Outpatient pharmacies. *See* Hospital pharmacies
Ova, 423
Ovaries, 265, 270
  hormones secreted and their uses, 279
Ovcon, 436
Over-the-counter medications. *See* OTC medications
Ovral, 437
Oxazepam, 256
Oxymetazoline, 325
Oxytocin, 267, 268t, 271

P
Pacemakers, 407
Package inserts. *See* Monographs
Packaging of drugs, 83
Paclitaxel, 531t
Paget's disease, 263, 273
Pain
  from inflammation, 477
  medications
    aspirin. *See* Aspirin
    cyclooxygenase, 480–481
    glucocorticoids, 481–483
    NSAIDS. *See* Nonsteroidal antiinflammatory drugs (NSAIDS)
    salicylates, 478, 479t
  skeletal muscle pain, 297
Palliative, 423
Palm pilot reference books, 94
Pamidronate, 274
Pancreas, 265, 269–270
  conditions and their treatment, 277–279
Pancuronium, 310
Pantoprazole, 366
Pantothenic acid, 501
Papillomavirus, 469
PAR level. *See* Periodic automatic replenishment (PAR) level
Paracelsus, 3, 5
Paracrine hormones, 266
Parafon Forte DSC, 298

Parasites, 447, 463. *See also specific parasite*
Parasympathetic nervous system (PNS), 283, 295–296
  GI system, control of, 357
Parathyroid glands, 265, 268–269
  conditions and their treatment, 273–274
Parathyroid hormone (PTH), 268, 269
Parenteral agents/medications, 29, 64, 76–77, 206–207. *See also* Aseptic technique
  additives, 220
  compatibility considerations, 222–223
  containers used for preparing, 208b
  controlled analgesia devices, 210
  delivery systems, 207, 209–213
  electrolytes, 220, 222
  filters, 212–213
  hyperalimentation, 29, 206, 220
  IV chambers, 210
  piggyback containers, 209
  preparation of. *See* Aseptic technique
  routes of administration, 208b
  solutions used/ordered for, 208b
  stock levels, 213
  supplies and equipment, 209b, 213
  "syringe" medications, 216–218
    analgesic intravenous preparations, 218–219
    chemotherapeutic agents, 219
    electrolytes and additives, 220, 222
    hyperalimentation, 29, 206, 220
  syringes. *See* Syringes
  terminology, 207, 208b
  vials, 211
Parenteral systems, 83
Parepectolin, 368t
Parkinson's disease, 306–308
  drug treatment, 306–308
Parlodel, 441
Parnate, 252
Paroxetine, 253
Passive immunity, 508, 511
Pastes, 72
Pasteur, Louis, 541, 543b
Patches, 69
Patient counseling, 9, 125, 127
  and OTC medications, 132
Patient-controlled analgesia (PCA), 210
Patients' rights, 125
Pavulon, 310
Paxil, 253
PCA, 210
Pediatric dosing, 50–52
Pediatric Handbook, 93t
Pellagra, 500
Penetrex, 392t

Penicillin, 455–456
  discovery of, 449–450, 552
  mechanism of action, 553
Penicillin V potassium, 456
Pentobarbital, 255t
Pentostatin, 528
Pepcid, 365
Peptic ulcers, 356, 363, 366–367
  diagnostic tests, 367t
  medications for, 367t
Peptidoglycan, 539
Pepto-Bismol, 369
Percentages, 45
Pergonal, 441
Periodic automatic replenishment (PAR) level,
    170, 179, 234
  hospital specialty areas, 181
  importance of maintaining, 235
Periodic table, 566f
Peripheral parenteral, 206
Peripheral parenteral nutrition (PPN), 220
Peristalsis, 356
Peritoneal dialysis, 386–387
Pernicious anemia, 501
Perphenazine, 247
Persantine, 418t
Petit mal seizures, 300, 301
Pharmacists
  defined, 3
  early American pharmacists, 7
  educational requirements, 8
  specializations, 9
  trust, 9
Pharmacokinetics, 64, 79
Pharmacology, 88
Pharmacy clerk, 3
Pharmacy technician, defined, 3
Pharmacy Technician Certification Board
    (PTCB), 13, 33, 583
Pharmacy Technician Certification Board
    (PTCB) examination, 33–34, 583
  laws, understanding of, 13
Pharyngitis, 320
Pheneizine, 252
Phenobarbital, 255t, 301
Phenol, 321
Phenylephrine, 325
Pheochromocytomas, 276
Phillips, 364
Phone calls
  etiquette, 106
  filtering of, 8
PhosLo, 274
Phospholide iodide, 342
Phyllocontin, 485
Physicians' Desk Reference (PDR), 13, 90, 93t

Physostigmine, 341
Phytonadione, 498
Piggyback containers, 209
Pilocar, 341
Pilocarpine, 341
Pimozide, 249
Pindolol, 414
Pineal gland, 265, 267
"Pink eye," 337, 453
  antiinfective agents for, 344–346
Pinworms, 465t
Pioglitazone, 278
Pituitary gland, 264, 267–268
  conditions and their treatment, 270–272
Placebo, 152
Placebo effect, 155
Plague vaccine, 517t
Plant cells, 544, 545f
Plantae kingdom, 542t, 544, 545f
Plasmodiumvivax, 547, 548f
Plendil, 415
Pleurisy, 323t
Plicamycin, 528
Pneumonia, 321
  vaccine, 516
Pneumothorax, 322
PNS. *See* Parasympathetic nervous system
    (PNS)
PO, 73
Pocket-sized reference books, 94
Point of sale (POS), 227, 235
Polarizing agents, 309–310
Polio vaccine, 514, 515
Polycillin, 456
POS, 227
Postcoidal contraceptives, 439–440
Potassium-sparing agents, 390
  for CHF-related edema, 410
Powders, 72
PPI, 366
PPN, 220
PPOs, 227, 230–231
Prandin, 278
Pravachol, 406
Pravastatin, 406
Prayer, healing through, 4
Precose, 278
Pred Forte (suspension), 344
Prednisolone, 344
Prednisone, 276, 482
Preferred provider organizations (PPOs), 227,
    230–231
Premarin, 433
Premphase, 433
Prempro, 433
Pre-op drugs, 170

Prescription Drug Marketing Act (1987), 15
Prescriptions
  asking for help, 117–118
  billing, 127
  calling-in, 115b
  childproof caps. *See* Childproof caps
  computer dispensing systems, 123–124
  controlled substances, 21
  counting the medication, 120
  current trends, 127
  DEA verification, 22
  doctor's orders
    errors in, 102–103
    translation of, 117–118
  faxing-in, 115b
  filling of, 114–127
  hard copy, 114, 126
  information
    database, entering into, 118–119
    inpatient settings, 116–117, 119
    outpatient settings, 115–116, 118
  initialing, 121
  inspection by pharmacist, 123
  labels, 21–22, 22b
    applying, 121
    auxiliary. *See* Auxiliary labels
    checking against the script, 120
    special, 22, 22b
  lids, 120–121. *See also* Childproof caps
  mailing medications, 23
  nonresistant bottles, use of, 22, 23t
  patients' rights, 125
  picking up medications, 127
  preparing, 8
  pulling the correct medication, 120
  "red flags," 125
  refilling, 126
    controlled substances, 19
    zero refill reorders, 126
  regulations, 20–23
  script processing, 119–125
  special labels, 22, 22b
  taking in, 115–116
  technician's initials, 122
  transfers, 126
  veterinarian, 15
  walking-in, 115b
  who can prescribe, 10, 20
  who can receive, 21
  zero refill reorders, 126
Prevacid, 366
Prilosec, 366
Primidone, 301
Prinivil, 412
Procainamide, 407
Procarbazine, 531t

Procardia, 414
Prochlorperazine, 247
Procrit, 388
Productive cough, 314
Profenal, 344
Professionalism, 100, 104, 107, 584–585
Progestasert, 438
Progesterone, 265, 270, 279, 431, 434, 438
Progestins, 433–434, 437
Prokaryotic organisms, 544, 551–552
Prolactin, 268t
Prolixin, 246, 248
Promethazine, codeine with, 323
Pronestyl, 407
Prophylaxis, 131, 314
Propine, 342
Proportion, 45–50
Propranolol, 413
Propylthiouracil, 272
Propylthiouracil (PTU), 272
Proscar, 430
Prostaglandin agonist, 339t, 342
Prostate gland, 425
  benign prostatic hypertrophy, 423
    medications for, 430–431
Prostigmin, 299
Protectants, 131
Protista kingdom, 542t, 549, 550f
Protocol, 3, 9, 100, 170
  hospital pharmacies, 171–172
  knowledge of, 101
Proton pump inhibitors (PPI), 366
Protonix, 366
Protons, 564
Protozoa, 447, 464, 539, 549, 550f
Proventil, 326
Provera, 434
Prozac, 253
Pruritus, 131, 244
Pseudoephedrine, 325
Psoriasis, 148
Psychiatrists, 245
Psychologists, 245
Psychosis, 244
  antipsychotic agents, 244, 246–249
Psychotherapeutic medications
  antidepressants. *See* Antidepressants
  antimanics, 249–250
  antipsychotic agents, 244, 246–249
  barbiturates, 255
  list of, 244
  sedative/hypnotic agents, 254–257
Psyllium powder, 371
PTH, 268, 269
PTU, 272
Pulling the correct medication, 120

Pulmonary edema, 323t
  zinc excess, 502
Pulmonary embolism, 322
Purple coneflower, 152, 161, 163
Pyelonephritis, 378
Pyrazinamide, 329t, 330
Pyridostigmine, 300
Pyridoxine, 501
PYXIS, 183, 236

Q

Qualifications. *See also* Competencies
Questran, 405
Quinalan (IV), 407
Quinidex (oral), 407
Quinidine gluconate, 407
Quinidine sulfate, 407
Quinidine/quinine, 103

R

Radiation therapy, 526
Radioactive isotopes, 526
Radiopharmaceuticals, 532b
Ranitidine, 365
Ratio/proportion, 45–50
Recalled drugs/devices, 23, 227
  inventory control, 238
  OTC medications, 136
Reconstituting suspensions, 196
Reconstitution, 188
Records and record keeping
  compounded products, nonsterile, 198
  controlled substances, 17
  medication administration record, 170
  prescription hard copy, 114, 126
  repackaged medications, 24, 192, 193b
  requirements, 23, 24t
Rectal agents
  over-the-counter, 73, 75
  suppositories, 72, 197
Red Book, 90–92, 93t
"Red flags," 125
Red sunflower, 161
Reference books, 88–89
  *American Hospital Formulary Service Drug
    Information*, 92, 93t
  choosing, 93–94
  Drug Topics Red Book, 90–92, 93t
  Facts and Comparisons, 89–90, 93t
  Geriatric Handbook, 93t
  *Goodman & Gilman's The Pharmacological
    Basis of Therapeutics*, 93t
  Ident-A-Drug, 92
  Injectable Drug Handbook, The, 92–93
  Pediatric Handbook, 93t
  Physicians' Desk Reference, 90, 93t

Reference books *(Continued)*
  pocket-sized, 94
  *Remington's Pharmaceutical Sciences: The
    Science and Practice of Pharmacy*, 93t
  *United States Pharmacopoeia Drug
    Information*, 92, 93t
Refilling prescriptions. *See* Prescriptions
Reglan, 373
Religious beliefs
  Aesculapius, 3, 5
  evil spirits, 3–4, 6
  prayer, healing through, 4, 156t, 166
*Remington's Pharmaceutical Sciences: The
    Science and Practice of Pharmacy*, 93t
Remission, 521
Renal failure, 384
  dialysis, 378, 386–388
Repackaged medications, 24
  containers used, 191–192, 191f
  dosage forms, 189
  equipment used, 190
  expiration date, 190–191
  FDA guidelines, 189
  good manufacturing practices, 189
  labels, 189
  preparation required, 192
  reasons for repackaging, 189
  records of, 24, 192, 193b
Repaglinide, 278
Reports and reporting
  competencies, 109
  FDA reporting process, 16
Reproductive system, 424–425
  contraceptives, 434–440
  female system, 426–427
  impotence, 441
  infertility medications, 440–441
  male system, 425–426
  medications for (or related to). *See also
    specific medication*
    female hormones, 431–440
    impotence, 441
    infertility, 440–441
    list of, 423t–424t
    male hormones, 427–431
Respiration, 317–318
Respiratory system, 315
  breathing, 318–319
  disorders. *See also specific disorder*
    lower respiratory system, 321–323
    upper respiratory system, 320–321
  exchange of gases, 318
  infections, 452–453
  inspiration/expiration, 317–318
  lower, 317
    disorders, 321–323

Respiratory system *(Continued)*
  medications for. *See also specific medication*
    chronic obstructive pulmonary disease,
      326–328
    colds and allergies, 323–325
    list of, 314
    tuberculosis, 329–330
  sneezing, 319
  structure of, 315–317
  terminology, 314
  upper, 316–317
    disorders, 320–321
Retrovir, 467
Returns
  to manufacturer or warehouse, 238–239
  nonreturnable drugs and their disposal, 239
  to stock, 114
Reye's syndrome, 137
Rhinitis, 320, 453, 474
Rhinorrhea, 320
Riboflavin, 500
Rifadin, 330
Rifampin, 329t, 330
Rilutek, 308
Riluzole, 308
Ringworm, 462
Risperdal, 249
Risperidone, 249
ROA (routes of administration), 73–78, 131
  abbreviations, 64
  for chemotherapeutic agents, 528t
  for parenteral agents/medications, 208b
Robaxin, 298
Robitussin, 324
Robot RX, 183
Rocuronium, 310
Rods, 333
Roman numerals, 58–59
Rosiglitazone, 278
Roundworms, 464, 539, 548, 549t
Routes of administration. *See* ROA (routes of
  administration)
RU-486, 440
Rx, 114, 131

S
St. John's wort, 152, 163
Salicylates, 478, 479t
Salmeterol, 326
Sampson root, 161
Sarcoma, 521
  Kaposi's, 525
Satellite pharmacies, 179–180
Schizophrenia, 244
  antipsychotic agents, 244, 246–249
Scopolamine, 373

Screening phone calls, 8
Script, 114. *See also* Prescriptions
  filling, 119–125
Scurvy, 502
Secobarbital, 255t
Seconal, 255t
Sectral, 414
Sedative/hypnotic agents, 254–257
Seizures, 300–302, 309t
  and vitamin B_6 deficiencies, 501
Selective serotonin reuptake inhibitors
  (SSRIs), 252–253
Selegiline, 306
Seminars, 96
Senna, 371
Senokot, 371
Sensory neurons, 290
Sepsis, 551
Serax, 256
Serevent, 326
Sertraline, 253
Sex hormones
  androgens, 269t, 279, 423, 425–426, 427–430
  estrogens, 265, 269, 270, 279, 431, 432, 437
  progesterone, 265, 270, 279, 431, 434, 438
  progestins, 433–434, 437
  testosterone, 265, 270, 279, 425, 427, 429
Sexually transmitted diseases (STDs), 451,
  452t
Shamans, 3–4
Shingles, 516
Sig, 114
Sildenafil, 441
Simethicone, 374
Simmonds' disease, 271
Simvastatin, 406
Sinemet, 307
Sinequan, 251
Singulair, 327, 485
Sio-Bid, 327, 485
Skeletal muscle pain, 297
Skeletal muscle relaxants (SMRs)
  central-acting medications, 297–299
  direct-acting medications, 299
Skin
  acne development, 145–146, 146
  acne treatments, 146
  anatomy, 142–143
  athlete's foot, 147
  canker sores, 147
  infectious conditions, 146, 453
  inflammation products, 147, 147t
  noninfectious conditions, 146
  OTC medications, 143t
    acne treatments, 146
    athlete's foot, 147

Skin (Continued)
   canker sores, 147
   inflammation products, 147, 147t
   sunscreen, 131, 144, 145t
   topical antibiotics, 148
   warts, 147
  psoriasis, 148
  sunscreen, 131, 144, 145t
  topical antibiotics, 148
  and vitamin B_2 deficiencies, 500
  and vitamin B_6 deficiencies, 501
  warts, 147
Skin protectant factor (SPF) agents, 144
Skin protectant factor (SPF) guide, 145t
Sleep aids
  over-the-counter, 140
  sedative/hypnotic agents, 254–257
Sleep disorders, 244
  and vitamin B_5 deficiencies, 501
SMRs. See Skeletal muscle relaxants (SMRs)
Sneezing, 319
Sodium bicarbonate, 364t
Sodium citrate, 364t
Sodium phosphates, 370t
Solu-Cortef, 483
Solu-Medrol, 276
Solute, 188
Solutions, 188, 202
Solvent, 188
Soma, 297
Soma compound, 299
Soma compound with codeine, 299
Somatic nervous system, 283, 293
Somatostatin, 269, 270
Sorbitrate, 416t
Sore throat products, 141, 320–321
Sound alike/look alike drugs, 103–104
Special labels, 22, 22b
Specialized technicians, 8
Species, 539
Spectrum, 447
Spermicides, 438
SPF agents, 144
SPF guide, 145t
Spinal cord, 290
Spiritual beliefs. See Religious beliefs
Spiritual healing, 4, 156t, 166
Spironolactone, 390, 410
Spironolactone/HCTZ, 390t
Spleen, 509
Sprays, 69–70
Sputum, 314
SSRIs, 252–253
Stanozolol, 430
STAT orders, 170, 174, 184
State laws, 24

Statins, 405–406
STDs, 451, 452t
Stelazine, 248
Steroids, 474. See also specific steroid
  adrenal effects of, 482–483
  corticosteroids. See Corticosteroids
  glucocorticoids, 481–483
  NSAIDS. See Nonsteroidal antiinflammatory
    drugs (NSAIDS)
Stock
  automated dispensing systems. See
    Automated dispensing systems
  damaged, 238
  expired, 239
  floor stock, 170, 181
  inventory control
    generally. See Inventory control
    technicians, 180–181
  new stock, 237–238
  ordering, 227, 236–237
    special considerations, 240
    suppliers, 239
  PAR level, 179, 235
    hospital specialty areas, 181
    importance of maintaining, 235
  parenteral agents/medications levels, 213
  returns to, 114
  suppliers, 239
Stomach conditions and remedies,
    362–367
  over-the-counter, 141–142, 362–363, 363,
    364–365
Stomatitis, 501
Storage of drugs, 83
Streptozocin, 530
Subcutaneous administrations, 76–77
Sublingual agents, 73
Subunit vaccines, 513b
Succinylcholine, 310
Sudafed, 325
Sulfacetamide sodium, 346
Sulfadiazine, 392t
Sulfamethoxazole, 392t
Sulfisoxazole, 392t
Sulfonamides, 345–346, 392t
Sunscreen, 131, 144, 145t
Supplies, ordering of, 109–110
Suppositories, 72
  preparation of, 197
Suprax, 457
Suprofen, 344
SUREMED, 183
Suspensions, 70–71, 188
  reconstituting, 196
Symbiotic, 447
Symmetrel, 306

Sympathetic nervous system, 283, 293–295
Sympathomimetics, 339t, 342
  for asthma, 483–484
Synthesis, 447
Synthetic medications, 152
Synthroid, 273
Syphilis, 452t
Syringes, 209–210
  needles, 212
  parenteral medications. *See* Parenteral
    agents/medications
  sizes of, 211
Syrups, 69, 188
Systemic, 474

T
T cells, 509–510, 511t
T lymphocytes, 509, 511t
Tablets, 66–67
TACE, 433
Tachycardia, zinc excess, 502
Tacrine, 303
Tagamet, 363, 365
Tagamet HB, 365
Tamsulosin, 430
Tapazole, 272
Tapeworms, 465t, 539, 549t
Tardive dyskinesia, 244
Taxonomy, 161–162, 539, 541
  Animalia kingdom, 542t, 545–548, 549t
  Fungi kingdom, 542t, 550–551
  Monera kingdom, 542t, 551–552, 553t
  Plantae kingdom, 542t, 544, 545f
  Protista kingdom, 542t, 549, 550f
  Whittaker's five kingdoms, 541, 542t,
    544–552
TB. *See* Tuberculosis (TB)
TCAs, 250–251
Tears products, 348
Tegretol, 301
Telephone calls
  etiquette, 106
  filtering of, 8
Teniposide, 528
Tenormin, 413
Terazosin, 430
Terminally ill patients, 110
Testes, 265, 270, 425
  conditions and their treatment, 279
Testex, 429
Testoderm, 429
Testosterone, 265, 270, 279, 425, 427, 429
Testosterone propionate, 429
Testred, 430
Tetanus immunization, 516, 517
Tetracycline, 367t

Thalidomide, 14–15
Theo-Dur, 327, 485
Theophylline, 327, 485
Therapeutic, 423
Thiamine, 499–500
Thiazides and thiazide-like agents, 388–389
  for CHF-related edema, 409
Thiethylperazine maleate, 373
Thioguanine, 527
Thioridazine, 247
Thioxanthene, 248
Third-party billing, 229
  HMOs, 229–230
  insurance companies, 232–235
  insurance types, 229
  Medicaid, 231
  Medicare, 231
  PPOs, 230–231
  workers' compensation, 231
Thoracic, 283
Thorazine, 248
Throlar, 273
Thrombin, 396
Thrombolytic, 396
Thrombosis, 400b, 404
  treatment of, 416–418
Thymus gland, 265, 509, 510f
Thyroid aplasia, 272
Thyroid desiccated, 273
Thyroid gland, 265, 268
  conditions and their treatment, 271–273
Thyroid-stimulating hormone (TSH), 268t
Thyroxine, 263, 268
Ticar, 456
Ticarcillin, 456
Ticlid, 418t
Ticlopidine, 418t
Tigan, 373
Timolol, 340
Timoptic, 340
Timoptic XE, 340
Tinctures, 152, 188
Tinea infections, 462
TOBI (inhalation), 460
Tobramycin, 346, 460
Tobrex (ophthalmic), 460
Tobrex (solution and ointment), 346
Tofranil-PM, 251
Tolazamide, 278t
Tolbutamide, 278t
Tolinase, 278t
Tonsils, 509
Topical antibiotics, 148
Topical treatments, 75–76
Torecan, 373
Torsemide, 389

Torts, 24

Total parenteral nutrition, 206, 220, 221f

Tourette's syndrome, 244

Toxoids, 508, 512–513

Toxoplasma gondii, 464

Trace elements, 493, 494, 495, 503t

Trade name drugs, 88, 227. *See also specific drug*

  generic *versus,* 229

Traditional medical treatment, 153

Training, 8, 584

Training programs, 34

Transderm, 416t

Transdermal, 432

Transdermal patches, 437

Transdermal preparations, 431

Transfers of prescriptions, 126

Tranxene, 257

Tranylcypromine, 252

Trasnderm-scop, 373

Trazodone, 253

Trephining, 3

Triamcinolone (#1), 276

Triamcinolone acetonide, 328, 483, 485

Triamcinolone acetonide (#3), 276

Triamcinolone hexacetonide (#2), 276

Triamterene, 390, 410

Triamterene/HCTZ, 390t

Trichomonas vaginalis, 464, 547

Trichomoniasis, 452t, 464

Tricyclic antidepressants (TCAs), 250–251

Tridil, 416t

Trifluoperazine, 248

Trifluridine, 348

Trihexyphenidyl, 308

Triiodothyronine, 263, 268

Trilafon, 247

Tri-Levlen, 437

Trimethobenzamide, 373

Tri-Norinyl, 437

Triphasic medications, 437–438

Triphasil, 437

Troches, 68

Trusopt, 340

Trust in technicians, 9

TSH, 268t

Tuberculosis (TB), 322, 457, 459

  medications for, 329–330, 459t

  vaccine, 517

Tumors growth, outcomes of, 523b

Tums, 274, 365

Tussionex, 324

Twenty-first century and beyond, 9–10

Tympanic membrane, 333

Typing skills, 109

Tyramine, foods containing, 251, 252t

U

Ulcers, 356, 362

  peptic ulcers, 356, 363, 366–367

Uni-Dur, 327

Unit doses, 188. *See also* Repackaged medications

United States Pharmacopoeia Drug Information (USP DI), 92, 93t

Universal precautions, 206

University of Sciences in Philadelphia (USP), 7

Uracil mustard, 530

Urea, 378, 391t

Ureaphil, 391t

Uremia, 378

Urinary retention, 378

Urinary system

  anatomy of, 379–380

  conditions affecting, 383–386. *See also specific condition*

    treatments for, 386–392

  drugs for. *See also specific drug*

    list of, 378

  kidneys, 379

    function of, 380–383

    nephron functions, 381–383

  terminology, 378

Urinary tract infections (UTI), 385

  treatment of, 391, 392t

Urofollitropin, 441

Urolithiasis, 378

Urticaria, 474

UTI. *See* Urinary tract infections (UTI)

V

Vaccines, 508

  acellular, 513b

  adult immunizations, 516–517

  anthrax, 517t

  antiidiotypic, 513b

  chicken pox, 516

  childhood immunization, 514–516

  cholera, 517t

  conjugated, 513b

  defined, 508

  development of, 513–514

  diptheria, 516

  diptheria, pertussis and tetanus, 514–515

  Haemophilus influenza type B, 515, 516

  hepatitis, 514, 516

  importance of immunizations, 510–511

  list of, 508

  measles, mumps and rubella, 515

  plague, 517t

  pneumonia, 516

  polio, 514, 515

Vaccines *(Continued)*
  preparation of
    bacterial vaccines, 512–513
      viral vaccines, 512
    subunit, 513b
    terminology, 508
    tuberculosis, 517
    yellow fever, 517t
Vaginal compounds, 197
Vaginal infections, 551
Vaginal rings, 432, 434
Valence, 564
Valerian, 152, 164
Valium, 256, 302
Valproic acid, 301
Valsartan, 413
Vancenase AQ, 327
Vanceril, 327, 485
Varicella vaccine, 516
Vasodilation, 474
Vasopressin, 267, 268t
Vasotec, 412
Vectors, 447, 539
Veetids, 456
Veins, 396
Venlafaxine, 254
Ventolin, 326
Verapamil, 414
Vertical flow hood, 206, 213, 215–216
Veterinarian prescriptions, 15
Viaflex bag, 209
Viagra, 441
Vials, 76f, 77f, 211
  lids, 120–121. *See also* Childproof caps
  multiple dose, 213
Vicks Chloraseptic mouth rinse, 321
Vicks Chloraseptic Sore Throat, 321
Vidarabine, 347
Villus, 356
Vinblastine, 528
Vincristine, 528
Vinorelbine, 528
Vira-A (ointment), 347
Viral vaccines, 512. *See also* Vaccines
Virology, 539, 540
Viroptic (solution), 348
Viruses, 447, 466–470, 539, 540, 555
  analysis of, 556–557, 558f
  antibody formation, 557, 558f
  characteristics of, 555, 556f
  classification of, 555
  composition of, 556f
  as disease fighters, 560
  infections. *See specific viral infection*
  inhibiting infection from, 559–560, 560b
  replication of, 555, 557f

Viscosity, 314
Vision, 337. *See also* Eyes
Visken, 414
Vistaril, 258
Vitamin A, 495, 497
Vitamin B, 498–499
Vitamin B_1, 499–500
Vitamin B_2, 500
Vitamin B_3, 500
Vitamin B_5, 501
Vitamin B_6, 501
Vitamin B_9, 501
Vitamin B_{12}, 501–502
Vitamin C, 502
Vitamin D, 497
Vitamin E, 498
Vitamin K, 498
Vitamins, 494–495. *See also specific vitamin*
  antioxidants, 502
    vitamin E, 498
  drug interactions, 496t
    vitamin B_6, 501
    vitamin D, 497
    vitamin E, 498
  fat-soluable, 493, 495–498
  FDA regulation, 495, 496t
  list of, 493
  recommended daily allowances, 500t
  terminology, 493
  water-soluable, 493, 494, 495, 496t, 498–502
Vivelle, 432
Voltaren, 344
Volume, 39
Vomiting, 356, 372
  treatment of, 373–374
  zinc excess, 502

W
Warfarin, 417
Warts, 147
Water-soluble vitamins. *See* Vitamins
Weight conversions, 52–53
Weight Watchers, 245
Wellbutrin, 253
Western medicine, 153–154
Whittaker, Robert, 541
Whooping cough, 323t
Winstrol, 430
Workers' compensation, 227, 231
Worms, 447, 464, 465t, 539, 548. *See also*
    specific type of worm
  antihelminthic agents, 466t
Writing skills, 107–108

X
Xalantan, 343

Xanax, 256
Xanthene bronchodilator agents,
    326–327
Xanthine agents, 485
Xylocaine, 408

Y
Yasmin, 436
Yeasts, 550
Yellow fever vaccine, 517t
Yin and yang, 156
Yoga, 153

Z
Zafirlukast, 327
Zantac OTC, 363, 365

Zaroxolyn, 389, 409
Zemuron, 310
Zero refill recorders, 125–126
Zidovudine, 467
Zileuton, 485
Zinacef (INJ), 457
Zinc combinations, 320
Zinc excess, 502
Zocor, 406
Zofran, 374
Zoloft, 253
Zolpidem, 257
Zovirax, 467
Zyban, 253
Zyflo, 485
Zyprexa, 249